Diseases of the Gallbladder

Jae Bock Chung · Kazuichi Okazaki
Editors

Diseases of the Gallbladder

Springer

Editors
Jae Bock Chung
Department of Internal Medicine
NHIS Ilsan Hospital
Goyang-si, Kyonggi-do
Korea (Republic of)

Kazuichi Okazaki
Department of Internal Medicine
Kouri Hospital, Kansai Medical
University
Neyagawa, Osaka, Japan

ISBN 978-981-15-6009-5 ISBN 978-981-15-6010-1 (eBook)
https://doi.org/10.1007/978-981-15-6010-1

This Springer imprint is published by the registered company Springer Nature Singapore Pte Ltd.
The registered company address is: 152 Beach Road, #21-01/04 Gateway East, Singapore 189721, Singapore

Preface

Diseases of the Gallbladder (GB) are relatively common, and the most common pathology is gallstone affecting 10–15% of the adult population. Most of the patients with GB diseases come to the hospital with RUQ pain or discomfort. We can diagnose most diseases of the GB (gallstone, inflammation, and cancer) by laboratory examinations and imaging (ultrasonography, CT, and MRI) along with endoscopic ultrasonography. However early diagnosis of gallbladder cancer is still difficult.

Our knowledge of the genetics and pathogenesis of various gallbladder diseases has expanded recently, and there are several guidelines for the management of diseases of the GB.

This book provides up-to-date information on all aspects of diseases of the GB. As an introduction, laboratory findings, diagnosis, and therapeutic methods on diseases of the GB are explained. Up-to-date knowledge regarding GB stones, acalculous cholecystitis, GB lesions associated with IgG4 related disease, and in patients with pancreaticobiliary maljunction, dyskinesia of the GB, and incidental GB cancer are described. All about GB cancer including epidemiology, risk factors, gene mutation, diagnostic methods, and various treatment modalities are explained. Current issues such as polypoid lesions and wall thickening of the GB, and prophylactic cholecystectomy in patients with concomitant gallstones after removal of CBD stone by ERCP are discussed. Furthermore, endoscopic drainage of the GB is compared with PTGBD.

The goals of this book are to provide those studying the GB with the opportunity to obtain a complete understanding, and to present the practicing physician with the principles of current diagnosis and treatment on diseases of the GB. We are deeply grateful to all the authors for their painstaking writing and contributions in preparing this informative book. The publisher has also made a significant contribution to this book and has turned out an impressive volume with illustrations of the highest quality.

Goyang-si, Korea (Republic of) — Jae Bock Chung
Neyagawa, Japan — Kazuichi Okazaki
March 2020

Contents

Introduction, Epidemiology, Laboratory Examinations, Diagnostic Methods and Pathology

Overview of Diseases of the Gallbladder

Jae Bock Chung and Jae Uk Chong

Introduction

The gallbladder (GB) is a small size, pear-shape, simple structure organ which temporarily stores bile. The GB lies on the inferior surface of the right lobe of the liver and has distinct anatomic zones (fundus, body/infundibulum, neck, and cystic duct). Histologically, the GB has four layers: mucosa, consisting of columnar epithelium and lamina propria; a thin layer of smooth muscle; a perimuscular layer of connective tissue; and a serosal layer [1]. The gallbladder, despite its simple structure and function, is a complex organ [2].

Diseases of the GB are relatively common, with the most common pathology, cholelithiasis, affecting 10–15% of the adult population, while the worldwide occurrence of gallbladder cancer is less than 2/100,000 individuals with a great geographic variation [3].

J. B. Chung (✉)
Department of Internal Medicine, NHIS Ilsan Hospital, Yonsei University College of Medicine, Goyang-si, Gyeonggi-do, Korea
e-mail: jbchung@yuhs.ac

J. U. Chong
Department of Surgery, NHIS Ilsan Hospital, Yonsei University College of Medicine, Goyang-si, Gyeonggi-do, Korea
e-mail: jaeuk1216@nhimc.or.kr

Currently, imaging studies such as ultrasonography (US), computerized tomography (CT) and magnetic resonance imaging (MRI), and endoscopic ultrasonography (EUS) can detect lesions in the lumen and the wall of GB. The contractile function of GB can be measured by cholecystokinin-cholescintigraphy (CCK-CS).

Almost all the patients come to the hospital with the symptoms (acute RUQ pain or recurrent RUQ vague discomfort to pain) or for evaluation of abnormal image findings (gallstone, polyp, wall thickening, and tumor) of the gallbladder.

RUQ Pain Suggesting Acute Cholecystitis

Differential Diagnosis

The differential diagnosis for RUQ pain suggesting acute cholecystitis should include diseases which simulate cholecystitis: gastrointestinal tract (perforated or penetrating ulcer and acute appendicitis), pancreas (acute pancreatitis and pseudocyst), kidney (acute pyelonephritis and renal colic), lung (pleurisy, right basilar pneumonia, empyema, and pleurodynia), heart (myocardial infarction and pericarditis), and pre-eruptive herpes zoster [4].

J. B. Chung and K. Okazaki (eds.), *Diseases of the Gallbladder*,
https://doi.org/10.1007/978-981-15-6010-1_1

Patients with acute cholecystitis may have a history of biliary colic attacks or remains asymptomatic until the presenting episode [5].

Plain abdominal radiographs can reveal radio-opaque gallstones in about 10% of cases of acute cholecystitis and gas within the gallbladder wall in emphysematous cholecystitis [5] Initial imaging modality considered for acute cholecystitis is ultrasonography. CT or MR imaging may be required for evaluating complications of acute cholecystitis and to exclude other pathologies that can present with right upper quadrant pain [6] (see chapter 'Imaging Diagnosis of Diseases of the Gallbladder: US, CT and MRI'). Biliary scintigraphy (hepato-iminodiacetic acid [HIDA] scan) is the gold standard when the diagnosis remains uncertain after ultrasonography [5].

Laboratory examinations of acute cholecystitis are CBC, liver function tests, amylase, and CRP (see chapter 'Laboratory Examinations of Diseases of the Gallbladder'). TG18/TG13 severity grading for acute cholecystitis is a useful indicator from the prognostic perspective [7].

Acute Calculous Cholecystitis

Acute cholecystitis is most often caused by gallstones. Gallstones are present in about 10–15% of adults, and more than 80% of them are asymptomatic. Acute cholecystitis develops in 1–3% of patients with symptomatic gallstones [3, 5, 8, 9].

As an initial examination, transabdominal ultrasonography can detect gallstones with distended GB, edematous GB wall, and pericholecystic fluid, and Murphy's sign can be elicited during the examination [5]. In addition, abnormal findings of the bile duct (dilatation and stone) and the pancreas (enlargement, peripancreatic fluid collection, and intrapancreatic parenchymal necrosis) can be detected.

If a stone in the common bile duct is highly suspected by liver function tests, MRCP may be helpful. When a CBD stone is found, preoperative ERCP with EST or intraoperative bile duct exploration can remove the stone.

About 20% of patients with acute cholecystitis need emergency surgery. Patients with acute cholecystitis who undergo early laparoscopic cholecystectomy (before symptoms have lasted for 72–96 hours) have lower complication rates, lower conversion rates, and shorter hospital stays than those undergoing interval surgery, which is performed 6–12 weeks after the acute episode to allow the inflammatory process to resolve [5].

Percutaneous cholecystostomy is a minimally invasive procedure that can benefit patients with high risk from surgery (see chapter 'Percutaneous Transhepatic Gallbladder Drainage (PTGBD)'). Endoscopic transpapillary and transmural gallbladder drainage are helpful in patients who are not good candidates for percutaneous therapy or surgery [5, 10] (see chapter 'Endoscopic Drainage of the Gallbladder').

Acute Acalculous Cholecystitis

Acute acalculous cholecystitis accounts for 5–14% of cholecystitis. Acalculous cholecystitis tends to occur in critically ill patients and results may be life-threatening. Risk factors include severe trauma or burns, major surgery (such as cardiopulmonary bypass), long term fasting, total parental nutrition, sepsis, diabetes mellitus, atherosclerotic disease, systemic vasculitis, acute renal failure, and AIDS [5, 11, 12].

The diagnosis of acute acalculous cholecystitis may be ambiguous in critically ill patients as Murphy's sign is difficult to elicit and many imaging findings are either insensitive or nonspecific [12].

Management involves percutaneous cholecystostomy, surgical cholecystectomy, or endoscopically placed metal stent through the gastrointestinal tract into the gallbladder [10, 12] (see chapter 'Acalculous Cholecystitis: Diagnosis and Treatment').

Unexplanied Recurrent RUQ Vague Discomfort or/and Pain

Differential Diagnosis

Diagnostic tests for differential diagnosis of a patient with recurrent unexplained RUQ vague discomfort or/and pain should focus on excluding more common diseases including malignancy, GB microlithiasis or sludge, GERD, peptic ulcer disease, functional dyspepsia, chronic pancreatitis, and musculoskeletal syndrome [13, 14].

Although initial ultrasound examination may show no abnormal findings, repeat examination may be of use for the evaluation of biliary colic. In a patient with suspected microlithiasis, EUS may be more valuable than ultrasonography (see chapter 'EUS of Diseases of the Gallbladder'). EGD is also essential to exclude common causes within GI tracts. Abdominal CT and MRI should be reserved for patients with persistent symptoms.

Gallbladder Dyskinesia

Gallbladder dyskinesia is a motility disorder characterized by biliary pain without structural and mechanical cause for the pain. Recently, diagnostic criteria for gallbladder dyskinesia was defined in Rome IV criteria [13, 14].

Although the etiology of GB dyskinesia is not known, there are several hypotheses. GB dyskinesia is a diagnosis of exclusion in patients with typical biliary pain. To exclude structural abnormality and malignancy of the biliary duct and pancreas, various laboratory tests including bile examination and imaging studies with EUS can be done. Cholecystokinin-cholescintigraphy (CCK-CS) is an important diagnostic tool for gallbladder ejection fraction (GBEF). A decreased GBEF (<40) is considered an objective measure of gallbladder disorder [13] (see chapter 'Dyskinesia of the Gallbladder').

Gallstone

Differential Diagnosis

Ultrasonography can detect almost all gallstones accurately except for microlithiasis. The lesions for differential diagnosis of gallstone include cholesterol polyp and small sludge ball. These lesions can be differentiated with EUS or other imaging studies such as CT or MRI.

Management

Gallstones are classified into cholesterol stones and pigment stones based on composition. Black pigment stones can be caused by chronic hemolysis; brown pigment stones typically develop in obstructed and infected bile ducts [15].

Risk factors for gallstones include female sex, age, pregnancy, physical inactivity, obesity, and overnutrition. Metabolic syndrome increases the risk of developing gallstones and forms the basis for primary prevention with lifestyle modifications [15]. There are studies about genetic background as a risk factor of gallstone (see chapter 'Pathogenesis and Treatment of Gallbladder Stones').

The therapeutic option for gallstone disease is based on a few crucial steps, i.e., presence/absence of typical symptoms such as colicky pain, presence of complications, and gallbladder function, as well as composition and size of gallstones [16].

Common bile duct (CBD) stones are found in 5–10% of patients undergoing cholecystectomy for symptomatic cholelithiasis [17–19]. Currently, cholecystectomy after removal of stone in the CBD with EST is the usual method for patients with stones in both GB and CBD. However, prophylactic cholecystectomy in patients with GB stones after CBD stones removal by EST remains controversial (see chapter 'Prophylactic Cholecystectomy in Patients with Concomitant Gallstones After Removal of CBD Stones by ERCP').

Gallbladder Polyp

Differential Diagnosis

The prevalence of gallbladder polyps varies from 0.3 to 12% in healthy adults who undergo abdominal ultrasonography. GB polyps are classified into two groups: neoplastic (adenoma and adenocarcinoma) and nonneoplastic (cholesterol polyps, inflammatory polyps, and adenomyomatosis). However, only 5% of polyps are considered to be true gallbladder polyps, meaning that they are malignant or have malignant potential [20, 21].

Adenomas have malignant potential, and there are reports suggesting adenoma–carcinoma sequence in the GB [21–23].

Transabdominal ultrasonography is the current mainstay for the radiological investigation of gallbladder polyps. In case of uncertainty, additional imaging modalities and EUS may be used for therapeutic decision (see chapters 'Differential Diagnosis by Imaging Between Benign and Malignant Lesion with Imaging' and 'Role of EUS').

Management and Follow-up

Retrospective studies have found the risk of malignancy for polyps rises sharply from 10 mm and upwards, and the general consensus is that patients with polyps of 10 mm or greater should be treated with cholecystectomy [24–26]. Polyps under 10 mm should undergo surveillance unless significant risk factors are present in which cholecystectomy should be offered [24].

A case report showed a malignant transformation of a 5 mm polyp into a 20 mm carcinoma over a period of two years [27]. Babu et al. [25] reviewed 10 studies which looked at the follow-up of gallbladder polyps between six months and seven years, and found that 7.6% of polyps increased in size during the follow-up.

The recommended follow-up for patients with gallbladder polyps depends on the size of the polyps and the presence of risk factors for malignancy (see chapter 'Diagnostic and Therapeutic Algorithm: Polypoid Lesions of the Gallbladder').

GB Wall Thickening

Differential Diagnosis

Diffuse GB wall thickening (>3 mm) can result from a broad spectrum of pathologic conditions, including surgical and nonsurgical diseases: cholecystitis (acute calculous and acalculous, and chronic), liver diseases (hepatitis, cirrhosis, and portal hypertension), extracholecystic inflammation (pancreatitis, colitis, peritonitis, and pyelonephritis), systemic diseases (congestive heart failure, renal failure, sepsis, and hypoalbuminemia), malignancy (primary GB carcinoma and lymphoma), adenomyomatosis, pseudothickening (contracted state), and atypical infection (tuberculosis and Dengue hemorrhagic fever) [28, 29].

Focal wall thickening of the GB can be seen in polyps (adenomas and cholesterol polyp), malignancy (primary GB carcinoma and metastases), focal adenomyomatosis, and focal xanthogranulomatous cholecystitis [28, 30].

Distinguishing early-stage cancer from benign wall thickening of GB is important. The contour of lesion, patterns of wall thickness, intramural cystic space, and patterns of GB wall enhancement are used as differential points [31, 32] (see chapter 'Diagnostic Strategies for Early Diagnosis').

Ultrasonography may be the initial imaging modality for GB wall thickening, but further evaluation with contrast-enhanced CT and/or MRI may be needed when the findings are equivocal. EUS can better define the characteristics of GB wall thickening. There are many reports on differentiating benign and malignant wall thickening using MRI (conventional and/or diffusion-weighted imaging), contrast-enhanced US, real-time GB elastography, multi-detector CT (MDCT), nuclear medicine and contrast-enhanced harmonic EUS (CEUS) [28,

33, 34] (see chapters ‘Differential Diagnosis by Imaging Between Benign and Malignant Lesion with Imaging’ and ‘Role of EUS’).

Management

Diffuse GB wall thickening can result from a broad spectrum of systemic pathological condition, and sometimes a short-term follow-up examination with ultrasonography, and inquiring the list of broad etiologies for difficult cases may prove to be helpful.

Corwin et al. [30] analyzed retrospectively 116 patients with incidental focal fundal GB wall thickening on contrast-enhanced CT, and found four cases (3.4%; 95% CI, 0.9–8.6%) of malignancy which showed characteristic findings of GB wall (hyperenhancing/heterogeneous enhancement in three cases and full thickness homogeneous enhancement in one case). The mean thickness of the malignant lesion was significantly greater than the benign lesion (15.8 ± 8.1 mm vs. 9.0 ± 3.1 mm, $p < 0.0001$, respectively).

For early detection of carcinoma of the gallbladder, it seemed essential to pay careful attention to mild mucosal changes, as more than 50% of early cancer did not show apparently protruding lesions [35].

The diagnostic and therapeutic algorithm of wall thickening of GB is discussed in chapter ‘Imaging Features of Gallbladder Lesions Manifesting Wall Thickening’.

GB Tumor

Differential Diagnosis

GB tumors are rare compared to gallstone disease, and its prevalence varies from 3 to 7% in the general population [36, 37].

GB tumors are classified as malignant and benign tumors. Malignant tumors include epithelial tumors (adenocarcinoma, undifferentiated carcinoma, adenosquamous carcinoma, squamous carcinoma, and neuroendocrine tumor), non-epithelial tumors (lymphomas and sarcomas), and metastatic tumors (melanoma, kidney, and breast). Benign tumors include epithelial tumors (adenoma, adenomyomatosis, papillomatosis, and heterotopic tissue), non-epithelial tumors (leiomyoma, lipoma, and neural tumors), and pseudotumors (cholecystitis, cholesterolosis, and inflammatory polyp) [36] (see chapter ‘Pathology: Non-neoplastic and Neoplastic Diseases of the Gallbladder’).

The most frequent benign tumors and pseudotumors of the gallbladder are cholestesterol polyp, adenoma, adenomyomatosis, and cholesterolosis [36–38].

Rare mass forming lesions mimicking neoplasm of GB include hematoma and tumefactive sludge [39, 40]. Mass forming lesion of GB can also be seen in patients with malakoplakia and IgG4-related sclerosing cholecystitis [41, 42] (see chapter ‘IgG4 Related Cholecystitis’).

The cross-sectional imaging patterns of gallbladder carcinoma have been described as a mass replacing the gallbladder in 40–65% of cases, focal or diffuse gallbladder wall thickening in 20–30%, and an intraluminal polypoid mass in 15–25% [43–47].

Ultrasonography, contrast-enhanced CT, and EUS may be valuable in the differential diagnosis of GB tumor. Tumor markers such as CA 19-9 and CEA should be checked. Serum IgG4 is helpful for the diagnosis of mass forming IgG4-related sclerosing cholecystitis. Equivocal mass lesions of the gallbladder can be diagnosed histologically by EUS-FNA or percutaneous needle biopsy (see chapters ‘Tissue Acquisition of Diseases of the Gallbladder: Percutaneous Ultrasound-Guided Biopsy’ and ‘Tissue Acquisition for Diagnosis of the Gallbladder Disease: EUS-Guided Biopsy’).

Gallbladder Cancer (GBC)

The worldwide occurrence of gallbladder cancer is less than 2/100,000 individuals, but this has been recorded with extensive variance in geography, ethnicity, and cultural differences [3, 48, 49] (see chapter 'Epidemiology').

The development of GBC has been linked to various genetic and environmental factors. Many studies concerning the genetic predisposition of GBC have been conducted (see chapter 'Gene Mutations and its Clinical Significance'). Well known GBC risk factors include advanced age, female sex, polyps greater than 1 cm, porcelain GB, anomalous pancreaticobiliary ductal union (APBDU), and gallstone [48–50]. Chronic infection of GB or/and environmental exposure to specific chemicals, heavy metals, and even many dietary factors have also been found to be associated with GBC formation [51, 52] (see chapters 'Gallbladder Lesions in Patients with Pancreaticobiliary Maljunction' and 'Risk Factors').

Preoperative imaging should include CT with MRI. PET may be of use in selected cases of suspected metastatic disease (see chapters 'Staging by Radiological Imaging' and 'Roles of PET/CT in Evaluating Gallbladder and Hepatobiliary Tumors'). Laboratory testing, including CBC, comprehensive metabolic panel including liver function tests, and coagulation factors, are appropriate [53]. Tumor markers currently used are CA 19-9 and CEA. Endoscopic ultrasonography can be useful for assessing depth of invasion and for fine-needle aspiration of the lesion in question [54, 55].

GB cancers identified incidentally on cholecystectomy account for less than 1% of cholecystectomy specimens. Incidentally discovered GB cancers after cholecystectomy have improved survival, because they are often diagnosed at an earlier stage. For incidental GBC after laparoscopic cholecystectomy, observation is recommended for pT1a and for pT1b or greater, more extensive resection is necessary [53, 56–58] (see chapter 'Incidental Gallbladder Carcinoma').

Patients with T2 or greater disease seem to benefit most from adjuvant therapy following definite resection [53, 59–61] (see chapter 'Recent Advances of Surgical Treatment for Gallbladder Carcinoma').

In order to improve survival in patients with locally advanced T3/T4 tumors and lymph node involvement, adjuvant chemotherapy and chemoradiotherapy following surgical resection are recommended [62, 63]. While neoadjuvant chemotherapy may increase resectability and survival, there are concerns regarding a delay in the surgical resection and disease progression. The results of neoadjuvant chemotherapy (NACT) or chemoradiotherapy (NACRT) in patients with GBC were reviewed recently [64] (see chapters 'Neoadjuvant and Adjuvant Chemotherapy' and 'Role of Radiation Therapy').

If jaundice is present, gallbladder drainage can be done via endoscopic (transpapillary or transmural), or percutaneous routes. Chemotherapy, radiation, or both may improve survival and palliation of symptoms. Patients who recur early should be managed similar to those with initial metastatic disease [53, 59, 65–67] (see chapter 'Patterns of Recurrence and its Effective Treatment').

Conclusion

Currently, we can diagnose most of the patients with diseases of the gallbladder using various imaging modalities (abdominal ultrasonography, CT, and MRI) and endoscopic ultrasonography. Patients are treated by laparoscopic cholecystectomy, percutaneous cholecystostomy or endoscopic drainage of gallbladder depending on the physical status without difficulties. However, the prognosis of gallbladder cancer is dismal due to delayed diagnosis and absence of adequate personalized target therapy. In the chapters of this book, up-to-date information on all aspects of diseases of the gallbladder will be described.

References

1. Behar J. Anatomy and anomalies of the bile duct. In: Haubrich WS, Schaffner F, Berk JE, editors. Bockus gastroenterology, 5th ed. Philadelphia, Pennsylvania: W.B. Saunders; 1995. p. 2547–8.

2. Maurer KJ, Carey MC, Fox JG. Role of infection, inflammation, and immune system in cholesterol gallstone formation. Gastroenterology. 2009;136(2):425–40.
3. Stinton LM, Shaffer EA. Epidemiology of gallbladder disease: cholelithiasis and cancer. Gut Liver. 2012;6(2):172–87.
4. Strasberg SM, Clavien P-A. Acute calculous cholecystitis. In: Haubrich WS, Schaffner F, Berk JE, editors. Bockus gastroenterology, 5th ed. Philadelphia, Pennsylvania: W.B. Saunders; 1995. p. 2647–8.
5. Indar AA, Beckingham IJ. Acute cholecystitis. BMJ. 2002;325:639–43.
6. Chawla A, Bosco JI, Lim TC, Srinivasan S, Teh HS, Shenoy JN. Imaging of acute cholecystitis and cholecystitis-associated complications in the emergency setting. Singapore Med J. 2015;56(8):438–44.
7. Yokoe M, Hata J, Takada T, Strasberg SM, Asbun HJ, Wakabayashi G, et al. Tokyo guidelines 2018: diagnostic criteria and severity grading of acute cholecystitis (with videos). J Hepatobiliary Pancreat Sci. 2018;25:41–54.
8. Ransohoff DF, Gracie WA, Wolfenson LB, Neuhauser D. Prophylactic cholecystectomy or expectant management for silent gallstones. A decision analysis to assess survival. Ann Intern Med. 1983;99(2):199–204.
9. Friedman GD. Natural history of asymptomatic and symptomatic gallstones. Am J Surg. 1993;165(4):399–404.
10. Baron TH, Grimm IS, Swanstrom LL. Interventional approaches to gallbladder disease. N Engl J Med. 2015;373(4):357–65.
11. Savoca PF, Longo WE, Pastemak B, Gusberg RJ. Does visceral ischemia play a role in the pathogenesis of acute acalculous cholecystitis? J Clin Gastroenterol. 1990;12(1):33–6.
12. Balmadrid B. Recent advances in management of acalculous cholecystitis. F1000Res. 2018;7:F1000 Faculty Rev-1660. http://doi.org/10.12688/f1000research.14886.1.
13. Clark CJ. An update on biliary dyskinesia. Surg Clin N Am. 2019;99:203–14.
14. Cotton PB, Elta GH, Carter CR, Pasricha PJ, Corazziari ES. Gallbladder and Sphincter of Oddi Disorders. Gastroenterology. 2016;150:1420–9.
15. Lammert F, Gurusamy K, Ko CW, Miquel JF, Mendez-Sanchez N, Portincasa P, et al. Gallstones. Nat Rev Dis Primers. 2016;2:16024. https://doi.org/10.1038/nrdp.2016.24.
16. Portincasa P, Ciaula AD, Bonfrate L, Wang DQ. Therapy of gallstone disease: what it was, what it is, what it will be. World J Gastrointest Pharmacol Ther. 2012;3(2):7–20.
17. O'Neil CJ, Gilles DM, Gani JS. Choledocholithiasis: overdiagnosed endoscopically and undertreated laparoscopically. ANZ J Surg. 2008;78(6):487–91.
18. Quispel R, van Driel LM, Veldt BJ, van Haard PM, Bruno MJ. The utility and yield of endoscopic ultrasonography for suspected choledocholithiasis in common gastroenterology practice. Eur J Gastroenterol Hepatol. 2016;28(12):1473–6.
19. Rahal MA, Rammal MO, karaoui W, Hallal A, Tamim H, Shaib Y. Predictors of bile tree pathology in patients presenting with gallbladder disease. Eur J Gastroenterol Hepatol. 2017;29:1017–21.
20. Vijayakumar A, Vijayakumar A, Patil V, Mallikarjuna MN, Shivaswamy BS. Early diagnosis of gallbladder carcinoma: an algorithm approach. ISRN Radiol. 2012;2013:239424. https://doi.org/10.5402/2013/239424. eCollection 2013.
21. McCain RS, Diamond A, Jones C, Coleman HG. Current practices and future prospects for the management of gallbladder polyps: a topical review. World J Gastroenterol. 2018;24(26):2844–52.
22. Aldridge MC, Bismuth H. Gallbladder cancer: the polyp-cancer sequence. Br J Surg. 1990;77(4):363–4.
23. Kozuka S, Tsubone N, Yasui A, Hachisuka K. Relation of adenoma to carcinoma in the gallbladder. Cancer. 1982;50(10):2226–34.
24. Wiles R, Thoeni RF, Barbu ST, Vashist YK, Rafaelsen SR, Dewhuest C, et al. Management and follow-up of gallbladder polyps: joint guidelines between the European Society of Gastrointestinal and Abdominal Radiology (ESGAR), European Association for Endoscopic Surgery and other Interventional Techniques (EAES), International Society of Digestive Surgery – European Federation (EFISDS) and European Society of Gastrointestinal Endoscopy (ESGE). Eur Radiol. 2017;27:3856–66.
25. Babu BI, Dennison AR, Garcea G. Management and diagnosis of gallbladder polyps: a systematic review. Langenbecks Arch Surg. 2015;400(4):455–62.
26. Bhatt NR, Gillis A, Smoothey CO, Awan FN, Ridgway PF. Evidence based management of polyps of the gallbladder: a systematic review of the risk factors of malignancy. Surgeon. 2016;14(5):278–86.
27. Lu D, Radian R, Yung E, Tchelepi H. Malignant transformation of a 5-mm gallbladder polyp over 2 years: a case report and review of current literature. Ultrasound Q. 2015;31(1):66–8.
28. Runner GJ, Corwin MT, Siewert B, Eisenberg RL. Gallbladder wall thickening. AJR Am J Roentgenol. 2014;202:W1–12.
29. van Breda Vriesman AC, Engelbrecht MR, Smithuis RH, Puylaert JB. Diffuse gallbladder wall thickening: differential diagnosis. AJR Am J Roentgenol. 2007;188(2):495–501.
30. Corwin MT, Khera SS, Loehfelm TW, Yang NT, Fananapazir G. Incidentally detected focal fundal gallbladder wall thickening at contrast-enhanced computed tomography: prevalence and computed tomography features of malignancy. J Comput Assist Tomogr. 2019;43(1):149–54.
31. Kim SJ, Lee JM, Lee JY, Kim SH, Han JK, Choi BI, et al. Analysis of enhancement pattern of flat gallbladder wall thickening on MDCT to differentiate

gallbladder cancer from cholecystitis. AJR Am J Roentgenol. 2008;191(3):765–71.
32. Tongdee R, Maroongroge P, Suthikeree W. The value of MDCT scans in differention between benign and malignant gallbladder wall thickening. J Med Assoc Thai. 2011;94(5):592–600.
33. Imazu H, Mori N, Kanazawa K, Chiba M, Toyoizumi H, Torisu Y, et al. Contrast-enhanced harmonic endoscopic ultrasonography in the differential diagnois of gallbladder wall thickening. Dig Dis Sci. 2014;59:1909–16.
34. Kang TW, Kim SH, Park HJ, Lim S, Jang KM, Choi D, et al. Differentiating xanthogranulomatous cholecystitis from wall-thickening type of gallbladder cancer: added value of diffusion-weighted MRI. Clin Radiol. 2013;68(10):992–1001.
35. Tsuchiya Y. Early carcinoma of the gallbladder: macroscopic features and US findings. Radiology. 1991;179(1):171–5.
36. Zemour J, Marty M, Lapuyade B, Collet D, Chiche L. Gallbladder tumor and pseudotumor: diagnosis and management. J Visc Surg. 2014;151:289–300.
37. Andren-Sandberg A. Diagnosis and management of gallbladder polyps. N Am J Med Sci. 2012;4(5):203–11.
38. Yang HL, Sun YG, Wang Z. Polypoid lesions of the gallbladder: diagnosis and indications for surgery. Br J Surg. 1992;79(3):227–9.
39. Jung YM, Son BK, Ahn SB, Kim DH, Kim EK. Intramural gallbladder hematoma mimicking gallbladder neoplasm in a 55-year-old male patient. J Korean Surg Soc. 2011;81(3):216–20.
40. Lee CC, Huang JC, Shin JS, Wu MJ. Tumefactive sludge mimicking gallbladder neoplasm: a case report and review of literature. J Med Ultrasound. 2018;26(2):103–6.
41. Singh K, Chatterjee T. A case of gallbladder mass: Malakoplakia (The tumor mimicker). Indian J Pathol Microbiol. 2017;60(1):122–4.
42. Ishigami K, Shitani M, Kimura Y, Hasegawa T, Masaki Y, Ito A, et al. Ectopic relapse of IgG4-related disease presenting as IgG4-related sclerosing cholecystitis: a case report and review of literature. Medicine (Baltimore). 2018;97(52):e13868.
43. Franquet T, Montes M, Ruiz de Azura Y, Jimenez FJ, Cozcolluela R. Primary gallbladder carcinoma: imaging findings in 50 patients with pathologic correlation. Gastrointest Radiol. 1991;16(2):143–8.
44. Lane J, Buck JL, Zeman RK. Primary carcinoma of the gallbladder: a pictorial essay. RadioGraphics. 1989;9(2):209–28.
45. Yeh HC. Ultrasonography and computed tomography of carcinoma of the gallbladder. Radiology. 1979;133:167–73.
46. Yum HY, Fink AH. Sonographic findings in primary carcinoma of the gallbladder. Radiology. 1980;134:693–6.
47. Levy AD, Murakata LA, Rohrmann CA. Gallbladder carcinoma: Radiologic-pathologic correlation. RadioGraphics. 2001;21:295–314.
48. Misra S, Chaturvedi A, Misra NC, Sharma ID. Carcinoma of the gallbladder. Lancet Oncol. 2003;4(3):167–76.
49. Shaffer EA. Gallbladder cancer: the basics. Gastroenterol Hepatol (N Y). 2008;4(10):737–41.
50. Pilgrim CH, Groeschl RT, Christians KK, Gamblin TC. Modern perspectives on factors predisposing to the development of gallbladder cancer. HPB (oxford). 2013;15:839–44.
51. Sharma A, Sharma KL, Gupta A, Yadav A, Kumar A. Gallbladder cancer epidemiology, pathogenesis and molecular genetics: recent update. World J Gastroenterol. 2017;23(22):3978–98.
52. Sharma V, Chauhan VS, Nath G, Kumar A, Shukla VK. Role of bile bacteria in gallbladder carcinoma. Hepatogastroenterology. 2007;54(78):1622–5.
53. Sachs TE, Akintorin O, Tseng J. How should gallbladder cancer be managed? Adv Surg. 2018;52:89–100.
54. Sadamoto Y, Kubo H, Harada N, Tanaka M, Eguchi T, Nawata H. Preoperative diagnosis and staging of gallbladder carcinoma by EUS. Gastrointest Endosc. 2003;58(4):536–41.
55. Costache M, Iordache S, Kartensen JG, Saftoiu A, Vilmann P. Endoscopic ultrasound-guided fine needle aspiration: from the past to the future. Endosc Ultrasound. 2013;2(2):77–85.
56. Dorobisz T, Dorobisz K, Chabowski M, Pawlowski W, Janczak D, Patrzalek D, et al. Incidental gallbladder cancer after cholecystectomy: 1990–2014. Onco Targets Ther. 2016;9:4913–6.
57. Soreide K, Guest RV, Harrison EM, Kendall TJ, Garden OJ, Wigmore SJ. Systematic review of management of incidental gallbladder cancer after cholecystectomy. Br J Surg. 2019;106(1):32–45.
58. Hickman L, Contreras C. Gallbladder cancer: diagnosis, surgical management, and adjuvant therapies. Surg Clin N Am. 2019;99:337–55.
59. Duffy A, Capanu M, Abou-Alfa GK, Huitzil D, Jarnagin W, Fong Y, et al. Gallbladder cancer (GBC): 10-year experience at memorial sloan-kettering cancer center (MSKCC). J Surg Oncol. 2008;98(7):485–9.
60. Kasumova GG, Tabatabaie O, Najarian RM, Callery MP, Ng SC, Bullock AJ, et al. Surgical management of gallbladder cancer: simple versus extended cholecystectomy and the role of adjuvant therapy. Am Surg. 2017;266:625–31.
61. Wang SJ, Lemieux A, Kalpathy-Cramer J, Ord CB, Walker GV, Fuller CD, et al. Nomogram for predicting the benefit of adjuvant chemoradiotherapy for resected gallbladder cancer. J Clin Oncol. 2011;29(35):4627–32. https://doi.org/10.1200/JCO.2010.33.8020 Epub 2011 Nov 7.

62. Verma V, Surkar SM, Brooks ED, Simone CB 2nd, Lin C. Chemoradiotherapy versus chemotherapy alone for unresected nonmetastatic gallbladder cancer: national practice patterns and outcomes. J Natl Compr Canc Netw. 2018;16(1):59–65.
63. Shroff RT, Knox J, Dixon E. Consensus conference on gallbladder cancer. HPB (Oxford). 2015;17(8):664–5.
64. Hakeem AR, Papoulas M, Menon KV. The role of neoadjuvant chemotherapy or chemoradiotherapy for advanced gallbladder cancer—a systematic review. Eur J Surg Oncol. 2019;45:83–91.
65. Houry S, Barrier A, Huguier M. Irradiation therapy for gallbladder carcinoma: recent advances. J Hepatobiliary Pancreat Surg. 2001;8(6):518–24.
66. Houry S, Haccart V, Huguier M, Schlienger M. Gallbladder cancer: role of radiation therapy. Hepatogastroenterology. 1999;46(27):1578–84.
67. Ishii H, Furuse J, Yonemoto N, Nagase M, Yoshino M, Sato T. Chemotherapy in the treatment of advanced gallbladder cancer. Oncology. 2004;66(2):138–42.

Laboratory Examinations of Diseases of the Gallbladder

Jae Bock Chung and Jae Uk Chong

Introduction

When patients present to the physician with abdominal pain in the right upper quadrant (RUQ), nausea, vomiting, and fever, we can diagnose the disease of the gallbladder (GB) with ease. However, if the symptom is vague RUQ discomfort, it is not easy to diagnose the problem, and several examinations are needed to solve the problem. Laboratory examinations for diseases of the GB include CBC, liver function tests including bilirubin, serum amylase, and CRP, and tumor markers such as CA 19-9 and CEA. In addition, there are stool examination for parasites, serum IgG4 for IgG4-related disease, bile examinations from duodenum or GB, and tests for *Helicobacter* sp. In this chapter, we describe laboratory examinations for diseases of the GB.

J. B. Chung (✉)
Department of Internal Medicine, NHIS Ilsan Hospital, Yonsei University College of Medicine, Goyang-si, Gyeonggi-do, Korea
e-mail: jbchung@yuhs.ac

J. U. Chong
Department of Surgery, NHIS Ilsan Hospital, Yonsei University College of Medicine, Goyang-si, Gyeonggi-do, Korea
e-mail: jaeuk1216@nhimc.or.kr

Tests of Acute Cholecystitis

White Blood Cell (WBC)

Mild acute cholecystitis (AC) produces only subtle abnormalities on routine laboratory investigations. The white blood cell count commonly ranges between 10,000 and 15,000/mm^3, usually with a preponderance of neutrophils, but counts may be normal [1]. Generally, the mean WBC count increases significantly with increasing clinical score of AC [mild, 10.4 ± 3.9/μL (range; 4–19.8/μL); moderate, 12.1 ± 5.1/μL (3.8–28/μL); severe, 18.8 ± 9.9/μL (3.1–53.8/μL)] [2].

WBC counts greater than 13,000–17,000/mm^3 suggest the possibility of more severe disease such as gangrene [3–5], but high counts may still occur in patients with uncomplicated disease [6].

According to the TG18/TG13 severity grading for AC, elevated WBC count (>18,000/mm^3) is associated with Grade II (moderate) AC; and presence of renal dysfunction (creatinine >2.0 mg/dl), hepatic dysfunction (PT-INR >1.5), or hematologic dysfunction (platelet count <100,000/mm^3) is regarded as Grade III (severe) AC [7].

Gallbladder (GB) perforation may also occur in patients with only mildly elevated or even normal WBC counts, especially in elderly patients [1, 8, 9]. Among the 90 patients with

J. B. Chung and K. Okazaki (eds.), *Diseases of the Gallbladder*,
https://doi.org/10.1007/978-981-15-6010-1_2

GB perforation due to AC, WBC counts were 5,000–10,000/mm^3 in 18.9%, 10,000–12,000/mm^3 in 20.0%, 12,000–20,000/mm^3 in 24.4%, and 20,000–37,000/mm^3 in 36.7% [10].

Recently, Sato et al. [11] reported that inflammation-based prognostic scores, such as the NLR (neutrophil-to-lymphocyte ratio), GPS (the Glasgow Prognostic Score), mGPS (modified Glasgow Prognostic Score) and the CRP/ALB (C-reactive protein/Albumin) ratio, could predict the severity grade independently in patients with AC, and may play a complementary role in predicting disease severity of AC in conjunction with the TG 13 severity grade.

Bilirubin

Jaundice is occasionally present in acute cholecystitis (AC) and is generally mild. Elevated serum bilirubin levels of up to 3.5 mg/dL are most frequently caused by extension of the inflammatory process to the common bile duct (CBD) or the hepatic parenchyma, rather than the CBD obstruction [1].

Twenty-five percent of patients with acute calculous cholecystitis had a serum bilirubin level between 2.0 and 5.0 mg/dL with no CBD abnormality. Over one-third of patients with acute acalculous cholecystitis had an elevated bilirubin level (greater than 2.0 mg/dL) with a normal CBD [12].

The serum total bilirubin (mg/dL) [mean ± SD (range)] level of patients with AC and concomitant CBD stone was significantly higher than those without CBD stone [4.08 ± 3.30 (0.6–23.0) vs. 1.72 ± 1.48 (0.2–8.6), $p < 0.001$] [13].

A rapid increase in serum bilirubin level of more than 4 mg/dL in a day should raise suspicions for GB perforation [1].

Liver Function Test (LFT)

About 70% of patients with acute cholecystitis (AC) showed some evidence of liver dysfunction [14]. Acute cholecystitis is associated with mild elevation of LFTs such as the serum transaminase and alkaline phosphatase, which rarely exceed two to three times the normal levels [1].

However, incidences of liver dysfunction were significantly increased when ductal calculi were present [15]. Choledocholithiasis is estimated to be present in 5–10% of patients undergoing cholecystectomy for symptomatic cholelithiasis [16, 17]. According to the recent report by Rahal et al. [18], the prevalence of CBD stone was 25% in patients with AC.

The proportions of abnormal LFTs were significantly higher in acute cholecystitis with CBD stone for total bilirubin (47.7% vs. 20.2%), SGOT (62.8% vs. 27.1%), and ALP (56.6% vs. 21.0%) ($p < 0.0001$) than those without CBD stone [19]. AC patients with any abnormal LFT, any two abnormal LFTs, and three abnormal LFTs, among total bilirubin >1.2 mg/dl, SGOT >40 U/L and ALP >120 IU/L, were found to be 2.23, 5.73, and 12.0 times more likely to have a simultaneous CBD stone, respectively [19].

A prospective study by Vildehult et al. [20] analyzed 1171 patients operated for gallstone disease and established ALP and bilirubin as the most reliable predictors of CBD stone, which were found in 4.2% of patients with elevated liver function values. However, false positive and false negative values were common, especially in patients with a history of cholecystitis or pancreatitis. Another study found a different liver enzyme, namely γ-glutamyl transpeptidase, as the most reliable predictor of CBD stone [13]. Many other studies evaluating LFTs for prediction of CBD stone only had limited results [18].

A scoring system integrating LFTs and clinical variables would be more informative in predicting the presence of CBD stone [19].

C-Reactive Protein (CRP)

The serum CRP, a well-known acute phase reactant that increases rapidly in inflammatory process, is included in the laboratory findings for the diagnosis of acute cholecystitis (AC) in Tokyo Guidelines [7], and reflects severity of the gallbladder inflammation and have been identified as a predictor for conversion from laparoscopic cholecystectomy (LC) to open procedure in several studies [21–24].

In general, the serum CRP levels <10 mg/L are clinically insignificant for diagnosis of AC and other acute inflammatory reactions. On the other hand, CRP levels >100 mg/L are strongly associated with local tissue necrosis, and bacterial infection rates are reported to be 80–85% [25, 26].

The serum CRP cutoff value in diagnosing AC was reported as 30.5 mg/L (95% CI, 10.2–50.8 mg/L) with 85% sensitivity, 92% specificity, and 89% AUC at the cutoff point [27]. Advanced inflammatory stages of GB were associated with significantly increased CRP values (mean; 42.1 mg/L [range; 2–227 mg/L] in mild AC, 91.0 mg/L [2–319 mg/L] in moderate AC and 146.4 mg/L [2–419 mg/L] in advanced AC) [24]. Mean CRP levels of groups according to Tokyo Guidelines were also found to be significantly different: 18.96 mg/L in Group I, 133.51 mg/L in Group II and 237.23 mg/L in Group III [28].

In a large-scale retrospective cohort study of 1843 patients, the optimal cutoff value of CRP in diagnosing mild AC was 26.5 mg/L (95% CI, 13.6–39.4 mg/L) with 84% sensitivity, 89% specificity, and 86% AUC at the cutoff point, and the cutoff point of CRP in diagnosing moderate and/or severe AC was 67 mg/L (95% CI, 61.9–72.1 mg/L) with 96% sensitivity, 100% specificity, and 97% AUC at the cutoff point [27].

The serum CRP levels can be a predictor of gangrenous cholecystitis. Patients with gangrenous cholecystitis had a greater CRP value (median; 94 mg/L, range; 0–500 mg/L, n = 106) than non-gangrenous acute cholecystitis (median; 17 mg/L, range; 1.0–380 mg/L, n = 184) [29].

An increase in the WBC count, LFT values (AST, ALT, ALP, GGT), and indices of inflammation (CRP, fibrinogen) reflect the severity of GB inflammation and have been identified as risk factors for conversion in several studies [30, 31]. Wevers et al. [23] found that older age (>65 years) and elevated CRP level (>165 mg/L) are independent factors for conversion in early LC for acute cholecystitis, and concluded that high risk of conversion should be informed during surgical planning for AC in patients with age >65 years and/or CRP level >165 mg/L.

Amylase

Hyperamylasemia occurring with GB disease in the absence of pancreatitis has been described by many authors [32–35]. Mild elevation of serum amylase activity is a frequent finding in acute cholecystitis, and amylase activity may increase by 3–5 times the normal values. Hyperamylasemia is especially common in gangrenous forms [1].

Hyperamylasemia without pancreatitis was found in 4% of acute calculous cholecystitis and 37% of acute acalculous cholecystitis, all without CBD abnormality [12].

In most of the patients (41 of 43 patients) who underwent cholecystectomy in presence of elevated amylase and/or lipase level without the evidence of clinical pancreatitis preoperatively or gross pancreatitis intraoperatively, the amylase and lipase levels returned to normal within 48 hours of cholecystectomy [36].

Geokas et al. [37] speculated that a normal pancreas in presence of cholecystitis may respond with a high output of amylase, whereas the output of amylase from a chronically inflamed, fibrotic pancreas may be much lower.

Bernard and associates [32] suggested that the hyperamylasemia seen in acute cholecystitis without pancreatic disease is caused by absorption of the enzyme via the biliary ducts and liver. Their experimental study showed that the injection of pancreatic juice into the obstructed common bile duct resulted in no change in serum amylase concentration, while concomitant ligation of the cystic duct increased the amylase several folds.

Although hyperamylasemia may result from associated pancreatic inflammation in AC, evidence of acute pancreatitis is often lacking and the source of the enzyme may be the GB itself.

Amylase is present in various concentrations in many tissues including the GB [38], and ectopic pancreatic tissue has been reported to be found in the GB [39].

Etiologic Pathogens

Acute cholecystitis (AC) is initially a chemical inflammation, but regularly complicated by bacterial invasion from the gut. Mixed infections are prevalent, bactibilia occurs in at least 60% of the early stage of AC. In a series of 515 patients with AC, GB bile culture was positive in 63% of cases operated within 24 hours of the onset of AC, while in the group receiving delayed surgery, after 11 days or more, the rate decreased to 31% [40]. A close relationship is found between the presence of bactibilia and infectious complications [41].

In ACC (acute calculous cholecystitis), the most commonly encountered pathogens are enteric origin (*Escherichia coli*, *Klebsiella* spp., *Enterococcus* spp. and anaerobes) regardless of the duration of ACC [42, 43]. The presence of bacteria in the gallbladder (GB) bile varies from 41 to 63% in patients who underwent cholecystectomy for ACC [40, 42, 43].

Among 139 eligible patients who underwent cholecystectomy for the treatment of ACC, 50.4% (79 pts) showed bactibilia and 21.6% (30 pts) showed bacteremia. In patients with both bactibilia and bacteremia, 50% (11/22 pts) showed concordant cultured organisms. Antimicrobial resistance rate of *E. coli* was 59.1% in bile specimens and 16.7% in blood samples [44].

Recurrence of ACC following antibiotic treatment was between 0 and 37% [45].

In AAC (acute acalculous cholecystitis), the reported pathogens are bacteria (*Brucella* spp., *Coxiella burnetii*, *Leptospira interrogans*, *Mycobacterium tuberculosis*, *Orientia tsutsugamushi*, *Salmonella* spp., and *Vibrio cholerae*), fungus (*Candida albicans*, *C. glabrata*, *C. parapsilosis*, *C. tropicalis*; *Histoplasma capsulatum*, and *Cryptococcus* spp.), parasite (*Cyclospora* spp., microsporidia, *Plasmodium falciparum*, *P. vivax*, and *Schistosoma mansoni*), and virus (Cytomegalovirus, Epstein-Barr virus, and Dengue virus) [46, 47].

There were some reports of patients with AAC from *Fusarium* spp., *Clostridia glycolicum*, *Actinomyces* spp., *Klebsiella ozaenae*, *Listeria monocytogenes*, *Staphylococcus aureus*, *Streptococcus bovis* and *Campylobacter* spp. [47–54].

Bile aspiration of the GB showed a limited role in the diagnosis of AC. Bile culture was not helpful in the prediction of AC, since results were not available until a minimum of 24–48 hours after the aspiration. In addition, gram-stained smears and bile cultures suffered from low sensitivity (48% and 38%, respectively); consequently, a negative test does not allow the diagnosis of AC to be excluded [55]. Interestingly, GB bile obtained after cholecystectomy for symptomatic cholelithiasis showed different culture positivity rate depending on the location acquired from (100.0% in neck, 64.5% in body, and 41.9% in fundus) [56]. Yoshida et al. [57] also recommend that a separate fragment of gallbladder wall should be sent for culture and histology, along with gallbladder bile for culture during cholecystectomy, especially in severe forms of AC.

Tumor Markers

Carbohydrate antigen 19-9 and carcinoembryonic antigen are tumor markers most commonly utilized in the diagnosis of gallbladder cancer (GBC). The sensitivity/specificity of CA 19-9, CA 125, CA 242 and CEA in diagnosis of GBC were 77.5%/68.7%, 64%/90%, 64%/83%, and 61%/44%, respectively [58–61].

Shukla et al. [58] reported that combination of CA 242 and CA 125 achieved best sensitivity (87.5%) and specificity (85.7%) among CA 242, CA 19-9, CA 15-3, and CA 125 in patients with GBC. Diagnostic accuracy (80.65%) was the highest in the combination of CA 19-9 and CA 125.

There are also case reports of unusual GBC producing α-fetoprotein, α-fetoprotein-L3, and human chorionic gonadotrophin, and α-fetoprotein and CEA [62–64].

Tunan et al. [65] evaluated the prognostic value of CA 19-9 and CEA in 73 patients who underwent radical resection for GBC. The cumulative 5-year survival rates in group I (patients with elevation of CEA), group II (patients with elevation of CA 19-9 but not CEA), and group III (patients without elevations of either CA 19-9 or CEA) were 0, 14.0%, and 42.8%, respectively ($P < 0.05$).

There are several reports investigating neutrophil/lymphocyte ratio (NLR), platelet/lymphocyte ratio (PLR), GPS, absolute neutrophil count, and absolute lymphocyte count in patients with GBC as a prognostic indicator [66–69].

Currently, many tumor diagnostic, prognostic, predictive, and therapeutic biomarkers are being evaluated for clinical applications, but the results are still unsatisfactory [70–75].

Parasite

Ascaris lumbricoides is the most frequent human intestinal nematode. Ascaris may enter the common bile duct and main pancreatic duct in 2.1% of cases [76]. In gallbladder ascariasis, fatal complications such as gallbladder empyema, septicemia, pericholecystic abscess, or perforation may ensue [76, 77].

In gallbladder ascariasis, the worms were expelled spontaneously with the resolution of symptoms and signs in 21% (10/47 patients) [77].

The parasites causing cholecystitis have been reported as following: *Taenia solium*, *T. saginata*, *Schistosoma mansoni*, *S. haematobium*, *Giardia lamblia*, *Leishmania* spp., *Plasmodium falciparum*, *Sarcocystis* spp., *Cryptosporidium* spp., *Cystoisospora belli*, *Echinococcus granulosus*, *Toxocara canis*, *T. cati*, *Clonorchis sinensis*, *Opisthorchis felineus*, *Fasciola hepatica*, *F. gigantica and Dicrocoelium dendriticum* [46, 78–97].

C. sinensis eggs were detected in 122 (66.7%) of 183 gallbladder stones (pigment stones; 115, cholesterol stones; 23, mixed stones; 45) based on morphologic characteristics and results from real-time fluorescent PCR. The positive rate of *C. sinensis* with light microscopy was 84.3% in pigment stones, 17.4% in cholesterol stones, and 46.7% in mixed stones [98]. Numerous calcified parasite eggs detected in the gallbladder wall were compatible with eggs from the liver fluke [99].

Parasite infection can be diagnosed by detecting eggs in stool and bile examinations. Serology test can also be informative. US guided gallbladder aspiration has been reported to be useful in diagnosis of biliary fascioliasis [100].

Immunoglobulin G4 (IgG4)

IgG4-related disease (RD) is a chronic inflammatory disorder characterized by high level of serum IgG4, tumefaction, or tissue infiltration by $IgG4^+$ plasma cells. A diagnosis of IgG4-RD is definite in patients with positive findings in following three features: (1) diffuse/localized swelling or masses in single or multiple organs, (2) elevated levels of serum IgG4 concentration (135 mg/dl or higher), and (3) histopathological study showing marked lymphocyte and plasmacyte infiltration and fibrosis, and IgG4-positive plasma cell infiltration (ratio of IgG4/IgG positive cell >40% and IgG4-positive plasma cells/HPF >10) [101, 102].

A serum IgG4 cut-off level of $\geq$135 mg/dl is considered a unique and reliable marker predictive of IgG4-RD [102]. The reported sensitivity of IgG4 for the diagnosis of IgG4-RD ranged from 52 to 97%, whereas the specificity ranged from 60 to 97% [103]. The IgG4 value was significantly higher in patients with multiorgan involvement than in those with a single manifestation (median; 629 mg/dl vs. 299 mg/dl, $p < 0.01$) [104].

IgG4-RD in the hepato-biliary pancreatic system are IgG4-related pancreatitis, IgG4-related sclerosing cholangitis, IgG4-related cholecystitis, and IgG4-related hepatopathy [105, 106].

IgG4-related cholecystitis has been reported to present as either diffuse gallbladder wall thickening or localized mass. Ishigami et al. [107] found 12 cases of IgG4-related cholecystitis after systemic review through PubMed search (1980 to February 2018), and analyzed 13 cases after adding their case. Among the 13 cases, 5 cases showed diffuse wall thickening, while remaining 8 cases presented with focal mass formation mimicking GB cancer. And only 6 of 13 cases showed serum IgG4 levels of ≥135 mg/dl at the time of diagnosis.

For early diagnosis of IgG4-related cholecystitis, we should keep in mind the radiologic findings which suggest IgG4-related cholecystitis, including diffuse wall thickening with intact mucosal layer [107]. And in the case presenting with a mass lesion of GB, consider a biopsy from the lesion if possible with a test of serum IgG4.

Bile

Microscopic examination of bile began in 1919, when Lyon used a magnesium sulfate solution instilled into the duodenum to cause contraction of the GB and relaxation of the sphincter of Oddi [108].

The criteria for microscopic examination of bile in diagnosis of cholecystolithiasis include the presence of at least one typical cholesterol crystal or bilirubinate granule according to Juniper and Burson [109] or in the presence of a large amount of spheroliths [109, 110].

Intermittent secretion of supersaturated bile was noticed by repeated sampling of hepatic bile from patients with T tubes [111]. And the intermittent presence of cholesterol crystals in duodenal bile is probably not due to dissolution of crystals or varying dietary cholesterol intake [112].

Microscopic examination of duodenal bile from nasoduodenal intubation predicted the gallstone composition correctly in 75% (21 of 42 patients); it predicted all four (100%) pigment stones, 50% (3 of 6) of calcium-containing cholesterol stones, and 78% (14 of 18) of cholesterol stones with pigment shells, and the prediction rate was similar to microscopic examination of bile aspirated directly from the gallbladder during surgery (75% vs. 82%; p=NS) [113].

Dahan et al. [114] reported on the prospective evaluation of endoscopic ultrasonography and microscopic examination of duodenal bile obtained under endoscopic control in 45 patients with suspected cholecystolithiasis and at least two normal transcutaneous ultrasonography for the diagnosis of cholecystolithiasis. The sensitivity of EUS was higher than that of microscopic examination of duodenal bile (96% vs. 67%, $p < 0.03$) with similar specificity (86% vs. 91%).

Itoi et al. [115] evaluated the efficacy of bile cytology using endoscopic transpapillary gallbladder drainage (ETGD) and CT in 85 patients (27 GB cancer and 58 benign GB diseases). Looking only at the 71 successful ETGD cases, ETGD cytology and CT had 100% and 82% sensitivity, 98% and 92% specificity, and 99% and 89% accuracy, respectively ($p = 0.036$ and 0.025, respectively). GB bile from percutaneous aspiration of the GB for gram-stained smear and culture in patients with acute cholecystitis showed a limited diagnostic role as mentioned earlier in this chapter [55].

At present, bile examination is not widely used clinically due to invasiveness of the procedure with relatively poor clinical benefits. However, further efforts in improving the methods of examination and discovery of novel targets to improve diagnosis may prove to be valuable in the future for treatment of diseases of the GB.

Helicobacter

H. pylori urease gene was demonstrated in three bile samples from patients with advanced gastric cancer and pancreatic head cancer by nested PCR using two sets of primers for the *H. pylori* urease A gene in 1995 [116], and Kawaguchi et al. [117] detected *H. pylori* in the gallbladder's mucosa of a patient with calculous cholecystitis in 1996.

The prevalence of *Helicobacter* species infection of the biliary tract has been reported from 0 to 70% in different studies from different regions [118–122].

Among 95 gallstone patients, serum *H. pylori* IgG was detected in 75 (79%) patients. Of the 75 IgG sero-positive patients, 26 (34.7%) were positive for *H. pylori* antigen in the bile samples [119]. *Helicobacter* genus DNA detected in bile ranged from 24.4 to 46% of cholecystolithiasis [118, 120, 121].

PCR for *H. pylori* DNA was positive in 32.6% of GB tissue specimens in 49 patients (GB stones in 43 patients, GB with CBD stone in 5 patients, and GB tuberculosis in one patient) [118].

In gallstones, *Helicobacter spp.* and *pylori* have been detected in the nucleus of gallstone but not in the envelope [122, 123]. *H. pylori* specific DNA was detected in 11 of 20 patients with cholesterol gallstones consisting of mixed bacterial population [123].

In gallbladder cancer (GBC), *H. pylori* was confirmed in 18 (33%) of 54 GBC tissue samples [124].

A meta-analysis study of 18 articles involving 1544 participants, of which 1061 biliary cases with chronic cholecystitis/cholelithia sis and 483 for control, showed significantly increased risk of chronic cholecystitis and cholelithiasis in the presence of *H. pylori* infection of the GB (OR = 3.022; 95% CI, 1.987–4.815) [125]. In contrast, Sanchez et al. [126] found *Helicobacter* sp. in only one of 95 Mexican patients with gallstone disease by immunohistochemistry analysis and in only one of 32 cases by PCR. Similar result was reported from Germany [127]. Among the 99 patients (57 cases of gallstone disease, 20 cases of GBC and 20 control patients), Helicobacteraceae was detected in only one patient (acute gallbladder disease with biliary colics) by PCR.

Recently and interestingly, Backert et al. [128] reported, for the first time, the identification and characterization of a community consisting of live *Staphylococcus saprophyticus*, *Corynebacterium urinapleomorphum*, and *H. pylori* in the gallbladder of a patient with acute cholecystitis.

In summary, *H. pylori* may have a role in the formation of gallstone and inflammation of the gallbladder, but further studies are warranted to prove the association.

Conclusion

Currently, we can diagnose the patients with typical manifestations of gallbladder diseases utilizing laboratory examinations described in this chapter along with imaging study. Nevertheless, diagnosis of patients with vague symptoms for suspected gallbladder disease and early gallbladder cancer is still challenging when evidences from laboratory examinations and the imaging study are uncertain. To overcome this challenge, discovery of novel laboratory tests and tumor markers that can enhance diagnostic accuracy are critically needed.

References

1. Strasberg SM, Clavien P-A. Acute calculous cholecystitis. In: Haubrich WS, Schaffner F, Berk JE, editors. Bockus gastroenterology, 5th ed. Philadelphia, Pennsylvania: W.B. Saunders Company; 1995. p. 2641–2
2. Ambe PC, Papadakis M, Zimgibl H. A proposal for a preoperative clinical scoring system for acute cholecystitis. J Surg Res. 2016;200(2):473–9.
3. Yacoub WN, Petrosyan M, Sehgal I, Ma Y, Chandrasoma P, Mason RJ. Prediction of patients with acute cholecystitis requiring emergent cholecystectomy: a simple score. Gastroenterol Res Pract. 2010;2010:901739. https://doi.org/10.1155/2010/901739.
4. Merriam LT, Kanaan SA, Dawes LG, Angelos P, Prystowsky JB, Rega RV, et al. Gangrenous cholecystitis: analysis of risk factors and experience with laparascopic cholecystectomy. Surgery. 1999;126:680–6.
5. Falor AE, Zobel M, Kaji A, Neville A, De Virgilio C. Admission variables predictive of gangrenous cholecystitis. Am Surg. 2012;78(10):1075–8.
6. McDonald JA. Perforation of the gallbladder associated with acute cholecystitis: 8-year review of 20 cases. Ann Surg. 1966;164:849–52.
7. Yokoe M, Hata J, Takada T, Strasberg SM, Asbun HJ, Wakabayashi G, et al. Tokyo guidelines 2018: diagnostic criteria and severity grading of acute cholecystitis (with videos). J Hepatobiliary Pancreat Sci. 2018;25:41–54.
8. Hoerr ST, Hazard JB. Acute cholecystitis without gallbladder stones. Am J Surg. 1966;111:47–55.
9. Lindberg EF, Grinnan GLB, Smith L. Acalculous cholecystitis in Viet Nam casualties. Ann Surg. 1970;171:152–7.
10. Pines B, Rabinovitch J. Perforation of the gallbladder in acute cholecystitis. Ann Surg. 1954;140(2):170–9.

11. Sato N, Kinoshita A, Imai N, Akau T, Yokota T, Iwaku A, et al. Inflammation-based prognostic scores predict disease severity in patients with acute cholecystitis. Eur J Gastroenterol Hepatol. 2018;30:484–9.
12. Kurzweil SM, Shapiro MC, Andrus CH, Wiittgen CM, Herrmann VM, Kaminski DL. Hyperbilirubinemia without common bile duct abnormalities and hyperamylasemia without pancreatitis with gallbladder disease. Arch Surg. 1994;129:829–33.
13. Ahn KS, Yoon Y-S, Han H-S, Cho JY. Use of liver function tests as first-line diagnostic tools for predicting common bile duct stones in acute cholecystitis. World J Surg. 2016;40:1925–31.
14. Dunlop MG, King PM, Gunn AA. Acute abdominal pain: the value of liver function tests in suspected cholelithiasis. J R Coll Surg Edinb. 1989;34(3):124–7.
15. Jarvinen H. Abnormal liver function tests in acute cholecystitis; the predicting of common duct stones. Ann Clin Res. 1978;10(6):323–7.
16. O'Neil CJ, Gilles DM, Gani JS. Choledocholithiasis: overdiagnosed endoscopically and untreated laparoscopically. ANZ J Surg. 2008;487–91.
17. Quispel R, van Driel LM, Veldt BJ, van Haard PM, Bruno MJ. The utility and yield of endoscopic ultrasonography for suspected choledocholithiasis in common gastroenterology practice. Eur J Gastroenterol Hepatol. 2016;28:1473–6.
18. Rahal MA, Rammal MO, karaoui W, Hallal A, Tamim H, Shaib Y. Predictors of bile tree pathology in patients with gallbladder disease. Eur J Gastroenterol Hepatol. 2017;29:1017–21.
19. Zgheib H, Wakil C, Shayya S, Maihac A, Al-Taki N, El Sayed M, et al. Utility of liver function tests in acute cholecystitis. Ann Hepatobiliary Pancreat Surg. 2019;23(3):219–27.
20. Vildehult P, Sandblom G, Rudberg C, Rasmussen IC. Are liver function tests, pancreatitis and cholecystitis predictors of common bile duct stones? Result of a prospective, population-based cohort study of 1171 patients undergoing cholecystectomy. HPB (Oxford). 2011;13:519–27.
21. Kim MS, Kwon HJ, Park HW, Park JY, Chung EC, Park HJ, et al. Preoperative prediction model for conversion of laparoscopic to open cholecystectomy in patients with acute cholecystitis: based on clinical, laboratory, and CT parameters. J Comput Assist Tomogr. 2014;38(5):727–32.
22. Ercan M, Bostanci EB, Teke Z, Karaman K, Dalgic T, Ulas M, et al. Predictive factors for conversion to open surgery in patients undergoing elective laparoscopic cholecystectomy. J Laparoendosc Adv Surg Tech A. 2010;20:427–34.
23. Wevers KP, van Westreenen HL, Patijn GA. Laparoscopic cholecystectomy in acute cholecystitis: C-reactive protein level combined with age predicts conversion. Surg Laparosc Endosc Percutan Tech. 2013;23(2):163–6.
24. Schafer M, Krahenbuhl L, Buchler MW. Predictive factors for the type of surgery in acute cholecystitis. Am J Surg. 2001;182(3):291–7.
25. Gabay C, Kushner I. Acute-phase proteins and other systemic responses to inflammation. N Engl J Med. 1999;340:448–54.
26. Moeley JJ, Kushner I. Serum C-reactive protein levels in disease. Ann NY Acad Sci. 1982;389:406–18.
27. Beliave AM, Marshall RJ, Booth M. C-reactive protein has a better discriminative power than white cell count in the diagnosis of acute cholecystitis. J Surg Res. 2015;198:66–72.
28. Gurbulak EK, Gurbulak B, Akgun IE, Duzkoylu Y, Battal M, Celayir MF, et al. Prediction of the grade of acute cholecystitis by plasma level of C-reactive protein. Iran Red Xrescent Med J. 2015;17(4):e28091.
29. Nikfarjam M, Niumsawatt V, Sethu A, Fink MA, Muralidharan V, Starkey G, et al. Outcomes of contemporary management of gangrenous and non-gangrenous acute cholecystitis. HPB (Oxford). 2011;13:551–8.
30. Lipman JM, Claridge JA, Haridas M, Marin MD, Yao DC, Grimes KL, et al. Preoperative findings predict conversion from laparoscopic to open cholecystectomy. Surgery. 2007;142:556–65.
31. Licciardello A, Arena M, Nicosia A, Di Stefano B, Cali G, Arena G, et al. Preoperative risk factors for conversion from laparoscopic to open cholecystectomy. Eur Rev Med Pharmacol Sci. 2014;18(2 Suppl):60–8.
32. Bernard HR, Criscione JR, Moyer CA. The pathologic significance of the serum amylase concentration; an evaluation with special reference to pancreatitis and biliary lithiasis. AMA Arch Surg. 1959;79:311–8.
33. Adams JT, Libertino JA, Schwartz SI. Significance of the elevated serum amylase. Surgery. 1968;63:877–84.
34. Parodi HC, Colombato LO, Gutierrez S, Lattanzi M. The pancreatic enzyme values in the diagnosis of acute pancreatitis and acute biliary tract diseases. Acta Gastroenterol Latinam. 1989;19:123–9.
35. Mackie CR, Wood RA, Preece PE, Cuschieri A. Surgical pathology at early elective operation for suspected acute gallstone pancreatitis: preliminary report of a prospective clinical trial. Br J Surg. 1985;72(3):179–81.
36. Vernava A, Andrus C, Hermann VM, Kaminski DL. Pancreatitis after biliary tract surgery. Arch Surg. 1987;122:575–80.
37. Geokas MC, Van Lancker JL, Kadell BM, Machleder HI. Acute pancreatitis. Ann Intern Med. 1972;76(1):105–17.
38. Whitten RO, Chandler WL, Thomas MGE, Clayson KJ, Fine JS. Survey of alpha-amylase activity and isoamylase in autopsy tissue. Clin Chem. 1988;34(8):1552–5.
39. Sanchiz Cardenas EM, Soler Humanes R, Lavado Fernandez AI, Diaz Nieto R, Suarez Munoz MA. Ectopic pancreas in gallbladder. Clinical significance, diagnostic and therapeutic implications. Rev Esp Enferm Dig. 2015;107:701–3.

40. Jarvinen HJ. Biliary bacteremia at various stages of acute cholecystitis. Acta Chir Scand. 1980;146:427–30.
41. Bjorvatn B. Cholecystitis-etiology and treatment-microbiological aspects. Scand J Gastroenterol Suppl. 1984;90:65–70.
42. Fuks D, Cosse C, Regimbeau J-M. Antibiotic therapy in acute calculous cholecystitis. J Visc Surg. 2013;150:3–8.
43. Csendes A, Burdiles P, Maluenda F, Diaz JC, Csendes P, Mitru N. Simultaneous bacteriologic assessment of bile from gallbladder and common bile duct in control subjects and patients with gallstones and common duct stones. Arch Surg. 1996;131:389–94.
44. Bang CS, Yoon JH, Kim YJ, Kim JB, Baik GH, Suk KT, et al. Clinical impact of body mass index on bactibilia and bacteremia. BMC Gastroenterol. 2014;14:104. https://doi.org/10.1186/1471-230X-14-104.
45. van Dijk AH, de Reuver PR, Tasma TN, van Dieren S, Hugh TJ, Boermeester MA. Systemic review of antibiotic treatment for acute calculous cholecystitis. Br J Surg. 2016;103:797–811.
46. Huffman JL, Schenker S. Acute acalculous cholecystitis: a review. Clin Gastroenterol Hepatol. 2010;8:15–22.
47. Szvalb AD, Kontoyiannis DP. Acute acalculous cholecystitis due to Fusarium species and review of the literature on fungal cholecystitis. Mycoses. 2019;62:847–53.
48. Cai D, Sorokin V, Lutwick L, Liu W, Dalal S, Sandhu K, et al. C. glycolicum as the sole cause pf bacteremia in a patient with acute cholecystitis. Ann Clin Lab Sci. 2012;42(2):162–4.
49. Santos LD, Roqan KA, Kennerson AR. Cytologic diagnosis of suppurative cholecystitis due to Candida albicans and actinomyces. A report of 2 cases. Acta Cytol. 2004;48(3):407–10.
50. Baig A, Gujral M, Hameed R, Borra S. Klebsiella ozaenae cholecystitis. Am J Med Sci. 2011;342(3):259–61.
51. Descy J, De Mol P, Hayette MP, Huynen P, Meex C, Melin P. Acute cholecystitis with Listeria monocytogenes. Acta Clin Belg. 2012;67(4):295–7.
52. Merchant SS, Falsey AR. Staphylococcus aureus cholecystitis: a report of three cases with review of the literature. Yale J Biol Med. 2002;75(5–6):285–91.
53. Deering EM, Muravec Z, Castineira CF, O'Donoghue G. Streptococcus bovis-related cholecystitis. BMJ Case Rep. 2013;2013:bcr2013008581. https://doi.org/10.1136/bcr-2013-008581.
54. Udayakumar D, Sanaullah M. Campylobacter cholecystitis. Int J Med Sci. 2009;42(2):162–4.
55. McGahan JP, Lindfors KK. Acute cholecystitis: diagnostic accuracy of percutaneous aspiration of the gallbladder. Radiology. 1988;167(3):669–71.
56. Manolis EN, Filippou DK, Papadopoulos VP, Katostaras T, Christianakis E, Bonatsos G, et al. The culture site of the gallbladder affects recovery of bacteria in symptomatic cholelithiasis. J Gastrointestin Liver Dis. 2008;17(2):179–82.
57. Yoshida M, Takada T, Kawarada Y, Tanaka A, Nimura Y, Gomi H, et al. Antimicrobial therapy for acute cholecystitis: Tokyo guidelines. J Hepatobiliary Pancreat Surg. 2007;14:83–90.
58. Shukla VK, Gurubachan, Sharma D, Dixit VK, Usha. Diagnostic value of serum CA 242, CA 19-9, CA 15-3 and CA 125 in patients with carcinoma of the gallbladder. Trop Gastroenterol. 2006;27(4):160-5.
59. Chaube A, Tewari M, Singh U, Shukla HS. CA 125: a potential tumor marker for gallbladder cancer. J Surg Oncol. 2006;93:665–9.
60. Rana S, Dutta U, Kochhar R, Rana SV, Gupta R, Pal R, et al. Evaluation of CA 242 as a tumor marker in gallbladder cancer. J Gastrointest Cancer. 2012;43:267–71.
61. Srivastava K, Srivastava A, Mittal B. Potential biomarkers in gallbladder cancer: present status and future directions. Biomarkers. 2013;18(1):1–9.
62. Sentani K, Uraoka N, Oue N, Yasui W. Alpha-fetoprotein-producing clear cell carcinoma of the gallbladder with neuroendocrine differentiation. Med Mol Morphol. 2014;47(1):54–6.
63. Sugaya Y, Sugaya H, Kuronuma Y, Hisauchi T, Harada T. A case of gallbladder carcinoma producing alpha-fetoprotein (AFP) and carcinoembryonic antigen (CEA). Gastroenterol Jpn. 1989;24(3):325–31.
64. Goto A, Ishimine Y, Hirata T, Naito T, Yabana T, Adachi T, et al. Gallbladder cancer with elevated serum α-fetoprotein, α-fetoprotein-L3, and human chorionic gonadotropin levels. Gan To Kagaku Ryoho. 2014;41(8):1021–5.
65. Tunan Y, Hong Y, Xiujun C. Preoperative prediction of survival in resectable gallbladder cancer by a combined utilization of CA 19-9 and carcinoembryonic antigen. Chin Med J. 2014;127(12):2299–303.
66. Zhang Y, Jiang C, Li J, Sun J, Qu X. Prognostic significance of preoperative neutrophil/lymphocyte ratio and platelet/lymphocyte ratio in patients with gallbladder carcinoma. Clin Transl Oncol. 2015;17:810–8.
67. Zhang L, Wang R, Chen W, Xu X, Dong S, Fan H, et al. Prognostic significance of neutrophil to lymphocyte ratio in patients with gallbladder carcinoma. HPB (Oxford). 2016;18:600–7.
68. Wu X-S, Shi L-B, Li M-L, Ding Q, Weng H, Wu WG, et al. Evaluation of two inflammation-based prognostic scores in patients with resectable gallbladder carcinoma. Ann Surg Oncol. 2014;21:449–57.
69. Zhnag Y, Ma C, Wang M, Hou H, Cui L, Jiang C, et al. Prognostic significance of immune cell in the tumor microenvironment and peripheral blood of gallbladder carcinoma patients. Clin Transl Oncol. 2017;19:477–88.

70. Zhang X, Niu Y, Wang X, Liu ZP, Liu T, Wang RT. Mean platelet volume and platelet distribution width are associated with gallbladder cancer. Asian Pac J Cancer Pre. 2018;19(2):351–5.
71. Xu WY, Zhang HH, Xiong JP, Yang XB, Bai Y, Kin JZ, et al. Prognostic significance of the fibrinogen-to-albumin ratio in gallbladder cancer patients. World J Gastroenterol. 2018;24(29):3281–92.
72. Vinocha A, Grover RK, Deepak R. Clinical significance of interleukin-6 in diagnosis of lung, oral, esophageal, and gall bladder carcinomas. J Cancer Res Ther. 2018;14(Suppl):S758–60.
73. Kumara S, Husain N, Agarwal A, Neyaz A, Gupta S, et al. Daignostic value of circulating free DNA integrity and global methylation status in gallbladder carcinoma. Pathol Oncol Res. 2018. https://doi.org/10.1007/s12253-017-0380-6.
74. Letelier P, Riquelme I, Hernandez AH, Guzman N, Farias JG, Roa JG. Circulating microRNAs as biomarkers in biliary tract cencers. Int J Mol Sci. 2016;17:791. https://doi.org/10.3390/ijms17050791.
75. Hu J, Yin B. Advances in biomarkers of biliary tract cancers. Biomed Pharmacother. 2016;81:128–35.
76. Sharma A, Jariwala P, Kaur N. Biliary ascariasis presenting with gangrenous perforation of the gall bladder: report of a case and brief review of literature. Trop Doct. 2018;48(3):242–5. https://doi.org/10.1177/0049475518768103 Epub 2018 Apr 13.
77. Javid G, Wani N, Gulzar GM, Javid O, Khan B, Shah A. Gallbladder ascariasis: presentation and management. Br J Surg. 1999;86:1526–7.
78. Yu HJ, Ahn CS, Lim S, Kim JG, Kim MS, Chae SW, et al. Cholecystitis: an unusual case of *Taenia solium* Infection with a literature review. Am J Trop Med Hyg. 2019;100(1):135–9. https://doi.org/10.4269/ajtmh.18-0633.
79. Malik AA, Wani RA, Bari S. Acute acalculous cholecystitis due to Taenia saginata. Ann Saudi Med. 2008;28(5):388–9.
80. Manes K, Chatzimargaritis K, Apessou D, Papastergiou V, Dervenis C. Granulomatous cholecystitis in a patient with Schistosoma mansoni infection: a case report. Int J Case Rep Imag. 2014;5:439–43.
81. Rappaport I, Albukerk J, Schneider IJ. Schistosomal cholecystitis. Arch Pathol. 1975;99(4):227–8.
82. Faisy C, Boye B, Douniama D, Iloumbou J. Gallbladder schistosomiasis haematobium. A case report. Med Trop (Mars). 1995;55(3):286–7.
83. Araki H, Shimizu S, Hayashi K, Yamada T, Kusakabe A, Kanie H, et al. Acute acalculous cholecystitis caused by Giardia lamblia. Intern Med. 2017;56:1657–62.
84. Cermano JR, Caraballo AJ, Gonzalez J. Acalculous cholecystitis in a patient with visceral leishmaniasis. Trans R Soc Trop Med Hyg. 2001;95(6):621–2.
85. Yombi JC, Meuris CM, Van Gompel AM, Ben Younes M, Vandercam BC. Acalculous cholecystitis in a patient with Plasmodium falciparum infection: a case report and literature review. J Travel Med. 2006;13(3):178–80.
86. Agholi M, Heidarian HR, Moghadami M, Hatam GR. First detection of acalculous cholecystitis associated with Sarcocystis infection in a patient with AIDS. Acta Parasitol. 2014;59(2):310–5.
87. Megremis S, Segkos N, Daskalaki M, Tzortzakakis E, Paspatis G, Zois E, et al. Gallbladder cryptosporidiosis in a patient with acquired immunodeficiency syndrome. J Ultrasound Med. 2004;23:137–40.
88. Martelli MG, Lee JY. Parasitic infection of the gallbladder: cystoisospora belli infection as a cause of chronic abdominal pain and acalculous cholecystitis. J Miss State Med Assoc. 2016;57(6):174–6.
89. Safioleas M, Stamoulis I, Theocharis S, Moulakakis K, Makris S, Kostakis A. Primary hydatid disease of the gallbladder: a rare clinical entity. J Hepatobiliary Pancreat Surg. 2004;11(5):352–6.
90. Strickler A, Vasquez N, Maggi L, Hernnandez J, Hidalgo X. Toxocarosis and acalculous cholecystitis: Consequence or coincidence? Rev Chilena Infectol. 2016;33(3):346–51.
91. Lai CH, Chin C, Chung HC, Liu H, Hwang JC, Lin HH. Clonorchiasis-associated perforated eosinophilic cholecystitis. Am J Trop Med Hyg. 2007;76(2):396–8.
92. Ziganshin RV, Shchopechkin VI. Rare case of the episthorchiasis of the liver and gallbladder. Klin Khir. 1973;7:63–5.
93. Mirer VI. The etiology and treatment of acute cholecystitis provoked by the Siberian liver fluke Opisthorochis felineus. Vestn Khir Im I I Grek. 1958;81(9):139–40.
94. Riedtmann HJ, Obeid T, Aeberhard P, Sakmann P. Fasciola Hepatica – a unusual cause of acute cholecystitis with cholestatic jaundice. Schweiz Med Wochenschr. 1995;125(35):1642–8.
95. Hong ST, Lee SH, Chi JG, Lee TS, Lee CY, Suh BY, et al. A human case of gallbladder fascioliasis in Korea. Kisaengchunghak Chapchi. 1896;24(1):89–94.
96. Gupta NM. Fasciola gigantica in gallbladder. Indian J Gastroenterol. 1987;6(2):113.
97. Soyer T, Turkmen F, Tatar N, Bozogan O, Kul O, Yagmurlu A, et al. Rare gallbladder parasitosis mimicking cholelithiasis: Dicrocoelium dendriticum. Eur J Pediatr Surg. 2008;18(4):280–1.
98. Qiao T, Ma RH, Luo XB, Luo ZL, Zheng PM. Cholecystolithiasis is associated with Clonorchiasis sinensis infection. PLoS ONE. 2012;7(8):e42471.
99. Antonsen A, Nielsen PL. Parasitic gallbladder infection. Ugeskr Laeger. 2001;164(1):64–5.
100. Kabaalioglu A, Apaydin A, Sindel T, Luleci E. US-guided gallbladder aspiration: a new diagnostic method for biliary fascioliasis. Eur Radiol. 1999;9:880–2.
101. Umehara H, Okazaki K, Masaki Y, Kawano M, Yamamoto M, Saeki T, et al. Comprehensive diagnostic criteria for IgG4-related disease (IgG4-RD), 2011. Mod Rheumatol. 2012;22(1):21–30.
102. Umehara H, Okazaki K, Nakamura T, Satoh-Nakamura T, Nakajima A, Kawano M, et al. Current approach to the diagnosis of IgG4-related

disease - Combination of comprehensive diagnostic and organ-specific criteria. Mod Rheumatol. 2017;27(3):381–91.
103. Yu KH, Chan TM, Tsai PH, Cheng CH, Chang PY. Diagnostic performance of serum IgG4 levels in patients with IgG4-related disease. Medicine (Baltimore). 2015;94(41):e1707. https://doi.org/10.1097/MD.0000000000001707.
104. Inoue D, Yoshida K, Yoneda N, Ozaki K, Matsubara T, Nagia K, et al. IgG4-related disease: dataset of 235 consecutive patients. Medicine (Baltimore). 2015;94(15):e680.
105. Okazaki K, Yanagawa M, Mitsuyama T, Uchida K. Recent advances in the concept and pathogenesis of IgG4-related disease in the Hepato-Bilio-Pancreatic system. Gut Liver. 2014;8(5):462–70.
106. Stone JH, Khosroshahi A, Deshpande V, Chan JK, Heathcote JG, Aalberse R, et al. Recommendations for the nomenclature of IgG4-related disease and its individual organ system manifestations. Arthritis Rheum. 2012;64:3061–7.
107. Ishigami K, Shitani M, Kimura Y, Hasegawa T, Masaki Y, Ito A, et al. Ectopic relapse of IgG4-related disease presenting as IgG4-related sclerosing cholecystitis: a case report and review of literature. Medicine (Baltimore). 2018;97(52):e13868. https://doi.org/10.1097/md.0000000000013868.
108. Lyon BBV. Diagnosis and treatment of diseases of the gallbladder and bile ducts. JAMA. 1919;73:980–2.
109. Juniper K Jr, Burson EN Jr. Biliary tract studies. II. The significance of biliary crystals. Gastroenterology. 1957;32(2):175–208.
110. Goodman AJ, Neoptolemos JP, Carr-Locke DL, Finlay DB, Fossard DP. Detection of gallstones after acute pancreatitis. Gut. 1985;26:125–32.
111. Smallwood RA, Jablonski P, Watts JM. Intermittent secretion of abnormal bile in patients with cholesterol gallstones. Br Med J. 1972;4(5835):263–6.
112. Marks JW, Bonorris G. Intermittency of cholesterol crystals in duodenal bile from gallstone patients. Gastroenterology. 1984;87(3):622–7.
113. Agarwal DK, Choudhuri G, Saraswat VA, Negi TS, Kapoor VK, Saxena R. Duodenal bile examination in identifying potential non-responders to bile salt treatment and its comparison with gall bladder bile examination. Gut. 1994;35(1):112–6.
114. Dahan P, Andant C, Levy P, Amouyal P, Amouyal G, Dumont M, et al. Prospective evaluation of endoscopic ultrasonography and microscopic examination of duodenal bile in the diagnosis of cholecystolithiasis in 45 patients with normal convential ultrasonography. Gut. 1996;38(2):277–81.
115. Itoi T, Sofuni A, Itokawa F, Kurihara T, Tsuchiya T, Moriyasu F, et al. Preoperative diagnosis and management of thick-walled gallbladder based on bile cytology obtained by endoscopic transpapillary gallbladder drainage. Gastrointest Endosc. 2006;64(4):512–9.
116. Lin TT, Yeh CT, Wu CS, Liaw YF. Detection and partial sequence analysis of Helicobacter pylori DNA in the bile samples. Dig Dis Sci. 1995;40:2214–9.
117. Kawaguchi M, Saito T, Ohno H, Midorikawa S, Sanji T, Hanada Y, et al. Bacteria closely resembling Helicobacter pylori detected immunohistologically and genetically in related gallbladder mucosa. J Gastroenterol. 1996;31:294–8.
118. Bansal VK, Misra MC, Chaubal G, Gupta SD, Das B, Ahuja V, Sagar S. Helicobacter pylori in gallbladder mucosa in patients with gallbladder disease. Indian J Gastroenterol. 2012;31(2):57–60.
119. Guraya SY, Ahmad AA, El-Ageery SM, Hemeg HA, Ozbak HA, Yousef K, et al. The correlation of Helicobacter Pylori with the development of cholelithiasis and cholecystitis: the results of a prospective clinical study in Saudi Arabia. Eur Rev Med Pharmacol Sci. 2015;19(20):3873–80.
120. Kobayashi T, Harada K, Miwa K, Nakanuma Y. Helicobacter genus DNA fragments are commonly detectable in bile from patients with extrahepatic biliary diseases and associated with their pathogenesis. Dig Dis Sci. 2005;50(5):862–7.
121. Hamada T, Yokota K, Ayada K, Hirai K, Kamada T, Haruma K, et al. Detection of helicobacter hepaticus in human bile samples of patients with biliary disease. Helicobacter. 2009;14:545–51.
122. Abayli B, Colakoglu S, Serin M, Erdogan S, Isiksal YF, Tuncer I, et al. Helicobacter pylori in the etiology of cholesterol gallstones. J Clin Gastroenterol. 2005;39(2):134–7.
123. Monstein HJ, Jonsson Y, Zdolsek J, Svanvik J. Identification of Helicobacter pylori DNA in human cholesterol gallstones. Scand J Gasdtroenterol. 2002;37:112–9.
124. Mishra RR, Tewari M, Shukla HS. Association of Helicobacter pylori infection with inflammatory cytokine expression in patients with gallbladder cancer. Indian J Gastroenterol. 2013;32(4):232–5.
125. Cen L, Pan J, Zhou B, Yu C, Li Y, Chen W, et al. Helicobacter Pylori infection of the gallbladder and the risk of chronic cholecystitis and cholelithiasis: a systematic review and meta-analysis. Helicobacter. 2018;23(1). https://doi.org/10.1111/hel.12457. Epub 2017 Dec 20.
126. Mendez-Sanchez N, Pichardo R, Gonzalez J, Sanchez H, Moreno M, Barquera F, et al. Lack of association between Helicobacter sp colonization and gallstone disease. J Clin Gastroenterol. 2001;32:138–41.
127. Bohr URM, Kuester D, Meyer F, Wex T, Stillert M, Csepregi A, et al. Low prevalence of Helicobacteraceae in gall-stone disease and gallbladder carcinoma in the German population. Clin Microbiol Infect. 2007;13:525–31.
128. Backert S, Tegtmeyer N, Oyarzabal OA, Osman D, Rohde M, Grutzmann R, et al. Unusual manifestation of live Staphylococcus saprophyticus, Corynebacterium urinapleomorphum, and Helicobacter pylori in the gallbladder with cholecystitis. Int J Mol Sci. 2018;19(7):E1826. https://doi.org/10.3390/ijms19071826.

Pathology: Non-neoplastic and Neoplastic Diseases of the Gallbladder

Kenji Notohara and Hirohisa Kitagawa

Introduction

The gallbladder is a unique saclike organ that is connected to the extrahepatic bile duct through a small tube called the cystic duct. The gallbladder is attached to the inferior surface of the liver, and it is filled with bile, which becomes congealed in the gallbladder. The mucosa of the gallbladder is always exposed to condensed bile. Thus, diseases of the gallbladder are closely related to the bile components.

Cholecystolithiasis is a typical example. Inflammatory lesions in the gallbladder are related mostly to cholecystolithiasis, but the exact mechanisms underlying how gallstones develop inflammation have not been elucidated.

Some inflammatory lesions—such as xanthogranulomatous cholecystitis and IgG4-related cholecystitis—clinically mimic gallbladder carcinomas. Gallbladder neoplasms are similar to those of the extrahepatic bile duct, except for pyloric gland adenoma (PGA), in which tumor occurrence is limited almost entirely to the gallbladder. Gallbladder carcinomas are clinically unique and are different from carcinomas in the extrahepatic bile duct as follows: jaundice is rare in the early stages of the gallbladder carcinomas, and gallbladder carcinomas can easily invade the liver due to the anatomical reasons. In this chapter, the pathogenesis of cholecystolithiasis is briefly described, and the pathological features of representative inflammatory, proliferative, and neoplastic diseases of the gallbladder are explained.

Cholecystolithiasis

Two types of gallstones are recognized: cholesterol gallstones and bilirubin gallstones. The pathogenesis of stone formation is different between these two types of stones. The majority of gallbladder calculi are cholesterol gallstones. Cholesterol is insoluble in the bile and is thus secreted as a micelle formed with bile salts and phospholipids. If the amount of cholesterol is too excessive to be dissolved in the bile in proportion to the amounts of bile salts and phospholipids, cholesterol crystals precipitate and give rise to cholesterol stones. In addition to the amount of cholesterol in the bile, other factors such as impaired motility of the gallbladder, pro-nucleating factors such as biliary glycoproteins and mucin [1], and some lithogenic genes

K. Notohara (✉)
Department of Anatomic Pathology, Kurashiki Central Hospital, Kurashiki, Japan
e-mail: notohara@kchnet.or.jp

H. Kitagawa
Department of Surgery, Kurashiki Central Hospital, Kurashiki, Japan
e-mail: hk16133@kchnet.or.jp

J. B. Chung and K. Okazaki (eds.), *Diseases of the Gallbladder*,
https://doi.org/10.1007/978-981-15-6010-1_3

[2–4] are also involved in the formation of cholesterol gallstones.

Black stones, a type of bilirubin gallstones without bacterial infection, are less frequent, but they have been observed in the gallbladder. The formation of black stones is related to excessive amounts of bilirubin in the settings of hemolysis, liver cirrhosis, Crohn's disease, and the formation of Rokitansky-Aschoff sinuses (RAS; see section 'Chronic Cholecystitis') [5–7].

Bilirubin calcium gallstones are rare in the gallbladder. The trigger for the formation of bilirubin calcium stones is a bacterial infection. Bacterial beta-glucuronidase degrades conjugated bilirubin and indirect bilirubin precipitate to form bilirubin calcium gallstones. This type of stone is thus common in the bile duct. Due to the improvement of hygienic environments, the number of patients with bilirubin calcium gallstones is low in developed countries.

Inflammatory and Circulatory Disorders

Acute Cholecystitis

Acute cholecystitis is an acute form of inflammation of the gallbladder. The two types of acute cholecystitis, i.e., acute calculous cholecystitis and acute acalculous cholecystitis, depend on the presence/absence of gallbladder calculi.

Acute Calculous Cholecystitis

Acute calculous cholecystitis is caused by impacted gallbladder stones at the cystic duct or gallbladder neck or biliary sludge at the neck [8, 9], which gives rise to stasis of the bile in the gallbladder and subsequent tissue damages. The exact mechanism by which tissue damages occur in the gallbladder with impacted gallbladder calculi or biliary sludge is not clear, given that impacted gallbladder stones do not necessarily cause acute cholecystitis. Theories about this include impaired blood flow and mechanical or chemical irritation by the components of stones or bile [10]. Impaired blood flow may be caused by the direct obstruction of the cystic artery and/or vein by the impacted stones or by the oppression caused by the increased innate pressure of the gallbladder. Because suppurative changes are not a basic or universal finding, infection does not seem to be the primary cause of acute cholecystitis in most cases.

Macroscopically, resected gallbladders are dilated, and the walls are edematous (Fig. 1). The yellow color of the subserosal adipose tissues is blurred. The mucosa may be necrotic, and sometimes pus is attached to the mucosal surface. In severe inflammatory lesions, the gallbladder walls are transmurally necrotic and hemorrhagic, and may even be accompanied by abscesses.

Histological features of acute calculous cholecystitis vary depending on the time course and the severity. Pathological changes are most common in the subserosal layer, where the adipose tissues disappear and are replaced by fibroblastic proliferation and fibrosis. The changes of adipose tissues are not typical of necrosis, because inflammatory reactions are absent in the lost adipose tissues. The changes in adipose tissues look more like a disappearance of the adipose tissues. In some cases, a ghost-like degeneration of adipose tissues can be identified by careful observation (Fig. 2a), but this finding is easily confused with simple edema. Moreover, degenerative adipose tissues often show myxoid changes, where plump fibroblasts proliferate at the early stage of the inflammation (Fig. 2b). In about a week, fine fibrosis consisting of delicate pale eosinophilic collagen fibers starts to develop around the fibroblasts (Fig. 2c). In older lesions, a fibrous scar with a decreased number of fibroblasts remains. Scar formation in the midst of subserosal adipose tissue can hardly be observed in chronic cholecystitis, and we regard such a finding as healed acute cholecystitis.

Mucosal necrosis is also commonly observed. The necrosis may be accompanied by neutrophilic infiltration due to the damaged mucosal barrier with a subsequent bacterial infection. In severe cases, necrosis can be found

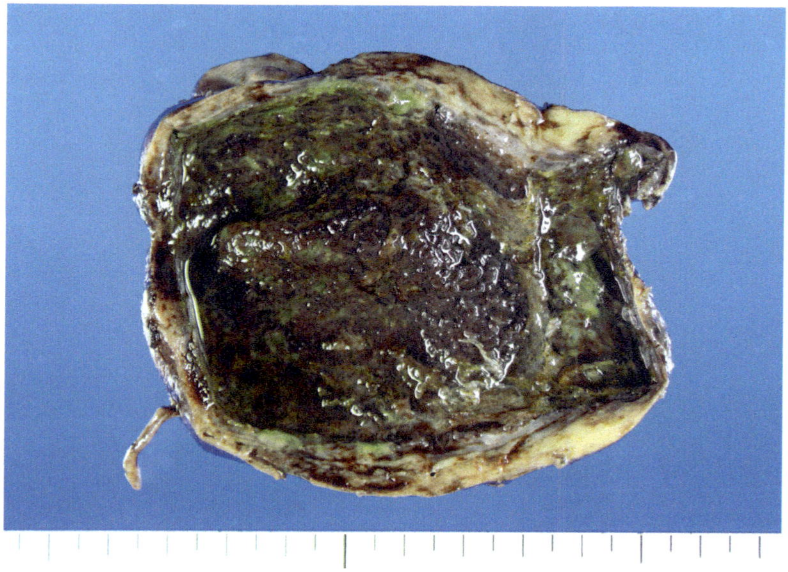

Fig. 1 A macroscopic picture of acute cholecystitis. The *green spots* on the mucosa represent necrosis. In the biliary tract, bile pigments attach to the mucosal necrosis and then reveal green spots after formalin fixation

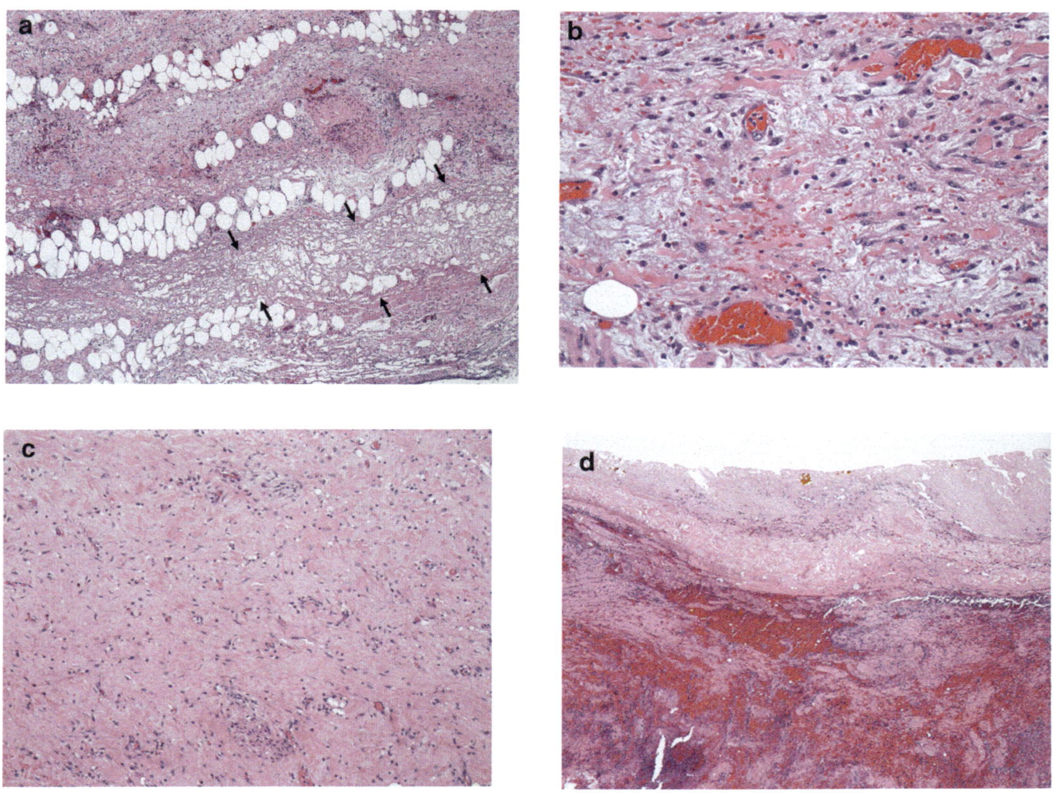

Fig. 2 Microscopic pictures of acute cholecystitis. **a** Typical findings are observed in the subserosal layer, where adipose tissues disappear and are replaced by fibroblastic proliferation. Some foci that look like ghosts of preexisting adipose tissues are indicated by the *arrows*. **b** Fibroblastic proliferation. **c** Over the time course, the number of fibroblasts decreases, and fibrosis appears. Finally, such foci will become a scar. **d** Transmural necrosis with hemorrhage is a severe form of acute cholecystitis

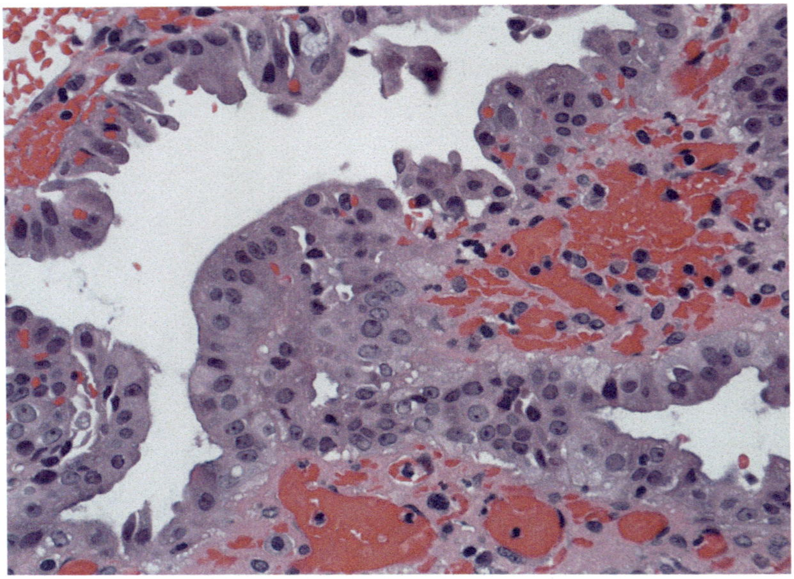

Fig. 3 Regenerative epithelium in acute cholecystitis. Such cells should not be confused with biliary intraepithelial neoplasia

diffusely and/or transmurally (Fig. 2d). When necrosis is transmural, the gallbladder walls are hemorrhagic and associated with marked neutrophilic infiltration. If neutrophilic infiltration is severe, it is a dangerous sign that may represent the development of a systemic infection.

Epithelial injuries give rise to epithelial regeneration within a few days. The regenerative epithelium reveals enlarged nuclei with prominent nucleoli (Fig. 3). These cells are sometimes misinterpreted as biliary intraepithelial neoplasia (BilIN). Given that acute cholecystitis may develop in a gallbladder with preexisting BilIN or even invasive carcinomas, this is a diagnostic dilemma. Compared to the cells in BilIN, regenerative cells have vesicular and round nuclei and lack nuclear hyperchromatism. Even so, the distinction is often difficult, and the diagnosis of BilIN must be rendered cautiously in the background of acute cholecystitis.

Among cases with a clinical diagnosis of acute calculous cholecystitis, a milder form of inflammation composed of neutrophilic infiltration in the epithelium may be observed. This type of inflammation also often involves RAS (see section 'Chronic Cholecystitis'), and in addition to neutrophils in the epithelium, fibroblasts proliferate at the bottom of RAS (Fig. 4). In contrast to the usual acute calculous cholecystitis, the structures of the gallbladder wall are usually well preserved.

Acute Acalculous Cholecystitis

Acute acalculous cholecystitis has been observed in the setting of severe traumas, burns, major surgeries, and sepsis [10]. Although the precise mechanisms are not yet clear, tissue damage is thought to occur in the gallbladder due to the dehydration of bile and/or blood flow disturbances [11]. The pathological features are similar to those of acute calculous cholecystitis, and acute calculous/acalculous cholecystitis is difficult to distinguish histologically. Subserosal fat degeneration is often the main finding, and mucosal necrosis is also commonly observed. Neutrophils are absent in genuine acute acalculous cholecystitis, but they may be observed once necrosis occurs in the mucosa.

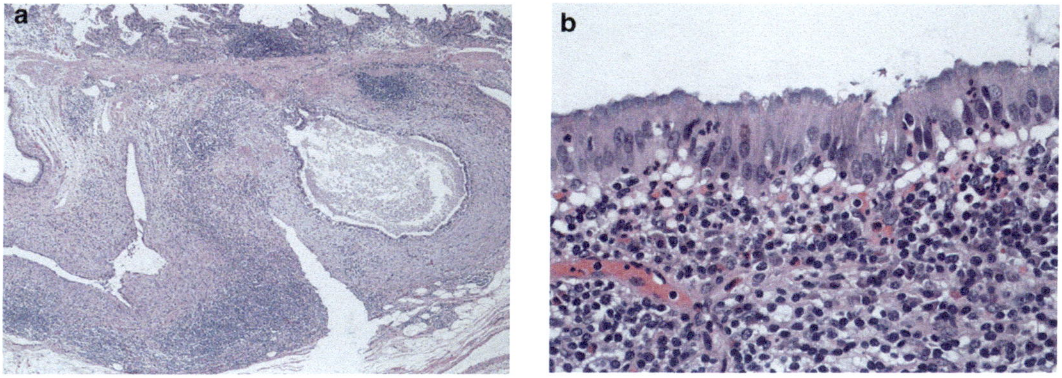

Fig. 4 A type of acute cholecystitis involving RAS. **a** Fibroblastic proliferation is observed around the RAS. **b** Neutrophils are numerous in the epithelium

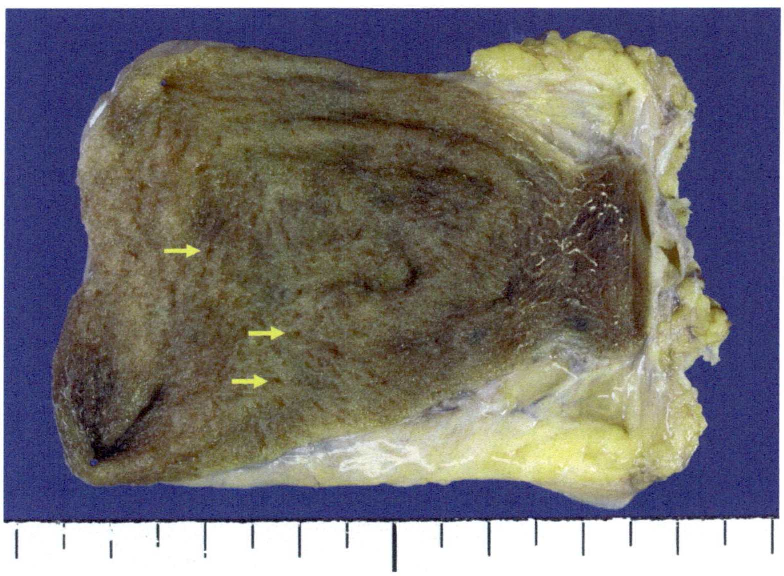

Fig. 5 A macroscopic picture of chronic cholecystitis. Sometimes orifices of RAS are observed (representative examples are indicated by *arrows*)

Chronic Cholecystitis

Chronic cholecystitis almost always occurs in gallbladders with cholecystolithiasis. It is suspected to be caused by chemical irritations of the mucosa by components of bile [10]. Chronic cholecystitis is not a focus of medical attention because it is clinically indolent and does not seem to increase the morbidity.

Macroscopically, gallbladders with chronic cholecystitis might show wall thickening with fibrosis but are unremarkable in most cases. Sometimes, small holes that correspond to the orifices of RAS are detected on the mucosa (Fig. 5), and RAS themselves are present in the walls.

RAS is a common finding in chronic cholecystitis [12]. Because the lamina muscularis propria (LMP) in the gallbladder is so thin (similar to the lamina muscular mucosae in the gastrointestinal tract), the mucosa can easily protrude outside of the LMP when the innate pressure increases, in a phenomenon called RAS formation. In this sense,

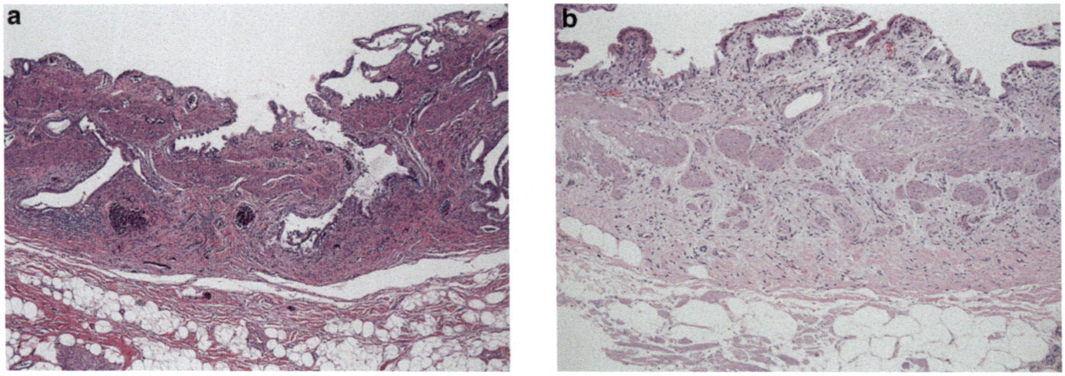

Fig. 6 Microscopic pictures of chronic cholecystitis. **a** RAS formation surrounded by fibrosis is a typical feature. **b** A layer of nearly uniform thickness of fibrosis and minimal inflammatory infiltration observed just beneath the lamina muscularis propria is a characteristic finding, and it may be continuous with the fibrosis in the mucosa

RAS simulate diverticulosis in the colon. Fibrosis with minimal lymphocytic infiltration can be observed at the bottom of RAS (Fig. 6a). In fact, a layer of nearly uniform thickness of fibrosis and mild inflammatory (usually lymphocytic) infiltration observed just beneath the LMP is usually identified in chronic cholecystitis, and it can be observed even in areas without RAS.

The fibrosis beneath the LMP may be continuous with the fibrosis in the mucosa (Fig. 6b). In fact, the mucosa is often affected by the inflammation, given that metaplastic changes such as mucus cells and pyloric glands are common in chronic cholecystitis. However, inflammatory cell infiltration in the mucosa is minimal, and if marked, an association of lymphoplasmacytic cholecystitis (see section 'Lymphoplasmacytic Cholecystitis') is more likely. As described in section 'Acute Calculous Cholecystitis', a fibrous scar in the subserosal adipose tissues is not a typical feature of chronic cholecystitis, and we regard such a case as healed acute cholecystitis unless it is associated with a continuous inflammation. However, some pathologists regard such a scar as a feature of chronic cholecystitis.

Xanthogranulomatous Cholecystitis

Xanthogranulomatous cholecystitis is a unique form of cholecystitis that is characterized by a marked destruction of the gallbladder walls and the aggregation of foamy macrophages. Xanthogranulomatous cholecystitis clinically resembles gallbladder cancers for the following reasons. First, because of marked tissue-destructive changes, imaging findings resemble those of gallbladder cancers. In addition, fluorodeoxyglucose-positron emission tomography scans may be positive [13]. Second, patients often reveal elevated serum CA19-9.

Xanthogranulomatous cholecystitis is often observed in the setting of stone impaction at the cystic duct or gallbladder neck. In addition to the aggregation of foamy macrophages, destructive tissue changes (i.e., the disappearance of the normal gallbladder structure), marked lymphoplasmacytic infiltration, and fibrosis is commonly observed (Fig. 7), and may even involve the surrounding tissues of the gallbladder.

It is unknown why foamy macrophages appear in xanthogranulomatous cholecystitis. Some researchers have speculated that this is a reaction against cholesterol in the bile leaking into the gallbladder walls. In fact, foci of bile leakage are commonly encountered in xanthogranulomatous cholecystitis. There are reports of the identification of proteins and genes of *E. coli* in the foamy macrophages [14, 15].

Another report indicated that xanthogranulomatous cholecystitis resembled IgG4-related disease (IgG4-RD) and contained numerous

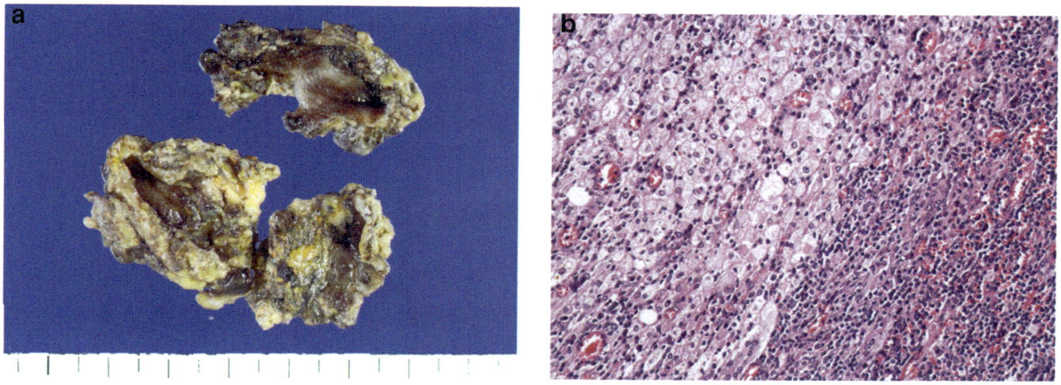

Fig. 7 Xanthogranulomatous cholecystitis. **a** Macroscopic findings. The gallbladder wall is damaged, and *yellow spots* that represent foci with foamy macrophages are identified. **b** Histological findings. A focus with aggregated foamy macrophages and surrounding lymphoplasmacytic infiltration

IgG4-positive cells and some histological features of IgG4-RD [16]. In fact, curiously, many xanthogranulomatous inflammations in the human body show numerous IgG4-positive cells. Some of these inflammations, for example, a case of autoimmune pancreatitis associated with a periorbital xanthogranuloma in the subsequent clinical course, may be true IgG4-RD [17], but other inflammations seem to be mimickers [18].

In the gallbladder, it is important to remember that IgG4-related cholecystitis (see section 'IgG4-Related Cholecystitis') is characterized by minimal tissue destruction, which is inconsistent with the marked tissue injuries in xanthogranulomatous cholecystitis. Numerous IgG4-positive cells observed in seriously injured tissues are nonspecific, and they are also reported in other destructive inflammatory diseases such as primary sclerosing cholangitis.

Porcelain Gallbladder

Porcelain gallbladder is a destructive inflammation of the gallbladder characterized by calcification in the background of the hyalinized gallbladder wall (Fig. 8). Cholecystolithiasis is found in most of the cases. Despite the drastic pathological changes of the gallbladder, most of the patients are asymptomatic. Porcelain gallbladder is reported to be a risk factor for gallbladder carcinomas, and when examined, pathologists should take care not to overlook co-existing carcinomas. Gallbladders with marked hyaline degeneration but with no or only scattered calcification also exist, and they seem similar to present a risk of carcinoma [19].

Lymphoplasmacytic Cholecystitis

Lymphoplasmacytic cholecystitis is characterized by a diffuse infiltration of lymphocytes and plasma cells in the mucosa (Fig. 9), and it was first reported as a gallbladder manifestation of primary sclerosing cholangitis [20]. In the later reports [21, 22], this finding was also observed in various conditions that cause an obstruction of the extrahepatic bile duct, such as bile duct cancers, pancreas head cancers, ampullary cancers, and choledocholithiasis. Similar diffuse lymphoplasmacytic infiltration is sometimes observed in the routine cases with cholecystolithiasis, but in our experience, such cases often show choledocholithiasis or gallstone impaction at the cystic duct or gallbladder neck. Thus, when the finding of lymphoplasmacytic cholecystitis is observed, obstructive changes in the extrahepatic bile duct and cystic duct should be considered.

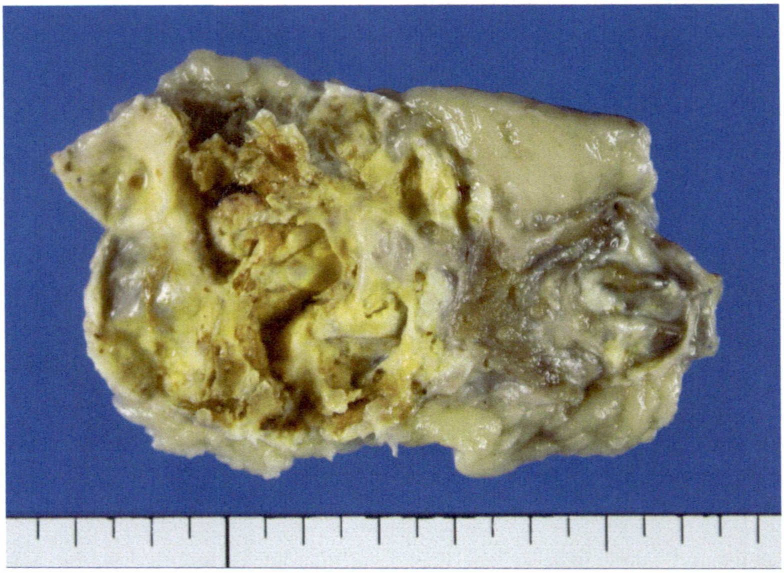

Fig. 8 Porcelain gallbladder. The inflammation is destructive, and calcification (*yellow portions*) is observed

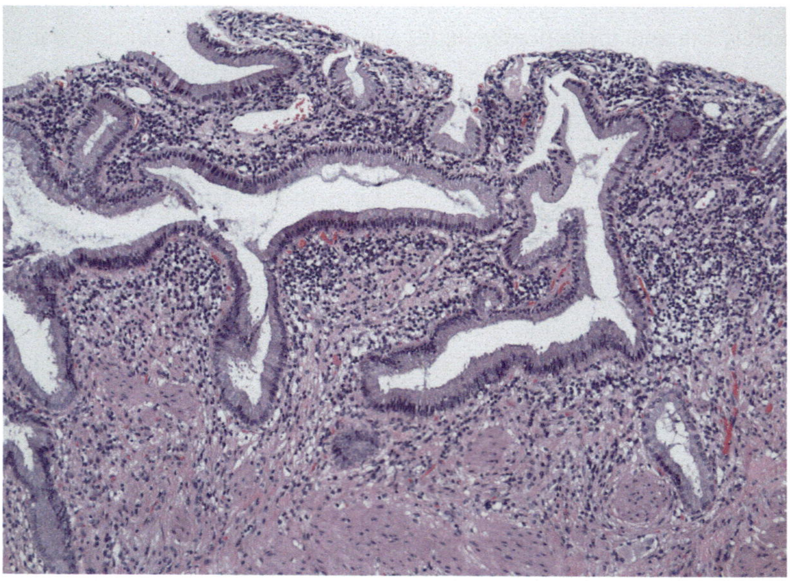

Fig. 9 Lymphoplasmacytic cholecystitis. Lymphocytes and plasma cells diffusely infiltrate in the mucosa

IgG4-Related Cholecystitis

IgG4-RD is a systemic inflammatory disease that is characterized by tumefactive lesions (organ swelling or mass formation) and an elevation of serum IgG4 [23, 24]. Histologically, lymphoplasmacytic infiltration with numerous IgG4-positive plasma cells but without neutrophils in the background of fibrosis is characteristic [23, 25]. In typical cases, storiform fibrosis and/or obliterative phlebitis are also observed [25–27]. In the pancreaticobiliary system, type 1 autoimmune pancreatitis [25] and IgG4-related sclerosing cholangitis [28, 29] is the well-known manifestations of IgG4-RD, but IgG4-related cholecystitis, a gallbladder manifestation of IgG4-RD, is also sporadically reported [30].

Macroscopically, the gallbladder wall is thickened and thus resembles carcinomas. The histological features of IgG4-related cholecystitis consist of a dense lymphoplasmacytic infiltration predominated by plasma cells observed in the subserosal layer (Fig. 10a). In typical cases, storiform fibrosis (Fig. 10b) and obliterative phlebitis are observed, but not in every case. Immunohistochemically, IgG4-positive cells are numerous (Fig. 10c); usually >50/high-power field (HPF) in the resected tissues. Eosinophils may be present and even numerous, but neutrophils are absent. Numerous IgG4-positive cells may also be present in the mucosa.

In contrast to autoimmune diseases, e.g., autoimmune hepatitis, tissue destruction is not remarkable in IgG4-RD despite the presence of dense inflammatory cell infiltration. In addition, tissue damage is observed in the confined tissues, such as acinar cell loss in the pancreatic lobules, and a loss of adipocytes in the adipose tissues. Steroid treatment is thus effective, and organ failures are rare in IgG4-RD. In IgG4-related cholecystitis, the gallbladder structure is usually well preserved. For example, the epithelium is intact (no destruction, no repairing features) and smooth muscle cells in the LMP are preserved, even though the LMP is affected by the inflammatory cells. The only exception is the subserosal adipose tissues, which disappear and are replaced by the histologically characteristic inflammation and may even give rise to hyalinization [31]. As mentioned in the text above about xanthogranulomatous cholecystitis (see section 'Xanthogranulomatous Cholecystitis'), it

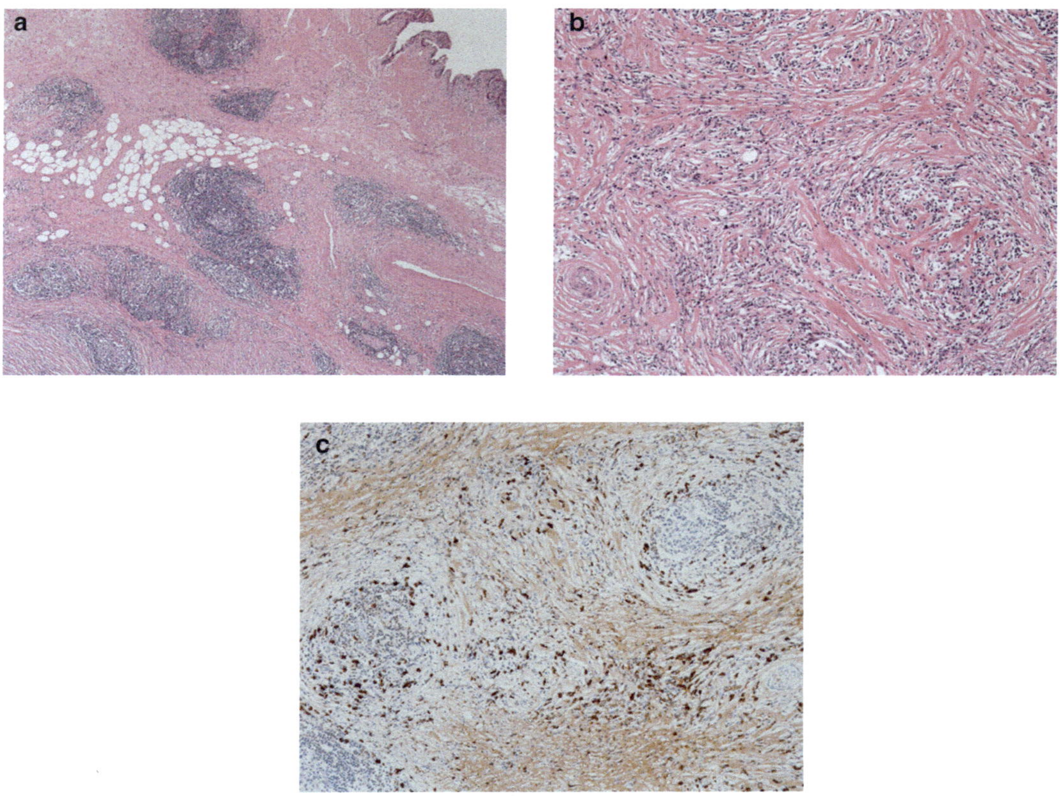

Fig. 10 IgG4-related cholecystitis. **a** The subserosal layer is diffusely affected by lymphoplasmacytic infiltration and fibrosis. **b** Storiform fibrosis is a characteristic finding. **c** Numerous IgG4-positive cells are observed (immunostaining for IgG4)

is unusual for the gallbladder wall and the surrounding structures to be markedly destroyed in IgG4-related cholecystitis.

Infarction

Infarction of the gallbladder can be caused by the torsion of the gallbladder [32] or embolization. The latter is common after therapeutic hepatic artery embolization for liver tumors [33]. Pathologically, a gallbladder infarction is characterized by transmural necrosis of the wall (Fig. 11). The contour of the lamina muscularis propria and adipose tissue may remain even though those tissues are necrotic. Although there are overlapping histological features between gallbladder infarction and acute calculous/acalculous cholecystitis, there are some differences. First, the lamina muscularis propria is also necrotic in gallbladder infarction, whereas it is relatively preserved in acute calculous/acalculous cholecystitis. Second, stromal reactive changes, such as fibroblastic proliferation, are absent in gallbladder infarction but present in acute calculous/acalculous cholecystitis. Inflammatory reactions are thus rare in gallbladder infarctions.

Non-neoplastic Proliferative Lesions

Adenomyomatosis

Adenomyomatosis (also called adenomyomatous hyperplasia) is a wall thickening lesion of the gallbladder. It occurs focally in any portion of the gallbladder and in some cases, involves the gallbladder diffusely (Fig. 12a). The patients are usually asymptomatic, and adenomyomatosis is incidentally detected by imaging studies. Adenomyomatosis usually reveals a submucosal tumor at the fundus and a stenotic lesion at the body and neck.

Histologically, the LMP is thickened, where hyperplastic epithelium invaginates similar to diverticulosis. Some glands protrude into the subserosal layer, are dilated cystically, and may contain black stones (Fig. 12b). Compared to the RAS, the glands in adenomyomatosis are more

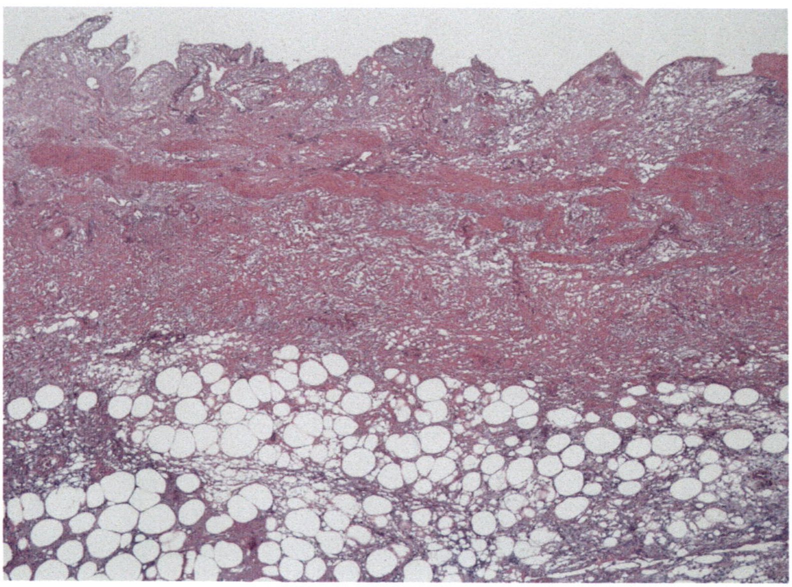

Fig. 11 Infarction of gallbladder. The gallbladder wall is transmurally necrotic, and no inflammatory reactions are observed

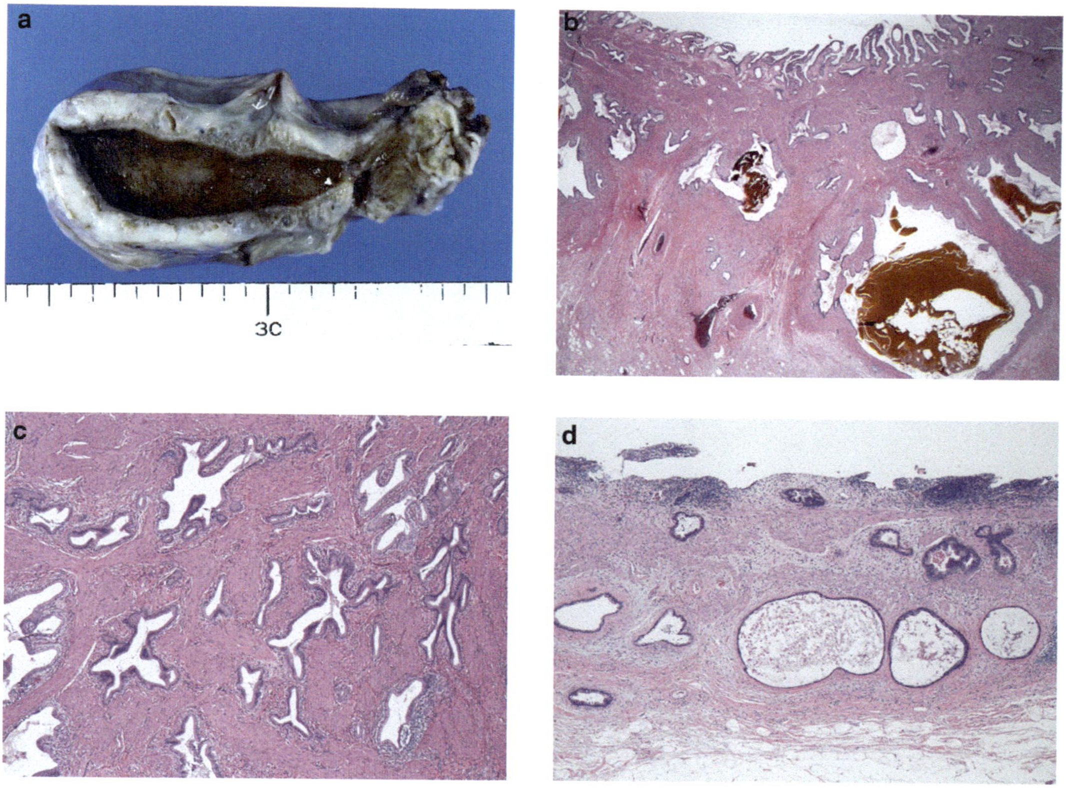

Fig. 12 Adenomyomatosis (**a**–**c**). **a** Macroscopic features of a case with diffuse adenomyomatosis. **b** The lamina muscularis propria is thickened and is affected by invaginated gallbladder mucosa. Black stones are often observed in the cystic lumen. **c** Glands in adenomyomatosis are tortuous but should not be confused with cancerous glands. **d** Invasive adenocarcinoma resembling adenomyomatosis. These cancerous glands are atypical and should be carefully distinguished from adenomyomatosis

tortuous and irregular in shape (Fig. 12c), and they often elongate laterally due to the interruption of smooth muscle cells. Adenomyomatosis may, therefore, be confused with carcinomas, or more often, carcinomas with mild atypia may be confused with adenomyomatosis (Fig. 12d).

Cholesterosis and Cholesterol Polyps

Cholesterosis (also called cholesterolosis) and cholesterol polyps consist of the accumulation of foamy macrophages in the mucosa, which macroscopically reveals yellow spots or polyps. Cholesterosis consists of multiple small spots that are flat or bumpy (Fig. 13a), and cholesterol polyps show a flat or ragged surface (Fig. 13b). Cholesterosis and cholesterol polyps are usually asymptomatic and are detected by imaging studies or incidentally identified in resected gallbladders.

Histologically, the difference between cholesterosis and cholesterol polyps depends on whether the epithelium is normal or proliferating (Fig. 13c, d). Cholesterol polyps are associated with the epithelial hyperplasia. Curiously, in the human body, foam cell accumulation is sometimes associated with epithelial proliferation, e.g., verruciform xanthoma observed in the skin and oral mucosa, and some xanthomas in the stomach [34]. In rare cases of cholesterol polyps, only epithelial hyperplasia remains with scarce foamy macrophages present in the stroma. The proliferating epithelium in the

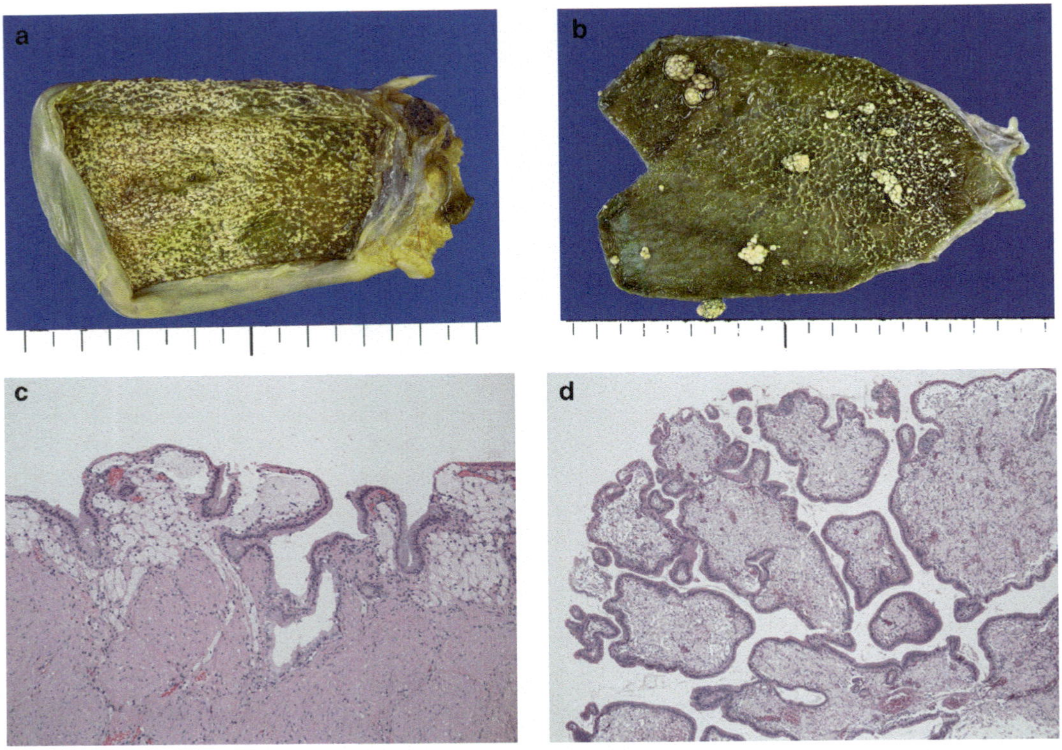

Fig. 13 Comparison of cholesterosis (**a**, **c**) and cholesterol polyps (**b**, **d**). Macroscopically, cholesterosis consists of *yellow spots* (**a**) that are histologically aggregations of xanthomas cells (**c**). Cholesterol polyps are macroscopically yellow polyps (**b**), and, in addition to aggregations of xanthoma cells, the covering epithelium is proliferative (**d**)

cholesterol polyps usually looks benign, but it may be atypical and look adenomatous in rare cases.

Neoplastic Diseases

Neoplastic diseases of the gallbladder and extrahepatic bile duct are classified together in the World Health Organization (WHO) Classification 2019 [35]. Among the entities listed in the WHO Classification 2019, those that arise in the gallbladder are listed in Table 1. Representative neoplasms are described next.

Adenocarcinoma

Macroscopically, gallbladder carcinomas show various features. They may be localized papillary or nodular masses, or ill-defined flat masses. They often show superficial extension laterally in the mucosa (Fig. 14a), which needs to be distinguished from intracystic papillary neoplasms (ICPNs) with invasive carcinoma. Gallbladder adenocarcinomas are occasionally multifocal. Adenocarcinomas of the gallbladder are sometimes associated with acute cholecystitis. In such a case, the lesion may be unclear due to the inflammation.

Histologically, biliary-type adenocarcinoma is the most common. This type is composed of cuboidal atypical carcinoma cells forming papillary, tubular, or poorly differentiated structures (Fig. 14b, c), and it resembles pancreatic ductal adenocarcinoma.

Precursor Lesions

Adenocarcinomas of the gallbladder arise in the background of BilIN. Based on the architectural

Table 1 WHO classification of the gallbladder (2019)

Benign epithelial tumors and precursors
Adenoma
Biliary intraepithelial neoplasia, low-grade
Biliary intraepithelial neoplasia, high-grade
Intracystic papillary neoplasm with low-grade intraepithelial neoplasia
Intracystic papillary neoplasm with high-grade intraepithelial neoplasia
Intracystic papillary neoplasm with associated invasive carcinoma
Malignant epithelial tumors
Adenocarcinoma NOS
Adenocarcinoma, intestinal type
Clear cell adenocarcinoma NOS
Mucinous cystic neoplasm with associated invasive carcinoma
Mucinous adenocarcinoma
Poorly cohesive carcinoma
Intracystic papillary neoplasm with associated invasive carcinoma
Squamous cell carcinoma NOS
Carcinoma, undifferentiated, NOS
Adenosquamous carcinoma
Neuroendocrine tumor NOS
Neuroendocrine tumor, grade 1
Neuroendocrine tumor, grade 2
Neuroendocrine tumor, grade 3
Neuroendocrine carcinoma NOS
Large cell neuroendocrine carcinoma
Small cell neuroendocrine carcinoma
Mixed neuroendocrine-non-neuroendocrine neoplasm (MiNEN)

and cytological atypia, BilIN is classified from low- to high-grade, and high-grade BilIN (Fig. 14d) corresponds to adenocarcinoma in situ. Some invasive adenocarcinomas also arise in the background of ICPN, mucinous cystic neoplasm, or pyloric gland adenoma (PGA).

Risk Factors and Genetic Abnormalities

Risk factors and genetic abnormalities for gallbladder carcinomas may differ among countries and regions. Gallstones are believed to be an important risk factor for gallbladder carcinomas, but a causal relationship of gallstones with gallbladder carcinomas has not been well established [36, 37]. A risk factor in Japan is a pancreaticobiliary maljunction [38], which seems to cause carcinomas through mucosal injuries and subsequent diffuse mucosal hyperplasia [39]. Smoking and alcohol are not convincingly related to gallbladder carcinomas [40]. Adiposity is a risk for gallbladder carcinomas [41].

No driver mutations have been reported in gallbladder adenocarcinoma, and an accumulation of multiple gene mutations is likely to be responsible for the carcinogenesis. Alterations of *TP53*, *CDKN2A*, *CDKN2B*, *ARID1A*, *PIK3CA*, or *CTNNB1* are relatively common [35]. Regional differences in genetic abnormalities are also reported and may explain the reasons why the patient demographics and clinical features of gallbladder carcinomas vary among countries [42]. Compared to pancreatic ductal adenocarcinoma, *K-ras* mutations are less common but have been reported in cases with a pancreaticobiliary maljunction in Japan [43]. Loss of mismatch-repair proteins that gives rise to high-frequent microsatellite instabilities was initially reported in 7.8% of gallbladder cancers [44], but a recent report described a lower frequency at 1.6% [45].

Variants

Squamous cell carcinoma arising in the gallbladder often has a component of adenocarcinoma and is, therefore, regarded as a variant of adenocarcinoma (adenosquamous carcinoma). A component of squamous cell carcinoma shows a huge and well-demarcated mass with prominent necrosis (Fig. 15a). Similarly, undifferentiated carcinoma (Fig. 15b) and neuroendocrine carcinoma (Fig. 15c) is observed in the background of adenocarcinoma. They often involve a large protruding mass in the gallbladder lumen and invade surrounding tissues. A direct invasion into the liver is commonly observed in these tumors. Although mucus production is commonly observed in adenocarcinoma of the gallbladder, mucinous adenocarcinoma (Fig. 15d) that reveals a predominant component of extracellular mucus production is rare.

Poorly cohesive carcinoma (signet-ring cell carcinoma) has been sporadically reported in the gallbladder, but it is more common to encounter a gallbladder invasion of gastric poorly cohesive carcinoma. It is important to remember that gastric poorly cohesive carcinoma often invades

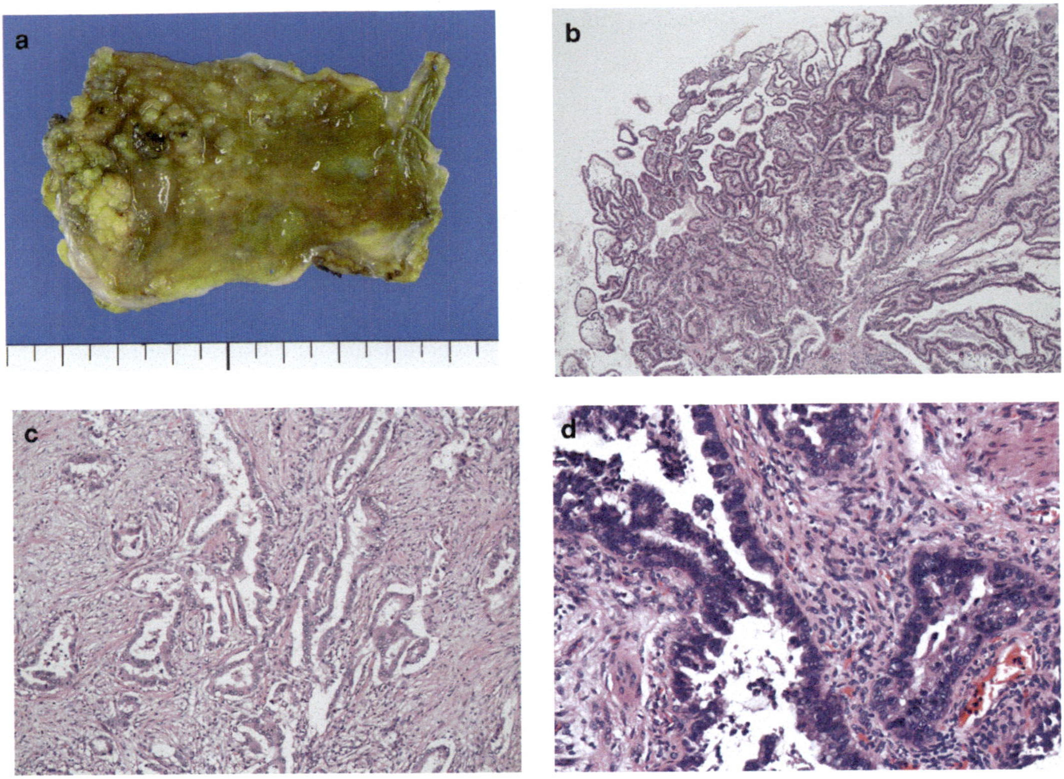

Fig. 14 Gallbladder adenocarcinoma. **a** A macroscopic picture of a papillary configuration. The lesion extends diffusely in the mucosa, and the border is not evident. **b**, **c** Microscopic pictures. The mucosal component often shows a papillary pattern (**b**), but the invasive portions are more often tubular (**c**). **d** High-grade biliary intraepithelial neoplasia arising in adenomyomatosis

the biliary tract without showing any imaging features of a mass. Because a primary gastric poorly cohesive carcinoma may be invisible endoscopically, the diagnosis of primary poorly cohesive carcinoma of the gallbladder must be cautiously rendered.

Intracystic Papillary Neoplasms

ICPN is a macroscopically identifiable papillary epithelial neoplasm without invasive growth (Fig. 16) [46]. ICPN is regarded as a counterpart of pancreatic intraductal papillary mucinous neoplasm (IPMN). There have been arguments regarding a similar concept in the bile duct, i.e., intraductal papillary neoplasm of the bile ducts (IPNB). The controversy is based on the issue of whether this is a biliary counterpart of pancreatic IPMN. Compared to pancreatic IPMN, IPNB often shows more high-grade morphology, a more frequent association with invasive carcinoma, and a lack of GNAS mutations [47]. IPNB was recently subclassified as types 1 and 2. A type 1 IPNB is similar to the gastric or intestinal types of IPMN and is characterized by frequent localization in the intrahepatic bile ducts, frequent excessive mucus production, and less frequent invasiveness. In contrast, type 2 IPNB seems more like de novo carcinoma and is characterized by localization in the extrahepatic bile ducts, scarce mucus production, more complex architecture, more prominent cytological atypia, and more frequent invasive growth.

ICPN seems to us to be more similar to type 2 IPNB, and genuine lesions resembling

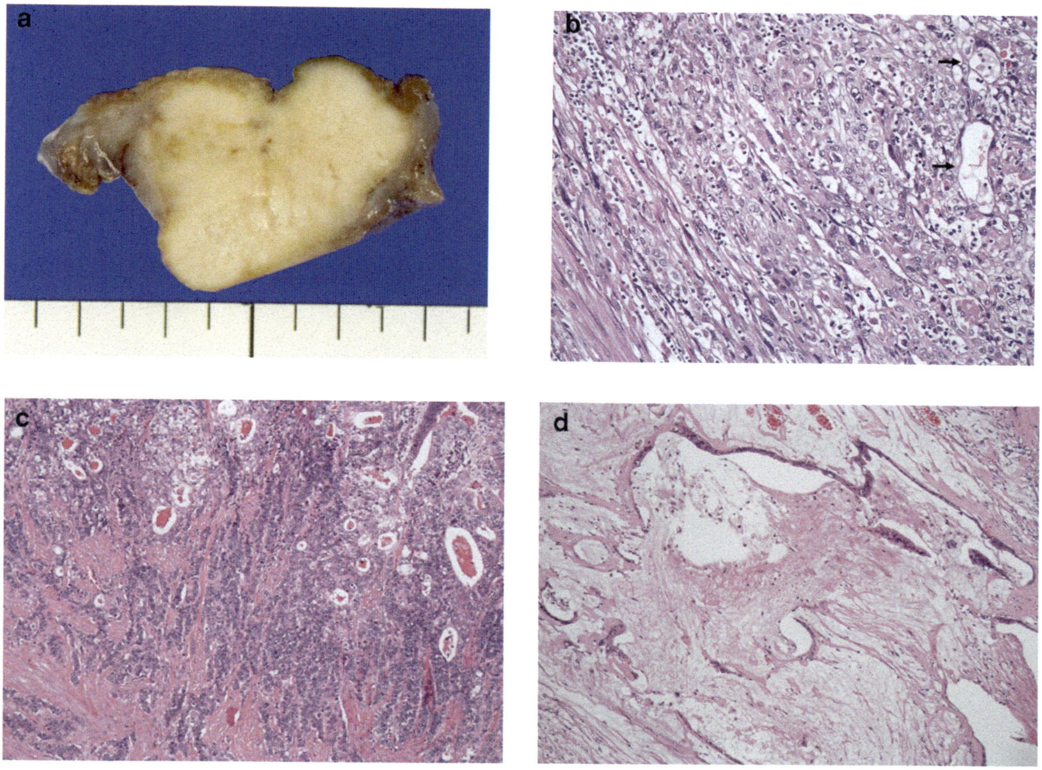

Fig. 15 Variants of adenocarcinoma and other types. **a** Adenosquamous carcinoma showing a clear border. **b** Undifferentiated carcinoma (*left portion*) with a component of adenocarcinoma (*arrows*). **c** Neuroendocrine carcinoma (*lower portion*) arising in adenocarcinoma (*upper portion*), which corresponds to mixed neuroendocrine-non-neuroendocrine neoplasm. **d** Mucinous adenocarcinoma

pancreatic IPMN are scarce in the gallbladder. A stringent histological distinction of ICPN and papillary adenocarcinoma was recently reported to be justified by differing genetic findings, and ICPNs more commonly revealed genetic abnormalities of the Wnt pathway [48]. More pathological discussions, as well as genetic studies, are necessary to place this category appropriately.

Adenomas

Pyloric gland adenoma (PGA) is a polypoid neoplasm of the gallbladder, and it consists of aggregates of small mucus glands that are reminiscent of pyloric glands. Macroscopically, PGA shows polypoid tumors that often connect to the gallbladder mucosa with a thin stalk (Fig. 17a). When resected gallbladders are opened, the polyps are often detached from the gallbladder wall. Histological features are characteristic. PGA is packed with small glands resembling pyloric glands with scarce intervening stroma (Fig. 17b). Larger glands are also intermingled in most of the cases. The cellular features are homogeneous and show mild atypia, but sometimes atypia is marked and corresponds to the high-grade.

Immunohistochemically, MUC6, which is a marker of pyloric glands, is diffusely positive in PGAs. Immunostaining for beta-catenin is often positive in the nuclei and cytoplasm (Fig. 17c), which represents *CTNNB1* (beta-catenin gene) mutation found in most of the cases of PGA [49]. In such cases, a morula consisting of nests

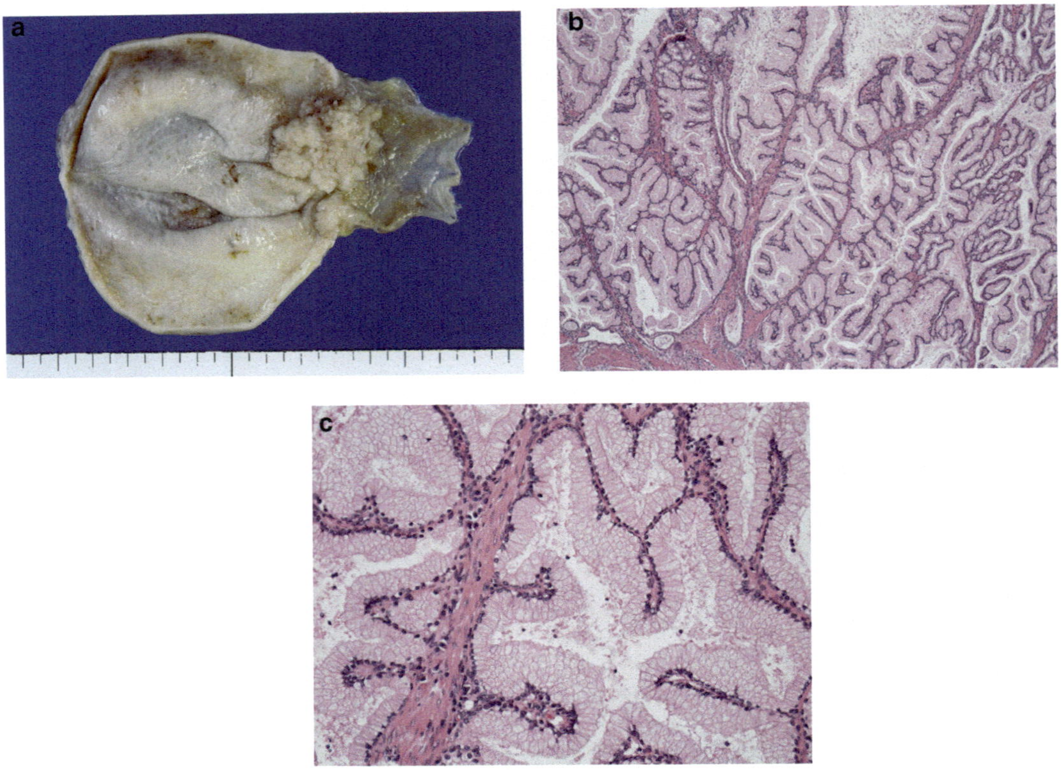

Fig. 16 Intracystic papillary neoplasm. **a** A macroscopic picture showing a papillary growth. **b** A papillary neoplasm showing histological features of gastric phenotype. **c** Nuclear atypia is mild

with spindle-shaped neoplastic cells may be identified by careful observation (Fig. 17d) [50]. CDX2 is a useful marker to identify a morula [51]. A lateral spread along the gallbladder mucosa is not a feature of PGA.

According to the WHO Classification 2019, macroscopic mass-forming, noninvasive tumors are categorized at ICPN except for PGA, and terms such as papillary/villous adenoma and papillary carcinoma are not recommended.

Concluding Remarks

At the beginning of this chapter, we mentioned the unique anatomy and functions of the gallbladder that may give rise to the unique diseases observed there. However, similar diseases may have different manifestations around the world. The incidence of cholecystolithiasis and the types of gallstones vary among different regions in the world. The clinicopathologic features and genetic abnormalities of gallbladder carcinomas also differ. Although some of these differences can plausibly be explained by different environmental factors and dietary habits, it is highly likely that genetic differences play an important role. Future studies of genetics are expected to increase our understanding of gallbladder diseases.

Acknowledgments The authors thank the following pathologists and a gastroenterologist who kindly provided pictures of IgG4-related cholecystitis (Fig. 10): Dr. Hiroshi Yamaguchi, Department of Pathology; Dr. Shuntaro Mukai, Department of Gastroenterology and Hepatology, Tokyo Medical University; Dr. Midori Wakiya, Department of Diagnostic Pathology, Tokyo Medical University Hachioji Medical Center, Hachiojishi, Tokyo, Japan.

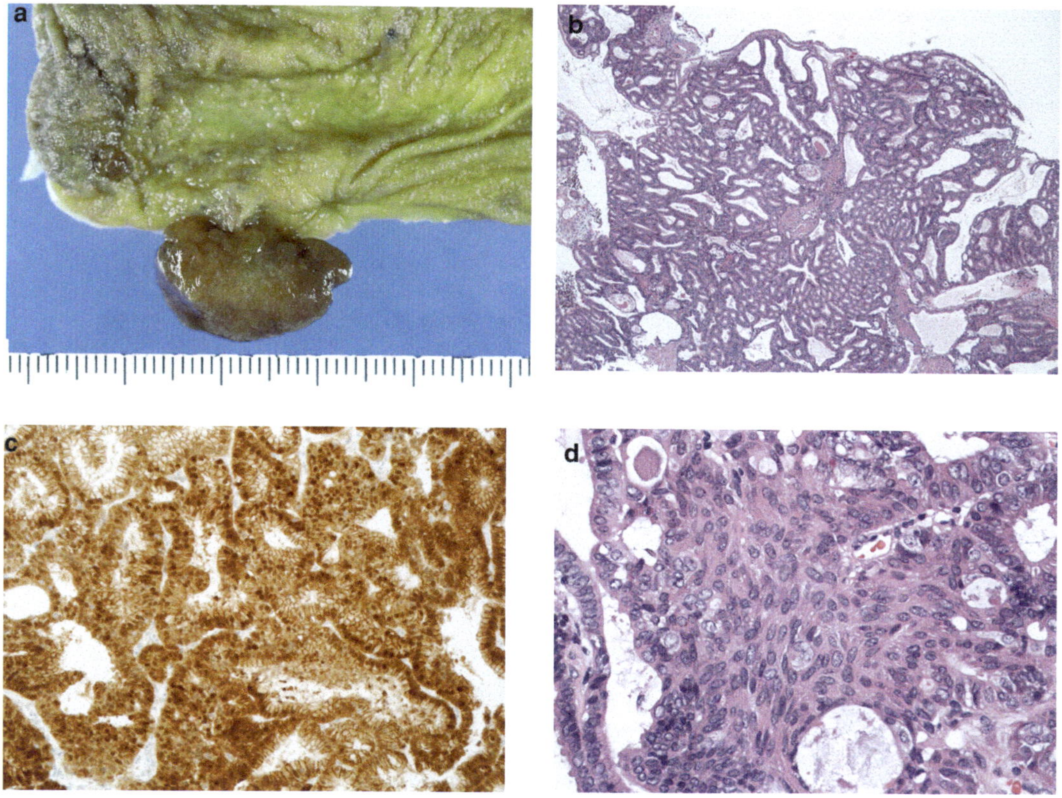

Fig. 17 Pyloric gland adenoma. **a** A polyp connected to the mucosa with a narrow stalk is a characteristic feature. **b** Packed small glands resembling pyloric glands with a mixture of larger glands. **c** Beta-catenin is positive within the nuclei and cytoplasm. **d** A morula consisting of spindle-shaped neoplastic cells

References

1. Jirsa M, Groen AK. Role of biliary proteins and non-protein factors in kinetics of cholesterol crystallisation and gallstone growth. Front Biosci. 2001;6:E154–67.
2. Wittenburg H, Lammert F. Genetic predisposition to gallbladder stones. Semin Liver Dis. 2007;27(1):109–21.
3. Wittenburg H. Hereditary liver disease: gallstones. Best Pract Res Clin Gastroenterol. 2010;24(5):747–56.
4. Di Ciaula A, Wang DQ, Portincasa P. An update on the pathogenesis of cholesterol gallstone disease. Curr Opin Gastroenterol. 2018;34(2):71–80.
5. Cariati A, Cetta F. Rokitansky-Aschoff sinuses of the gallbladder are associated with black pigment gallstone formation: a scanning electron microscopy study. Ultrastruct Pathol. 2003;27(4):265–70.
6. Nishimura A, Shirai Y, Hatakeyama K. Segmental adenomyomatosis of the gallbladder predisposes to cholecystolithiasis. J Hepatobiliary Pancreat Surg. 2004;11(5):342–7.
7. Vitek L, Carey MC. New pathophysiological concepts underlying pathogenesis of pigment gallstones. Clin Res Hepatol Gastroenterol. 2012;36(2):122–9.
8. Jessurun J, Pambuccian S. Infectious and inflammatory disorders of the gallbladder and extrahepatic biliary tract. In: Odze RD, Goldblum JR, editors. Odze and Goldlum surgical pathology of the GI tract, liver, biliary tract, and pancreas. 3rd ed. Philaderphia, PA, USA: Elsevier Saunders; 2015.
9. Indar AA, Beckingham IJ. Acute cholecystitis. BMJ (Clin Res Ed). 2002;325(7365):639–43.
10. Theise ND. Liver and gallbladder. In: Kumar V, Abbas AK, Aster JC, editors. Robbins basic pathology. 10th ed. Philaderphia, PA, USA: Elsevier; 2018.
11. Huffman JL, Schenker S. Acute acalculous cholecystitis: a review. Clin Gastroenterol Hepatol. 2010;8(1):15–22.
12. Lack EE. Pathology of the pancreas, gallbladder, extrahepatic biliary tract, and ampullary region. New York, NY, USA: Oxford University Press; 2003.

13. Sawada S, Shimada Y, Sekine S, Shibuya K, Yoshioka I, Matsui K, et al. Expression of GLUT-1 and GLUT-3 in xanthogranulomatous cholecystitis induced a positive result on (1)(8)F-FDG PET: report of a case. Int Surg. 2013;98(4):372–8.
14. Mori M, Watanabe M, Sakuma M, Tsutsumi Y. Infectious etiology of xanthogranulomatous cholecystitis: immunohistochemical identification of bacterial antigens in the xanthogranulomatous lesions. Pathol Int. 1999;49(10):849–52.
15. Sawada S, Harada K, Isse K, Sato Y, Sasaki M, Kaizaki Y, et al. Involvement of Escherichia coli in pathogenesis of xanthogranulomatous cholecystitis with scavenger receptor class A and CXCL16-CXCR6 interaction. Pathol Int. 2007;57(10):652–63.
16. Hong SA, Sung YN, Kim HJ, Lee SS, Lee JH, Ahn CS, et al. Xanthogranulomatous cholecystitis shows overlapping histological features with IgG4-related cholecystitis. Histopathology. 2018;72(4):569–79.
17. Roggin KK, Rudloff U, Klimstra DS, Russell LA, Blumgart LH. Adult-onset asthma and periocular xanthogranulomas in a patient with lymphoplasmacytic sclerosing pancreatitis. Pancreas. 2007;34(1):157–60.
18. Verdijk RM, Heidari P, Verschooten R, van Daele PL, Simonsz HJ, Paridaens D. Raised numbers of IgG4-positive plasma cells are a common histopathological finding in orbital xanthogranulomatous disease. Orbit. 2014;33(1):17–22.
19. Patel S, Roa JC, Tapia O, Dursun N, Bagci P, Basturk O, et al. Hyalinizing cholecystitis and associated carcinomas: clinicopathologic analysis of a distinctive variant of cholecystitis with porcelain-like features and accompanying diagnostically challenging carcinomas. Am J Surg Pathol. 2011;35(8):1104–13.
20. Jessurun J, Bolio-Solis A, Manivel JC. Diffuse lymphoplasmacytic acalculous cholecystitis: a distinctive form of chronic cholecystitis associated with primary sclerosing cholangitis. Hum Pathol. 1998;29(5):512–7.
21. Abraham SC, Cruz-Correa M, Argani P, Furth EE, Hruban RH, Boitnott JK. Diffuse lymphoplasmacytic chronic cholecystitis is highly specific for extrahepatic biliary tract disease but does not distinguish between primary and secondary sclerosing cholangiopathy. Am J Surg Pathol. 2003;27(10):1313–20.
22. Hammer ST, Appelman HD. Sporadic lymphoplasmacytic cholecystitis: a clinicopathologic entity. Am J Clin Pathol. 2014;142(2):209–12.
23. Umehara H, Okazaki K, Masaki Y, Kawano M, Yamamoto M, Saeki T, et al. Comprehensive diagnostic criteria for IgG4-related disease (IgG4-RD), 2011. Mod Rheumatol. 2012;22(1):21–30.
24. Stone JH, Khosroshahi A, Deshpande V, Chan JK, Heathcote JG, Aalberse R, et al. Recommendations for the nomenclature of IgG4-related disease and its individual organ system manifestations. Arthritis Rheum. 2012;64(10):3061–7.
25. Shimosegawa T, Chari ST, Frulloni L, Kamisawa T, Kawa S, Mino-Kenudson M, et al. International consensus diagnostic criteria for autoimmune pancreatitis: guidelines of the International Association of Pancreatology. Pancreas. 2011;40(3):352–8.
26. Kawaguchi K, Koike M, Tsuruta K, Okamoto A, Tabata I, Fujita N. Lymphoplasmacytic sclerosing pancreatitis with cholangitis: a variant of primary sclerosing cholangitis extensively involving pancreas. Hum Pathol. 1991;22(4):387–95.
27. Notohara K, Burgart LJ, Yadav D, Chari S, Smyrk TC. Idiopathic chronic pancreatitis with periductal lymphoplasmacytic infiltration: clinicopathologic features of 35 cases. Am J Surg Pathol. 2003;27(8):1119–27.
28. Ohara H, Okazaki K, Tsubouchi H, Inui K, Kawa S, Kamisawa T, et al. Clinical diagnostic criteria of IgG4-related sclerosing cholangitis 2012. J Hepatobiliary Pancreat Sci. 2012;19(5):536–42.
29. Kamisawa T, Nakazawa T, Tazuma S, Zen Y, Tanaka A, Ohara H, et al. Clinical practice guidelines for IgG4-related sclerosing cholangitis. J Hepatobiliary Pancreat Sci. 2019;26(1):9–42.
30. Ishigami K, Shitani M, Kimura Y, Hasegawa T, Masaki Y, Ito A, et al. Ectopic relapse of IgG4-related disease presenting as IgG4-related sclerosing cholecystitis: a case report and review of literature. Medicine. 2018;97(52):e13868.
31. Gupta RK, Patton KT. Hyalinizing cholecystitis with features of immunoglobulin G4-related disease-coincidence or an unrecognized association? A case report. Hum Pathol. 2015;46(4):625–8.
32. Ahmed M, Alibhai M, Samee A. Torsion of the gallbladder. BMJ case reports; 2011:bcr0620103116.
33. Takayasu K, Moriyama N, Muramatsu Y, Shima Y, Ushio K, Yamada T, et al. Gallbladder infarction after hepatic artery embolization. AJR Am J Roentgenol. 1985;144(1):135–8.
34. Bassullu N, Turkmen I, Uraz S, Yagiz Korkmaz P, Memisoglu R, Gultekin OS, et al. Xanthomatous hyperplastic polyps of the stomach: clinicopathologic study of 5 patients with polypoid gastric lesions showing combined features of gastric xanthelasma and hyperplastic polyp. Ann Diagn Pathol. 2013;17(1):72–4.
35. WHO Classification of Tumours Editorial Board. WHO Classification of tumours series, 5th ed.: Digestive system tumours. Lyon, France: International Agency for Research on Cancer; 2019.
36. Misra S, Chaturvedi A, Misra NC, Sharma ID. Carcinoma of the gallbladder. Lancet Oncol. 2003;4(3):167–76.
37. Goldin RD, Roa JC. Gallbladder cancer: a morphological and molecular update. Histopathology. 2009;55(2):218–29.
38. Chijiiwa K, Kimura H, Tanaka M. Malignant potential of the gallbladder in patients with anomalous pancreaticobiliary ductal junction. The difference in risk between patients with and without choledochal cyst. Int Surg. 1995;80(1):61–4.

39. Muraki T, Memis B, Reid MD, Uehara T, Ito T, Hasebe O, et al. Reflux-associated cholecystopathy: analysis of 76 gallbladders from patients with Supra-Oddi union of the pancreatic duct and common bile duct (Pancreatobiliary Maljunction) elucidates a specific diagnostic pattern of mucosal hyperplasia as a prelude to carcinoma. Am J Surg Pathol. 2017;41(9):1167–77.
40. McGee EE, Jackson SS, Petrick JL, Van Dyke AL, Adami HO, Albanes D, et al. Smoking, alcohol, and biliary tract cancer risk: a pooling project of 26 prospective studies. J Natl Cancer Inst. 2019;111(12):1263–78.
41. Jackson SS, Van Dyke AL, Zhu B, Pfeiffer RM, Petrick JL, Adami HO, et al. Anthropometric risk factors for cancers of the biliary tract in the biliary tract cancers pooling project. Cancer Res. 2019;79(15):3973–82.
42. Narayan RR, Creasy JM, Goldman DA, Gonen M, Kandoth C, Kundra R, et al. Regional differences in gallbladder cancer pathogenesis: insights from a multi-institutional comparison of tumor mutations. Cancer. 2019;125(4):575–85.
43. Iwase T, Nakazawa S, Yamao K, Yoshino J, Inui K, Yamachika H, et al. Ras gene point mutations in gallbladder lesions associated with anomalous connection of pancreatobiliary ducts. Hepatogastroenterology. 1997;44(17):1457–62.
44. Moy AP, Shahid M, Ferrone CR, Borger DR, Zhu AX, Ting D, et al. Microsatellite instability in gallbladder carcinoma. Virchows Arch. 2015;466(4):393–402.
45. Goeppert B, Roessler S, Renner M, Loeffler M, Singer S, Rausch M, et al. Low frequency of mismatch repair deficiency in gallbladder cancer. Diagn Pathol. 2019;14(1):36.
46. Adsay V, Jang KT, Roa JC, Dursun N, Ohike N, Bagci P, et al. Intracholecystic papillary-tubular neoplasms (ICPN) of the gallbladder (neoplastic polyps, adenomas, and papillary neoplasms that are>/=1.0 cm): clinicopathologic and immunohistochemical analysis of 123 cases. Am J Surg Pathol. 2012;36(9):1279–301.
47. Matthaei H, Wu J, Dal Molin M, Debeljak M, Lingohr P, Katabi N, et al. GNAS codon 201 mutations are uncommon in intraductal papillary neoplasms of the bile duct. HPB (Oxford). 2012;14(10):677–83.
48. Akita M, Fujikura K, Ajiki T, Fukumoto T, Otani K, Hirose T, et al. Intracholecystic papillary neoplasms are distinct from papillary gallbladder cancers: a clinicopathologic and Exome-sequencing study. Am J Surg Pathol. 2019;43(6):783–91.
49. He C, Fukumura Y, Toriyama A, Ogura K, Sasahara N, Mitani K, et al. Pyloric Gland Adenoma (PGA) of the gallbladder: a unique and distinct tumor from PGAs of the Stomach, Duodenum, and Pancreas. Am J Surg Pathol. 2018;42(9):1237–45.
50. Kushima R, Remmele W, Stolte M, Borchard F. Pyloric gland type adenoma of the gallbladder with squamoid spindle cell metaplasia. Pathol Res Pract. 1996;192(9):963–9.
51. Wani Y, Notohara K, Fujisawa M. Aberrant expression of an "intestinal marker" Cdx2 in pyloric gland adenoma of the gallbladder. Virchows Arch. 2008;453(5):521–7.

Imaging Diagnosis of Diseases of the Gallbladder: US, CT, and MRI

Jin-Young Choi and Dong Ryul Chang

Introduction

The importance of imaging tests is increasing for accurate diagnosis of gallbladder disease. Plain radiography is rarely used in the assessment of gallbladder disease, because it provides little diagnostic information. Ultrasound and CT are commonly used imaging modalities for evaluating gallbladder abnormalities. MRI is used as a secondary or problem solving exam to obtain more information when a diagnosis cannot be reached by ultrasound or CT. In this chapter, we describe techniques, important anatomy, and imaging features of various gallbladder diseases on ultrasound, CT, and MRI.

Imaging Modalities for Diagnosing Diseases of the Gallbladder

Ultrasound

Ultrasonography is the first screening and diagnostic tool to be used when a patient is suspected of having bile duct or gallbladder disease because it is non-invasive and can be readily performed without any extra preparation other than fasting. In addition, ultrasonography images can be obtained from various planes as intended by the operator (Table 1).

Technique

Patients need to fast at least 6–8 hours before gallbladder ultrasound to allow maximal distention of the gallbladder and to enhance the detectability of gallstones. For most adult patients, a curved probe with frequencies between 1 and 5 megahertz (MHz) is most commonly used. If the gallbladder is close to the abdominal wall or if the patient is underweight, a high-resolution image can be obtained with a higher frequency transducer (Fig. 1). A patient is first asked to lie in the supine position for the ultrasound examination, and the right subcostal or lower intercostal spaces should be scanned along the anterior axillary line. Longitudinal and transverse plane views should be obtained to evaluate the entire gallbladder. For further evaluation, the patient may be asked to change into other positions, such as the left lateral decubitus, upright, and Trendelenburg position. Deep breathing or increasing the intraperitoneal pressure (Valsalva maneuver) will move the gallbladder down into the ribs for easier examination. Using harmonic and compound imaging, high-quality ultrasound images can be obtained. Harmonic imaging detects the harmonic frequencies created by the non-linear propagation of

J.-Y. Choi (✉) · D. R. Chang
Department of Radiology, Severance Hospital, Yonsei University College of Medicine, 50-1 Yonsei-ro, Seodaemun-gu, Seoul 03722, Korea
e-mail: gafield2@yuhs.ac

D. R. Chang
e-mail: rarara419@yuhs.ac

J. B. Chung and K. Okazaki (eds.), *Diseases of the Gallbladder*,
https://doi.org/10.1007/978-981-15-6010-1_4

Table 1 Imaging modalities for gallbladder evaluation

Modalities	Main purposes	Advantages
Ultrasound	First screening and diagnostic tool to evaluate gallbladder disease Diagnosis of gallstones, polyp, and acute cholecystitis	Non-invasive Easy to perform without complex preparation Can be performed in real-time and various planes can be obtained as intended by the operator
CT	Diagnosis and staging of gallbladder carcinoma Diagnosis of cholecystitis complications such as emphysematous cholecystitis, gangrenous cholecystitis, and gallbladder perforation	Evaluation of other organs in the abdominal cavity is possible in addition to the gallbladder within a short time frame
MRI	Modality for problem solving rather than for screening Evaluation of the gallbladder and biliary system Staging of gallbladder carcinoma	Superior evaluation of cystic ductal pathology than CT and ultrasound

ultrasound through body tissue. It reduces reverberation artifacts, side lobe artifacts, and noise, and thus, increases tissue contrast. Compound imaging incorporates ultrasound beams that are steered electronically from an array transducer to rapidly acquire several overlapping scans of an object from different view angles. These single-angle scans are averaged to form a multi-angle compound image. Image quality improves because speckle, clutter, and other acoustic artifacts are reduced with compound imaging.

Normal Anatomy

The gallbladder is a pear-shaped organ that is located under the liver. On the longitudinal scan, the gallbladder of a sufficiently fasted patient presents as an anechoic, oval structure (Fig. 2). A normal gallbladder is about 40–50 mm wide and 80–100 mm in length. The thickness of the normal gallbladder wall is about 2–3 mm. The outer strong echogenic line is the perimuscular layer, the middle hypoechoic line is the muscular layer, and the inner slightly hyperechoic line is the mucosa. The gallbladder lies beneath the major hepatic interlobar fissure, which is apparent as a highly echogenic line always adjacent to the gallbladder neck [1].

Computed Tomography (CT)

CT is not commonly used when screening for gallbladder disease because it does not show higher sensitivity for gallstones than ultrasound. Rather, CT is more useful for the diagnosis and staging of gallbladder cancer, and for the evaluation of complications from cholecystitis, such as gallbladder perforation or pericholecystic abscess, porcelain gallbladder, and emphysematous cholecystitis (Table 1).

Technique

If gallbladder or biliary disease is suspected, unenhanced and contrast-enhanced studies during the hepatic arterial and portal venous phases are obtained without an oral contrast agent. The use of a positive oral contrast agent may interfere with the detection of choledocholithiasis due to the oral contrast agent refluxing into the biliary tree. A hepatic arterial phase image can be obtained 20–25 seconds after the intravenous injection of contrast media, and a portal venous phase image can be obtained 60–70 seconds after the injection. Multiphase images obtained with contrast material during the hepatic arterial and portal venous phases may improve visualization of hypovascular tumors involving the gallbladder, bile ducts, and surrounding tissue. Reconstruction of multiple planes and different slice thicknesses can be obtained for further lesion characterization. Images of 2–4 mm slice thickness with axial and coronal planes are commonly used.

Normal Anatomy

The gallbladder presents as a low-attenuation, fluid-filled, oval structure on CT. The normal

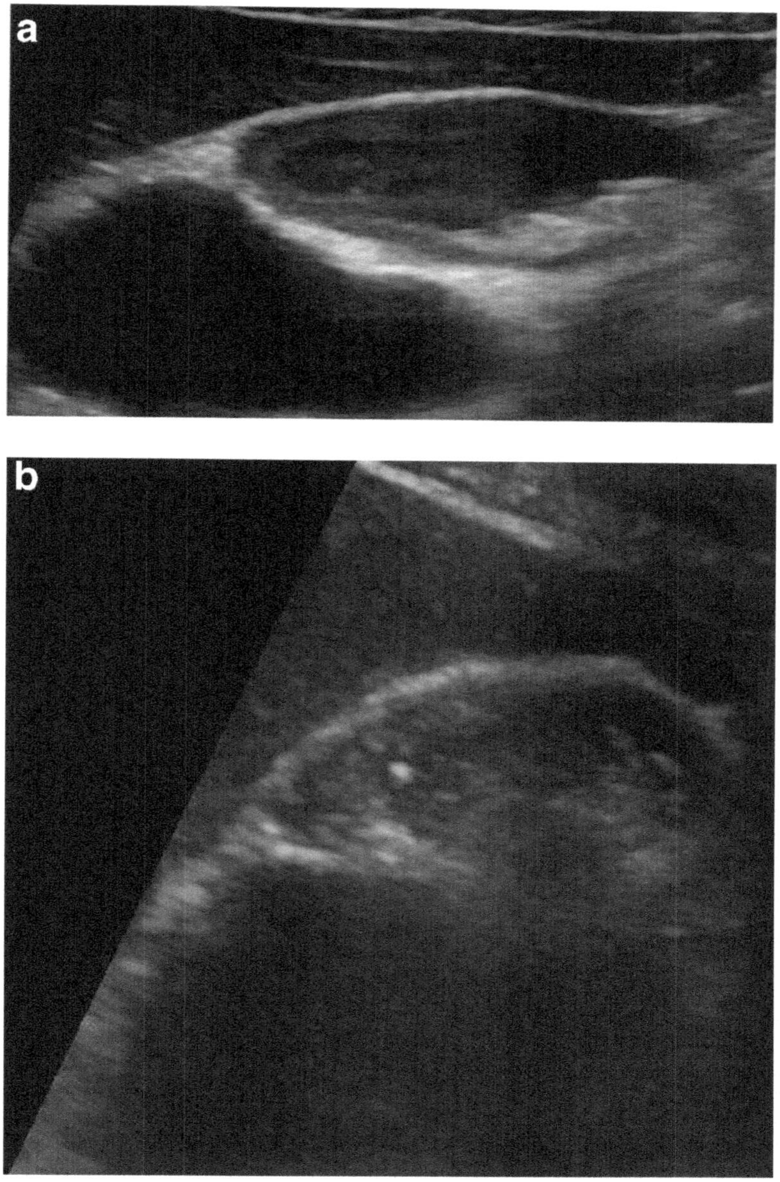

Fig. 1 Gallbladder ultrasound image, using **a** a high frequency probe (9 MHz), and **b** a conventional frequency probe (1–5 MHz) in a 55-year-old male. Thickening of the gallbladder fundal wall and layers are observed more accurately and clearly with the high frequency probe (**a**) than the conventional probe (**b**)

gallbladder wall can be seen as a thin line (2–3 mm) and may show contrast enhancement (Fig. 3). The collapsed gallbladder may be more difficult to identify on CT [2].

Magnetic Resonance Imaging (MRI)

MRI is used less than ultrasound or CT when evaluating the gallbladder. Rather, MRI is performed to gather additional information of

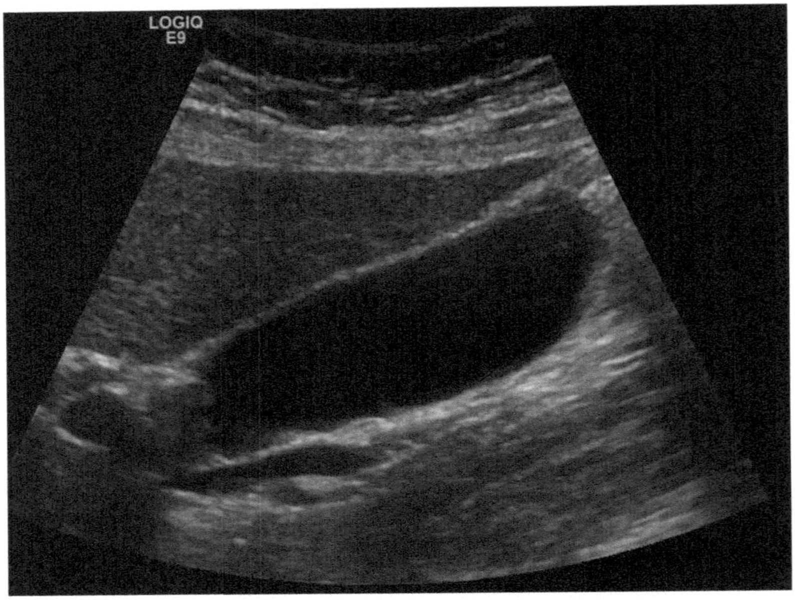

Fig. 2 Normal gallbladder on ultrasound after fasting. Note the anechoic, oval structure with a thin echogenic wall (2–3 mm) under the liver

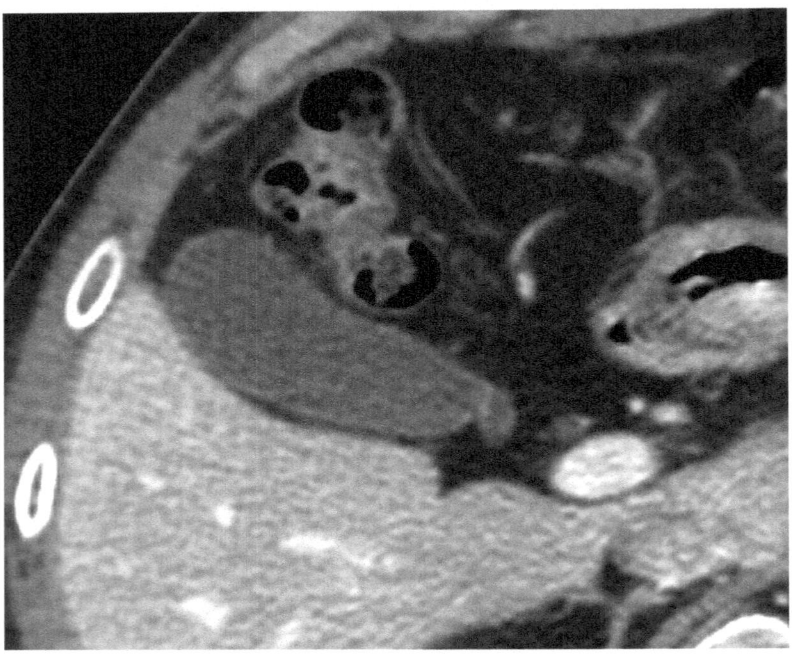

Fig. 3 Normal gallbladder on CT in a fasting 58-year-old male. Note the fluid-filled oval structure with enhancing thin wall (2–3 mm) on the under surface of the liver

diseases that are difficult to diagnose on US or CT. It is also used to evaluate cystic ducts or the biliary system (Table 1).

Technique

Conventional MRI of the gallbladder and bile ducts comprises T1- and T2-weighted sequences. T1-weighted fat suppression sequences can be used to demonstrate the lumen as well as the gallbladder wall and the bile ducts. The use of contrast material improves the delineation of the gallbladder wall and bile ducts, and helps clinicians diagnose disease entities for both benign and malignant disease. T2-weighted sequences, usually fast spin-echo (FSE) sequences with respiratory gating, are optimal for evaluating the surrounding soft tissue abnormalities involving the gallbladder wall. Magnetic resonance cholangiopancreatography (MRCP) is a technique that distinguishes bile ducts and the surrounding tissue as bile ducts appear as bright signals on T2-weighted images. It is very useful for evaluating the gallbladder and biliary system because it is a non-invasive exam, unlike endoscopic retrograde cholangiopancreatography. The insertion site for the cystic duct and common hepatic duct is clearly visible on MRCP, therefore allowing an easy diagnosis of cystic ductal obstructive pathology.

Normal Anatomy

On T2-weighted images, the gallbladder wall has low signal intensity and stands out against bright visceral fat (Fig. 4). The gallbladder lumen appears as high or low signal intensity depending on bile juice concentrations, and the pulse sequence is used. Bile is concentrated during the fasting period, and usually shows high signals on T1-weighted images.

Inflammatory Diseases of the Gallbladder

Gallstones

Ultrasonography is the most important imaging tool for evaluating gallstones. The sensitivity of ultrasonography for gallstones is up to 95% [3]. On ultrasonography, gallstones appear as highly echogenic and mobile lesions, accompanied by posterior acoustic shadowing (Fig. 5). The right anterior oblique position is the best position to find gallstones, as it allows gallstones in the neck to flow out to the fundus and be easily observed. If the gallbladder is contracted and the lumen is filled with shadowing gallstones, it is observed with a double-arc appearance on ultrasonography. On ultrasonography, the perceivable gallbladder wall is separated from the intraluminal stones, a finding called the wall-echo-shadow sign that is specific for chronic cholecystitis [4]. Bile sludge has no or weak posterior acoustic shadowing, and it does not move easily due to its viscosity, even when a patient changes position. When the bile sludge clumps together, it is called a tumefactive sludge and may be misdiagnosed as a polyp or tumor. Thus, checking for changes in the shape or mobility of sludge after position changes can help make an accurate diagnosis.

The ability to detect gallstones on CT depends on the differing density of the stones with respect to bile. CT is known to diagnose only about 80% of the gallstones identified by ultrasonography. Calcified stones are easily detected because they are denser than bile and appear as hyperdense foci in the gallbladder lumen. One study found that the sensitivity for in vitro gallstone detection is significantly higher at 140 kVp than at lower voltage settings [5]. Recently, another study suggested that cholesterol stones are more clearly seen in virtual unenhanced images using dual-energy CT rather than true unenhanced CT [6].

Gallstones are best recognized on T2-weighted MR imaging. On T2-weighted MRI, gallstones are visualized as signal voids within the high signal intensity bile. Cholesterol stones are generally isointense or hypointense on T1-weighted images, whereas pigment stones usually show increased signal intensity on T1-weighted images due to paramagnetic substances such as calcium gluconate or calcium bilirubinate [7]. The presence of protein within gallstones may sometimes be responsible for central hyperintensity with a

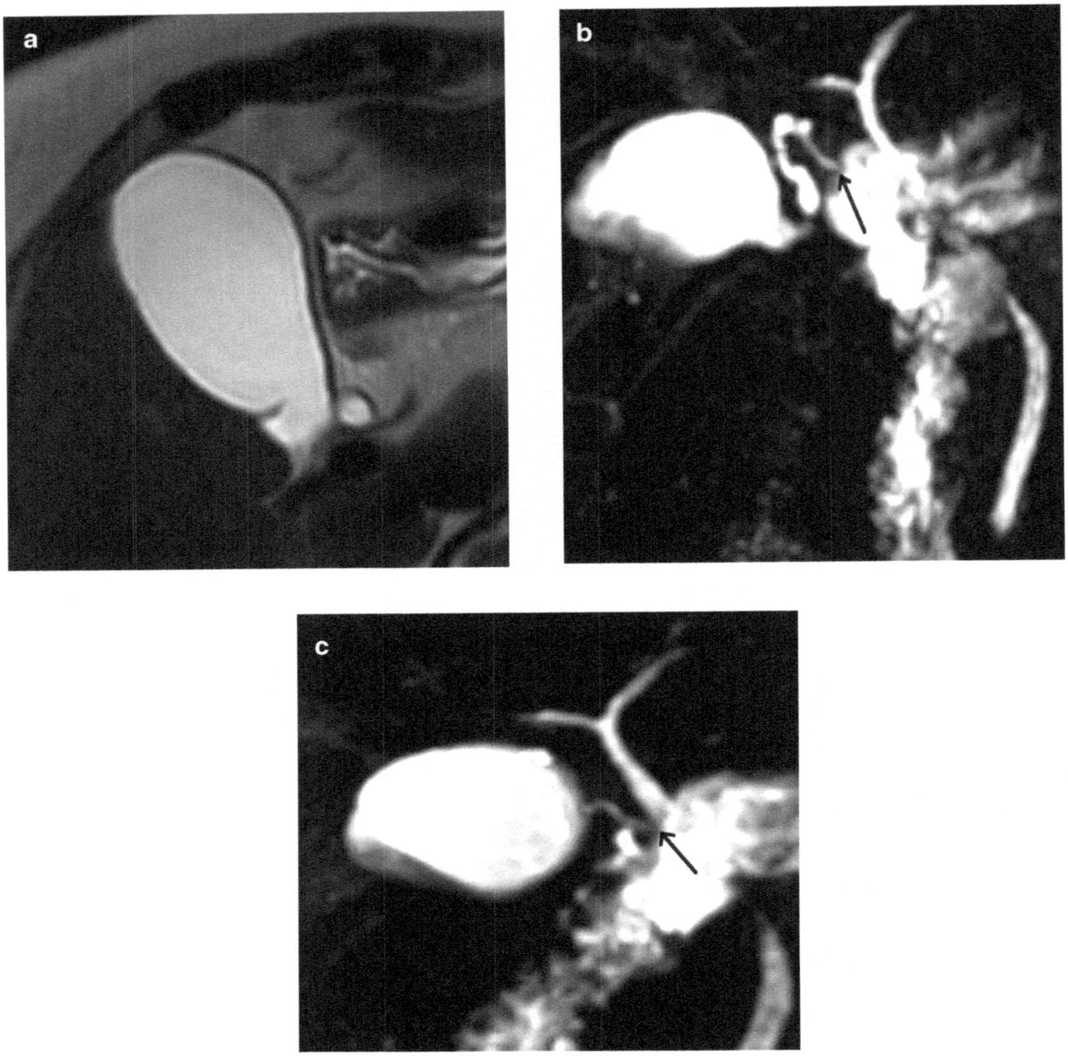

Fig. 4 Normal gallbladder on T2-weighted sequences (**a**) and MRCP (**b**, **c**) after fasting. **a** Axial T2-weighted image shows a hyperintense fluid-filled oval structure with a hyperintense thin wall. **b**, **c** 2-dimensional MRCP clearly demonstrates a cystic duct (arrow) and insertion to the common hepatic duct

peripheral rim of hypointensity seen on T1- or T2-weighted images, or for the predominant hyperintensity seen on T1-weighted images [8, 9].

Acute Cholecystitis

The ultrasonographic findings of acute calculous cholecystitis include gallstones, sonographic Murphy's sign, gallbladder distension, wall thickening, and pericholecystic fluid in severe cases (Fig. 6) [10]. On Doppler ultrasonography, increased blood flow may be observed in the gallbladder wall, but not always [11]. The CT findings of acute calculous cholecystitis are similar to those found on ultrasonography including gallstones, gallbladder distention, thickening of the gallbladder wall and pericholecystic fluid,

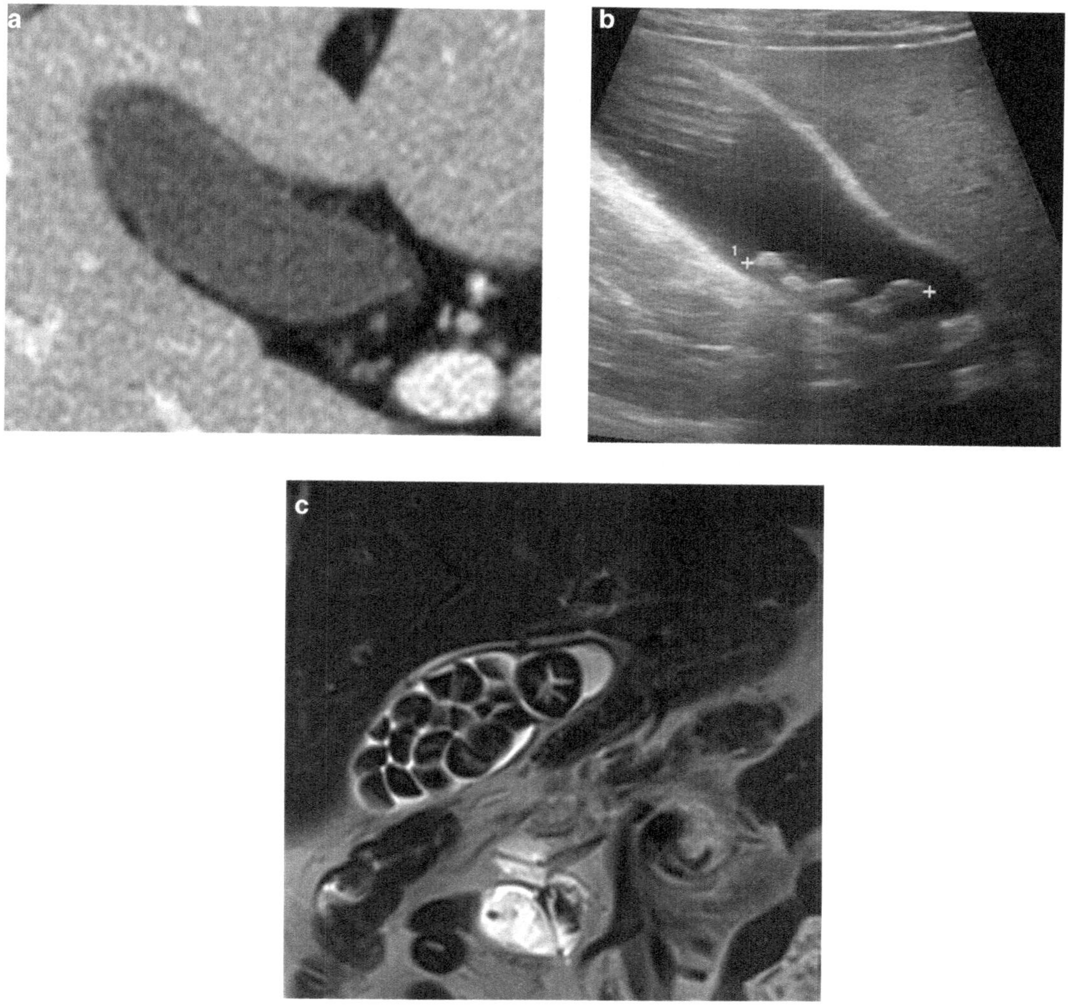

Fig. 5 CT, US and MRI findings of gallstones. (**a**, **b**) CT and US images of gallstones in a 35-year-old male. **a** No stones in the gallbladder on CT. **b** Multiple gallstones are clearly demonstrated on US and present as highly echogenic foci with posterior acoustic shadowing. **c** Coronal T2-weighted image of a 52-year-old male. Multiple filling defects and signal voids can be observed within the hyperintense bile

and inflammation [12]. In addition, it is easy to detect congestion or hyperemia of the adjacent liver parenchyma caused by inflammation around the gallbladder on CT [13]. This could be an early sign of acute cholecystitis. Generally, CT is recommended when complications from cholecystitis are suspected or if ultrasonography results are not conclusive.

Complication of Acute Cholecystitis

Emphysematous Cholecystitis

Emphysematous cholecystitis is characterized by the presence of gas in the gallbladder wall, lumen, or pericholecystic tissue without a fistulous tract between gastrointestinal tracts. On ultrasonography, posterior acoustic shadowing

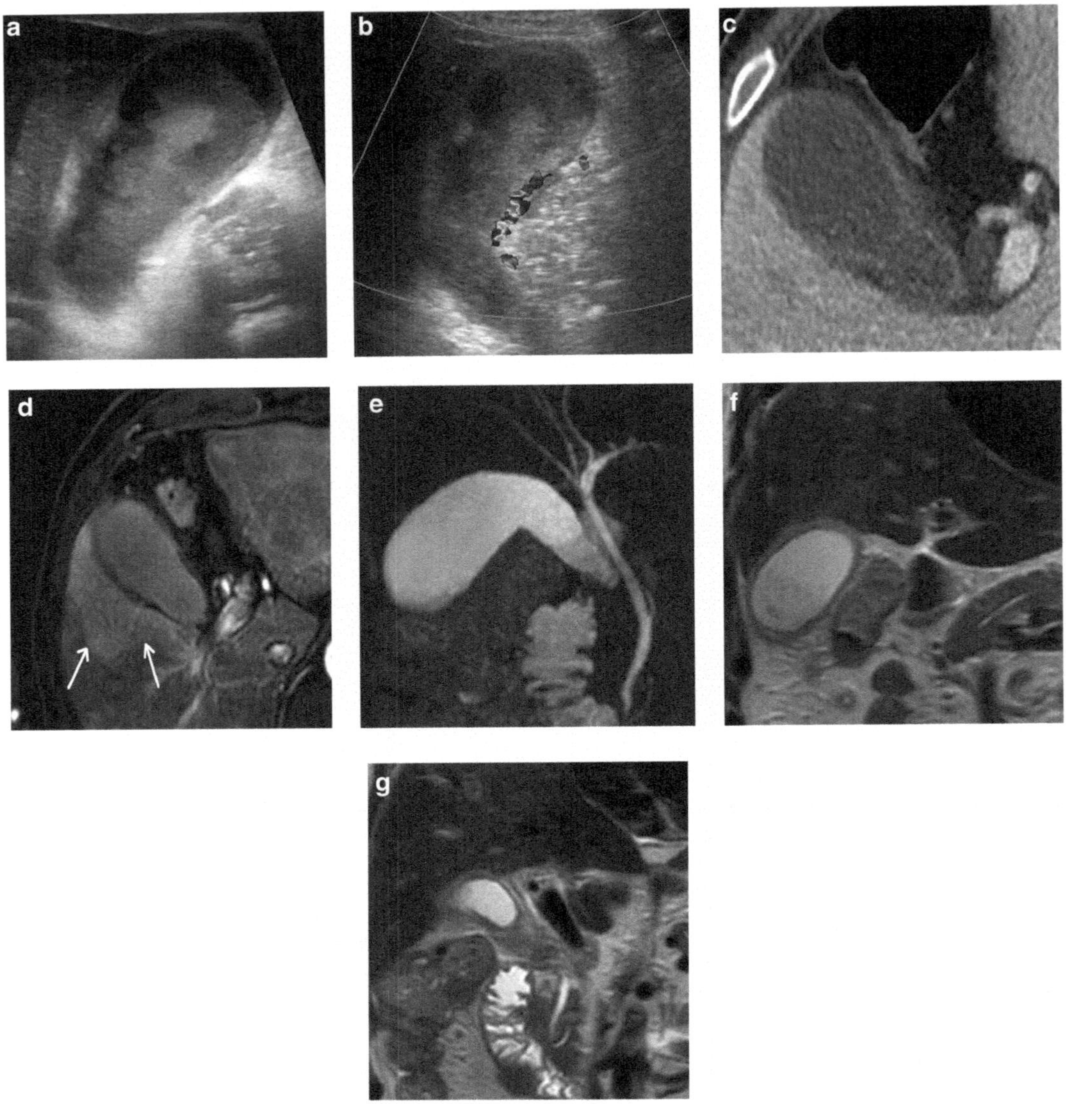

Fig. 6 Image findings of acute cholecystitis in a 63-year-old male. **a** Gray-scale ultrasonography shows gallbladder distension and wall thickening with sludge in the gallbladder lumen. **b** Increased blood flow is seen on Doppler ultrasonography. **c** Contrast-enhanced CT demonstrates gallbladder distention, wall thickening and pericholecystic fluid. **d** Contrast-enhanced axial T1-weighted image shows increased enhancement of the adjacent liver parenchyma (arrow). **e** The cystic duct is not visible on MRCP. **f**, **g** Coronal and axial T2-weighted images show thickened cystic ductal walls and lumen obstruction which are the reason for the gallbladder distention and inflammatory change

due to intraluminal or intramural air is observed, making it sometimes difficult to differentiate emphysematous cholecystitis from calcifications [14]. CT is a more sensitive and specific technique for detecting intraluminal or intramural gas [15].

Gangrenous Cholecystitis

Gangrenous cholecystitis results from prolonged distention of the gallbladder which if left untreated can lead to intramural hemorrhage, ischemia, and necrosis. On ultrasonography, the gallbladder wall appears as heterogeneous, striated, or irregular thickening. Intraluminal septae or membrane may be detected, resulting from the desquamation of the necrotic gallbladder mucosa [16]. On CT, asymmetric gallbladder wall thickening due to intramural microabscesses and discontinuous and/or irregular mucosal enhancement are specific findings of gangrenous cholecystitis [17]. A hyperdense gallbladder wall on unenhanced CT is also regarded as a sign of acute gangrenous cholecystitis.

Perforation of Gallbladder

Gallbladder perforation can be divided into three phases. In the acute phase, it appears as diffuse peritonitis, and in the subacute phase, a pericholecystic abscess is formed. In the chronic phase, a fistula tract may develop between the gallbladder and adjacent bowel loops.

Chronic Cholecystitis

Imaging findings of chronic cholecystitis include gallstones, wall thickening, and contracted or not distended gallbladder, without pericholecystic inflammation (Fig. 7) [18, 19]. A thickened gallbladder wall with a preserved normal wall layer is observed in chronic cholecystitis, which is not normally seen with gallbladder carcinoma. However, sometimes a thickened wall is not enough to distinguish chronic cholecystitis and gallbladder carcinoma [19]. The differential diagnostic imaging findings for chronic cholecystitis and gallbladder cancer will be discussed later on in this chapter.

Xanthogranulomatous cholecystitis is an uncommon form of chronic cholecystitis, which shows closely similar imaging features with gallbladder carcinoma. With xanthogranulomatous, multiple intramural nodules are present as

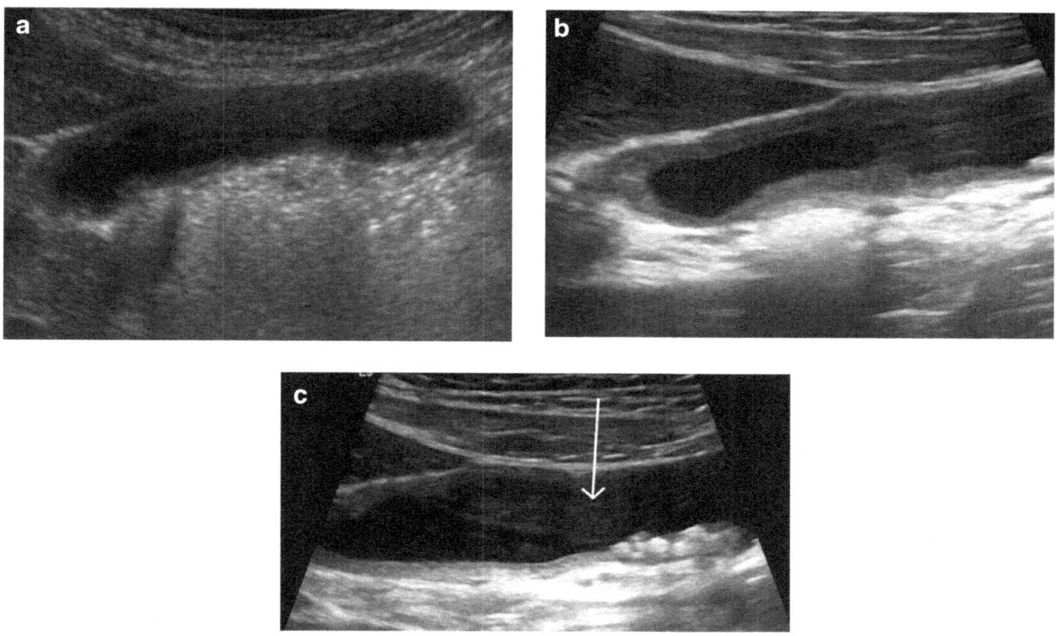

Fig. 7 Image findings of chronic cholecystitis in a 32-year-old female. **a** Gray-scale ultrasonography shows diffuse wall thickening of the gallbladder without significant distention. **b**, **c** Gallbladder wall thickening and gallstones are clearly visible on high resolution gray-scale ultrasonography. Note the reverberation artifact within the gallbladder lumen which is caused by the abdominal wall (arrows)

hypoattenuation on CT and hyperintensity on T2-weighted MRI, which helps differentiate it from gallbladder carcinoma [20, 21].

Mirizzi Syndrome

Mirizzi syndrome occurs when an impacted gallstone in the gallbladder neck or cystic duct compresses the common hepatic duct, leading to obstruction. Imaging findings of Mirizzi syndrome on ultrasonography, CT, or MRI include a collapsed gallbladder, stones in the cystic duct or gallbladder neck, and dilated intrahepatic bile ducts and common hepatic duct without common bile duct dilatation (Fig. 8) [22]. On MRCP, a more accurate evaluation of the nature of the obstruction, burden of gallstones in the biliary tree, and cystic duct obstruction is possible. Anatomical variants that predispose to Mirizzi syndrome are also better detected with MRCP, such as low insertion of the cystic duct or long parallel cystic duct.

Adenomyomatosis

Gallbladder adenomyomatosis is classified into three types according to gross findings: *focal, segmental, and diffuse types* (Fig. 9). The diffuse type appears as diffuse wall thickening involving the entire gallbladder. The focal type presents itself as focal wall thickening or nodule, frequently observed at the fundus. Segmental adenomyomatosis usually occurs at the body, causing annular narrowing or stricture of the gallbladder lumen.

On ultrasonography, wall thickening with a large number of strong and immobile echogenic foci is specific for adenomyomatosis. The foci themselves are associated with comet tail artifacts, which are indicative of cholesterol crystals in the Rokitansky–Aschoff sinuses [23–25]. Sometimes twinkle artifacts on color Doppler, due to the interaction of the ultrasound beam with a rough acoustic interface composed by calcifications or cholesterol depositions in the Rokitansky–Aschoff sinuses, may help diagnose adenomyomatosis [26].

On CT, the common findings of adenomyomatosis are diffuse or focal gallbladder wall thickening or diverticula with bile juice or stones [27]. The segmental and focal forms of adenomyomatosis are particularly difficult to differentiate from carcinoma because they appear as focal thickening of the gallbladder wall or a fundal intraluminal mass. Since the Rokitansky–Aschoff sinuses are also located in the muscularis layer, it is sometimes difficult to differentiate gallbladder carcinoma from adenomyomatosis.

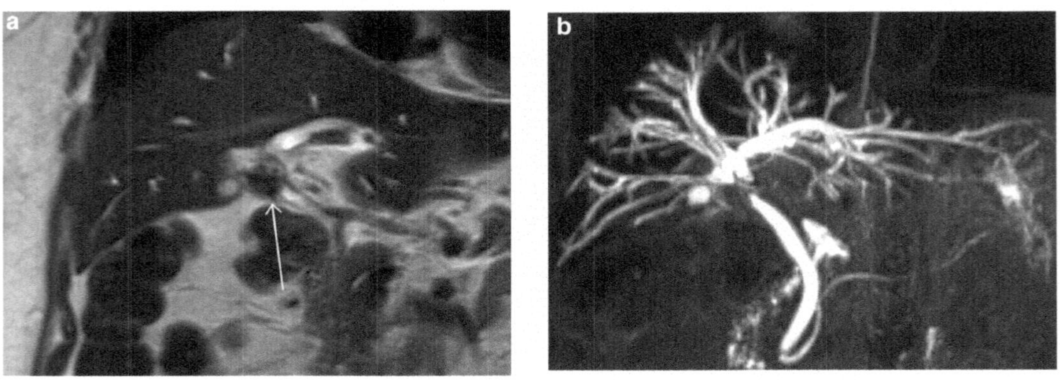

Fig. 8 Image findings of Mirizzi syndrome in a 71-year-old male. **a** Coronal T2-weighted image shows an impacted gallstone in the gallbladder neck (arrow) compressing the common hepatic duct. **b** On MRCP, diffuse dilatation of the intrahepatic duct and extrinsic compression of the common hepatic duct is observed

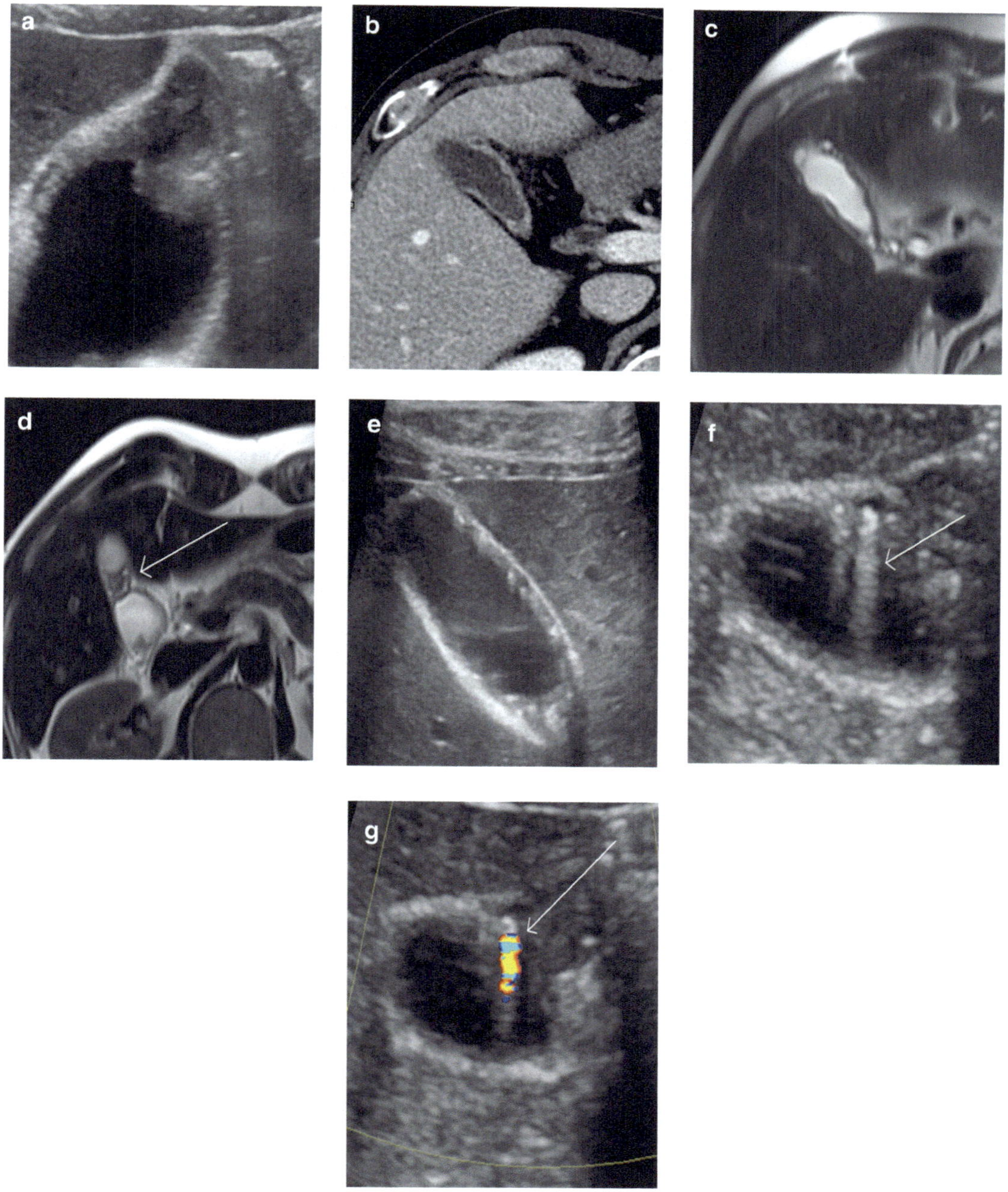

Fig. 9 Image findings of adenomyomatosis. **a** A typical example of focal fundal adenomyomatosis on ultrasonography in a 65-year-old female. Focal nodular wall thickening with an intramural cyst is observed on gray-scale ultrasonography. **b, c** Diffuse adenomyomatosis is observed on CT and T2-weighted MR. **b** Contrast-enhanced CT shows mild diffuse wall thickening, enhancement, and intramural low attenuating foci. **c** Axial T2-weighted image demonstrates multiple small intramural cysts which make up the signature pearl-necklace sign of adenomyomatosis. **d** Axial T2-weighted image reveals segmental adenomyomatosis in the body of the gallbladder (arrow). Note annular wall thickening with multiple intramural cysts in the gallbladder. **e** Diffuse adenomyomatosis on ultrasonography. Ultrasonography shows diffuse wall thickening with multiple small intramural echogenic foci. Note the **g** comet-tail artifact (arrow) and **h** twinkle artifact (arrow) on Doppler ultrasound

On T2-weighted images of MRI, the gallbladder wall shows low signal intensity, and the bile filling the gallbladder appears to be hyperintense. A curvilinear arrangement of multiple small, rounded, high signal intensity foci representing Rokitansky–Aschoff sinuses can be seen within the thickened wall of the gallbladder. This pearl necklace sign is highly specific for adenomyomatosis and differentiates it from gallbladder carcinoma [28].

Cholesterolosis

Cholesterolosis or cholesterol polyps is a disease entity in which lipid, such as cholesterol esters and triglyceride, accumulates in the gallbladder epithelium. On ultrasonography, cholesterol polyps are represented as single or multiple immobile, non-shadowing projections from the gallbladder wall (Fig. 10). On contrast-enhanced CT, cholesterol polyps may be seen as floating lesions within the gallbladder lumen. They may show contrast enhancement due to vascularity within the polyp [29].

Neoplastic Diseases of the Gallbladder

Gallbladder Cancer

Morphologic Classification

Gallbladder carcinomas are classified into three types according to gross morphology and imaging findings: (1) focal or diffuse thickening, (2) polypoid mass protruding into lumen, and (3) mass replacing the gallbladder [30, 31] (Fig. 11) (Table 2).

Focal or Diffuse Thickening

This type of gallbladder carcinoma is more difficult to diagnose preoperatively than other types of gallbladder cancers, especially in its early stages. Gallbladder carcinoma presents as mild to marked asymmetric mural thickening in either a focal or diffuse pattern and shows enhancement after contrast injection. Diagnosis is especially difficult if chronic cholecystitis, gallstones, or gallbladder wall calcifications accompany the findings. According to a report by Kim and colleagues, the following CT findings for

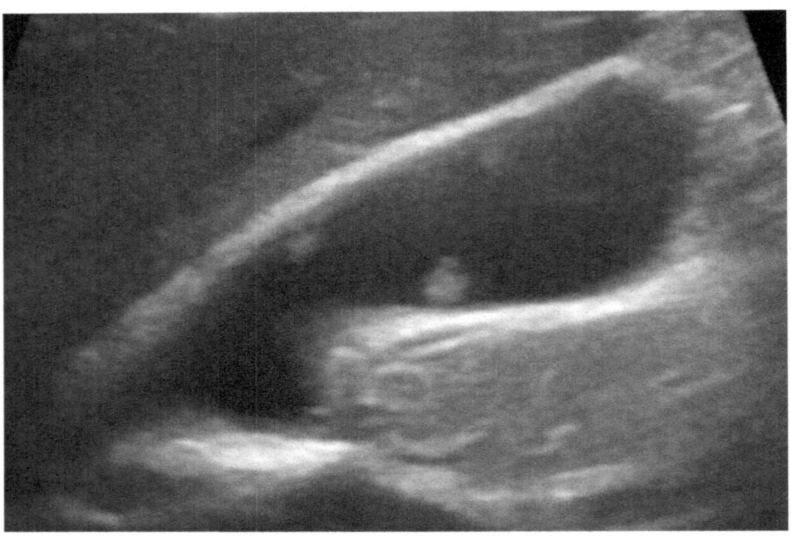

Fig. 10 Typical cholesterol polyp on ultrasonography in a 44-year-old female. Ultrasonography shows several immobile, non-shadowing projections attached to the gallbladder wall

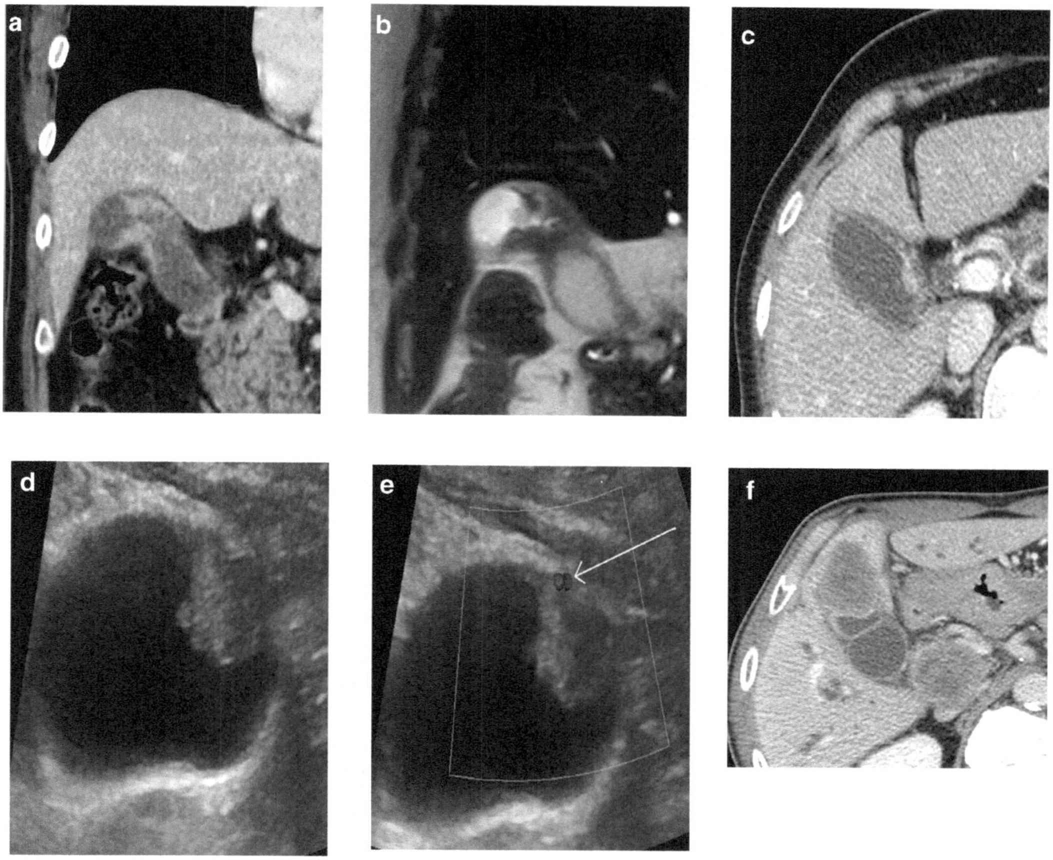

Fig. 11 Different image features of gallbladder cancer. **a**, **b** *Focal or diffuse thickening type in a 57-year-old male.* Contrast-enhanced coronal CT and coronal T2-weighted images show irregular wall thickening in the gallbladder body. **c**, **d**, **e** *Polypoid mass protruding into lumen type.* **c** Contrast-enhanced axial CT shows an enhancing mass, broadly based on the gallbladder wall. **d** Ultrasonography reveals a heterogeneous polypoid mass without posterior shadowing at the gallbladder fundus. **e** Increased vascularity (arrow)is observed in the stalk of the polyp on Doppler ultrasound. **f** *Mass replacing the gallbladder type in a 57-year-old male.* Contrast-enhanced axial CT shows a heterogeneously enhancing solid mass arising from the gallbladder fundus, invading the adjacent hepatic parenchyma. Note the metastatic lymph node at the portacaval space

Table 2 Morphological classification of gallbladder carcinomas

Types	Imaging features
Focal or diffuse thickening	Mild to marked asymmetric mural thickening Focal or diffuse contrast enhancement on CT or MRI *Note—often difficult to distinguish from inflammatory wall thickening
Polypoid mass	Enhancing polypoid mass The larger the size, the higher the potential for malignancy
Mass replacing the gallbladder	Ill-defined, heterogeneously enhancing solid mass invading the adjacent liver parenchyma

the gallbladder wall suggest malignant causes rather than benign: (1) hyperenhancing thick inner wall ≥2.6 mm during the portal venous phase, (2) weakly enhancing or nonenhancing thin outer wall ≤3.4 mm, and (3) irregular and focal wall thickening [32].

Polypoid Mass Protruding into Lumen

On ultrasound, polypoid masses appear as variable echoes with clear boundaries, broadly based on the gallbladder wall and no posterior acoustic shadows. On Doppler ultrasound, vascular signals within the polypoid mass may be observed, which can be distinguished from tumefactive sludge or blood clots [33]. This is due to the enhancing polypoid mass. Necrosis and calcifications are not common. The size of the polypoid mass is directly related to its malignant potential. If the polypoid mass is more than 1 cm in size, its probability of malignancy increases, and if it is larger than 2 cm, the mass is almost definitely a malignant lesion [34].

Mass Replacing the Gallbladder

On imaging, the third type of gallbladder carcinoma manifests as an infiltrative mass with or without necrosis replacing the entire gallbladder. It is an ill-defined, heterogeneously enhancing solid mass, often invading the adjacent hepatic parenchyma, hepatoduodenal ligament, and bile ducts, resulting in bile duct dilatation. Regional lymph node enlargement is another common finding observed when mass infiltrates the gallbladder.

Pathways of the Spreading Tumor

Gallbladder carcinomas can spread by several routes: direct invasion of the liver, hepatoduodenal ligament, duodenum, or colon; lymphatic spread to regional lymph nodes; hematogenous spread to the liver; intraductal tumor extension; and metastasis to the peritoneum. Distant metastases are relatively uncommon. Direct invasion of the liver occurs relatively quickly in the early stages of gallbladder carcinoma because the gallbladder wall is composed of only a single muscle layer without a submucosal layer. On ultrasound, the boundaries of the gallbladder become indistinct as mass invades the adjacent liver parenchyma. The portions of the tumor invading into the liver will show contrast enhancement on CT or MRI [35]. On T2-weighted MR images, tumor invasion shows high signal intensity, similar to the signal intensity of primary gallbladder cancer [36]. Lymphatic spread is also common in gallbladder carcinoma. Lymph node metastasis begins from the gallbladder fossa, follows the hepatoduodenal ligament, proceeds near the pancreas head, and eventually spreads to the abdominal para-aortic area and retroperitoneum (Fig. 12). Imaging findings suggestive of lymph node metastasis are anteroposterior diameter of 10 mm or more and a ring-shaped or heterogeneous contrast enhancement pattern [35].

Other Gallbladder Tumors

Metastatic neoplasm of the gallbladder results from direct invasion or hematogeneous metastasis. Direct invasion is often from malignancies of the stomach, pancreas, and bile duct. Imaging findings of these metastatic tumors are difficult to distinguish from primary gallbladder carcinoma. In addition, other primary malignancies of the gallbladder have been reported such as neuroendocrine tumors, lymphomas, and sarcomas those presented as polypoid masses.

Benign Gallbladder Tumors

Benign gallbladder tumors include adenomas, gastric heterotopias, cystadenomas, granular cell tumors, hemangiomas, lipomas, and leiomyomas [37]. Most benign gallbladder tumors are adenomas. On ultrasound, adenomas appear as small, broad-based, non-shadowing, sessile, or pedunculated polypoid filling defects that do not move with gravitational maneuvers. It is difficult to differentiate adenomas from other polypoid tumors such as primary or metastatic neoplasm by imaging studies. Therefore, polyp size is the most important factor to consider when deciding on the method of treatment. Polyps more than

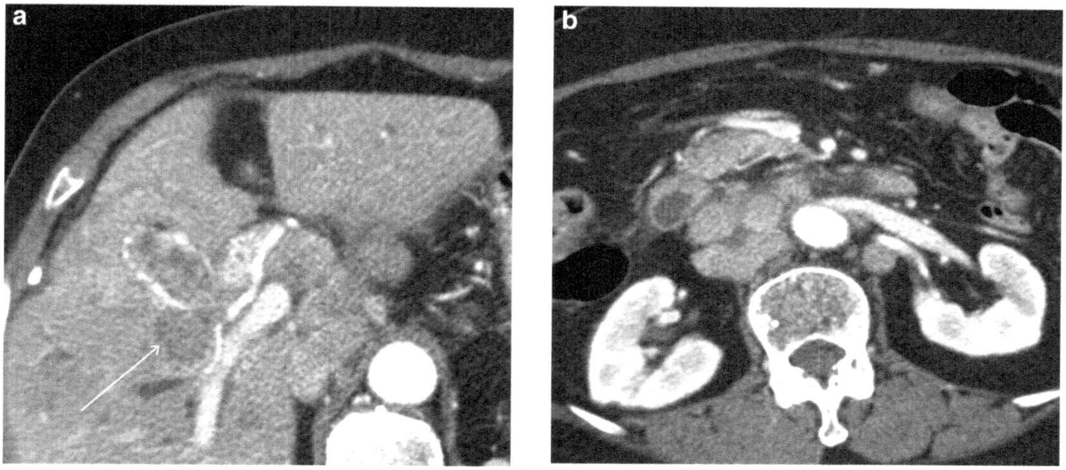

Fig. 12 Image findings of spread pathway of gallbladder cancer in a 75-year-old female **a** Irregular wall thickening and enhancement extending to gallbladder and cystic duct. Note the tumor invasion to the adjacent liver (arrow) and right intrahepatic duct dilatation. Spreading tumor along hepatoduodenal ligament is represented as common bile duct wall thickening. Multiple, conglomerated metastatic lymph nodes are also noted along hepatoduodenal ligament and peripancreatic area. **b** Lymph node metastasis spreads to the abdominal para-aortic area

10 mm in size are at increased risk for malignancy, and prophylactic cholecystectomy is recommended [38].

Conclusion

The accurate diagnosis of gallbladder disease must be preceded in order to choose the appropriate treatment. Gallbladder imaging is important because it can make more accurate diagnosis through the combination of image findings and laboratory result. The new imaging technique needs to be developed to help differential diagnosing of the gallbladder diseases.

References

1. Callen PW, Filly RA. Ultrasonographic localization of the gallbladder. Radiology. 1979;133(3 Pt 1):687–91.
2. Yeh BM, Liu PS, Soto JA, Corvera CA, Hussain HK. MR imaging and CT of the biliary tract. Radiographics. 2009;29(6):1669–88.
3. McIntosh DM, Penney HF. Gray-scale ultrasonography as a screening procedure in the detection of gallbladder disease. Radiology. 1980;136(3):725–7.
4. MacDonald FR, Cooperberg PL, Cohen MM. The WES triad—a specific sonographic sign of gallstones in the contracted gallbladder. Gastrointest Radiol. 1981;6(1):39–41.
5. Chan WC, Joe BN, Coakley FV, Prien EL Jr, Gould RG, Prevrhal S, et al. Gallstone detection at CT in vitro: effect of peak voltage setting. Radiology. 2006;241(2):546–53.
6. Lee HA, Lee YH, Yoon KH, Bang DH, Park DE. Comparison of virtual unenhanced images derived from dual-energy CT with true unenhanced images in evaluation of gallstone disease. AJR Am J Roentgenol. 2016;206(1):74–80.
7. Tsai HM, Lin XZ, Chen CY, Lin PW, Lin JC. MRI of gallstones with different compositions. AJR Am J Roentgenol. 2004;182(6):1513–9.
8. Moriyasu F, Ban N, Nishida O, Nakamura T, Soh Y, Kawasaki T, et al. Central signals of gallstones in magnetic resonance imaging. Am J Gastroenterol. 1987;82(2):139–42.
9. Baron RL, Shuman WP, Lee SP, Rohrmann CA, Jr., Golden RN, Richards TL, et al. MR appearance of gallstones in vitro at 1.5 T: correlation with chemical composition. AJR Am J Roentgenol. 1989;153(3):497–502.
10. Ralls PW, Colletti PM, Lapin SA, Chandrasoma P, Boswell WD, Jr., Ngo C, et al. Real-time sonography in suspected acute cholecystitis. Prospective evaluation of primary and secondary signs. Radiology. 1985;155(3):767–71.
11. Draghi F, Ferrozzi G, Calliada F, Solcia M, Madonia L, Campani R. Power Doppler ultrasound of gallbladder wall vascularization in

inflammation: clinical implications. Eur Radiol. 2000;10(10):1587–90.
12. Fidler J, Paulson EK, Layfield L. CT evaluation of acute cholecystitis: findings and usefulness in diagnosis. AJR Am J Roentgenol. 1996;166(5):1085–8.
13. Yamashita K, Jin MJ, Hirose Y, Morikawa M, Sumioka H, Itoh K, et al. CT finding of transient focal increased attenuation of the liver adjacent to the gallbladder in acute cholecystitis. AJR Am J Roentgenol. 1995;164(2):343–6.
14. Konno K, Ishida H, Naganuma H, Sato M, Komatsuda T, Sato A, et al. Emphysematous cholecystitis: sonographic findings. Abdom Imaging. 2002;27(2):191–5.
15. Gill KS, Chapman AH, Weston MJ. The changing face of emphysematous cholecystitis. Br J Radiol. 1997;70(838):986–91.
16. Jeffrey RB, Laing FC, Wong W, Callen PW. Gangrenous cholecystitis: diagnosis by ultrasound. Radiology. 1983;148(1):219–21.
17. Bennett GL, Rusinek H, Lisi V, Israel GM, Krinsky GA, Slywotzky CM, et al. CT findings in acute gangrenous cholecystitis. AJR Am J Roentgenol. 2002;178(2):275–81.
18. Grand D, Horton KM, Fishman EK. CT of the gallbladder: spectrum of disease. AJR Am J Roentgenol. 2004;183(1):163–70.
19. Yun EJ, Cho SG, Park S, Park SW, Kim WH, Kim HJ, et al. Gallbladder carcinoma and chronic cholecystitis: differentiation with two-phase spiral CT. Abdom Imaging. 2004;29(1):102–8.
20. Chun KA, Ha HK, Yu ES, Shinn KS, Kim KW, Lee DH, et al. Xanthogranulomatous cholecystitis: CT features with emphasis on differentiation from gallbladder carcinoma. Radiology. 1997;203(1):93–7.
21. Shuto R, Kiyosue H, Komatsu E, Matsumoto S, Kawano K, Kondo Y, et al. CT and MR imaging findings of xanthogranulomatous cholecystitis: correlation with pathologic findings. Eur Radiol. 2004;14(3):440–6.
22. Koehler RE, Melson GL, Lee JK, Long J. Common hepatic duct obstruction by cystic duct stone: Mirizzi syndrome. AJR Am J Roentgenol. 1979;132(6):1007–9.
23. Ghersin E, Soudack M, Gaitini D. Twinkling artifact in gallbladder adenomyomatosis. J Ultrasound Med. 2003;22(2):229–31.
24. Yoon JH, Cha SS, Han SS, Lee SJ, Kang MS. Gallbladder adenomyomatosis: imaging findings. Abdom Imaging. 2006;31(5):555–63.
25. Raghavendra BN, Subramanyam BR, Balthazar EJ, Horii SC, Megibow AJ, Hilton S. Sonography of adenomyomatosis of the gallbladder: radiologic-pathologic correlation. Radiology. 1983;146(3):747–52.
26. Kim HC, Yang DM, Jin W, Ryu JK, Shin HC. Color Doppler twinkling artifacts in various conditions during abdominal and pelvic sonography. J Ultrasound Med. 2010;29(4):621–32.
27. Gerard PS, Berman D, Zafaranloo S. CT and ultrasound of gallbladder adenomyomatosis mimicking carcinoma. J Comput Assist Tomogr. 1990;14(3):490–1.
28. Yoshimitsu K, Honda H, Jimi M, Kuroiwa T, Hanada K, Irie H, et al. MR diagnosis of adenomyomatosis of the gallbladder and differentiation from gallbladder carcinoma: importance of showing Rokitansky-Aschoff sinuses. AJR Am J Roentgenol. 1999;172(6):1535–40.
29. Furukawa H, Takayasu K, Mukai K, Inoue K, Kyokane T, Shimada K, et al. CT evaluation of small polypoid lesions of the gallbladder. Hepatogastroenterology. 1995;42(6):800–10.
30. Soyer P, Gouhiri M, Boudiaf M, Brocheriou-Spelle I, Kardache M, Fishman EK, et al. Carcinoma of the gallbladder: imaging features with surgical correlation. AJR Am J Roentgenol. 1997;169(3):781–5.
31. Levy AD, Murakata LA, Rohrmann CA, Jr. Gallbladder carcinoma: radiologic-pathologic correlation. Radiographics. 2001;21(2):295–314; questionnaire, 549–55.
32. Kim SJ, Lee JM, Lee JY, Kim SH, Han JK, Choi BI, et al. Analysis of enhancement pattern of flat gallbladder wall thickening on MDCT to differentiate gallbladder cancer from cholecystitis. AJR Am J Roentgenol. 2008;191(3):765–71.
33. Wilbur AC, Sagireddy PB, Aizenstein RI. Carcinoma of the gallbladder: color Doppler ultrasound and CT findings. Abdom Imaging. 1997;22(2):187–9.
34. Koga A, Watanabe K, Fukuyama T, Takiguchi S, Nakayama F. Diagnosis and operative indications for polypoid lesions of the gallbladder. Arch Surg. 1988;123(1):26–9.
35. Ohtani T, Shirai Y, Tsukada K, Muto T, Hatakeyama K. Spread of gallbladder carcinoma: CT evaluation with pathologic correlation. Abdom Imaging. 1996;21(3):195–201.
36. Tseng JH, Wan YL, Hung CF, Ng KK, Pan KT, Chou AS, et al. Diagnosis and staging of gallbladder carcinoma. Evaluation with dynamic MR imaging. Clin Imaging. 2002;26(3):177–82.
37. Levy AD, Murakata LA, Abbott RM, Rohrmann CA, Jr. From the archives of the AFIP. Benign tumors and tumorlike lesions of the gallbladder and extrahepatic bile ducts: radiologic-pathologic correlation. Armed Forces Institute of Pathology. Radiographics. 2002;22(2):387–413.
38. Wiles R, Thoeni RF, Barbu ST, Vashist YK, Rafaelsen SR, Dewhurst C, et al. Management and follow-up of gallbladder polyps: joint guidelines between the European Society of Gastrointestinal and Abdominal Radiology (ESGAR), European Association for Endoscopic Surgery and other Interventional Techniques (EAES), International Society of Digestive Surgery – European Federation (EFISDS) and European Society of Gastrointestinal Endoscopy (ESGE). Eur Radiol. 2017;27(9):3856–66.

EUS of Diseases of the Gallbladder

Kazuo Inui, Hironao Miyoshi, and Satoshi Yamamoto

Introduction

Gallbladder diseases represent a variety of lesions including gallstones, cholesterol polyps, adenomyomatosis, and gallbladder carcinoma. Most importantly, clinicians need a precise diagnosis to guide decisions as to whether to resect the gallbladder, thus avoiding unnecessary surgery. The first modality used to detect a gallbladder lesion usually is transabdominal ultrasonography (TAUS). Further imaging modalities available for refining the diagnosis include endoscopic ultrasonography (EUS), multi-detector-row computed tomography, magnetic resonance imaging, and contrast-enhanced TAUS or EUS. Since the introduction of EUS in 1980 [1, 2], numerous clinical applications have been reported, and this modality has significantly increased diagnostic accuracy among gallbladder diseases. This chapter outlines the usefulness and limitations of EUS for gallbladder diseases.

K. Inui (✉) · H. Miyoshi · S. Yamamoto
Department of Gastroenterology, Bantane Hospital, Fujita Health University School of Medicine, Aichi, Japan
e-mail: kinui@fujita-hu.ac.jp

H. Miyoshi
e-mail: hmiyoshi@fujita-hu.ac.jp

S. Yamamoto
e-mail: syama@fujita-hu.ac.jp

Detection and Differential Diagnosis of Polypoid Gallbladder Lesions

Detection of Gallbladder Polypoid Lesions

Mass screening for hepato-pancreatobiliary cancers using TAUS has been promoted throughout Japan. Recently a Manual for Abdominal Ultrasound in Cancer Screening and Health Checkups, a publication of the Ultrasonic Screening Committee of the Japanese Society of Gastrointestinal Cancer Screening, has become generally available on the Internet [3]. A variety of gallbladder lesions have been detected by mass screening. In asymptomatic populations, gallbladder polyps were found at a prevalence of 4.3–6.9% [4]. Based on six studies involving 16,260 participants in various countries, a recent Cochrane report [5] found the median prevalence of gallbladder polyps to be 6.4% (interquartile range or IQR, 2.4–18.8%).

Polypoid gallbladder lesions include a variety of pathologic entities that can be divided into true neoplasms and pseudotumors. The latter group includes cholesterol polyps, inflammatory polyps, and hyperplasia. True neoplasms, including both adenomas and malignant lesions, should be treated by surgical resection, while pseudotumors can be observed serially. A common rule maintains that polypoid lesions larger than 10 mm should be resected. However, in

J. B. Chung and K. Okazaki (eds.), *Diseases of the Gallbladder*,
https://doi.org/10.1007/978-981-15-6010-1_5

the experience of Kubota et al. [6], only 57% of cholesterol polyps measured less than 10 mm, while 75% of adenomas and 13% of cancers were smaller than 10 mm. On the other hand, Akatsu et al. [7] reported that 20/29 of gallbladder polyps larger than 10 mm (69%) that were preoperatively suspected of malignancy proved to be non-neoplastic. Thus, lesion size alone cannot predict the histopathologic nature of a polyp.

Differential Diagnosis with EUS

EUS is recommended for close examination after TAUS, because images obtained are more distinct than those obtained with TAUS. Using high ultrasound frequencies, EUS can visualize the layered structure of the gallbladder and provide high-resolution images [8]. Several studies have evaluated EUS in the differential diagnosis of polypoid gallbladder lesions [9–12]. EUS depicts a cholesterol polyp as a pedunculated mass with a nodular surface overlying hyperechoic foci (Fig. 1). In particular, EUS can differentiate cholesterol polyps, which have slender stalks and produce homogeneous echoes (except for pedunculated, highly echogenic areas) from early gallbladder carcinomas, which have thick stalks and shows heterogeneous echoes. Overall accuracy of EUS in differentiating neoplastic from non-neoplastic masses has been reported as 91.1–97% [9, 10]. When Sugiyama et al. [10] compared the diagnostic accuracy of EUS with that of TAUS for polypoid gallbladder lesions in a surgical series, EUS (97%) differentiated polypoid lesions more precisely than TAUS (76%). Although the accuracy of EUS in differentiating neoplastic from non-neoplastic polypoid lesions smaller than 10 mm was reported to be low [11]. EUS is considered useful for guiding treatment of larger pedunculated polyps [12]. Sadamoto

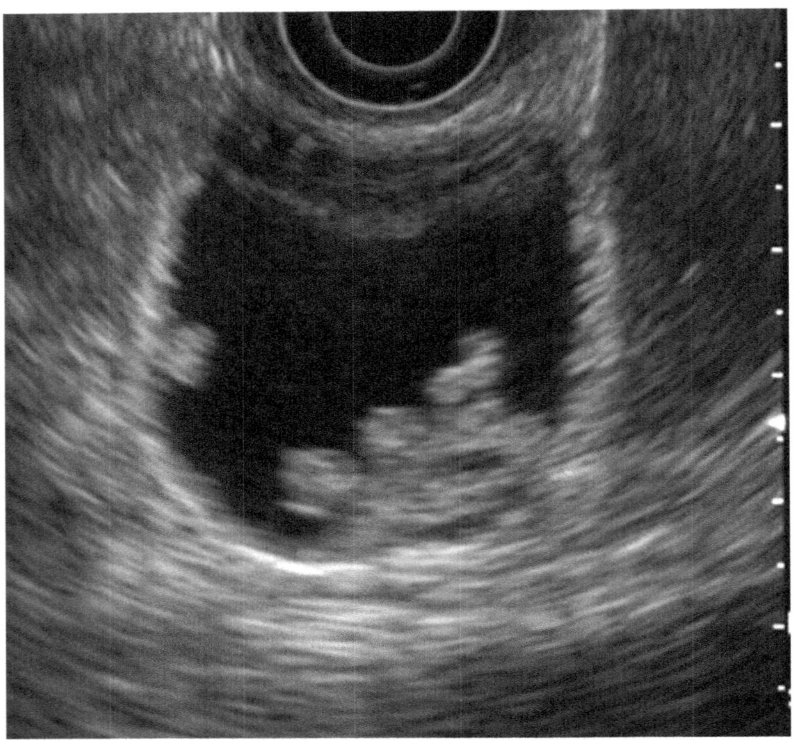

Fig. 1 EUS shows a cholesterol polyp of the gallbladder as a nodular-surfaced pedunculated mass with hyperechoic foci

et al. [13] reported usefulness of an EUS score based on a coefficient of multivariate analysis: (maximum diameter in mm) + (internal echo pattern score, where heterogeneous = 4 and homogeneous = 0) + (hyperechoic spot score, present = −5 and absence = 0). Those authors regarded polyp size, heterogeneous internal echo pattern, and absence of hyperechoic foci as important indicators that a polyp is neoplastic.

EUS visualizes localized adenomyomatosis as a non-sessile polypoid lesion with small cystic areas corresponding to proliferation of Rokitansky–Aschoff sinuses (Fig. 2). EUS is highly accurate in the diagnosis of cholesterol polyp and adenomyomatosis [7], which represent the most common types of gallbladder polyps.

EUS shows an adenoma as a homogeneously isoechoic pedunculated mass with a granular or smooth surface (Fig. 3) and an adenocarcinoma as a heterogeneously echogenic pedunculated mass with a granular or smooth surface (Fig. 4). Cho et al. [14] focused on relatively hypoechoic areas at the cores of polyps, reporting the presence of such hypoechoic cores on EUS to be a strong predictive factor for neoplastic polyps.

EUS also can delineate connections between pancreatobiliary ducts in the pancreatic parenchyma of the pancreas as clearly as endoscopic retrograde cholangiopancreatography (ERCP) [15], abnormal connections between pancreatobiliary ducts are closely associated with gallbladder carcinoma because they permit reflux of pancreatic juice into the bile duct [16, 17]. When EUS shows abnormal connections between pancreatobiliary ducts, gallbladder lesions should be suspected to be malignant.

Differential Diagnosis of Gallbladder Wall Thickening Lesions

Gallbladder wall thickening poses difficulty in differentiating between benign processes such as inflammation and malignant tumor. Diffuse adenomyomatosis sometimes can mimic

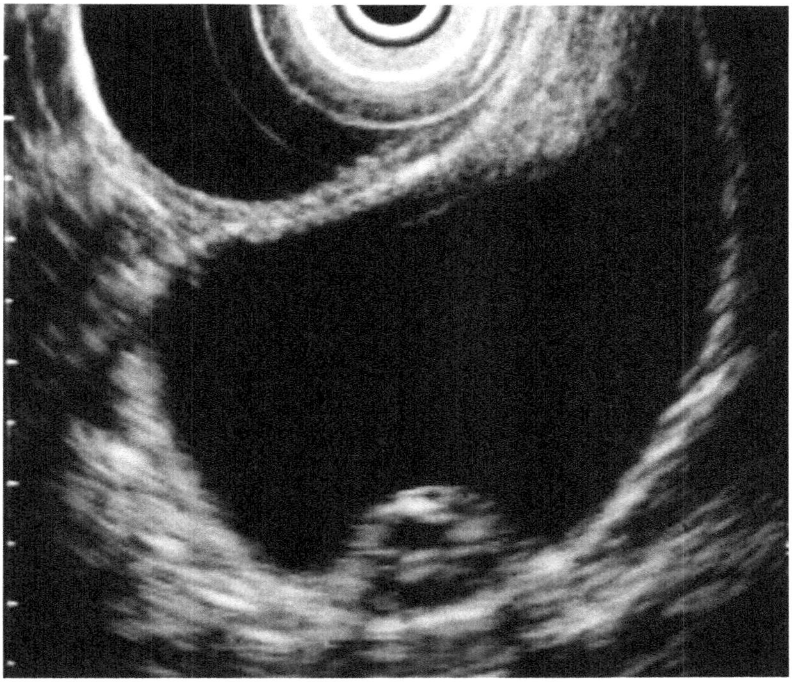

Fig. 2 EUS shows localized adenomyomatosis as a non-sessile polypoid lesion with small cystic areas corresponding to proliferation of Rokitansky–Aschoff sinuses (RAS)

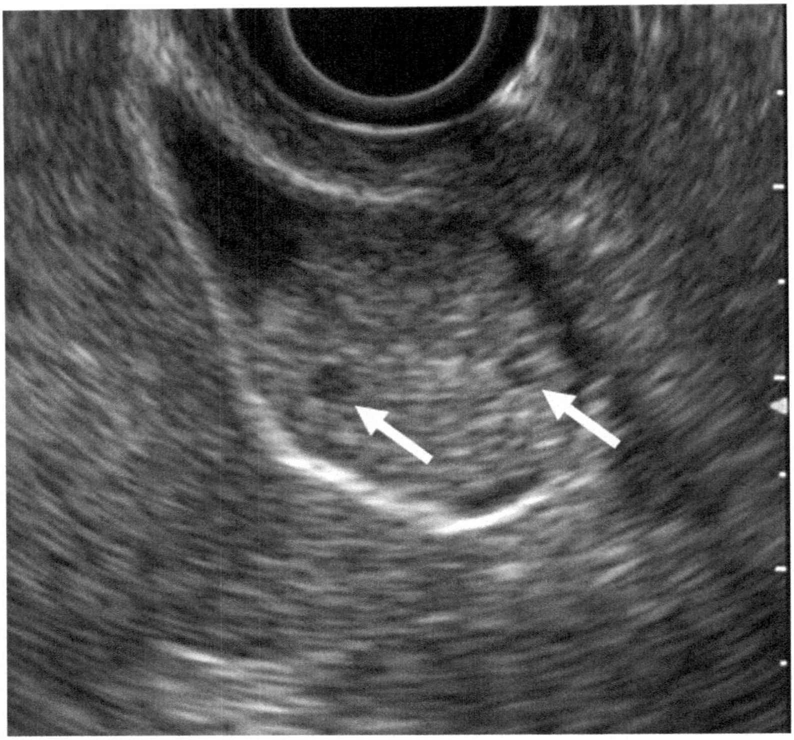

Fig. 3 EUS shows an adenoma as a pedunculated, homogeneously isoechoic mass with a smooth surface. In the core of the polyp, relatively hypoechoic areas compared with general background echogenicity are shown by arrows

gallbladder carcinoma. Xanthogranulomatous cholecystitis (XGC) can be particularly difficult to differentiate from gallbladder cancer using EUS alone, given possible loss of the multilayered structure of the gallbladder wall and infiltration of the inflammatory process into adjacent organs [18]. Kim et al. [19] noted EUS findings of gallbladder wall thickness exceeding 10 mm and reduced internal echogenicity as independent predictive factors for neoplasm. However, differentiating malignant lesions from benign gallbladder wall thickening remains to be difficult. Recent refinements of EUS instruments and use of an ultrasonographic contrast agent can improve diagnostic accuracy. Imazu et al. [20] reported that overall sensitivity, specificity, and accuracy for diagnosing malignant gallbladder wall thickening for EUS and contrast-enhanced EUS, respectively, were 83.3% versus 89.6%, 65% versus 98% ($p < 0.001$), and 73.1% versus 94.4% ($p < 0.001$). In the same study, an inhomogeneous enhancement pattern in contrast-enhanced EUS was a strong predictive factor for malignant gallbladder wall thickening.

Staging of Gallbladder Carcinoma

Mitake et al. [21] reported the effectiveness of EUS in determining the extent of tumor invasion; differentiation between early and advanced-stage tumors was 79.5% accurate, and the overall accuracy for tumor invasion depth assessment was 76.9%. Tumor infiltration can be visualized as hypoechoic tumor disrupting the layers of the gallbladder wall. In patients with an T2-stage adenocarcinoma, EUS can demonstrate a hypoechoic tumor at the base of a non-sessile polypoid lesion even when invasion is only as deep as the second or third hyperechoic layer of the gallbladder wall (Fig. 5). Kimura et al. [22] also reported EUS to

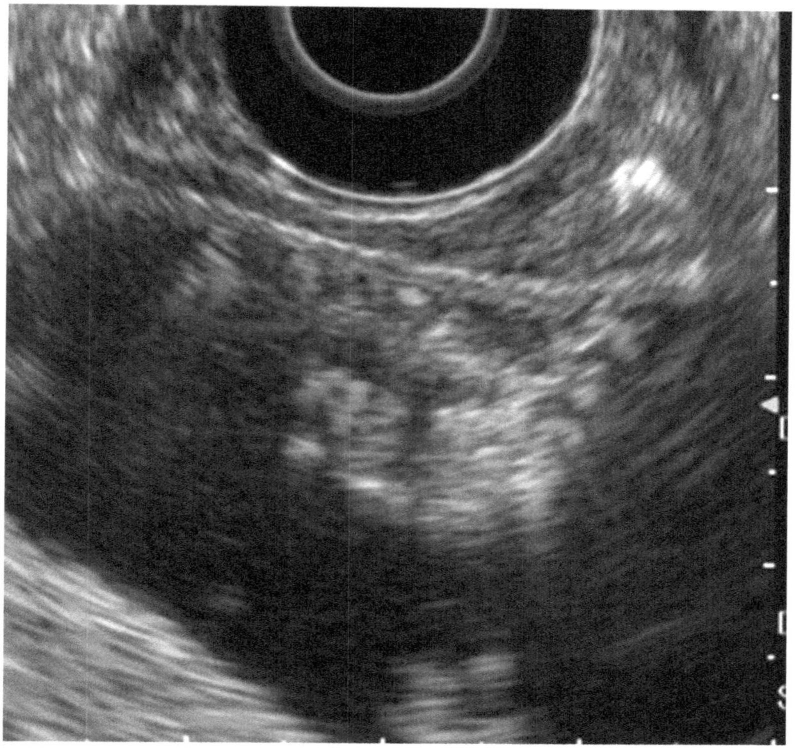

Fig. 4 EUS shows an adenocarcinoma as a pedunculated, heterogeneously echogenic mass with a granular surface

be useful for diagnosis of T2 gallbladder cancer. Fujita et al. [23] classified EUS images into four categories: type A, a pedunculated mass with a finely nodular surface and without abnormality of the neighboring gallbladder wall; type B, a broad-based mass with an irregular surface and no disruption of the outer hyperechoic layer of the gallbladder wall; type C, irregularity of the outer hyperechoic layer due to mass echo; and type D, disruption of the outer hyperechoic layer by mass echo. They then assigned the image types EUS to T stages for gallbladder carcinoma. Type A would be tumor in situ (Tis); type B, T1 or possibly T2; type C, T2; and type D, T3 or higher. Each of the four EUS image categories correlated well with the histologic depth of invasion.

Developments of contrast agents may increase the usefulness of EUS for tumor assessment. Hirooka et al. [24] reported that in non-contrast EUS, depth of tumor invasion was assessed accurately in 11 of 14 cases (78.6%), while assessment was accurate in 13 of 14 cases (92.9%) using contrast-enhanced EUS.

Diagnosis of Cholelithiasis and Gallbladder Microlithiasis in Patients with Acute Pancreatitis

Acute pancreatitis may be either idiopathic or a complication of alcoholism, gallstones, medication, hyperglycemia, or post endoscopic retrograde cholangiopancreatography (ERCP). In Japan, gallstones are responsible for about one-quarter of cases, while in Europe and North America they account for about half. Neoptolemos et al. [25] reported that endoscopic sphincterotomy (EST) with stone extraction performed within 72 hours of admission decreased morbidity and shortened hospital stays in patients with acute pancreatitis. However, ERCP

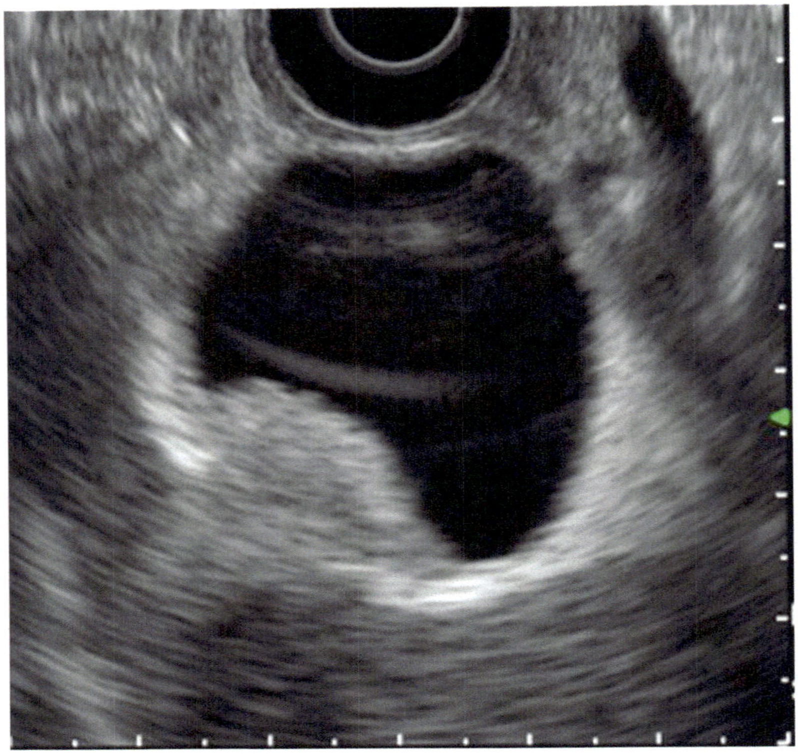

Fig. 5 EUS demonstrates a hypoechoic lesion at the base of a non-sessile polypoid lesions invading only as deeply as the second hyperechoic layer of the gallbladder

and EST occasionally can themselves cause acute pancreatitis, so such treatment should be considered cautiously for patients suspected to have biliary pancreatitis. In such patients, EUS can reliably identify cholelithiasis with greater sensitivity than TAUS [26]. Furthermore, EUS sometimes can detect microlithiasis in the gallbladder in patients with grossly non-calculous biliary colic and normal TAUS findings [27]. EUS has been recommended as part of the diagnostic assessment in patients with unexplained acute pancreatitis [28].

Conclusions

EUS, recommended as the second examination for gallbladder lesions after TAUS, is highly useful for differential diagnosis of polypoid gallbladder lesions. EUS also is important in staging gallbladder carcinoma. While pedunculated carcinomas have been correctly diagnosed using EUS in essentially all cases, this modality is far less reliable in assessing broad-based carcinomas, whether elevated or flat. Further developments are awaited for more accurate diagnosis of such cancers and for more precise determination of the depth of invasion by gallbladder carcinomas.

References

1. DiMagno EP, Buxton JL, Regan PT, James EM, Buxton JL. Ultrasonic endoscope. Lancet. 1980;1:629–31.
2. Strohm WD, Phillip J, Hagenmuller F, Classen M. Ultrasonic tomography by means of an ultrasonic fiberendoscope. Endoscopy. 1980;12:241–4.
3. https://www.ningen-dock.jp/wp/wp-content/uploads/2018/06/Abdominal-Ultrasound.pdf.
4. Inui K, Yoshino J, Miyoshi H. Diagnosis of gallbladder tumors. Intern Med. 2011;50:1133–6.

5. Wennmacker SZ, Lamberts MP, Di Martino M, Drenth JP, Gurusamy KS, van Laarhoven CJ. Transabdominal ultrasound and endoscopic ultrasound for diagnosis of gallbladder polyps. Cochrane Database Syst Rev. 2018;15:8.
6. Kubota K, Bandai Y, Noie T, Ishizaki Y, Teruya M, Makuuchi M. How should polypoid lesions of the gallbladder be treated in the era of laparoscopic cholecystectomy? Surgery. 1995;117:481–7.
7. Akatsu T, Aiura K, Shimazu M, Ueda M, Wakabayashi G, Tanabe M, et al. Can endoscopic ultrasonography differentiate nonneoplastic from neoplastic gallbladder polyps? Dig Dis Sci. 2006;51:416–21.
8. Chantarojanasiri T, Hirooka Y, Kawashima H, Ohno E, Kongkam P, Goto H. The role of endoscopic ultrasound in the diagnosis of gallbladder diseases. J Med Ultrasonics. 2017;44:63–70.
9. Kimura K. Diagnosis for pedunculated polypoid lesions of the gallbladder by endoscopic ultrasonography. Nippon Shokakibyo Gakkai Zasshi. 1997;94:249–60. (in Japanese, Abstract in English).
10. Sugiyama M, Atomi Y, Yamato T. Endoscopic ultrasonography for differential diagnosis of polypoid gall bladder lesions: analysis in surgical and follow up series. Gut. 2000;46:250–4.
11. Cheon YK, Cho WY, Lee TH, Cho YD, Moon JH, Lee JS, et al. Endoscopic ultrasonography does not differentiate neoplastic from non-neoplastic small gallbladder polyps. World J Gastroenterol. 2009;15:2361–6.
12. Kimura K, Fujita N, Noda Y, Kobayashi G, Ito K. Differential diagnosis of large-sized pedunculated polypoid lesions of the gallbladder by endoscopic ultrasonography: a prospective study. J Gastroenterol. 2001;36:619–22.
13. Sadamoto Y, Oda S, Tanaka M, Harada N, Kubo H, Eguchi T, et al. A useful approach to the differential diagnosis of small polypoid lesions of the gallbladder, utilizing an endoscopic ultrasound scoring system. Endoscopy. 2002;34:959–65.
14. Cho JH, Park JY, Kim YJ, Kim HM, Kim HJ, Hong SP, et al. Hypoechoic foci on EUS are simple and strong predictive factors for neoplastic gallbladder polyps. Gastrointest Endosc. 2009;69:1244–50.
15. Mitake M, Nakazawa S, Naitoh Y, Kimoto E, Tsukamoto Y, Yamao K, et al. Value of endoscopic ultrasonography in the detection of anomalous connection of the pancreatobiliary duct. Endoscopy. 1991;23:117–20.
16. Kimura K, Ohto M, Saisho H, Unozawa T, Tsuchiya Y, Morita M, et al. Association of gallbladder carcinoma and anomalous pancreatobiliary ductal union. Gastroenterology. 1985;89:1258–65.
17. Yamauchi S, Koga A, Matsumoto S, Tanaka M, Nakayama F. Anomalous junction of pancreaticobiliary duct without congenital choledocal cyst: a possible risk factor for gallbladder cancer. Am J Gastroenterol. 1987;82:20–4.
18. Muguruma N, Okamura S, Ichikawa S, Tsujigami K, Suzuki M, Tadatsu M, et al. Endoscopic sonography in the diagnosis of gallbladder wall lesions in patients with gallstones. J Clin Ultrasound. 2001;29:395–400.
19. Kim HJ, Park JH, Park DI, Cho YK, Sohn CI, Jeon WK, et al. Clinical usefulness of endoscopic ultrasonography in the differential diagnosis of gallbladder wall thickening. Dig Dis Sci. 2012;57:508–15.
20. Imazu H, Mori N, Kanazawa K, Chiba M, Toyoizumi H, Torisu Y, et al. Contrast-enhanced harmonic endoscopic ultrasonography in the differential diagnosis of gallbladder wall thickening. Dig Dis Sci. 2014;59:1909–16.
21. Mitake M, Nakazawa S, Naitoh Y, Kimoto E, Tsukamoto Y, Asai T, et al. Endoscopic ultrasonography in diagnosis of the extent of gallbladder carcinoma. Gastrointest Endosc. 1990;36:562–6.
22. Kimura K, Fujita N, Noda Y, Kobayashi G, Ito K. Diagnosis of pT2 gallbladder cancer by serial examinations with endoscopic ultrasound and angiography. J Gastroenterol. 2002;37:200–3.
23. Fujita N, Noda Y, Kobayashi G, Kimura K, Yago A. Diagnosis of the depth of invasion of gallbladder carcinoma by EUS. Gastrointest Endosc. 1999;50:659–63.
24. Hirooka Y, Naitoh Y, Goto H, Ito A, Hayakawa S, Watanabe Y, et al. Contrast-enhanced endoscopic ultrasonogramphy in gallbladder diseases. Gastrointest Endosc. 1998;48:406–10.
25. Neoptolemos JP, Carr-Locke DL, London NJ, Baily LA, James D, Fossard DP. Controlled trial of urgent endoscopic retrograde cholangiopancreatography and endoscopic sphincterotomy versus conservative treatment for acute pancreatitis due to gallstones. Lancet. 1988;2:979–83.
26. Chak A, Hawes RH, Cooper GS, Hoffman B, Catalano MF, Wong RC, et al. Prospective assessment of the utility of EUS in the evaluation of gallstone pancreatitis. Gastrointest Endosc. 1999;49:599–604.
27. Thorbøll J, Vilmann P, Jacobsen B, Hassan H. Endoscopic ultrasonography in detection of cholelithiasis in patients with biliary pain and negative transabdominal ultrasonography. Scand J Gastroenterol. 2004;39:267–9.
28. Ardengh JC, Malheiros CA, Rahal F, Pereira V, Ganc AJ. Microlithiasis of the gallbladder: role of endoscopic ultrasonography in patients with idiopathic acute pancreatitis. Rev Assoc Med Bras. 2010;56:27–31.

Tissue Acquisition of Diseases of the Gallbladder: Percutaneous Ultrasound-Guided Biopsy

Toshiharu Ueki, Toru Maruo, and Ken Kinjyo

Introduction

In general, collected specimens are subjected to cytology and histology; however, histology that can be diagnosed by taking into account structural variants in addition to cell variants has higher diagnostic ability.

Regarding the biliary tract, the usefulness of cytology and histology of bile ducts and the gallbladder under endoscopic retrograde cholangiography (ERC) has been reported, but the accuracy of diagnoses is not satisfactory [1, 2]. Pathological diagnosis plays a major role in definitive and qualitative diagnosis of gallbladder disease, surgical indication, and determination of surgical procedure. Recently, there have been reports of endoscopic ultrasound-guided fine needle aspiration (EUS-FNA) [3–5]. Moreover, the usefulness of percutaneous ultrasound-guided pancreas core biopsy has been reported [6, 7], but there are few reports of percutaneous gallbladder biopsy [8]. Therefore, this study aimed to report the actual conditions and problems of percutaneous ultrasound-guided gallbladder biopsy.

T. Ueki (✉) · T. Maruo · K. Kinjyo
Department of Gastroenterology, Fukuoka University Chikushi Hospital, 1-1-1 Zokumyoin, Chikushino, Fukuoka 818-8502, Japan
e-mail: tosiueki@fukuoka-u.ac.jp

T. Maruo · K. Kinjyo
Department of Pathology, Fukuoka University Chikushi Hospital, 1-1-1 Zokumyoin, Chikushino, Fukuoka 818-8502, Japan

Methods

Instrument

There are linear, sector, and convex types of ultrasound puncture probes that can be used for collecting tissues. The linear type is only used for punctures, and there is a groove for passing a puncture needle in section of the probe. It has the advantage that the needle can penetrate straight to the target directly under the probe, and deflection of the needle can be reduced. A sector type and microconvex type are used with a detachable guide attachment. The microconvex type is often used, and during applications, there are a few blind spots and its direction can be freely changed in close contact with the recessed abdominal wall. Therefore, it can puncture the target site avoiding relatively large blood vessels in the puncture path (Fig. 1 Canon Medical Systems Corporation, Japan).

A percutaneous transhepatic cholangiography (PTC) needle that is used for cytology is used as a puncture needle, and a biopsy needle is used for histology. The biopsy needles are cutting needle and suction biopsy needle. Cutting needles include Tru cut needle and Quick-Core® Coaxial Needle (Cook Medical Holdings LLC,

J. B. Chung and K. Okazaki (eds.), *Diseases of the Gallbladder*,
https://doi.org/10.1007/978-981-15-6010-1_6

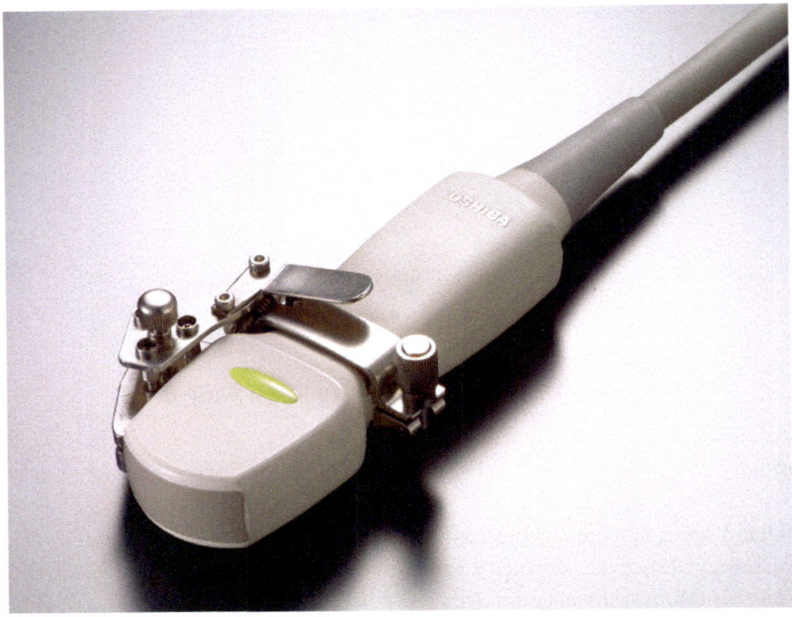

Fig. 1 Microconvex probe of ultrasound (Canon Medical Systems Corporation, Japan)

USA). In addition, there are products such as Sonoguide biopsy needle (Fig. 2 Sonopsy-C1, Hakkou Co., Ltd. Japan) and Surecut needle (Task Laboratory, Japan), but we choose to use a 21-gauge, 17-cm-long Sonoguide biopsy needle.

Preparation Before Percutaneous Ultrasound-Guided Gallbladder Biopsy

It is important to obtain an image of the puncture site and puncture route using ultrasonography before the procedure. It needed to be confirmed that the target site can be punctured without involving the gallbladder lumen and that there is no large blood vessel in the puncture route, as assessed with the color Doppler method of ultrasound. A contrast method of ultrasound is used to check the blood flow at the target site, i.e., the gallbladder (Fig. 3a, b). As a general rule, percutaneous ultrasound-guided gallbladder biopsy is not performed in patients with ascites.

If percutaneous ultrasound-guided biopsy is planned, platelet count, prothrombin time, and activated partial thromboplastin time are evaluated to check for a bleeding tendency. The patient fasts on the day of biopsy, but a small amount of water is allowed.

Percutaneous Ultrasound-Guided Gallbladder Biopsy

Disinfection and Local Anesthesia

After confirming the puncture site with a microconvex probe, the skin is disinfected around the puncture site and a local anesthetic is administered. A gel is placed in a sterilized disposable probe cover (CIV-FlexTM General Purpose Ultrasound Probe Covers, CIVCO Medical Solutions, USA), and the probe and cable are covered by it. Subsequently, a sterilized guide attachment is attached to the probe. Isodine disinfectant is used as an echo-transmitter on the skin surface.

Biopsy Technique

First, gallbladder puncture is approached transhepatically mainly from the intercostal space.

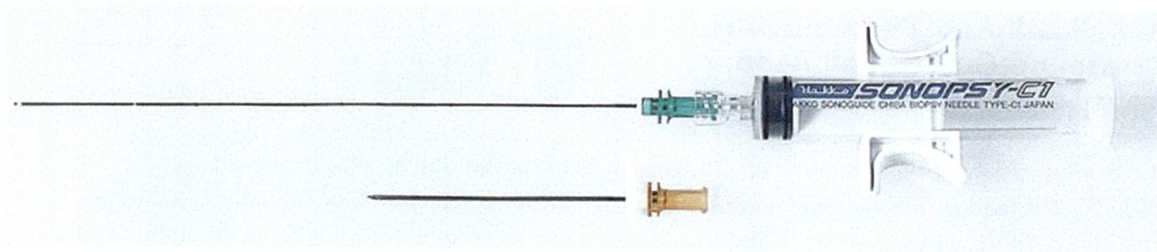

Fig. 2 Sonoguide biopsy needle (Sonopsy-C1, Hakko Co., Ltd., Japan)

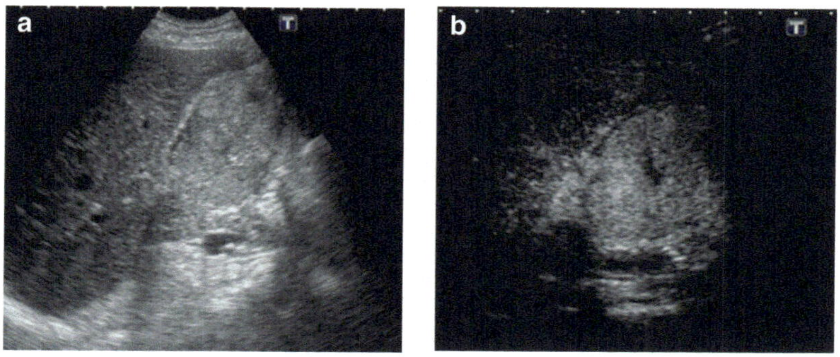

Fig. 3 Ultrasonographic findings in gallbladder bladder carcinoma (case 1). The tumor occupies the entire gallbladder (**a**) and is associated with abundant blood flow on color contrast method (**b**)

When puncturing with deep inspiration, the puncture needle may be considerably displaced while breathing. Therefore, the patient must breathe as shallowly as possible, and the position of the probe must be determined so that the target site enters the puncture line during inspiration or expiration. A guide needle is inserted into the puncture opening of the guide attachment attached to the probe. Next, a biopsy needle (Sonoguide biopsy needle) is slowly inserted while confirming the target site using ultrasound.

A microconvex probe has a small echo beam surface, so it is easy to check whether the tip of the biopsy needle can reliably puncture the target site. When the tip of the needle is confirmed in the target site, the tip of the needle is returned to the abdominal wall side in the target site, the suction piston is fully pulled, and then, the needle is reciprocated a few times in the target site. The needle is pulled out after manually rotating it. When the puncture needle is placed in a bottle containing 20% formalin and the negative pressure of the puncture needle is released, the tissue inside the puncture needle is pushed out naturally. If macroscopic white-colored tissue is sufficiently collected, it is often completed with single puncture. If initial puncture was insufficient, it can be repunctured 2–3 times (Fig. 4a, b).

Post-biopsy Procedure

A small pillow is placed on the patient's abdomen wall over the puncture site, and wrapped around the compression band for 6 hours after biopsy. Blood pressure and body temperature are measured over time whiling paying attention to clinical symptoms such as abdominal pain. The next day after biopsy, a blood biochemistry test is performed. If there is a change in clinical findings, abdominal ultrasonography or enhanced CT is performed.

Complications of Percutaneous Ultrasound-Guided Gallbladder Biopsy

The complications of percutaneous ultrasound-guided gallbladder biopsy are mainly bleeding, cholecystitis, bile leakage, and intraperitoneal infection. Bleeding may be caused by vascular injury of the puncture route in the liver or from the gallbladder. Intrahepatic vascular injury can be avoided using the ultrasonic color Doppler method for relatively large blood vessels. To avoid bleeding from the gallbladder, a site with poor blood flow in the target site is punctured. The biopsy needle may be damaged in the gallbladder owing to the patient's breathing; therefore, it is important for patient to hold the breath firmly so that the gallbladder itself does not move during breathing. Although we have experienced a small number, there were no cases in which bleeding was evident after the examination.

In addition, we have had no experience with cholecystitis after biopsy, which may be caused by bile leakage from the gallbladder after puncture of the gallbladder.

Among the complications associated with biopsy, the problem of tumor dissemination is controversial. The most common purpose of biopsy is the pathological confirmation of malignant tumors, such as cancer. Although the frequency of tumor seeding is low, the possibility must always be considered [9]. The possibility of cancer is high as a result of imaging examination. Moreover, regardless of the results of pathological diagnosis via biopsy, in principle, if resection is indicated, a biopsy is not considered. Additionally, as the number of punctures increases, the risk of tumor dissemination increases. Therefore, efforts must be made to ensure that samples are collected with a small number of punctures.

Results of Percutaneous Ultrasound-Guided Gallbladder Biopsy in Our Hospital

The results of five cases of percutaneous ultrasound-guided gallbladder biopsy for gallbladder masses are shown in Table 1. The average age was 74 years, and there are four males and one female. In the three cases, the tumors were localized entirely within the gallbladder; there was one tumor in the neck, and one in the fundus. All patients underwent biopsy using a 21-guage, 17-cm-long Sonopsy needle. The number of punctures was one in four cases and two in one case. Pathological diagnosis was an adenocarcinoma in four cases and invasion by hepatocellular carcinoma in one case. One patient experienced nausea after biopsy, but it improved with follow-up.

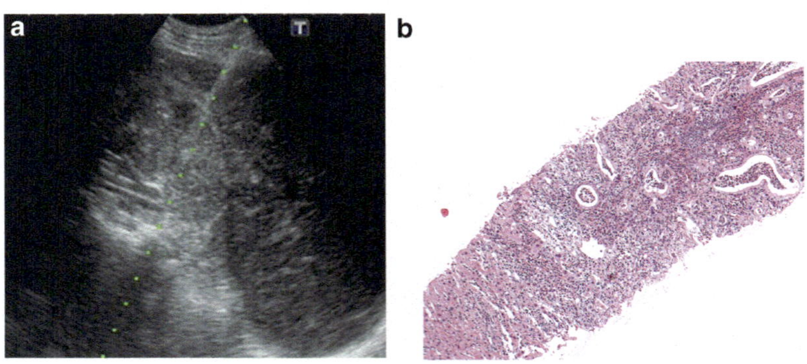

Fig. 4 Histological feature of gallbladder carcinoma (case 1). Gallbladder core tissue was acquired by percutaneous ultrasound-guided gallbladder biopsy (**a**). Moderated-poorly adenocarcinoma is shown (**b**)

Table 1 Clinical findings in gallbladder diseases with percutaneous ultrasound-guided biopsy

Case.	Age/Gender	Tumor site	Number of punctures	Pathological diagnosis
1	57/Male	Hole	One	Adenocarcinoma
2	80/Female	Hole	One	Adenocarcinoma
3	83/Male	Neck	One	Adenocarcinoma
4	80/Male	Fundus	Two	Adenocarcinoma
5	72/Male	Hole	One	Hepatocellular carcinoma

Indications of EUS-FNA and Percutaneous Ultrasound-Guided Biopsy in Gallbladder Disease

Recently, the usefulness of EUS-FNA for gallbladder masses and thickened gallbladder walls was reported [2]. The advantage of EUS-FNA over percutaneous gallbladder biopsy is that it can be used to perform biopsy for small lesions in the neck of the gallbladder, which is difficult to perform with percutaneous ultrasound-guided gallbladder biopsy. EUS-FNA can avoid relatively small blood vessels when performed with a color Doppler method, reducing complications such as bleeding. However, although EUS-FNA is more popular presently than it was previously, there are still few facilities that can implement this procedure. Furthermore, although there are few cases that require gallbladder biopsy, percutaneous ultrasound-guided gallbladder biopsy is a desirable investigation technique owing to its simplicity and versatility.

Conclusion

Percutaneous ultrasound-guided gallbladder biopsy can safely and adequately collect gallbladder tissue. It is an alternative test in facilities where EUS-FNA can't be performed, or when the gallbladder diseases can't be histologically diagnosed by EUS-FNA and ERC.

References

1. Weilert F, Bhat YM, Binmoeller KF, Kane S, Jaffee IM, Shaw RF, et al. EUS-FNA is superior to ERCP-based tissue sampling in suspected malignant biliary obstruction: results of a prospective, single-blind, comparative study. Gastrointest Endosco. 2014;80:97–104.
2. Jo JH, Cho CM, Jun JH, Chung MJ, Kim TH, Seo DW, et al. Same-session endoscopic ultrasound-guided fine needle aspiration and endoscopic retrograde cholangiopancreatography-based tissue sampling in suspected malignant biliary obstruction: a multicenter experience. J Gastroenterol Hepatol. 2019;28:799–805.
3. Jacobson BC, Pitman MB, Brugge WR. EUS-guided FNA for the diagnosis of gallbladder masses. Gastrointest Endosco. 2003;57:251–4.
4. Varadarajulu S, Eloubeidi MA. Endoscopic ultrasound-guided fine-needle aspiration in the evaluation of gallbladder masses. Endoscopy. 2005;37:751–4.
5. Singla V, Agarwal R, Anikhindi SA, Puri Pankaj, Kumar M, Ranjan P, et al. Role of EUS-FNA for gallbladder mass lesions with biliary obstruction: a large single-center experience. Endosc Int Open. 2019;7:E1403–E9.
6. Ueki T, Kawamoto K, Otsuka Y, Minoda R, Maruo T, Matsumera K, et al. Prevalence and clinicopathological features of autoimmune pancreatitis in Japanese Patients with inflammatory bowel disease. Pancreas. 2015;44:434–40.
7. Huang Y, Shi J, Chen YY, Li Kao. Ultrasound-guided percutaneous core needle biopsy for the diagnosis of pancreatic disease. Ultrasound Med Biol. 2018;44:1145–54.
8. Zargar SA, Khuroo MS, Mahajan R, Jan GN, Shah P. US-guided fine-needle aspiration biopsy of gallbladder masses. Radiology. 1991;179:275–8.
9. Matsui T, Nishikawa K, Yukimoto H, Katsuta K, Nakamura Y, Tanaka S, et al. Needle tract seeding following endoscopic ultrasound-guided fine-needle aspiration for pancreatic cancer: a report of two cases. World J Surg Oncol. 2019;17:134. https://doi.org/10.1186/s12957-019-1681-x.

Tissue Acquisition for Diagnosis of the Gallbladder Diseases: EUS-Guided Biopsy

Masayuki Kitano and Takashi Tamura

Introduction

Obtaining pathological evidence of gallbladder carcinoma (GBC) is necessary for patients with operable tumors prior to resection and non-operable tumors before chemotherapy. Malignant tumors of the gallbladder include not only adenocarcinomas but also other types such as neuroendocrine cancer [1], making histological diagnosis of unresectable malignant gallbladder tumors necessary for determining chemotherapy regimens. Traditionally, tissue samples from gallbladder mass lesions have been obtained by fine needle aspiration (FNA), guided by transabdominal ultrasound (US) or computed tomography (CT), or by surgery [1–3]. These methods have reported sensitivity of>88% and specificity of nearly 100%. Percutaneous aspiration, however, may have suboptimal performance in patients with smaller gallbladder lesions [1–6], as well as being associated with risks of abdominal pain (4.5%), bile peritonitis (1–6%), and needle tract seeding [5, 6].

Alternatively, gallbladder masses with biliary obstruction can be diagnosed by endoscopic retrograde cholangiography (ERC)-guided biopsy and brushing, which has an accuracy of 60–80% in the diagnosis of gallbladder cancer [7]. Although this method is satisfactory for obtaining tissue from gallbladder cancers extending to the biliary duct, this method has difficulty in obtaining adequate tissue samples from gallbladder tumors that do not extend to the bile duct. Gallbladder cytology has been assessed by endoscopic transpapillary gallbladder drainage (ETGBD), in which a drainage tube is inserted into the gallbladder using a catheter and guidewire [7–9]. Although this innovative technique shows high rates of sensitivity (59–81%) and success (83–100%), it requires the skills of expert endoscopists and may not be technically feasible for all patients with gallbladder carcinoma [7, 10]. In addition, insertion of an ETGBD tube into the gallbladder may increase the risk of complications such as gallbladder perforation and bile leakage compared with conventional ERC [7–9]. In recent years, endoscopic ultrasound-guided fine needle aspiration (EUS-FNA) has been used increasingly to obtain tissue samples from various organs [11]. EUS-FNA is reported to safely obtain sufficient tissue to diagnose gallbladder mass lesions [10–15].

M. Kitano (✉) · T. Tamura
Second Department of Internal Medicine, Wakayama Medical University, 811-1, Kimiidera, Wakayama City, Wakayama 641-8509, Japan
e-mail: kitano@wakayama-med.ac.jp

J. B. Chung and K. Okazaki (eds.), *Diseases of the Gallbladder*,
https://doi.org/10.1007/978-981-15-6010-1_7

Effectiveness and Safety of EUS-FNA for Gallbladder Tumors

EUS-FNA is performed in patients with gallbladder tumors to distinguish malignant from benign lesions. In six studies involving a total of 101 patients with gallbladder lesions, EUS-FNA showed a sensitivity of 91.7% and a specificity of 100% [10–15] (Table 1). EUS-FNA was first reported useful for diagnosing gallbladder tumors in six patients, with five having GBC and one having xanthogranulomatous cholecystitis (XGC), resulting in an 83% accuracy rate [12]. An assessment of six patients found that five had GBC and one had chronic cholecystitis, with EUS-FNA having an accuracy rate of 100% [14]. Although none of these patients experienced complications, the gallbladder tumor in one patient could not be punctured, with this patient requiring puncture of the lymph nodes [14]. Another study, which assessed seven patients with GBC by EUS-FNA, reported a sensitivity rate of 80%, as high as that of EUS-FNA in biliary duct [11]. EUS-FNA can distinguish between GBC and XGC, types of tumors difficult to differentiate by imaging methods. An assessment of 15 patients by EUS-FNA found that 10 had GBC and five had XGC, with an accuracy rate of 86.6% [13]. Five of six patients avoided surgery or major resection after EUS-FNA, indicating the usefulness of EUS-FNA when XGC is suspected.

Most previous reports describing the use of EUS-FNA for gallbladder lesions have included rapid on-site evaluation (ROSE) [10–15]. The diagnostic accuracy of EUS-FNA is dependent on the volume of samples [16, 17]. The presence of a ROSE, as determined by a cytopathologist, in the room from which the sample was obtained, has been shown to improve the diagnostic yield of the procedure [17]. ROSE may allow fewer needle passes and ensure the adequacy of the obtained sample, as shown by onsite staining prior to the completion of the procedure.

To date, no significant complications of EUS-FNA have been reported, such as bleeding, bile peritonitis, and needle track seeding. However, most studies to date have included few patients, and all of these studies were performed retrospectively. Larger scale studies also had limitations, in that they only included patients with gallbladder tumors accompanied by biliary obstruction.

Indications of EUS-FNA for Gallbladder Tumors

At present, there are no clear indications for EUS-FNA in the diagnosis of gallbladder tumors. Two studies to date have evaluated indications of EUS-FNA for gallbladder tumors. In

Table 1 Reports of endoscopic ultrasound guided-fine needle aspiration for gallbladder mass lesion

Study	Year published	Number of patients	Final diagnosis	Sensitivity (%)	Specificity (%)	Complications (%)
Jacobson et al. [12]	2003	6	Malignant 5 Benign 1	83.3	100	0
Varadarajulu et al. [14]	2005	6	Malignant 5 Benign 1	100	N/A	0
Meara et al. [11]	2006	7	Malignant 7	85.7	100	0
Hijioka et al. [13]	2010	15	Malignant 10 Benign 5	90	100	0
Hijioka et al. [10]	2011	50	Malignant 49	96	100	0
Singla et al. [15]	2019	101	Malignant 98 Benign 1	90.8	100	0
Total		185	Malignant 174 Benign 8	92.1	100	0

one, 50 patients underwent EUS-FNA for gallbladder tumors [10]. Because EUS-FNA of gallbladder tumors carries a risk of biliary peritonitis and needle track seeding, the liver and/or lymph node metastasis was punctured before the gallbladder tumor was punctured in patients with the liver and/or lymph node metastasis. EUS-FNA had a higher sensitivity rate than ERC sampling in patients with GBC (96% versus 47.4%, $p<0.001$) [10]. Gallbladder tumors were directly punctured in 10 patients, whereas lymph nodes were punctured in 37 and metastatic liver lesions in two to diagnose gallbladder tumors [10]. In the second large clinical trial, 101 patients with gallbladder mass lesions with biliary obstruction underwent EUS-FNA [15]. Gallbladder tumors were punctured in 58 patients, lymph nodes in 23, and both in 16. The sensitivity and specificity of EUS-FNA were 90.8% and 100%, respectively, with no patients experiencing serious adverse events [15].

Based on these findings, indications of EUS-FNA of gallbladder mass lesions should include the following:

① EUS-FNA is indicated for large tumors extending into the bile duct and tumors infiltrating the liver because it is easy to puncture the tumor while avoiding gallbladder lumen.

② Although ETGBD can assess the cytology of tumors localized to the gallbladder, ETGBD has drawbacks, including its insufficient diagnostic accuracy and the requirement for an expert endoscopist. In case of failure of ETGBD, EUS-FNA can be an alternative option for pathological diagnosis of gallbladder tumors.

③ In patients with gallbladder tumors accompanied by liver and/or lymph node metastasis, the liver and/or lymph node metastasis should be punctured before the gallbladder tumor is punctured.

EUS-FNA Technique for Gallbladder Mass Lesions

The routes for EUS puncture of gallbladder tumors include those from the duodenal bulb, the stomach vestibule, and the stomach body. Following EUS detection of a gallbladder mass lesion, the puncture site that avoids fluid space can be determined, thereby avoiding the risks of bile leakage and needle track seeding associated with direct puncture of the lesion (Fig. 1a). To avoid puncturing the gallbladder mass through any intervening layer of fluid or potential space while targeting the mass, the probe can be enfaced by changing the position of the EUS. In patients with GBC and liver and/or lymph node metastasis, the liver and/or lymph node metastasis should be punctured prior to puncturing the gallbladder tumor. However, in patients with tumors localized to the gallbladder, it is necessary to puncture the gallbladder tumor for pathologic diagnosis. Direct puncture of the tumor through the gallbladder wall should be in a tangential direction, increasing the stroke distance associated with needle movement (Fig. 1b). In patients with lesions known or suspected of infiltrating the liver parenchyma, part of the infiltrating liver parenchyma or the gallbladder wall in contact with the liver parenchyma should be punctured. It is frequently difficult to puncture gallbladder tumors in patients with preserved gallbladder lumen. After puncture, the inner cylinder of the FNA needle should be pulled out while applying a syringe with a suction pressure of 10–20 mL to the FNA needle (Fig. 1c), with the inside of the mass penetrated 10–20 times to collect cells. After the needle is withdrawn from the endoscope channel, the stylet should be reintroduced, and the specimens transferred to glass slides (Fig. 1d). The specimens obtained by EUS-FNA are subsequently analyzed cytologically and histologically, with part of the specimens used for ROSE. When the cytopathologist indicates that a sufficient number of cells have been obtained, the procedure is stopped (Fig. 1e).

Typical Patients Who Underwent EUS-FNA for Diagnosis of a Gallbladder Tumor

Patient 1

A 60-year-old man presenting with abdominal pain was evaluated by contrast-enhanced computed tomography (CECT). CECT showed a

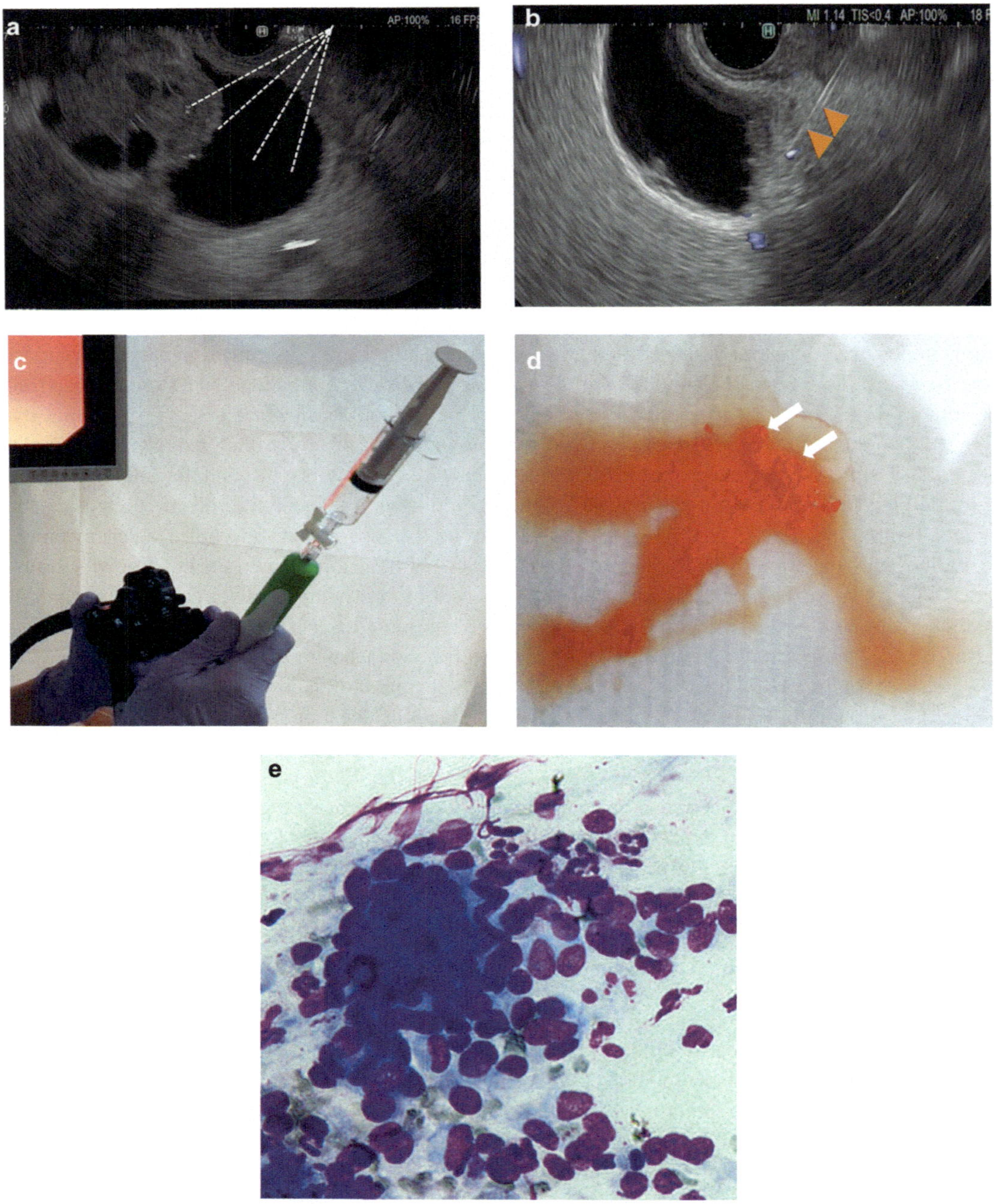

Fig. 1 EUS-FNA technique for gallbladder mass lesions. **a** Intervening layer of fluid space exists on puncture line (dotted lines). In this position of endoscopic ultrasound (EUS), the gallbladder tumor should not be punctured with a needle. **b** Gallbladder tumor is depicted on a punctured line without any intervening layer of fluid space. The gallbladder tumor is punctured with a needle (red arrowhead) through the gallbladder wall in a tangential direction. **c** A syringe with a suction pressure of 10–20 mL is applied to the needle. **d** After the needle is withdrawn from the endoscope channel, the specimens of gallbladder tumor (white arrow) are transferred from the needle tip to glass slides by reintroducing the stylet. **e** There are cohesive group of epithelial cells with altered nuclear (cytoplasmic ratio, cytoplasmic mucin, and nuclear membrane irregularity) in the smear (Stain: Diff Quik; magnification: ×20)

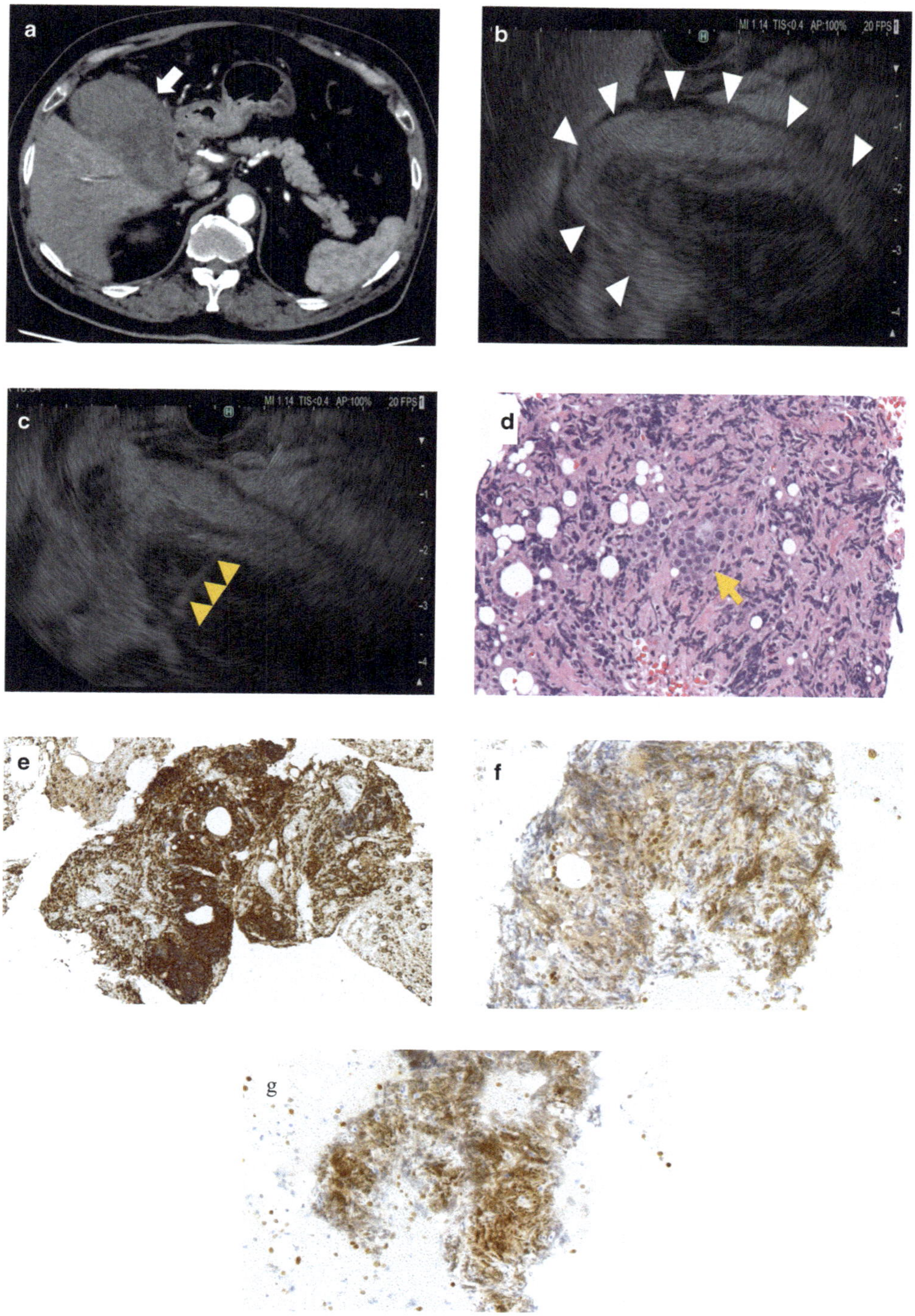

Fig. 2 A patient with a primary diffuse large B-cell lymphoma of the gallbladder. **a** Contrast-enhanced computed tomography, showing the hypovascular diffuse irregular wall of a thickened gallbladder (white arrow). **b** Endoscopic ultrasound, showing thickening of the gallbladder wall and a low echoic mass involving the entire lumen of the gallbladder (white arrowhead). **c** Endoscopic ultrasound-guided fine needle aspiration (EUS-FNA) of a gallbladder mass lesion. The arrowhead shows the FNA needle inside the lesion. **d** Histological examination of the lesion, showing atypical cells with a high N/C ratio and medium to large nuclei (yellow arrow). (Hematoxylin-eosin staining × 400). **e–g** Immunohistochemical staining with antibodies to CD20 (**e**), bcl6 (**f**), and MUM-1 (**g**), showing that the cells were positive for all three (× 200)

hypovascular gallbladder tumor with irregular borders, thickening of the gallbladder wall, and partial liver invasion. A preliminary diagnosis indicated that the gallbladder tumor was an unresectable GBC (Fig. 2a). EUS-FNA of the gallbladder tumor was performed for pathological diagnosis. EUS showed that the gallbladder wall was thickened, with an all-around low echoic mass inside the gallbladder lumen (Fig. 2b). The low echoic mass in the neck of the gallbladder was punctured from the duodenal bulb with a 22G needle (Fig. 2c). Hematoxylin and eosin staining showed atypical cells with a high N/C ratio and medium to large nuclei (Fig. 2d). Immunohistochemical staining showed that these cells were positive for CD20,

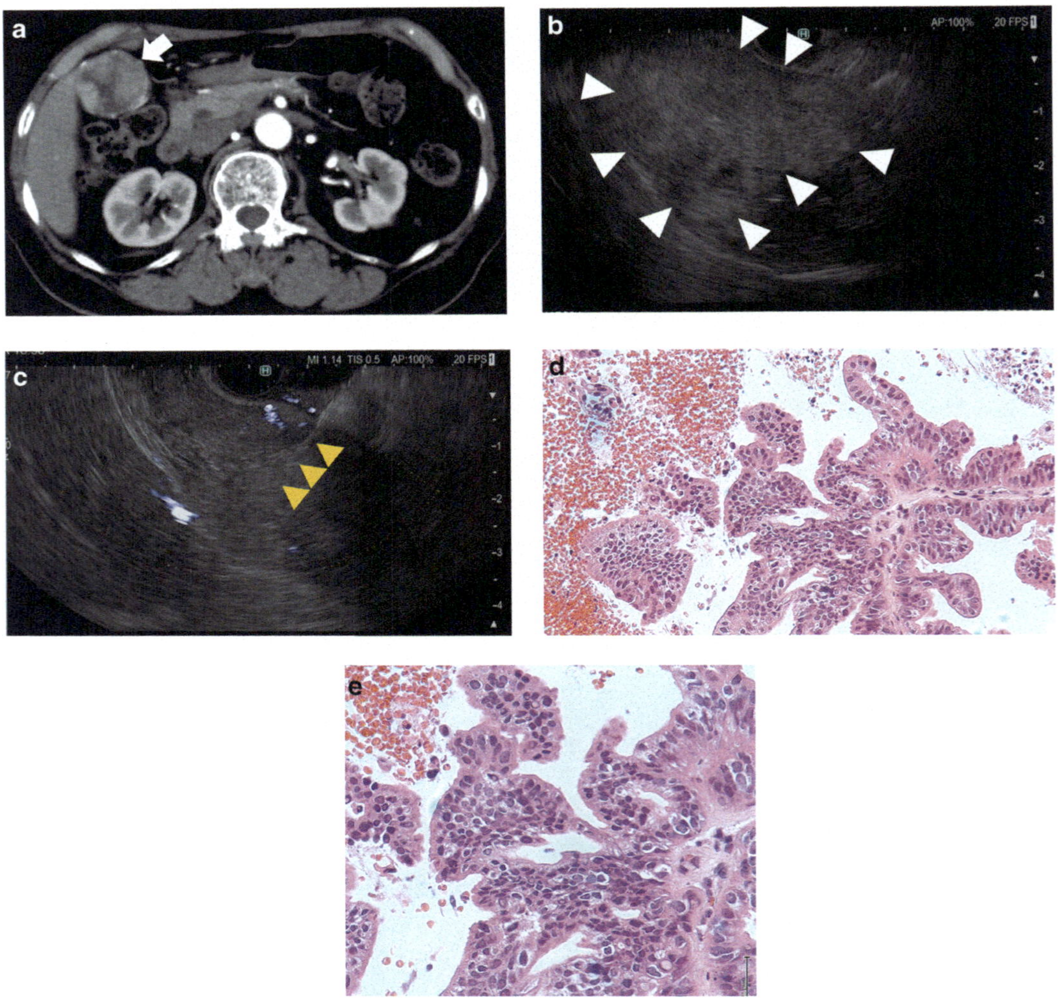

Fig. 3 A patient with a primary gallbladder adenocarcinoma. **a** Contrast-enhanced computer tomography, showing a hypervascular gallbladder tumor (white arrow) developing a papillary shape on the fundus gallbladder wall. **b** Endoscopic ultrasound, showing an iso-echoic mass developing an irregular papillary shape in the gallbladder (white arrowhead). **c** Endoscopic ultrasound-guided fine needle aspiration (EUS-FNA) of a gallbladder mass lesion. The arrowhead shows the FNA needle inside the lesion under guided EUS-e flow imaging. **d** Histological examination, showing atypical epithelium of the gallbladder wall with an irregular tubular structure (Hematoxylin-eosin staining × 100). **e** Histological examination, showing atypical cells with irregular nuclear enlargement. (Hematoxylin-eosin staining × 400)

bcl6, and MUM1 (Fig. 2e–g). Based on these findings, the gallbladder tumor was diagnosed as a primary diffuse large B-cell lymphoma of the gallbladder. The patient was therefore treated with R-CHOP (cyclophosphamide, doxorubicin, vincristine, and prednisolone in combination with rituximab) chemotherapy.

Patient 2

A 79-year-old woman presenting with abdominal pain was evaluated by CECT, which showed a hypervascular gallbladder tumor with a papillary shape on the fundus gallbladder wall. A preliminary diagnosis indicated that the gallbladder tumor was an unresectable GBC (Fig. 3a). EUS scanning from the duodenal bulb showed an iso-echoic mass developing into an irregular papillary shape (Fig. 3b). Under Doppler guidance, the mass was punctured in the fundus gallbladder with a 22 G needle (Fig. 3c). Hematoxylin and eosin staining showed atypical epithelium of the gallbladder wall with an irregular tubular structure and atypical cells with irregular nuclear enlargement (Fig. 3d, e). The gallbladder tumor was diagnosed as an adenocarcinoma.

Conclusion

Although EUS-FNA of the gallbladder is useful for diagnosing gallbladder tumors, it is not the initial method of choice because of its associated risks of bile leakage and needle track seeding. Also, the efficacy and safety of EUS-FNA for tumors localized in the gallbladder remain uncertain. Large clinical studies, including randomized controlled clinical trials, are needed to test the efficacy and safety of EUS-FNA in patients with gallbladder tumors.

References

1. Kumar R, Srinivasan R, Gupta N, Dey P, Rajwanshi A, Nijhawan R, Lal A, et al. Spectrum of gallbladder malignancies on fine-needle aspiration cytology: 5 years retrospective single institutional study with emphasis on uncommon variants. Diagn Cytopathol. 2017;45:36–42.
2. Das DK, Tripathi RP, Bhambhani S, Chachra KL, Sodhani P, Malhotra V. Ultrasound-guided fine-needle aspiration cytology diagnosis of gallbladder lesions: a study of 82 cases. Diagn Cytopathol. 1998;18:258–64.
3. Venkataramu NK, Sood BP, Gupta S, Gulati M, Khandelwal N, Suri S. Ultrasound-guided fine needle aspiration biopsy of gall bladder malignancies. Acta Radiol. 1999;40:436–9.
4. Kumar A, Aggarwal S, Berry M, Sawhney S, Kapur BM, Bhargava S. Ultrasonography of carcinoma of the gallbladder: an analysis of 80 cases. J Clin Ultrasound. 1990;18:715–20.
5. Wu SS, Lin KC, Soon MS, Yeh KT. Ultrasound-guided percutaneous transhepatic fine needle aspiration cytology study of gallbladder polypoid lesions. Am J Gastroenterol. 1996;91:1591–4.
6. Zargar SA, Khuroo MS, Mahajan R, Jan GM, Shah P. US-guided fine-needle aspiration biopsy of gallbladder masses. Radiology. 1991;179:275–8.
7. Itoi T, Sofuni A, Itokawa F, Kurihara T, Tsuchiya T, Moriyasu F, et al. Preoperative diagnosis and management of thick-walled gallbladder based on bile cytology obtained by endoscopic transpapillary gallbladder drainage tube. Gastrointest Endosc. 2006;64:512–9.
8. Naito Y, Okabe Y, Kawahara A, Taira T, Isida Y, Kaji R, et al. Usefulness of lavage cytology during endoscopic transpapillary catheterization into the gallbladder in the cytological diagnosis of gallbladder disease. Diagn Cytopathol. 2009;37:402–6.
9. Itsuki H, Serikawa M, Sasaki T, Ishii Y, Tsushima K, Furukawa Y, et al. Indication and usefulness of bile juice cytology for diagnosis of gallbladder cancer. Gastroenterol Res Pract. 2018;5410349.
10. Hijioka S, Hara K, Mizuno N, Imaoka H, Ogura T, Haba S, et al. Diagnostic yield of endoscopic retrograde cholangiography and of EUS-guided fine needle aspiration sampling in gallbladder carcinomas. J Hepatobiliary Pancreat Sci. 2012;19:650–5.
11. Meara RS, Jhala D, Eloubeidi MA, Eltoum I, Chhieng DC, Crowe DR, et al. Endoscopic ultrasound-guided FNA biopsy of bile duct and gallbladder: analysis of 53 cases. Cytopathology. 2006;17:42–9.
12. Jacobson BC, Pitman MB, Brugge WR. EUS-guided FNA for the diagnosis of gallbladder masses. Gastrointest Endosc. 2003;57:251–4.
13. Hijioka S, Mekky MA, Bhatia V, Sawaki A, Mizuno N, Hara K, et al. Can EUS-guided FNA distinguish between gallbladder cancer and xanthogranulomatous cholecystitis? Gastrointest Endosc. 2010;72:622–7.
14. Varadarajulu S, Eloubeidi MA. Endoscopic ultrasound-guided fine-needle aspiration in the evaluation of gallbladder masses. Endoscopy. 2005;37:751–4.

15. Singla V, Agarwal R, Anikhindi SA, Puri P, Kumar M, Ranjan P, et al. Role of EUS-FNA for gallbladder mass lesions with biliary obstruction: a large single-center experience. Endosc Int Open. 2019;7:E1403–9.
16. Hammoud GM, Almashhrawi A, Ibdah JA. Usefulness of endoscopic ultrasound-guided fine needle aspiration in the diagnosis of hepatic, gallbladder and biliary tract lesions. World J Gastrointest Oncol. 2014;6:420–9.
17. Matynia AP, Schmidt RL, Barraza G, Layfield LJ, Siddiqui AA, Adler DG. Impact of rapid on-site evaluation on the adequacy of endoscopic-ultrasound guided fine-needle aspiration of solid pancreatic lesions: a systematic review and meta-analysis. J Gastroenterol Hepatol. 2014;29:697–705.

Up-to-Date Knowledges

Pathogenesis and Treatment of Gallbladder Stone

Dong Ki Lee and Sung Ill Jang

Introduction

Various genetic and environmental factors are involved in the formation of gallbladder (GB) stones. Understanding the pathogenesis of GB stone formation can help in the prevention of GB stone and the development of future treatment methods. The treatment for GB stone has been performed by surgical and medical treatments depending on the patient's condition and clinical situation. We describe the pathogenesis and treatment of GB stone in this chapter.

Pathogenesis

Cholesterol Gallstone

Cholesterol gallbladder stones are formed in the gallbladder, due to changes in the bile-lipid composition in hepatocytes. As many metabolic diseases, the pathogenesis of the metabolic abnormalities underlying the formation of gallbladder stones involves both acquired and genetic factors.

Genetic Risk Factors

The prevalence of cholesterol gallstones varies among populations: specifically, it is extremely low in Asian and African populations in the equatorial regions, intermediate in North European and North American populations, and extremely high (30–70%) in populations of Native-American ancestry [1]. The prevalence of gallstones is high in Hispanic populations of Central and South America, Hispanic Americans from South America, and Hispanic Americans of Native-American ancestry [2–4]. Native populations of North and South America are the groups at the highest risk of gallstones worldwide. In these populations, genetic risk factors lead to lithogenic bile and gallstones early in life (<30 years of age) [3, 5], resulting in a gallstone prevalence of>50% at 50 years of age in both men and women [3, 4, 6, 7]. One hypothesis to explain this high prevalence is that exposure of their ancestors to Ice Age conditions of food deprivation favored selection for thrifty genes that confer predisposition to gallstones and obesity under conditions of caloric abundance [8]. The gene encoding 3-hydroxy-3-methyl-glutaryl-coenzyme A (HMG-CoA) reductase, which is involved in the de novo synthesis of cholesterol, was

D. K. Lee (✉) · S. I. Jang
Department of Internal Medicine, Institute of Gastroenterology, Gangnam Severance Hospital, Yonsei University College of Medicine, 211 Eonjuro, Gangnam-Gu, Seoul, South Korea
e-mail: dklee@yuhs.ac

S. I. Jang
e-mail: aerojsi@yuhs.ac

J. B. Chung and K. Okazaki (eds.), *Diseases of the Gallbladder*,
https://doi.org/10.1007/978-981-15-6010-1_8

upregulated; in contrast, the gene encoding 7-α-hydroxylase, which converts cholesterol to bile acid, was downregulated. These changes resulted in an increased level of free cholesterol in hepatocytes and increased cholesterol saturation index in excreted bile [6]. The associations between multiple lithogenic gene variants and gallstone formation indicate that the contributing genes are highly heterogenous [9, 10]. This may be due to genetic drift over many thousands of years, resulting in changes in the body to preserve energy sources in a manner involving cholesterol metabolism in the liver. Therefore, we call the gallstone that came in from the cold [8].

The effects of genetic factors on gallstone formation are supported by familial clustering within populations [11] and the identification of several lithogenic genes in an inbred mouse model [12]. A study of Swedish twin pairs with gallstone disease indicated that up to 25% of the risk of gallstone disease is determined by genetic factors [13]. Genome-wide association studies identified a variant of the hepatobiliary cholesterol transporter (*ABCG8* p.D19H) as the most frequent genetic risk factor in humans [10, 14, 15]. Combined with findings regarding *UGT1A1*, which is a risk factor predominantly in men, the data thus far indicate that genetic factors contribute up to 15% of the population-attributable gallstone risk [16]. Mutations in some lithogenic genes may cause gallstone formation; these genes include the common gallstone-associated variants of *ABCG4* and *ABCG8*, as well as *UGT1A1* [15, 16]. In addition, rare mutations in *ABCB4* (encoding hepatobiliary floppase), *ABCB11* (encoding a bile salt export pump), *CFTR* (encoding cystic fibrosis transmembrane conductance regulator), and *CYP7A1* (encoding cholesterol 7α-hydroxylase) each promote gallstone formation by directly altering the composition of bile [17]. In contrast, polymorphisms in other lithogenic genes (e.g., those encoding apolipoproteins, cholesteryl ester transfer protein, and adrenergic and nuclear receptors) might exert a lithogenic effect only in the presence of primary genetic risk factors [10, 17].

Metabolic and Exogenous Risk Factors

In addition to the above mentioned genetic factors, several conditions lead to cholesterol hypersecretion into bile, triggering the formation of gallstones. Epidemiological studies have identified a large number of risk factors for cholesterol stones (Table 1) [18, 19]. Obesity confers predisposition to gallstone formation [20], symptomatic gallstones [21], and the need for cholecystectomy. Hyperinsulinemia is associated with increased hepatic cholesterol uptake [22], and biliary secretion [23], as well as hyposecretion of biliary bile acids [24]. In addition, insulin resistance and type 2 diabetes mellitus are independently associated with cholesterol gallstone formation and associated disease [25, 26]. Obesity and rapid weight loss are associated with an extremely high incidence of gallstones [27]. Cholesterol synthesis is increased in obesity, reportedly because of increased HMG-CoA reductase activity [28]. The resulting expansion of the hepatic free cholesterol pool leads to an increase in biliary cholesterol saturation [29]. During weight loss, the lithogenicity of bile is further enhanced by net excretion of cholesterol; in circumstances involving severely fat-restricted diets or bariatric surgery causing rapid weight loss, the lithogenicity of bile is enhanced by gallbladder stasis [27, 30]. Rapid weight loss (more than 1.5 kg weekly) leads to the formation of gallstones in up to 30% of individuals and increases the risk of biliary symptoms and need for cholecystectomy [27, 31–33]. Omental and mesenteric fats consumed during weight loss enter the blood and increase the free cholesterol level in hepatocytes, leading to cholesterol gallstone formation.

Endogenous estrogens at puberty or during pregnancy, as well as exogenous estrogens (e.g., in the form of contraceptives, postmenopausal medication, or other pharmacological treatments), increase biliary cholesterol saturation and are associated with gallstone formation [34]. Input to the hepatic free cholesterol pool is increased by upregulation of the low-density lipoprotein receptor. Estrogen enhances hepatic synthesis and secretion of cholesterol; it also

Table 1 Major risk factors for gallbladder stones (adapted from Ref. [18])

Risk factor	Cholesterol gallstones	Black pigment gallstones
Family history/ethnicity	•	
Increasing age	•	
Female gender	•	
Obesity, especially central adiposity	•	
Rapid weight loss/bariatric surgery	•	
Physical inactivity	•	
Metabolic syndrome	•	
Dyslipidemia (↑TG, ↓HDL-C), Insulin resistance, diabetes		
Diet	•	
High calorie		
High refined carbohydrate/glycemic load		
Low fiber		
Prolonged TPN	•	
Drugs	•	
Estrogen therapy (HRT)		
Somatostatin analogue-octreotide		
Calcineurin inhibitors		
Fibrates		
Spinal cord injury	•	
Chronic HCV infection	•	
Enterohepatic bacteria (Helicobacter spp.)	•	
Vitamin B_{12} and folic acid deficiency		•
Anemia (haemolytic, sickle cell)		•
Ileal resections		•
Cystic fibrosis		•
Gastrectomy	•	•
Liver cirrhosis	•	•

HDL-C = high-density lipoprotein cholesterol; HCV = hepatitis C virus; HRT = hormone replacement therapy; TG = triglycerides; TPN = total parenteral nutrition

reduces bile salt synthesis by upregulation of estrogen receptor 1 and G protein-coupled receptor 30 (corresponding to lithogenic gene cluster 18 in inbred mice) [35]. This may partially explain the higher prevalence of gallstones in women than in men. Interestingly, in up to 60% of women, gallstones can disappear postpartum, indicating that pregnancy is associated with transient lithogenicity [14]. Notably, while estrogens increase the synthesis and secretion of hepatic cholesterol, progesterone causes gallbladder hypomotility [36].

Fibric acid derivatives increase biliary cholesterol saturation and reduce the serum cholesterol level. HMG-CoA reductase inhibitors reduce low-density lipoprotein receptor uptake, thereby reducing the hepatic free cholesterol pool and biliary cholesterol saturation [37]. Most cholesterol is endogenously synthesized; dietary cholesterol has a limited impact on cholesterol saturation. However, vegetable protein intake is negatively correlated with the incidence of gallstones. Patients with spinal cord injury have an extremely high prevalence of gallstones [38]. Biliary cholesterol saturation and the prevalence of gallstones increase with age, irrespective of sex. A decline in cholesterol 7-α-hydroxylase activity with age contributes to the increased cholesterol saturation [39, 40], as does a reduction in the bile-salts-to-cholesterol ratio.

Cholesterol gallstone formation is influenced by acquired and genetic factors. As the most representative case is described above, Africans living near the equator have a low prevalence of gallstone, whereas African-Americans have a high prevalence. This difference suggests that genetic adaptation over many thousands of years has led to a wide variety of acquired lifestyles, which can dramatically alter the prevalence of disease.

Pathogenic Mechanism

Cholesterol gallstone formation is the net result of a complex series of events in lipid metabolism and interactions in the hepatobiliary system. Cholesterol hypersecretion is essential for the development of cholesterol gallstones (Fig. 1). Although either an excess of cholesterol or a lack of bile salts could theoretically produce biliary cholesterol supersaturation, an excess of cholesterol is typically the primary cause, as discussed above. Most patients with gallstones have a normal rate of bile acid secretion [41]. The cholesterol-to-phosphatidylcholine ratio in the bile of patients with gallstones is elevated, compared to that in normal individuals [42]. The free cholesterol pool is a major determinant of biliary cholesterol saturation. Increases in the free cholesterol pool can occur through a number of mechanisms, which may have obscured attempts to identify common changes in the enzymes that mediate cholesterol and bile salt synthesis. Furthermore, synchronized changes in these regulated enzymes may lead to secondary changes [43]. Cholesterol secreted in bile is derived mainly from hepatic de novo synthesis; high-density lipoprotein cholesterol is generated by reverse cholesterol transport and chylomicrons

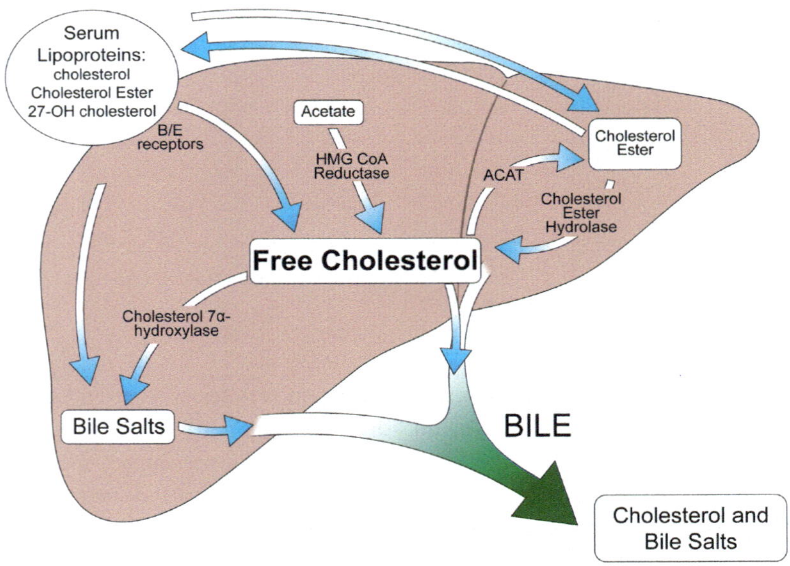

Fig. 1 Metabolic pathways in cholesterol and bile salt synthesis. The hepatocyte is a central regulator of cholesterol homeostasis and is the only site for major synthetic pathways of bile synthesis. Cholesterol gallstone formation is the result of a complex series of events in lipid metabolism and interactions in the hepatobiliary system. Cholesterol hypersecretion is essential for the development of cholesterol gallstones. Although either an excess of cholesterol or a lack of bile salts could theoretically produce biliary cholesterol supersaturation (adapted from Ref. [37])

(lipoprotein particles that transport cholesterol from the intestine, primarily to the liver). The contribution of each of these pathways to the formation of lithogenic bile is unclear. Insulin resistance promotes biliary cholesterol secretion by inducing *ABDG5* and *ABCG8* through dysregulation of the transcription factor forkhead box protein O1 in hepatocytes [44]. This might explain the high prevalence of gallstones in patients with diabetes.

Direct consequences of cholesterol-supersaturated bile include gallbladder hypomotility and mucin hypersecretion. In animal models, hypomotility precedes the development of gallstones [45]. In humans, gallbladder filling is impaired due to a substantial reduction in the flux of bile into the gallbladder [46]. Cholesterol-supersaturated bile directly depresses contractility [47] due to the increased cholesterol content of the epithelial cells that line the gallbladder [48, 49]. Excess cholesterol is converted to cholesteryl esters and stored in the mucosa and lamina propria; this storage of cholesteryl esters stiffens the sarcolemmal membrane of smooth-muscle cells, disrupts cholecystokinin 1 receptor signaling, and decouples the signal transduction mediated by G proteins, (e.g., $G_{q/11\alpha}$, $G_{i\alpha 1-2}$, and $G_{i\alpha 3}$) [50]. This causes dysfunction of the cholecystokinin receptor of muscle cells and gallbladder hypomotility; the residence time of bile within the gallbladder then increases, allowing sufficient time for nucleation. A greater fraction of newly secreted bile is also diverted directly to the intestine to undergo bacterial metabolism. Moreover, mucin secretion is increased, mediated by cholesterol supersaturation and increased levels of hydrophobic secondary bile acids [36].

An intermediate stage is the formation of biliary sludge, a viscous mixture of mucin glycoproteins, and cholesterol crystals. Formation of biliary sludge, gallbladder mucin and microscopic precipitates of multilamellar cholesterol-rich vesicles, and cholesterol monohydrate appears to precede the development of macroscopic cholesterol gallstone [1, 51]. The mucin gel matrix accelerates cholesterol crystallization and stone growth [52]. In practice, both sludge and formed stones can cause cholangitis or gallstone pancreatitis.

Cholesterol gallstone formation is the net result of a complex series of events. Cholesterol hypersecretion by hepatocytes leads to gallbladder hypomotility and increased mucin secretion by the gallbladder epithelium. Loss of the gallbladder reservoir function then leads to increased degradation of bile salts by intestinal bacteria, with resultant changes in the composition of bile. An increased proportion of hydrophobic secondary bile acids causes increased mucin secretion in the gallbladder. Cholesterol hypersecretion, increased mucin production, and increased deoxycholate content promote rapid cholesterol crystal formation, aggregation, and stone formation. Therefore, reduced gallbladder motility and prolongation of nucleation time are secondary and tertiary phenomena associated with cholesterol hypersecretion by the liver.

Black Pigment Stone

Increased production of unconjugated bilirubin can result from increased secretion of conjugated bilirubin, as observed in patients with hemolysis or alcoholism; this increased production of unconjugated bilirubin is associated with a high risk of black pigment gallstones (Fig. 2) [53]. Conditions that increase the colonic bile salt concentration, such as ileal disease, are presumed to favor the resorption of unconjugated bilirubin and subsequent hypersecretion into bile. Patients with Crohn's disease and total parenteral nutrition are at increased risk of black pigment stones [54], potentially because they exhibit increased levels of biliary calcium and unconjugated bilirubin.

Black pigment stones contain calcium bilirubinate, calcium phosphate, and calcium carbonate in a mucin glycoprotein matrix, with a small amount of cholesterol [37]. The solubility of the calcium salt of unconjugated bilirubin is extremely low, although bile salt micelles provide partial solubilization [55]. After deconjugation of conjugated bilirubin by intestinal bacteria, a fraction of unconjugated bilirubin is

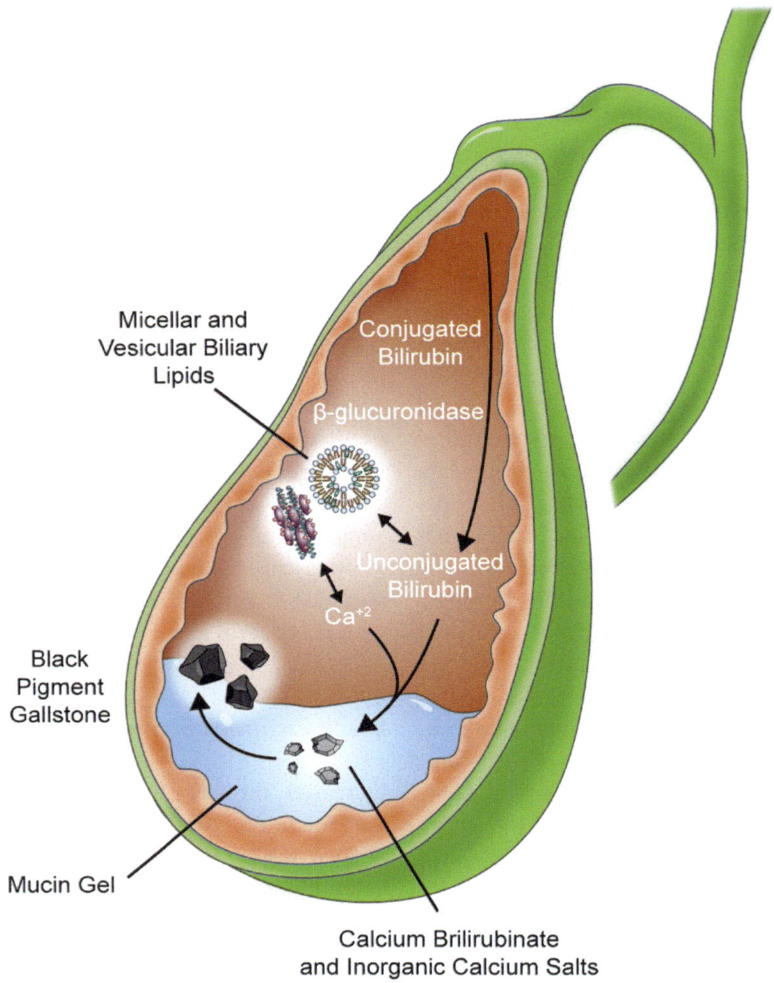

Fig. 2 Pathogenesis of black pigment gallstones. The major initiating event is an increase in conjugated bilirubin secretion. Deconjugation produces unconjugated bilirubin. The extreme insolubility of calcium bilirubinate promotes precipitation. In conjunction with calcium-binding protein, mucin promotes formation of black pigment gallstones (modified from Ref. [121])

reabsorbed in the colon in the presence of bile salts and undergoes enterohepatic circulation [56]. Increases in the unconjugated bilirubin concentration or reductions in the abundance of solubilizing micelles and vesicles contribute to biliary unconjugated bilirubin supersaturation [37]. Elevations in calcium ion concentration, possibly caused by bile salt hyposecretion, further accelerate calcium bilirubinate precipitation. Ionized calcium is partially bound by micelles and vesicles in bile [57]; reductions in the bile salt concentration diminish the calcium-buffering capacity of bile. Calcium bilirubinate undergoes free radical polymerization and possibly oxidation and, in the presence of gallbladder mucin, forms a mature black pigment gallstone [58]. Thus, black pigment gallstones are not hard, unlike cholesterol gallstones, and break when rubbed.

Brown Pigment Stone

Bile is generally sterile, but may briefly contain bacteria. In some clinical situations, the bile duct can be colonized by bacteria. The first prerequisite for brown pigment stone formation is bacterial colonization (Fig. 3) of the bile duct, especially by *Escherichia coli* [36]. Formation of brown pigment stones is associated with periampullary diverticula, presumably because of the increased rate of bacterial colonization of the distal common bile duct, rather than metabolic alterations in bile composition [59]. Therefore, brown pigment stones can form in all parts of the biliary tree; they typically form in the bile duct, so-called primary choledocholithiasis.

Bacterial infection of bile alters its tenuous solubilization balance, leading to precipitation of intact and degraded biliary lipids. Bacterial β-glucuronidases cleave conjugated bilirubin to its insoluble unconjugated form, which precipitates as the calcium salt [60]. Bacterial A1 phospholipases hydrolyze phosphatidylcholine to form lysolecithin and fatty acids, which precipitate as calcium salts. Bile salts are deconjugated to free bile acids by bile acid hydroxylase, and their calcium salts have been identified in stones. Loss of the cholesterol-solubilizing potency of bile due to the depletion of phosphatidylcholine and bile salts also leads to precipitation of cholesterol [37]. Central to the pathogenesis of brown pigment stones is the presence of bacterial cytoskeletons in the core, as demonstrated by scanning electron microscopy [61, 62]. The glycoprotein matrix of stones is derived both from synthetic bacterial products and from the mucin secreted by the biliary epithelium [37]. Brown pigment stones that develop from migrated cholesterol gallbladder stones are termed secondary choledocholithiasis. The cholesterol stone is the nidus, and the outer portion of the brown pigment stone grows by the same pathogenic mechanism involved in primary choledocholithiasis.

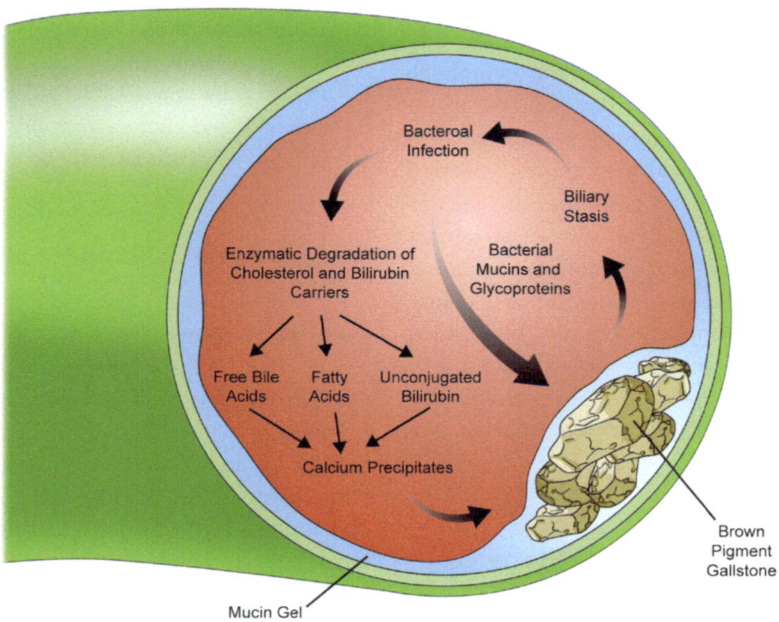

Fig. 3 Pathogenesis of brown pigment gallstones. Bacterial enzymes degrade biliary lipids and produce insoluble calcium salts of fatty acids and unconjugated bilirubin, typically in bile ducts. Degradation of biliary solubilizing agents, bile salts, and phosphatidylcholine exacerbates precipitation of these compounds and reduces cholesterol solubility (adapted from Ref. [37])

Treatment

Biliary Colic

Treatment of gallbladder stones depends on the presence of symptoms. Abdominal pain caused by gallstones is known as biliary colic; in affected patients, gallstones temporarily block the gallbladder neck or gallbladder ducts, inducing rigid spasms and causing visceral pain. Biliary colic can occur with or without inflammation. Biliary colic lasts for at least 30 minutes to several hours in the upper or right upper abdomen, and is typically of at least moderate intensity [63]. Pain often occurs at night, radiating to the back or right shoulder; it manifests at irregular intervals, from months to years [64]. In addition, biliary colic can cause symptoms after eating (especially fatty foods), but this symptom is not observed in all affected patients [65].

In patients with biliary colic, the recurrence rate of pain is 58–72% and the risk of complications is 1–2%, higher than in asymptomatic patients (0.1–0.2%) [66, 67]. Therefore, the standard indication for treatment of gallbladder stones is biliary colic. Indigestion, abdominal bloating, and burping are common complaints in patients with gallstones; however, the causal relationship of these complaints with gallstone formation is unclear, and they are not generally regarded as symptoms of gallstones. It is important to evaluate the characteristics of abdominal pain and determine whether the pain is caused by gallstones, because gallstone-related pain is an indication for cholecystectomy. If a patient with gallstones complains of abdominal pain rather than biliary colic, cholecystectomy may not be required, and the pain may persist after surgery.

Asymptomatic Gallbladder Stone

In general, asymptomatic gallbladder stones can be monitored without treatment [36, 68, 69]. Until the early 1980s, nearly all gallstones were presumed to cause symptoms; however, subsequent studies of the natural history of gallbladder stones have revealed the risks associated with asymptomatic gallstones [70]. In a 24-year follow-up of patients with asymptomatic gallbladder stones, the cumulative risks of symptoms were 10% after 5 years, 15% after 10 years, and 18% after 15 years [70]. In an Italian study that followed 580 patients with asymptomatic gallbladder stones for 8.7 years, 21.9% underwent cholecystectomy due to pain or complications [71]. In Denmark, 664 patients with asymptomatic gallbladder stones were followed for 17.4 years; 19.6% developed symptoms or complications [72]. The incidence of symptoms in patients with asymptomatic gallbladder stones is 1–4% per year [36], and the overall frequency of symptoms is 10–25% [70, 73–76]. The incidence of a serious complication as the first symptom in these patients is very low (0.1%) [77, 78].

Biliary colic is preceded by complications in patients with asymptomatic gallbladder stones. In 80% of patients with asymptomatic gallbladder stones, complications do not develop; biliary colic occurs as a prognostic symptom when complications occur, such that observation is recommended for patients with biliary colic [36, 69, 79]. Overall, asymptomatic gallbladder stones should be observed, and cholecystectomy should be performed if biliary colic or complications occur.

Symptomatic Gallbladder Stone

Surgical Treatment

Cholecystectomy is the principle treatment in patients with gallbladder stones who have typical biliary colic or complications such as cholecystitis (Fig. 4) [36, 69, 79–82]. Open cholecystectomy was performed in the past, but laparoscopic cholecystectomy is now the typical surgical treatment method. Laparoscopic cholecystectomy has the advantages of smaller surgical wounds, less pain after surgery, and shorter hospitalization and recovery times, compared to open cholecystectomy [80].

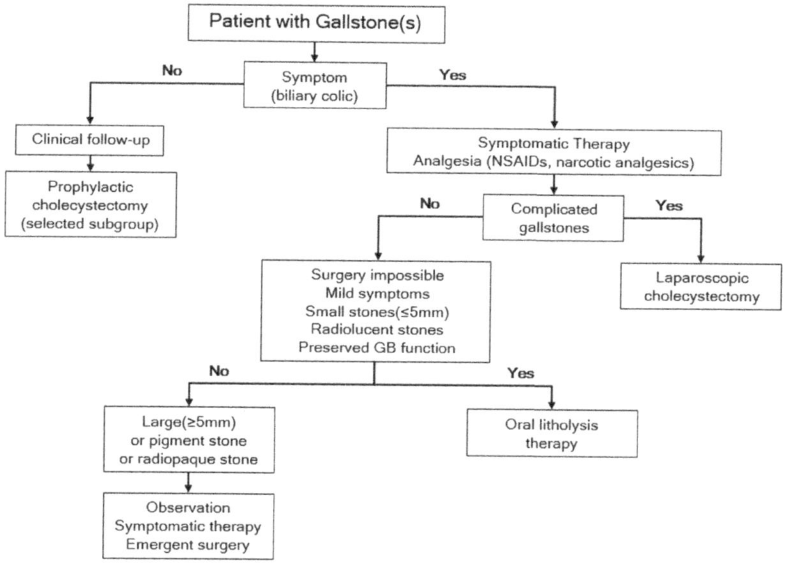

Fig. 4 Flowchart of the management of patients with gallstones (modified from Ref. [82])

Laparoscopic cholecystectomy has a 2–4% complication rate and a 0.04–0.08% mortality rate [83, 84]. Mortality rates of 0.1–0.7% have been reported among patients undergoing small incision cholecystectomy [80], which is superior in cost-effectiveness to both open cholecystectomy and laparoscopic cholecystectomy [81].

Advances in laparoscopic cholecystectomy and accumulation of surgical experience have led to reductions in complication rates, but prophylactic cholecystectomy is not recommended [36, 79]. However, prophylactic cholecystectomy can be considered if the risk of gallbladder cancer is high or if the risk of complications is expected to be high [79]. The risk factors for gallbladder cancer are as follows [85, 86]: large gallstones greater than 3 cm, gallbladder polyps greater than 1 cm, anomalous pancreaticobiliary ductal union, and porcelain gallbladder. The risk factors for complications of gallbladder stones are as follows [87]: transplantation, chronic hemolytic anemia, and common bile duct stone.

Medical Treatment

Medical treatment may be considered for patients with mild symptoms, those in whom it is difficult to confirm the presence of typical biliary colic, those with difficult surgery, or those who refuse surgery. The non-surgical treatment of gallbladder stones includes litholysis by oral gallstone-dissolving agents or intra-gallbladder drug injection, pulverization by extracorporeal shock wave lithotripsy, and removal by transcutaneous gallbladder cholangioscopy. Because laparoscopic cholecystectomy has become increasingly common in the past 20 years, the frequency of medical treatment has decreased. Other methods are rarely used because of the high cost and risk of complications.

Oral Litholytic Agents

Oral bile acid preparations are currently most commonly used for the treatment of gallstones; the preparations most frequently used are ursodeoxycholic acid (UDCA) and chenodeoxycholic acid (CDCA). CDCA was first used in 1972 to dissolve radiolucent gallstones [88]; in 1975, the hydrophilic UDCA was used to dissolve gallbladder gallstones [89]. Oral administration of bile acid preparations increases the capacity of bile acid reservoirs and inhibits the secretion of cholesterol into the bile, thereby reducing cholesterol saturation in the bile.

Cholesterol-unsaturated bile transfers cholesterol from gallstones into micelles, allowing gallstones to dissolve in the gallbladder.

UDCA is a hydrophilic tertiary bile acid formed in the liver or by members of the *Enterobacteriaceae* family. UDCA can reduce cholesterol saturation in the bile by 40–60% through inhibition of cholesterol absorption in the intestine and inhibition of the secretion of cholesterol into the bile [78, 90]. UDCA is less hepatotoxic than CDCA, does not raise blood cholesterol, and causes diarrhea in less than 1% of patients [91]. In contrast, CDCA alone has side effects such as diarrhea, liver failure, and an elevated serum cholesterol level. CDCA alone is no longer recommended as a treatment for gallstones. CDCA and UDCA combination therapy is used to reduce CDCA complications and increase treatment effectiveness [92].

Oral bile acid supplement therapy is effective for treatment of radiopaque cholesterol gallstones with normal gallbladder function [69]. Gallstone dissolution effects can be assessed by imaging modalities (e.g., ultrasound, endoscopic ultrasound, and computed tomography) after 6–12 months. Computed tomography can be used for prediction of the dissolution effect; dissolution is expected to be optimal for gallstones with a signal of less than 60 Hounsfield units on computed tomography [93–95]. The dissolution rate of gallbladder stones is 24–38% in UDCA monotherapy, whereas that of UDCA and CDCA combinations is 52–62.8% for gallstones smaller than 15 mm [92, 96–98].

The limitations of oral bile acid supplement therapy include its long treatment duration, low success rate, and high recurrence rate. After successful gallstone treatment, the recurrence rate of oral bile acid supplement therapy is 10% within 5 years [99]. For multiple gallstones, the recurrence rates are 30–50% within 5 years and 50–70% within 12 years [79, 100, 101]. Oral bile acid preparations can dissolve only cholesterol gallstones; increased calcium content is associated with greater difficulty in achieving effective dissolution. In addition, the dissolution rate is highest for gallstones smaller than 5 mm; larger gallstones are associated with lower dissolution rates. The cystic duct must be open to allow bile acids to enter the gallbladder and gallbladder motility should be normal. This therapy is not an indication for severe or frequent recurrence of biliary colic, nor for complications such as acute cholecystitis or acute cholangitis. Therefore, before initiating oral bile acid replacement, the symptoms, type (component) of gallstones, size and number of gallstones, gallbladder function, and patency of the cystic duct should be considered.

Terpene

Terpenes are volatile unsaturated hydrocarbon organic compounds found in essential oils extracted from plants, such as conifers and citrus trees. These compounds dissolve other lipid components and are used for dissolving gallstones. A mixture of cyclic monoterpenes (Rowachol®, Rowa Pharmaceuticals Ltd., Bantry, Ireland) is commercially available for medical treatment. Rowachol dissolves cholesterol gallstones by reducing cholesterol saturation in the bile [102]. In addition, it increases bile flow and reduces smooth-muscle contraction to relieve biliary pain.

Other Experimental Drugs

A variety of drugs have been used to treat gallstones. In the animal study reported by Wang et al. [103], ezetimibe reduced cholesterol absorption in the intestines and lowered biliary cholesterol secretion, thereby preventing gallstone formation and conserving gallbladder motility. Ezetimibe was also reported to increase gallstone dissolution and reduce biliary cholesterol saturation, thereby decreasing the formation of cholesterol crystals.

Epidemiological studies have investigated the therapeutic effect of omega-3 polyunsaturated fatty acids on cholesterol gallstones. For instance, Eskimo populations have a diet rich in fish oil; they have a lower prevalence of cholesterol gallstones than that of Western populations [104]. Polyunsaturated fatty acids prevent the formation of gallstones by increasing the levels of bile phospholipids and suppressing bile mucin production [105]. Combination treatment with polyunsaturated fatty acids and UDCA has been shown to dissolve cholesterol gallstones in mice by reducing mucin production and cholesterol saturation, as well as increasing the levels of phospholipids and bile acids in bile [106]. Further studies of the therapeutic effects of combination polyunsaturated fatty acids and UDCA treatment in patients with cholesterol gallstones are warranted.

Myriocin has been reported to reduce the serum and biliary ceramide concentrations and inhibit phosphorylation of p38, thereby reducing gallstone formation in C57BL/6 J mice; however, the mechanisms underlying this effect are not yet known [107]. Capsaicin and curcumin, extracted from spices in singular or combined forms, also lowered biliary cholesterol and increased phospholipid levels, thereby suppressing biliary gallstone formation in mice by increasing the cholesterol: phospholipid ratio [108]. However, UDCA is currently the only widely accepted medical agent for the treatment of cholesterol gallstones.

Pregnancy

The hormonal changes that occur during pregnancy increase the risk of gallstone formation [109]. Biliary cholesterol concentrations in gallbladder bile increase gradually from the first to the third trimester of pregnancy, in accordance with a progressive increase in the incidence of biliary sludge (a precursor to gallstones) and gallstones; moreover, the incidences of biliary sludge and/or gallstones are 30% and 12% during pregnancy and postpartum, respectively [110, 111]. Although most pregnant women remain asymptomatic, 1–3% undergo cholecystectomy due to clinical symptoms or complications within the first year postpartum [14, 111, 112].

Expectant management is the general policy and litholysis is not indicated in asymptomatic pregnant women with gallbladder gallstones. However, in symptomatic pregnant women, there are several management methods for gallstones during pregnancy [79, 113]. If possible, supportive management is highly recommended; curative treatment is ideally administered after delivery. Pain control is required during pregnancy. True biliary pain should be distinguished from nonspecific abdominal discomfort in a pregnant woman presenting with abdominal pain. Laparoscopic or open cholecystectomy performed for true biliary pain is essential, but symptoms may persist when the procedure is performed in pregnant women with nonspecific dyspepsia and gallstones. Uncomplicated biliary pain can be managed with intravenous hydration and narcotic pain control. The use of analgesics has successfully ameliorated biliary symptoms in 64% of symptomatic pregnant women [113].

Laparoscopic or open cholecystectomy is generally reserved for pregnant women with recurrent or unrelenting biliary pain that is refractory to medical management, or for pregnant women with gallstone-related complications [110]. Elective laparoscopic cholecystectomy is relatively safe and is the first-line option; however, it is recommended after the second trimester to reduce the rates of spontaneous abortion and preterm labor [36, 69, 110, 114]. If the condition of a pregnant woman with a complicated gallstone is too poor for surgery, percutaneous cholecystostomy with drainage may be considered [115, 116]. However, the long-term efficacy of these methods has not been proven by clinical trials; therefore, these approaches should be used only in pregnant women who require emergency therapy and are not good candidates for cholecystectomy.

Rapid Weight Loss

The risk of gallstone formation is higher during a period of acute weight loss [117]. The incidence of gallstone formation ranges from 10 to 38%, while the incidence of sequential cholecystectomy due to gallstones ranges from 6.2 to 14.7% after bariatric surgery [118]. Notably, 10–25% of obese men and women develop gallstones within a few months of beginning a very low-calorie diet [27]. Rapid weight loss (more than 1.5 kg weekly), leads to the formation of gallstones in up to 30% of individuals and increases the risks of biliary symptoms and need for cholecystectomy [27, 31–33]

UDCA is a secondary bile acid that has been used to prevent gallstone formation in obese patients undergoing acute weight loss. The administration of UDCA as a preventive agent for gallstone formation during weight loss was first reported in 1998 [118, 119]. A large amount of cholesterol can be mobilized from adipose tissue in obese individuals undergoing weight loss. During weight loss, UDCA decreases biliary cholesterol and glycoprotein secretion to reduce biliary cholesterol saturation and nucleating factors [120]. Concurrently, UDCA also reduces the intestinal absorption and biliary secretion of cholesterol.

The main advantages of UDCA therapy are its short treatment duration and its safety. Postoperative administration of UDCA did not cause mortality and the average incidence of adverse events was low [118]. The main adverse events were constipation, nausea, vomiting, and inconvenience. In addition, urgent cholecystectomy was required in fewer patients taking UDCA, compared to patients not taking UDCA. Administration of 500–600 mg of UDCA once daily or 250–300 mg twice daily for 6 months was associated with a reduced risk of postoperative gallstone formation [118].

Summary

A variety of genetic and environmental factors are involved in the pathogenesis of GB stone. A complete understanding of pathogenesis can help in the development of therapies as well as the prevention of GB stones. Currently, surgery is a gold standard for symptomatic GB stone treatment, but various medical treatments have been studied in patients with high morbidity. However, UDCA with or without CDCA is commonly used, and other drugs have only experimental results, and future clinical studies should demonstrate their safety and efficacy.

References

1. Carey MC, O'Donovan MA. Gallstone disease: current concepts on the epidemiology, pathogenesis, and management. In: Perersdorf RG, Adams RD, Braunwald E, editors. Harrison's principles of internal medicine, update V. New York: McGraw-Hill; 1984. p. 139–68.
2. Everhart JE, Ruhl CE. Burden of digestive diseases in the United States part III: liver, biliary tract, and pancreas. Gastroenterology. 2009;136:1134–44.
3. Miquel JF, Covarrubias C, Villaroel L, Mingrone G, Greco AV, Puglielli L, et al. Genetic epidemiology of cholesterol cholelithiasis among Chilean Hispanics, Amerindians, and Maoris. Gastroenterology. 1998;115:937–46.
4. Everhart JE, Yeh F, Lee ET, Hill MC, Fabsitz R, Howard BV, et al. Prevalence of gallbladder disease in American Indian populations: findings from the strong heart study. Hepatology. 2002;35:1507–12.
5. Sampliner RE, Bennett PH, Comess LJ, Rose FA, Burch TA. Gallbladder disease in pima indians. Demonstration of high prevalence and early onset by cholecystography. N Engl J Med. 1970;283:1358–64.
6. Carey MC, Paigen B. Epidemiology of the American Indians' burden and its likely genetic origins. Hepatology. 2002;36:781–91.
7. Nervi F, Miquel JF, Marshall G. The Amerindian epidemics of cholesterol gallstones: the North and South connection. Hepatology. 2003;37:947–8; author reply 948–9.
8. Lowenfels AB. Gallstones and glaciers: the stone that came in from the cold. Lancet. 1988;1:1385–6.
9. Wang DQ, Cohen DE, Carey MC. Biliary lipids and cholesterol gallstone disease. J Lipid Res. 2009;50(Suppl):S406–11.
10. Lammert F, Sauerbruch T. Mechanisms of disease: the genetic epidemiology of gallbladder stones. Nat Clin Pract Gastroenterol Hepatol. 2005;2:423–33.
11. Sarin SK, Negi VS, Dewan R, Sasan S, Saraya A. High familial prevalence of gallstones in the first-degree relatives of gallstone patients. Hepatology. 1995;22:138–41.
12. Khanuja B, Cheah YC, Hunt M, Nishina PM, Wang DQ, Chen HW, et al. Lith1, a major gene affecting cholesterol gallstone formation among inbred strains of mice. Proc Natl Acad Sci U S A. 1995;92:7729–33.
13. Katsika D, Grjibovski A, Einarsson C, Lammert F, Lichtenstein P, Marschall HU. Genetic and environmental influences on symptomatic gallstone disease: a Swedish study of 43,141 twin pairs. Hepatology. 2005;41:1138–43.
14. Valdivieso V, Covarrubias C, Siegel F, Cruz F. Pregnancy and cholelithiasis: pathogenesis and natural course of gallstones diagnosed in early puerperium. Hepatology. 1993;17:1–4.

15. Buch S, Schafmayer C, Volzke H, Becker C, Franke A, von Eller-Eberstein H, et al. A genome-wide association scan identifies the hepatic cholesterol transporter ABCG8 as a susceptibility factor for human gallstone disease. Nat Genet. 2007;39:995–9.
16. Buch S, Schafmayer C, Volzke H, Seeger M, Miquel JF, Sookoian SC, et al. Loci from a genome-wide analysis of bilirubin levels are associated with gallstone risk and composition. Gastroenterology. 2010;139(e1942):1942–51.
17. Wang DQ, Afdhal NH. Sleisenger and Fordtran's gastrointestinal and liver disease 10th edition. In: Feldman M, Friedman LS, Brandt L, editors. Elsevier Saunders; 2014. p. 1100–33.
18. Stokes CS, Krawczyk M, Lammert F. Gallstones: environment, lifestyle and genes. Dig Dis. 2011;29:191–201.
19. Paigen B, Carey MC. The genetic basis of common diseases. Oxford: Oxford University Press; 2002.
20. Mendez-Sanchez N, Chavez-Tapia NC, Motola-Kuba D, Sanchez-Lara K, Ponciano-Rodriguez G, Baptista H, et al. Metabolic syndrome as a risk factor for gallstone disease. World J Gastroenterol. 2005;11:1653–7.
21. Tsai CJ, Leitzmann MF, Willett WC, Giovannucci EL. Central adiposity, regional fat distribution, and the risk of cholecystectomy in women. Gut. 2006;55:708–14.
22. Chait A, Bierman EL, Albers JJ. Low-density lipoprotein receptor activity in cultured human skin fibroblasts. Mechanism of insulin-induced stimulation. J Clin Invest. 1979;64:1309–19.
23. Nepokroeff CM, Lakshmanan MR, Ness GC, Dugan RE, Porter JW. Regulation of the diurnal rhythm of rat liver beta-hydroxy-beta-methylglutaryl coenzmye A reductase activity by insulin, glucagon, cyclic AMP and hydrocortisone. Arch Biochem Biophys. 1974;160:387–96.
24. Subbiah MT, Yunker RL. Cholesterol 7 alpha-hydroxylase of rat liver: an insulin sensitive enzyme. Biochem Biophys Res Commun. 1984;124:896–902.
25. Weikert C, Weikert S, Schulze MB, Pischon T, Fritsche A, Bergmann MM, et al. Presence of gallstones or kidney stones and risk of type 2 diabetes. Am J Epidemiol. 2010;171:447–54.
26. Nervi F, Miquel JF, Alvarez M, Ferreccio C, Garcia-Zattera MJ, Gonzalez R, et al. Gallbladder disease is associated with insulin resistance in a high risk Hispanic population. J Hepatol. 2006;45:299–305.
27. Everhart JE. Contributions of obesity and weight loss to gallstone disease. Ann Intern Med. 1993;119:1029–35.
28. Angelin B, Backman L, Einarsson K, Eriksson L, Ewerth S. Hepatic cholesterol metabolism in obesity: activity of microsomal 3-hydroxy-3-methylglutaryl coenzyme A reductase. J Lipid Res. 1982;23:770–3.
29. Ahmed HA, Jazrawi RP, Goggin PM, Dormandy J, Northfield TC. Intrahepatic biliary cholesterol and phospholipid transport in humans: effect of obesity and cholesterol cholelithiasis. J Lipid Res. 1995;36:2562–73.
30. Marks JW, Bonorris GG, Albers G, Schoenfield LJ. The sequence of biliary events preceding the formation of gallstones in humans. Gastroenterology. 1992;103:566–70.
31. Weinsier RL, Wilson LJ, Lee J. Medically safe rate of weight loss for the treatment of obesity: a guideline based on risk of gallstone formation. Am J Med. 1995;98:115–7.
32. Moon RC, Teixeira AF, DuCoin C, Varnadore S, Jawad MA. Comparison of cholecystectomy cases after Roux-en-Y gastric bypass, sleeve gastrectomy, and gastric banding. Surg Obes Relat Dis. 2014;10:64–8.
33. Tsirline VB, Keilani ZM, El Djouzi S, Phillips RC, Kuwada TS, Gersin K, et al. How frequently and when do patients undergo cholecystectomy after bariatric surgery? Surg Obes Relat Dis. 2014;10:313–21.
34. Donovan JM, Carr-Locke DL. Gallstones. In: Eisenstat S, carlson K, editors. Primary Care of Women. St. Louis: Mosby; 1995. p. 86–97.
35. de Bari O, Wang TY, Liu M, Portincasa P, Wang DQH. Estrogen induces two distinct cholesterol crystallization pathways by activating ER and GPR30 in female mice. J Lipid Res. 2015;56:1691–700.
36. Lammert F, Gurusamy K, Ko CW, Miquel JF, Mendez-Sanchez N, Portincasa P, et al. Gallstones. Nat Rev Dis Prim. 2016;2:16024.
37. Donovan JM. Physical and metabolic factors in gallstone pathogenesis. Gastroenterol Clin North Am. 1999;28:75–97.
38. Hayes KC, Livingston A, Trautwein EA. Dietary impact on biliary lipids and gallstones. Annu Rev Nutr. 1992;12:299–326.
39. Einarsson K, Nilsell K, Leijd B, Angelin B. Influence of age on secretion of cholesterol and synthesis of bile acids by the liver. N Engl J Med. 1985;313:277–82.
40. Jorgensen T. Prevalence of gallstones in a Danish population. Am J Epidemiol. 1987;126:912–21.
41. Bennion LJ, Grundy SM. Effects of obesity and caloric intake on biliary lipid metabolism in man. J Clin Invest. 1975;56:996–1011.
42. Hofmann AF, Grundy SM, Lachin JM, Lan SP, Baum RA, Hanson RF, et al. Pretreatment biliary lipid composition in white patients with radiolucent gallstones in the national cooperative gallstone study. Gastroenterology. 1982;83:738–52.
43. Reihner E, Angelin B, Bjorkhem I, Einarsson K. Hepatic cholesterol metabolism in cholesterol gallstone disease. J Lipid Res. 1991;32:469–75.

44. Biddinger SB, Haas JT, Yu BB, Bezy O, Jing E, Zhang W, et al. Hepatic insulin resistance directly promotes formation of cholesterol gallstones. Nat Med. 2008;14:778–82.
45. Doty JE, Pitt HA, Kuchenbecker SL, DenBesten L. Impaired gallbladder emptying before gallstone formation in the prairie dog. Gastroenterology. 1983;85:168–74.
46. Jazrawi RP, Pazzi P, Petroni ML, Prandini N, Paul C, Adam JA, et al. Postprandial gallbladder motor function: refilling and turnover of bile in health and in cholelithiasis. Gastroenterology. 1995;109:582–91.
47. Behar J, Lee KY, Thompson WR, Biancani P. Gallbladder contraction in patients with pigment and cholesterol stones. Gastroenterology. 1989;97:1479–84.
48. Xu QW, Shaffer EA. The potential site of impaired gallbladder contractility in an animal model of cholesterol gallstone disease. Gastroenterology. 1996;110:251–7.
49. Yu P, Chen Q, Biancani P, Behar J. Membrane cholesterol alters gallbladder muscle contractility in prairie dogs. Am J Physiol. 1996;271:G56–61.
50. Wang DQ, Schmitz F, Kopin AS, Carey MC. Targeted disruption of the murine cholecystokinin-1 receptor promotes intestinal cholesterol absorption and susceptibility to cholesterol cholelithiasis. J Clin Invest. 2004;114:521–8.
51. Carey MC, Small DM. The physical chemistry of cholesterol solubility in bile. Relationship to gallstone formation and dissolution in man. J Clin Invest. 1978;61:998–26.
52. Smith BF. Human gallbladder mucin binds biliary lipids and promotes cholesterol crystal nucleation in model bile. J Lipid Res. 1987;28:1088–97.
53. Crawford JM, Mockel GM, Crawford AR, Hagen SJ, Hatch VC, Barnes S, et al. Imaging biliary lipid secretion in the rat: ultrastructural evidence for vesiculation of the hepatocyte canalicular membrane. J Lipid Res. 1995;36:2147–63.
54. Magnuson TH, Lillemoe KD, Pitt HA. How many americans will be eligible for biliary lithotripsy. Arch Surg. 1989;124:1195–200.
55. Ostrow JD, Celic L, Mukerjee P. Molecular and micellar associations in the Ph-dependent stable and metastable dissolution of unconjugated bilirubin by bile-salts. J Lipid Res. 1988;29:335–48.
56. Brink MA, MendezSanchez N, Carey MC. Bilirubin cycles enterohepatically after ileal resection in the rat. Gastroenterology. 1996;110:1945–57.
57. Donovan JM, Leonard MR, Batta AK, Carey MC. Calcium affinity for biliary lipid aggregates in model biles—complementary importance of bile-salts and lecithin. Gastroenterology. 1994;107:831–46.
58. Cahalane MJ, Neubrand MW, Carey MC. Physical-chemical pathogenesis of pigment gallstones. Semin Liver Dis. 1988;8:317–28.
59. Sandstad O, Osnes T, Skar V, Urdal P, Osnes M. Common bile duct stones are mainly brown and associated with duodenal diverticula. Gut. 1994;35:1464–7.
60. Schoenfield LJ, Sjovall J, Sjovall K. Bile acid composition of gallstones from man. J Lab Clin Med. 1966;68:186–94.
61. Kaufman HS, Magnuson TH, Lillemoe KD, Frasca P, Pitt HA. The role of bacteria in gallbladder and common duct stone formation. Ann Surg. 1989;209:584–92.
62. Stewart L, Smith AL, Pellegrini CA, Motson RW, Way LW. Pigment gallstones form as a composite of bacterial microcolonies and pigment solids. Ann Surg. 1987;206:242–50.
63. Diehl AK, Sugarek NJ, Todd KH. Clinical evaluation for gallstone disease: usefulness of symptoms and signs in diagnosis. Am J Med. 1990;89:29–33.
64. Gibney EJ. Asymptomatic gallstones. Br J Surg. 1990;77:368–72.
65. Rigas B, Torosis J, McDougall CJ, Vener KJ, Spiro HM. The circadian rhythm of biliary colic. J Clin Gastroenterol. 1990;12:409–14.
66. Thistle JL, Cleary PA, Lachin JM, Tyor MP, Hersh T. The natural history of cholelithiasis: the national cooperative gallstone study. Ann Intern Med. 1984;101:171–5.
67. Friedman GD, Raviola CA, Fireman B. Prognosis of gallstones with mild or no symptoms: 25 years of follow-up in a health maintenance organization. J Clin Epidemiol. 1989;42:127–36.
68. Portincasa P, Moschetta A, Palasciano G. Cholesterol gallstone disease. Lancet. 2006;368:230–9.
69. Tazuma S, Unno M, Igarashi Y, Inui K, Uchiyama K, Kai M, et al. Evidence-based clinical practice guidelines for cholelithiasis 2016. J Gastroenterol. 2017;52:276–300.
70. Gracie WA, Ransohoff DF. The natural history of silent gallstones: the innocent gallstone is not a myth. N Engl J Med. 1982;307:798–800.
71. Festi D, Reggiani ML, Attili AF, Loria P, Pazzi P, Scaioli E, et al. Natural history of gallstone disease: expectant management or active treatment? Results from a population-based cohort study. J Gastroenterol Hepatol. 2010;25:719–24.
72. Shabanzadeh DM, Sorensen LT, Jorgensen T. A prediction rule for risk stratification of incidentally discovered gallstones: results from a large cohort study. Gastroenterology. 2016;150(e151):156–67.
73. Attili AF, De Santis A, Capri R, Repice AM, Maselli S. The natural history of gallstones: the GREPCO experience. The GREPCO Group. Hepatology. 1995;21:655–60.
74. McSherry CK, Ferstenberg H, Calhoun WF, Lahman E, Virshup M. The natural history of diagnosed gallstone disease in symptomatic and asymptomatic patients. Ann Surg. 1985;202:59–63.
75. Cucchiaro G, Rossitch JC, Bowie J, Branum GD, Niotis MT, Watters CR, et al. Clinical significance

of ultrasonographically detected coincidental gallstones. Dig Dis Sci. 1990;35:417–21.
76. Zubler J, Markowski G, Yale S, Graham R, Rosenthal TC. Natural history of asymptomatic gallstones in family practice office practices. Arch Fam Med. 1998;7:230–3.
77. Sakorafas GH, Milingos D, Peros G. Asymptomatic cholelithiasis: is cholecystectomy really needed? A critical reappraisal 15 years after the introduction of laparoscopic cholecystectomy. Dig Dis Sci. 2007;52:1313–25.
78. Guarino MP, Cocca S, Altomare A, Emerenziani S, Cicala M. Ursodeoxycholic acid therapy in gallbladder disease, a story not yet completed. World J Gastroenterol. 2013;19:5029–34.
79. Portincasa P, Ciaula AD, Bonfrate L, Wang DQ. Therapy of gallstone disease: What it was, what it is, what it will be. World J Gastrointest Pharmacol Ther. 2012;3:7–20.
80. Keus F, de Jong JA, Gooszen HG, van Laarhoven CJ. Laparoscopic versus small-incision cholecystectomy for patients with symptomatic cholecystolithiasis. Cochrane Database Syst Rev. 2006. https://doi.org/10.1002/14651858.CD006229.CD006229.
81. Keus F, de Jong JA, Gooszen HG, van Laarhoven CJ. Laparoscopic versus open cholecystectomy for patients with symptomatic cholecystolithiasis. Cochrane Database Syst Rev. 2006. https://doi.org/10.1002/14651858.CD006231.CD006231.
82. Di Ciaula A, Wang DQ, Wang HH, Bonfrate L, Portincasa P. Targets for current pharmacologic therapy in cholesterol gallstone disease. Gastroenterol Clin North Am. 2010;39:245–64, viii–ix.
83. Deziel DJ, Millikan KW, Economou SG, Doolas A, Ko ST, Airan MC. Complications of laparoscopic cholecystectomy: a national survey of 4,292 hospitals and an analysis of 77,604 cases. Am J Surg. 1993;165:9–14.
84. Scott TR, Zucker KA, Bailey RW. Laparoscopic cholecystectomy: a review of 12,397 patients. Surg Laparosc Endosc. 1992;2:191–8.
85. Lowenfels AB, Lindstrom CG, Conway MJ, Hastings PR. Gallstones and risk of gallbladder cancer. J Natl Cancer Inst. 1985;75:77–80.
86. Randi G, Franceschi S, La Vecchia C. Gallbladder cancer worldwide: geographical distribution and risk factors. Int J Cancer. 2006;118:1591–602.
87. Bonatsos G, Birbas K, Toutouzas K, Durakis N. Laparoscopic cholecystectomy in adults with sickle cell disease. Surg Endosc. 2001;15:816–9.
88. Danzinger RG, Hofmann AF, Schoenfield LJ, Thistle JL. Dissolution of cholesterol gallstones by chenodeoxycholic acid. N Engl J Med. 1972;286:1–8.
89. Makino I, Shinozaki K, Yoshino K, Nakagawa S. Dissolution of cholesterol gallstones by long-term administration of ursodeoxycholic acid. Nihon Shokakibyo Gakkai Zasshi. 1975;72:690–702.
90. Roma MG, Toledo FD, Boaglio AC, Basiglio CL, Crocenzi FA, Sanchez Pozzi EJ. Ursodeoxycholic acid in cholestasis: linking action mechanisms to therapeutic applications. Clin Sci (Lond). 2011;121:523–44.
91. Bachrach WH, Hofmann AF. Ursodeoxycholic acid in the treatment of cholesterol cholelithiasis. part I. Dig Dis Sci. 1982;27:737–61.
92. Podda M, Zuin M, Battezzati PM, Ghezzi C, de Fazio C, Dioguardi ML. Efficacy and safety of a combination of chenodeoxycholic acid and ursodeoxycholic acid for gallstone dissolution: a comparison with ursodeoxycholic acid alone. Gastroenterology. 1989;96:222–9.
93. Caroli A, Del Favero G, Di Mario F, Spigariol F, Scalon P, Meggiato T, et al. Computed tomography in predicting gall stone solubility: a prospective trial. Gut. 1992;33:698–700.
94. Petroni ML, Jazrawi RP, Grundy A, Lanzini A, Pigozzi MG, Biasio A, et al. Prospective, multicenter study on value of computerized tomography (CT) in gallstone disease in predicting response to bile acid therapy. Dig Dis Sci. 1995;40:1956–62.
95. Pereira SP, Veysey MJ, Kennedy C, Hussaini SH, Murphy GM, Dowling RH. Gallstone dissolution with oral bile acid therapy. Importance of pretreatment CT scanning and reasons for nonresponse. Dig Dis Sci. 1997;42:1775–82.
96. May GR, Sutherland LR, Shaffer EA. Efficacy of bile acid therapy for gallstone dissolution: a meta-analysis of randomized trials. Aliment Pharmacol Ther. 1993;7:139–48.
97. Fromm H, Roat JW, Gonzalez V, Sarva RP, Farivar S. Comparative efficacy and side effects of ursodeoxycholic and chenodeoxycholic acids in dissolving gallstones. A double-blind controlled study. Gastroenterology. 1983;85:1257–64.
98. Erlinger S, Le Go A, Husson JM, Fevery J. Franco-Belgian cooperative study of ursodeoxycholic acid in the medical dissolution of gallstones: a double-blind, randomized, dose-response study, and comparison with chenodeoxycholic acid. Hepatology. 1984;4:308–14.
99. Rabenstein T, Radespiel-Troger M, Hopfner L, Benninger J, Farnbacher M, Greess H, et al. Ten years experience with piezoelectric extracorporeal shockwave lithotripsy of gallbladder stones. Eur J Gastroenterol Hepatol. 2005;17:629–39.
100. Villanova N, Bazzoli F, Taroni F, Frabboni R, Mazzella G, Festi D, et al. Gallstone recurrence after successful oral bile acid treatment. A 12-year follow-up study and evaluation of long-term postdissolution treatment. Gastroenterology. 1989;97:726–31.
101. Petroni ML, Jazrawi RP, Pazzi P, Zuin M, Lanzini A, Fracchia M, et al. Risk factors for the development of gallstone recurrence following medical dissolution. The British-Italian Gallstone Study Group. Eur J Gastroenterol Hepatol. 2000;12:695–700.

102. Doran J, Keighley MR, Bell GD. Rowachol–a possible treatment for cholesterol gallstones. Gut. 1979;20:312–7.
103. Wang HH, Portincasa P, Mendez-Sanchez N, Uribe M, Wang DQ. Effect of ezetimibe on the prevention and dissolution of cholesterol gallstones. Gastroenterology. 2008;134:2101–10.
104. Simopoulos AP. Importance of the ratio of omega-6/omega-3 essential fatty acids: evolutionary aspects. World Rev Nutr Diet. 2003;92:1–22.
105. Kim JK, Cho SM, Kang SH, Kim E, Yi H, Yun ES, et al. N-3 polyunsaturated fatty acid attenuates cholesterol gallstones by suppressing mucin production with a high cholesterol diet in mice. J Gastroenterol Hepatol. 2012;27:1745–51.
106. Jang SI, Fang S, Kim KP, Ko Y, Kim H, Oh J, et al. Combination treatment with n-3 polyunsaturated fatty acids and ursodeoxycholic acid dissolves cholesterol gallstones in mice. Sci Rep. 2019;9:12740.
107. Lee BJ, Kim JS, Kim BK, Jung SJ, Joo MK, Hong SG, et al. Effects of sphingolipid synthesis inhibition on cholesterol gallstone formation in C57BL/6 J mice. J Gastroenterol Hepatol. 2010;25:1105–10.
108. Shubha MC, Reddy RR, Srinivasan K. Antilithogenic influence of dietary capsaicin and curcumin during experimental induction of cholesterol gallstone in mice. Appl Physiol Nutr Metab. 2011;36:201–9.
109. Scragg RK, McMichael AJ, Seamark RF. Oral contraceptives, pregnancy, and endogenous oestrogen in gall stone disease–a case-control study. Br Med J (Clin Res Ed). 1984;288:1795–9.
110. de Bari O, Wang TY, Liu M, Paik CN, Portincasa P, Wang DQ. Cholesterol cholelithiasis in pregnant women: pathogenesis, prevention and treatment. Ann Hepatol. 2014;13:728–45.
111. Ko CW, Beresford SA, Schulte SJ, Matsumoto AM, Lee SP. Incidence, natural history, and risk factors for biliary sludge and stones during pregnancy. Hepatology. 2005;41:359–65.
112. Maringhini A, Ciambra M, Baccelliere P, Raimondo M, Orlando A, Tine F, et al. Biliary sludge and gallstones in pregnancy: incidence, risk factors, and natural history. Ann Intern Med. 1993;119:116–20.
113. Glasgow RE, Visser BC, Harris HW, Patti MG, Kilpatrick SJ, Mulvihill SJ. Changing management of gallstone disease during pregnancy. Surg Endosc. 1998;12:241–6.
114. Lu EJ, Curet MJ, El-Sayed YY, Kirkwood KS. Medical versus surgical management of biliary tract disease in pregnancy. Am J Surg. 2004;188:755–9.
115. Caliskan K. The use of percutaneous cholecystostomy in the treatment of acute cholecystitis during pregnancy. Clin Exp Obstet Gynecol. 2017;44:11–3.
116. Allmendinger N, Hallisey MJ, Ohki SK, Straub JJ. Percutaneous cholecystostomy treatment of acute cholecystitis in pregnancy. Obstet Gynecol. 1995;86:653–4.
117. Worobetz LJ, Inglis FG, Shaffer EA. The effect of ursodeoxycholic acid therapy on gallstone formation in the morbidly obese during rapid weight-loss. Am J Gastroenterol. 1993;88:1705–10.
118. Magouliotis DE, Tasiopoulou VS, Svokos AA, Svokos KA, Chatedaki C, Sioka E, et al. Ursodeoxycholic acid in the prevention of gallstone formation after bariatric surgery: an updated systematic review and meta-analysis. Obes Surg. 2017;27:3021–30.
119. Broomfield PH, Chopra R, Sheinbaum RC, Bonorris GG, Silverman A, Schoenfield LJ, et al. Effects of ursodeoxycholic acid and aspirin on the formation of lithogenic bile and gallstones during loss of weight. N Engl J Med. 1988;319:1567–72.
120. Williams C, Gowan R, Perey BJ. A double-blind placebo-controlled trial of ursodeoxycholic acid in the prevention of gallstones during weight loss after vertical banded gastroplasty. Obes Surg. 1993;3:257–9.
121. Donovan JM, Carey MC. Physical-chemical basis of gallstone formation. Gastroenterol Clin North Am. 1991;20:47–66.

Acalculous Cholecystitis: Diagnosis and Treatment

Seung Woo Yi and Don Haeng Lee

Introduction

Acute acalculous cholecystitis (AAC) is an acute necroinflammatory condition of the gallbladder (GB) that occurs in the absence of cholelithiasis and is attributable to a multifactorial pathogenesis. AAC accounts for approximately 10% (2–15%) of all cases of acute cholecystitis and is associated with high morbidity and mortality.

In this chapter, we review the pathophysiology, epidemiology, clinical manifestations, diagnosis, and treatment of AAC.

Pathogenesis

To date, the pathogenesis of AAC remains unclear. This condition may result from bile stasis or GB ischemia; however, several factors have been implicated in its aetiopathogenesis. Bile stasis can occur secondary to fasting, obstruction, postoperative/procedural irritation, or ileus (associated with total parenteral nutrition), which can lead to bile injection directly toxic to the GB epithelium. Ischemia of GB may occur at many risks associated with systemic inflammation and can have a direct detrimental effect on all layers of the GB wall [1, 2].

AAC is characterized by the following findings: (1) increased leucocyte margination (corresponding to ischemia and reperfusion injury), (2) increased focal lymphatic dilatation with interstitial edema associated with local microvascular occlusion (ischemia-induced) and, (3) increased and deeper bile infiltration into the GB wall suggesting bile stasis and increased epithelial permeability with consequent epithelial damage.

These features corroborate the hypothesis that implicates bile stasis and ischemia as aetiopathogenetic contributors to AAC.

Previous studies have discussed microvascular involvement associated with bile stasis, hypoperfusion, and ischemia in patients with AAC. The usual trend observed is progression to hypoperfusion and ischemia (which could be associated with any cause, usually sepsis), and GB inflammation, with consequent cholestasis and bacterial invasion culminating in AAC. This natural progression of the pathological process explains the frequent complications such as gangrene, empyema, and perforation caused by local microvascular occlusion, secondary infection, and a weakened GB wall, respectively [3, 4].

S. W. Yi (✉)
Division of Gastroenterology, Department of Internal Medicine, Yong-in Severance Hospital, Yonsei University College of Medicine, Yong-in, South Korea
e-mail: yiseungwoo@yuhs.ac

D. H. Lee
Division of Gastroenterology, Department of Internal Medicine, Inha University Hospital, Inha University School of Medicine, Incheon, South Korea

J. B. Chung and K. Okazaki (eds.), *Diseases of the Gallbladder*,
https://doi.org/10.1007/978-981-15-6010-1_9

However, this model does not explain the occurrence of AAC in an outpatient setting or AAC in the absence of known risk factors. Despite much research regarding this topic, the pathogenesis of AAC remains unclear.

Epidemiology

AAC most often occurs in critically ill patients and is particularly associated with trauma, surgery, shock, burns, sepsis, total parenteral nutrition, and/or prolonged fasting (Table 1).

A study compared the clinicopathological features and results of treatment in patients with AAC and acute calculous cholecystitis (ACC) and reported the following findings: Patients with AAC were older (69 years vs. 61 years) and were more likely to be febrile (46% vs. 21%) and hypotensive (23% vs. 5%) at initial presentation. Cerebrovascular accidents were significantly more common in patients with AAC than in those with ACC (15.9% vs. 6.7%). The incidence of chronic obstructive airway disease was higher in the AAC group (26% vs. 6%) in addition to a higher incidence of gangrenous cholecystitis (31.2 vs. 5.6%). Cerebrovascular accidents were significantly more frequent in patients with AAC than in those with ACC (15.9 vs. 6.7%).

No statistically significant intergroup difference was observed in the overall operative outcomes, regardless of treatment modalities. However, the length of postoperative hospitalization was higher in the AAC group (5 days vs. 3 days). Moreover, the recurrence rate after non-surgical treatment was significantly lower in the AAC group (2.7 vs. 23.2%) [5, 6].

Postoperative AAC is most commonly associated with gastrointestinal surgery, particularly gastric and colorectal procedures. Following a review of the English literature, we identified 28

Table 1 Risk factors of acute acalculous cholecystitis

Relatively common risk factors		
Sepsis		
	Bacterial	Brucellosis, Q fever, Leptospirosis, Tuberculosis, Scrub typhus, Salmonellosis, Cholera
	Fungal	Candida species
	Parasite	Cyclospora, Microsporidia, *Plasmodium falciparum*, *Plasmodium vivax*, *Schistosoma mansoni*
	Viral	Cytomegalovirus, Epstein-Barr virus, Dengue virus, Hepatitis
Critical illness (Requiring ICU care)		
Total parenteral nutrition		
Shock		
Recent general surgery		
Trauma	Injury severity score >12, and tachycardia >120 bpm	
Burn		
Relatively rare risk factors		
Hypovolemia		
Post-endoscopic retrograde cholangiopancreatography		
Immunodeficiency	Acquired immune deficiency syndrome, Transplant, Post-chemotherapy	
Chronic illness	Diabetes, Hypertension, Atherosclerotic disease, Chronic obstructive pulmonary disease	
Bile duct obstruction	Ampullary tumor, Metastasis, Sphincter of Oddi dysfunction	

articles that report 76 cases of AAC after gastrointestinal operations; 52.4% of patients developed gangrenous AAC with a mortality rate of 21.1% significantly higher than that associated with postoperative calculous cholecystitis [7].

Most patients showed known risk factors for AAC, including blood transfusion (56.6%), sepsis (52.2%), mechanical ventilation (45.5%), prolonged fasting or total parenteral nutrition (44.4%), and narcotic medication use (10%). Studies have reported that AAC is a rare life-threatening condition that may also occur and complicate recovery in patients with large thermal burns. The incidence of AAC in patients with burns ranges between 0.4 and 3.5%, and it typically affects men (82.4%) with a mean age of 35 years. Notably, 97.8% of burns involved >30% of the total body surface area. Improvements in critical care rendered to patients with burns have improved the management of known risk factors and reduced the incidence of this condition over recent decades [8].

AAC is the most frequent form of acute cholecystitis observed in children. Most cases of AAC in children occur in critically ill or post-surgical patients (similar to AAC in adults); however, most pediatric cases are associated with infectious diseases. In addition to bacterial and parasitic infections, most recent studies report AAC in children with viral illnesses, particularly, Epstein–Barr and hepatitis A virus infections [9, 10].

Notably, a few reports describe AAC in children with non-infectious disorders, such as immune-mediated conditions. Therefore, the medical management protocol for children with AAC significantly differs from that implemented in adults [11].

Diagnosis

Acute cholecystitis was diagnosed based on the Tokyo guidelines; diagnostic criteria included a combination of typical clinical symptoms (right upper quadrant pain/mass, tenderness, fever, positive Murphy's sign, and leukocytosis or elevated serum C-reactive protein levels) and radiological findings consistent with acute cholecystitis (an enlarged GB, thickened GB wall, or pericholecystic fluid collection observed on computed tomography [CT] or ultrasonography [US]) [12] (Table 2).

Compared with ACC, AAC is diagnostically challenging owing to the lack of specific clinical findings such as symptom review, physical examination, and laboratory tests. Notably, several confounding factors have been implicated in this condition; AAC usually occurs in critically ill patients in whom it is difficult to confirm the diagnosis during sedation, intubation, and/or an unconscious state in the intensive care unit. Furthermore, right upper quadrant pain, fever, leukocytosis, and abnormal liver function tests observed in these patients are not specific to AAC.

Although a combination of clinical factors may not conclusively establish the diagnosis, AAC should be suspected in all critically ill patients with no specific etiology to explain their condition.

The optimal diagnostic imaging modality for AAC remains controversial. Furthermore, the modality that should be used first in such cases is debatable. Most retrospective and prospective studies that have investigated this issue are small-scale studies, which limit the critical assessment of the role of radiological diagnosis. Radiological criteria for the diagnosis of AAC have been developed for the use of US, CT, and a hepatobiliary iminodiacetic acid scan (HIDA). Magnetic resonance imaging offers no benefit over other imaging modalities and is therefore not recommended.

Ultrasonography

Usually, US is the first-choice imaging modality for evaluation of suspected AAC owing to advantages such as rapidity, repeatability, and portability. The most studied diagnostic criteria for US are GB wall thickness, pericholecystic fluid or subserosal edema, intramural gas, coarse mucosa, sludge, and hydrops. The major and minor criteria for US-based diagnosis of AAC are listed in Table 2. GB wall thickness (3.5–4 mm) is

Table 2 Diagnostic criteria by imaging

Modality	Criteria		Diagnosis
US	Major	3.5–4-mm (or more)-thick wall (if at least 5 cm distended longitudinally with no ascites of hypoalbuminemia)	2 major or 1 major and 2 minor (most studies have favored the diagnostic triad—wall thickness, sludge, hydrops)
		Pericholecystic flud (halo)/subserosal edema	
		Intramural gas	
		Sloughed mucosal membrane	
	Minor	Echogenic bile (sludge)	
		Hydrops = distension greater than 8 cm longitudinally or 5 cm transversely (with clear fluid)	
CT	Major	3–4-mm wall thickness	2 major or 1 major and 2 minor
		Pericholecystic fluid	
		Subserosal edema	
		Intramural gas	
		Sloughed mucosa	
	Minor	Hyperdense bile (sludge)	
		Subjective distension (hydrops)	
HIDA	Nonvisualization of the gallbladder 1 hour after an injection of radiolabeled technetium (this is RC)		RC alone or RC and MC have been used
	Nonvisualization of the gallbladder 30 minutes after injection of morphine (after initial radiolabeled technetium) (this is MC)		

RC: radionuclide cholescintigraphy, MC: morphine cholescintigraphy considered an important component of the diagnostic criteria for AAC. The most researched and cited criterion is the diagnostic triad of GB wall thickness, sludge, and hydrops. However, this triad is not absolute. A few studies have reported that some or all criteria comprising the triad may be present in a few patients in the intensive care unit who may not show AAC. This does not mean that US findings are not useful or that they do not suggest a diagnosis of AAC. The finding only shows that these results may be nonspecific and should therefore not be considered alone, without correlation with patients' clinical features and results of other imaging modalities.

A meta-analysis that compared various diagnostic imaging modalities for acute cholecystitis reported that US showed 81% sensitivity and 83% specificity; the differences in sensitivity and specificity could be attributable to the fact that this meta-analysis included small-sized retrospective studies that used diverse criteria to investigate the rarity and US-aided diagnosis of AAC [13, 14].

Computed Tomography

Typical CT findings in patients with AAC include GB distension, wall thickening, mucosal hyperenhancement, pericholecystic fat stranding or fluid collection, no gallstones, and reactive hyperemia surrounding the GB fossa within the liver parenchyma adjacent to the inflamed GB (CT rim sign). Many mixed cholesterol or pigment stones show attenuation patterns similar to those of bile and are not clearly identifiable using standard CT kilovoltage settings; therefore, distinguishing these cases from gallstone cholecystitis is challenging.

Moreover, diffuse thickening of the GB wall is a nonspecific finding associated with a wide range of inflammatory conditions, such as hypoalbuminemia, ascites, chronic cholecystitis, hepatitis, and pancreatitis. The negative predictive value of CT is lower than that of US (approximately 89% vs. 97%). CT is most often used in patients with abdominal pain, which is not specific for acute cholecystitis. Therefore, negative CT findings can rule out or at least suggest acute cholecystitis. CT diagnostic criteria are similar to those applicable for US [15, 16].

HIDA Scan

Nuclear medicine hepatobiliary imaging (HIDA scan) is a time-proven imaging methodology that uses radioactive drugs and specialized cameras for diagnostic imaging based on the body's physiological processes. HIDA radiopharmaceuticals are extracted by hepatocytes and cleared through the biliary system similar to bilirubin elimination.

The most common indication for HIDA imaging is acute cholecystitis, diagnosed by non-filling of the GB secondary to cystic duct obstruction. HIDA scanning can detect high-grade biliary obstruction prior to ductal dilatation; images reveal a persistent hepatogram without biliary clearance owing to the high backpressure. HIDA imaging also aids in the diagnosis of partial biliary obstruction caused by stones, biliary stricture, and sphincter of Oddi obstruction and can also confirm biliary leakage post-cholecystectomy and hepatic transplantation. Calculation of the GB ejection fraction after cholecystokinin (CCK) infusion is commonly used to diagnose chronic acalculous GB disease. In patients who undergo a CCK-HIDA scan, the GB ejection fraction is measured following CCK-induced GB contraction. Nuclear medicine procedures are time-consuming. This test needs to be performed over several hours; therefore, it is only suitable for selected patients. A GB ejection fraction <35% indicates GB dysfunction and AAC. Studies have reported that HIDA imaging showed sensitivity and specificity of 67–100% and 58–88%, respectively [17, 18].

Treatment

The administration of intravenous antibiotics is the first-line treatment for AAC in a hospital setting. The Surgical Infection Society and the Infectious Diseases Society of America guide whether antibiotic recommendations were a community or a hospital in 2010, but will focus on the therapies obtained in the hospital. The carbapenems and piperacillin/tazobactam constitute first-line antimicrobial monotherapy in these patients. The duration of antibiotic administration depends on control of the infection source, and antibiotics can be discontinued 4–5 days after the subsidence of infection. In patients in whom the source of infection cannot be controlled, the duration of antibiotic therapy should be based on the reduction in inflammatory biomarker levels, elimination of fever, and clinical improvement. No previous research and definitive guidelines are available in this regard; therefore, clinicians should determine the duration of antibiotic therapy on a case-by-case basis [19, 20].

Currently, there is a lack of consensus regarding cholecystectomy vs. percutaneous cholecystostomy (PC) as the therapy of choice for AAC. Cholecystectomy is the mainstay of treatment for AAC, particularly in patients with suspected perforation or gangrene. Although cholecystectomy is usually recommended for AAC, nonsurgical management may be feasible in patients who are deemed hemodynamically unstable to tolerate general anesthesia. PC is the recommended treatment for critically ill patients who show further deterioration or are deemed unfit for surgery. PC in critically ill patients with acute cholecystitis was first reported by Radder in 1980. It was mainly used as a bridging procedure that was followed by interval cholecystectomy after stabilization of the patient. Recently, several studies have reported the efficacy and safety of PC to definitively treat acute cholecystitis; it is usually considered definitive treatment for selected patients with high postoperative mortality and significant comorbidities. However, whether subsequent cholecystectomy is warranted in these patients remains controversial [21, 22].

PC used for definitive treatment of AAC reduces surgery-related mortality and other costs. Despite these advantages of PC, recurrent AAC cannot be avoided in all cases. Previous studies have shown that recurrence rates of cholecystitis after PC range from 4 to 22%. Therefore, it is necessary to assess the risk of recurrent AAC to determine the need for interval cholecystectomy in patients who undergo initial PC [23].

A study that investigated the role of interval cholecystectomy after PC in patients with AAC reported the following findings: PC was successfully performed in all 271 patients at diagnosis. The overall PC-induced complication rate was 2.2%, and the 30-day mortality rate was 8.4%. Notably, 46.8% of patients underwent interval cholecystectomy mostly during the index admission, early cholecystectomy during the index admission (111 patients), and interval cholecystectomy (16 patients) at a mean of 294 days after PC. In the remaining 44.6% (121 patients) who underwent only PC, the percutaneous drain was removed successfully in 72.7% of patients following a successful trial of catheter clamping, and an indwelling catheter was maintained in the remaining patients. The recurrence rate after drain removal was only 2.3% [24].

Although interval cholecystectomy is useful to prevent recurrence after resolution of AAC, the recurrence-free survival rate was good in most patients who did not undergo interval cholecystectomy. An increasing number of studies report that PC not only serves as a bridge for cholecystectomy but can also be considered definitive treatment for AAC, particularly in high-risk surgical patients [25, 26].

Although current guidelines discuss the role of PC in patients with AAC, these recommendations are based on limited Level II evidence. Based on the guidelines established by the American Gastrointestinal and Endoscopic Surgeon Association, PC is an effective temporary measure for critically ill patients with AAC. The Tokyo 2018 guidelines recommend PC at moderate acute cholecystitis in patients showing a significant GB inflammation. Moderate acute cholecystitis is usually characterized by ≥ 1 of the following findings: leukocytosis >18,000, a painful and noticeable upper right quadrant mass, symptoms lasting >72 hours, and local inflammation (defined as GB wall thickness of 8 mm) [12].

The optimal timing of PC catheter removal is controversial. Some authors prefer removal of the catheter during hospitalization after the resolution of sepsis; the mean duration reported in the literature is 4–6 weeks. In contrast, other studies have reported that PC tube drainage is continued over >2 weeks and is an independent risk factor associated with early relapse [27, 28]. Previous animal studies have shown that irritation of the GB mucosa could precipitate AAC [29].

Usually, PC drainage is maintained for at least 6 weeks, and the PC catheter is clamped for 1–2 weeks before the removal to reduce the risk of recurrence. The PC catheter needs to be maintained for a longer duration in patients with common bile duct stones, calculous cholecystitis, and underlying malignant tumors, and patients' symptoms and signs should be closely monitored after catheter removal [30, 31].

Endoscopic ultrasound-guided transmural GB drainage is an alternative to PC in patients with acute, high-risk, or advanced-stage cholecystitis who are refractory to initial medical treatment and cannot undergo cholecystectomy. A variety of stents have been described, including plastic stents, self-expandable metal stents, and lumen-apposing metal stents (LAMS). LAMS represent the only specifically designed model for transmural GB drainage. LAMS placement is not associated with external drainage, and the technical and clinical success rates are nearly similar, which serve as advantages of this device. An appropriate stent selection is important, and research is warranted to develop next-generation dedicated devices to further improve the feasibility and safety of these stents. Comparative controlled studies are necessary to confirm these results with regard to long-term outcomes and cost-effectiveness of these devices [32, 33].

Prognosis

The high incidence of gangrene of the GB in patients with AAC implicates ischemia as an etiopathogenetic contributor to this condition and explains the rapidity of disease progression and poor prognosis. Morbidity and mortality rates are higher in patients with AAC than in those with calculous cholecystitis. The mortality rate in critically ill patients with AAC is as high as 30%, although this rate can range from 6.7% (if diagnosed at an early stage) to 90% (if diagnosed during the late stages of pathological disease progression). The disparity in mortality rates could be attributed to patients' underlying condition, age, diagnostic delay, and therapeutic modalities used across different study populations [34, 35].

Therefore, early diagnosis and prompt treatment are essential to avoid a fulminant course and complications. In fact, necrosis, emphysema, and perforation are often reported in patients with AAC. This constitutes a high-risk group of patients in whom intervention would not alter the disease course. These results suggest that AAC is not only an indicator of a fatal condition but also a factor that affects mortality from severe systemic inflammatory reactions [36].

Conclusion

Early diagnosis and prompt treatment of AAC are essential to avoid a fulminant course and complications, such as GB gangrene or perforation associated with high mortality rates. This emphasizes the need for a high index of clinical suspicion among clinicians for early diagnosis postoperatively. This is because of the complex clinical setting in which AAC occurs, the lack of large prospective controlled trials evaluating the various diagnostic modalities for AAC, and the consequent dependence on a small database for clinical decision making. PC may be feasible in patients with AAC; it is associated with low mortality rates and reduces the need for future cholecystectomy. Moreover, the endoscopic approach using LAMS is useful for safe and effective transmural GB drainage in patients with AAC.

References

1. Kaminski DL, Amir G, Deshpande YG, Beck D, Li AP. Studies on the etiology of acute acalculous cholecystitis: the effect of lipopolysaccharide on human gallbladder mucosal cells. Prostaglandins. 1994;47:319–30.
2. Kaminski DL, Andrus CH, German D, Deshpande YG. The role of prostanoids in the production of acute acalculous cholecystitis by platelet-activating factor. Ann Surg. 1990;212:455–61.
3. Laurila JJ, Ala-Kokko TI, Laurila PA, Saarnio J, Koivukangas V, Syrjälä H, et al. Histopathology of acute acalculous cholecystitis in critically ill patients. Histopathology. 2005;47:485–92.
4. McChesney JA, Northup PG, Bickston SJ. Acute acalculous cholecystitis associated with systemic sepsis and visceral arterial hypoperfusion: a case series and review of pathophysiology. Dig Dis Sci. 2003;48:1960–7.
5. Nikfarjam M, Manya K, Fink MA, Hadj AK, Muralidharan V, Starkey G, et al. Outcomes of patients with histologically proven acute acalculous cholecystitis. ANZ J Surg. 2012;82:918–22.
6. Gu MG, Kim TN, Song J, Nam YJ, Lee JY, Park JS. Risk factors and therapeutic outcomes of acute acalculous cholecystitis. Digestion. 2014;90:75–80.
7. Crichlow L, Walcott-Sapp S, Major J, Jaffe B, Bellows CF. Acute acalculous cholecystitis after gastrointestinal surgery. Am Surg. 2012;78:220–4.
8. Walsh K, Goutos I, Dheansa B. Acute acalculous cholecystitis in burns: a review. J Burn Care Res. 2018;39:724–8.
9. Tsakayannis DE, Kozakewich HP, Lillehei CW. Acalculous cholecystitis in children. J Pediatr Surg. 1996;31:127–30.
10. Poddighe D, Tresoldi M, Licari A, Marseglia GL. Acalculous acute cholecystitis in previously healthy children: general overview and analysis of pediatric infectious cases. Int J Hepatol. 2015;2015:459608.
11. Murphy PB, Vogt KN, Winick-Ng J, McClure JA, Welk B, Jones SA. The increasing incidence of gallbladder disease in children: A 20 year perspective. J Pediatr Surg. 2016;51:748–52.
12. Yokoe M, Hata J, Takada T, Strasberg SM, Asbun HJ, Wakabayashi G, et al. Tokyo Guidelines 2018: diagnostic criteria and severity grading of acute cholecystitis (with videos). J Hepatobiliary Pancreat Sci. 2018;25:41–54.
13. Kiewiet JJ, Leeuwenburgh MM, Bipat S, Bossuyt PM, Stoker J, Boermeester MA. A systematic review and meta-analysis of diagnostic performance of imaging in acute cholecystitis. Radiology. 2012;264:708–20.
14. Huffman JL, Schenker S. Acute acalculous cholecystitis: a review. Clin Gastroenterol Hepatol. 2010;8:15–22.
15. Shakespear JS, Shaaban AM, Rezvani M. CT findings of acute cholecystitis and its complications. AJR Am J Roentgenol. 2010;194:1523–9.
16. McGillicuddy EA, Schuster KM, Brown E, Maxfield MW, Davis KA, Longo WE. Acute cholecystitis in the elderly: use of computed tomography and correlation with ultrasonography. Am J Surg. 2011;202:524–7.
17. Ziessman HA. Nuclear medicine hepatobiliary imaging. Clin Gastroenterol Hepatol. 2010;8:111–6.
18. Mariat G, Mahul P, Prévt N, De Filippis JP, Cuilleron M, Dubois F, et al. Contribution of ultrasonography and cholescintigraphy to the diagnosis of acute acalculous cholecystitis in intensive care unit patients. Intensive Care Med. 2000;26:1658–63.
19. Sawyer RG, Claridge JA, Nathens AB, Rotstein OD, Duane TM, Evans HL, et al. Trial of short-course antimicrobial therapy for intraabdominal infection. N Engl J Med. 2015;372:1996–2005.
20. Solomkin JS, Mazuski JE, Bradley JS, Rodvold KA, Goldstein EJ, Baron EJ, et al. Diagnosis and management of complicated intra-abdominal infection in adults and children: guidelines by the surgical infection society and the infectious diseases society of America. Surg Infect (Larchmt). 2010;11:79–109.
21. Radder RW. Ultrasonically guided percutaneous catheter drainage for gallbladder empyema. Diagn Imaging. 1980;49:330–3.
22. de Mestral C, Gomez D, Haas B, Zagorski B, Rotstein OD, Nathens AB. Cholecystostomy: a bridge to hospital discharge but not delayed cholecystectomy. J Trauma Acute Care Surg. 2013;74:175–9.
23. McGillicuddy EA, Schuster KM, Barre K, Suarez L, Hall MR, Kaml GJ, et al. Non-operative management of acute cholecystitis in the elderly. Br J Surg. 2012;99:1254–61.
24. Noh SY, Gwon DI, Ko GY, Yoon HK, Sung KB. Role of percutaneous cholecystostomy for acute acalculous cholecystitis: clinical outcomes of 271 patients. Eur Radiol. 2018;28:1449–55.
25. Zerem E, Omerovic S. Can percutaneous cholecystostomy be a definitive management for acute cholecystitis in high-risk patients? Surg Laparosc Endosc Percutan Tech. 2014;24:187–91.
26. Chang YR, Ahn YJ, Jang JY, Kang MJ, Kwon W, Jung WH, et al. Percutaneous cholecystostomy for acute cholecystitis in patients with high comorbidity and re-evaluation of treatment efficacy. Surgery. 2014;155:615–22.
27. Gumus B. Percutaneous cholecystostomy as a first-line therapy in chronic hemodialysis patients with acute cholecystitis with midterm follow-up. Cardiovasc Intervent Radiol. 2011;34:362–8.
28. Yun SS, Hwang DW, Kim SW, Park SH, Park SJ, Lee DS, et al. Better treatment strategies for patients with acute cholecystitis and American society of anesthesiologists classification 3 or greater. Yonsei Med J. 2010;51:540–5.
29. Morse BC, Smith JB, Lawdahl RB, Roettger RH. Management of acute cholecystitis in critically ill patients: contemporary role for cholecystostomy and subsequent cholecystectomy. Am Surg. 2010;76:708–12.

30. Park JK, Yang JI, Wi JW, Park JK, Lee KH, Lee KT, et al. Long-term outcome and recurrence factors after percutaneous cholecystostomy as a definitive treatment for acute cholecystitis. J Gastroenterol Hepatol. 2019;34:784–90.
31. Abbas SH, Ghazanfar MA, Gordon-Weeks AN, Reddy SR, Soonawalla Z, Silva MA. Acalculous cholecystitis: is an elective interval cholecystectomy necessary. Dig Surg. 2018;35:171–6.
32. Jang JW, Lee SS, Song TJ, Hyun YS, Park DY, Seo DW, et al. Endoscopic ultrasound-guided transmural and percutaneous transhepatic gallbladder drainage are comparable for acute cholecystitis. Gastroenterology. 2012;142:805–11.
33. Higa JT, Sahar N, Kozarek RA, La Selva D, Larsen MC, Gan SI, et al. EUS-guided gallbladder drainage with a lumen-apposing metal stent versus endoscopic transpapillary gallbladder drainage for the treatment of acute cholecystitis (with videos). Gastrointest Endosc. 2019;90:483–92.
34. Treinen C, Lomelin D, Krause C, Goede M, Oleynikov D. Acute acalculous cholecystitis in the critically ill: risk factors and surgical strategies. Langenbecks Arch Surg. 2015;400:421–7.
35. Kirkegård J, Horn T, Christensen SD, Larsen LP, Knudsen AR, Mortensen FV. Percutaneous cholecystostomy is an effective definitive treatment option for acute acalculous cholecystitis. Scand J Surg. 2015;104:238–43.
36. Barie PS, Eachempati SR. Acute acalculous cholecystitis. Curr Gastroenterol Rep. 2003;5:302–9.

IgG4-Related Cholecystitis

Takahiro Nakazawa, Shuya Simizu, Katsuyuki Miyabe, and Itaru Naitoh

Introduction

IgG4-related disease (IgG4-RD) is a chronic, relapsing, multi-organ fibro-inflammatory syndrome of presumed autoimmune etiology. The typical presentation and imaging findings include mass-forming synchronous or metachronous lesions; these can occur in almost any organ, including the retroperitoneum, kidneys, lungs, salivary glands, and lacrimal glands, but are seen most commonly in the pancreas and bile duct. IgG4-RD is characterized by increased serum levels of IgG4 and tissue infiltration by IgG4-positive plasma cells. Despite the relapsing–remitting course of IgG4-RD, patients tend to have a good response to steroid therapy and an excellent prognosis [1, 2].

IgG4-related cholecystitis, whether occurring as diffuse or localized disease, is a manifestation of IgG4-RD in the gallbladder. Diffuse IgG4-related cholecystitis is sometimes detected as diffuse thickness of the gallbladder wall in a patient being evaluated for autoimmune pancreatitis (AIP) or IgG4-related sclerosing cholangitis (IgG4-SC) [3, 4]. However, localized IgG4-related cholecystitis is difficult to diagnose because it must be distinguished from gallbladder cancer, which is often challenging [5].

In this study, we describe the characteristic features of diffuse and localized IgG4-related cholecystitis and present a challenging case as an example.

Diffuse IgG4-Related Cholecystitis

Frequency and Clinical Characteristics

The association of diffuse thickening of the gallbladder wall with AIP was reported by Abraham et al. [3]. They noted intense inflammatory infiltration of the gallbladder wall in 12 of 20 cases (60%) and transmural chronic cholecystitis in 7 of 20 cases (35%). In addition, Kamisawa et al. [2] reported severe or moderate thickening of the gallbladder wall, observed on radiological examination, including ultrasound (US) and/or computed tomography (CT), in 10 of 19 patients (53%) with AIP. In the same study, among eight patients (75%) with AIP who were undergoing surgery, the histological examinations showed gallbladder wall thickening in six patients, including four with fibrosis, IgG4-positive plasma cells, and transmural inflammation of lymphocytes.

T. Nakazawa (✉) · S. Simizu · I. Naitoh
Department of Gastroenterology and Metabolism, Nagoya City University Graduate School of Medical Sciences, Nagoya, Japan
e-mail: nakazawax3@gmail.com

K. Miyabe
Department of Gastroenterology, Japanese Red Cross Nagoya Daini Hospital, Nagoya, Japan

J. B. Chung and K. Okazaki (eds.), *Diseases of the Gallbladder*,
https://doi.org/10.1007/978-981-15-6010-1_10

In a report of 43 patients with AIP and biliary lesions [6], no gallbladder wall thickening or bile duct lesion was noted in 9 patients, whereas in 69% (9/13) and 19% (4/21) of the patients with extensive bile duct involvement and lower bile duct involvement, respectively, the only finding was gallbladder wall thickening. In the above-mentioned study of 19 patients with AIP [2], all patients with gallbladder wall thickening also had severe stenosis of the extrahepatic bile duct. Abraham et al. [3] concluded that mucosal inflammation of the gallbladder in AIP correlated significantly with the presence of inflammation in the extrapancreatic portion of the common bile duct.

Pathology

The above-cited study of Abraham et al. [3] also included the pathological findings of 20 gallbladders in patients with AIP. A high frequency of inflammation and lymphoid nodules was noted. According to their scoring system, the scores were similar to those for primary sclerosing cholangitis (PSC) and significantly higher than those for uncomplicated chronic cholelithiasis. However, the pattern of inflammation and cellular composition of the inflammatory infiltrates were somewhat more varied than in PSC gallbladders. For example, the most common pattern of inflammation in patients with AIP was transmural (35%) rather than mucosal (25%), whereas 50% of PSC gallbladders were characterized by mucosal-based infiltrates and only 10% by transmural infiltrates. The scores for deep inflammation were higher in AIP than in control gallbladders, and the composition of the inflammatory infiltrates was more varied.

A Typical Case of Diffuse IgG4-Related Cholecystitis

A 56-year-old male patient was referred to our hospital for further examination of pancreatic enlargement. His serum IgG4 level was 2,020 mg/dl. Abdominal CT showed diffuse pancreatic enlargement and diffuse thickness in the whole gallbladder (Fig. 1a). Endoscopic US (EUS) revealed thickening of the walls of the bile duct and gallbladder (4.5 and 6.5 mm, respectively; Fig. 1b, arrowhead, arrow). In both structures, the epithelium was preserved. Endoscopic retrograde pancreatography (ERP) showed diffuse narrowing of the main pancreatic duct (Fig. 1c), and endoscopic retrograde cholangiography revealed diffuse narrowing of the intrahepatic and lower common bile ducts (Fig. 1d). The diagnosis was diffuse IgG4-related cholecystitis associated with AIP and type 2b IgG4-SC. Pancreatic enlargement, as well as the thickened bile duct and gallbladder walls, were dramatically reduced by steroid therapy.

Localized IgG4-Related Cholecystitis

Frequency and Clinical Characteristics

In most patients with IgG4-related cholecystitis, diffuse, circumferential thickening of the gallbladder wall is associated with IgG4-SC or AIP. Therefore, confirmation of the diagnosis is not difficult in typical cases of IgG4-related cholecystitis. However, in patients with localized gallbladder lesions or inflammation, sometimes extending to the surrounding tissue in the gallbladder (mimicking the appearance of a malignant tumor), exclusion of gallbladder cancer can be challenging.

Fifteen cases of IgG4-related cholecystitis that were difficult to differentiate from gallbladder cancer have been reported [5, 7–17] (Table 1). Eleven were eventually determined to be localized gallbladder lesions, including 9 with fundus involvement, 2 with neck involvement, and 3 with both fundus and body. Eight cases were associated with AIP and six with IgG4-SC. Thirteen of the respective patient underwent surgical resection. The patients in the other two cases were treated by steroid administration. In 3 of 11 cases of localized IgG4-related cholecystitis, the serum IgG4 level was low. No association of one of AIP or

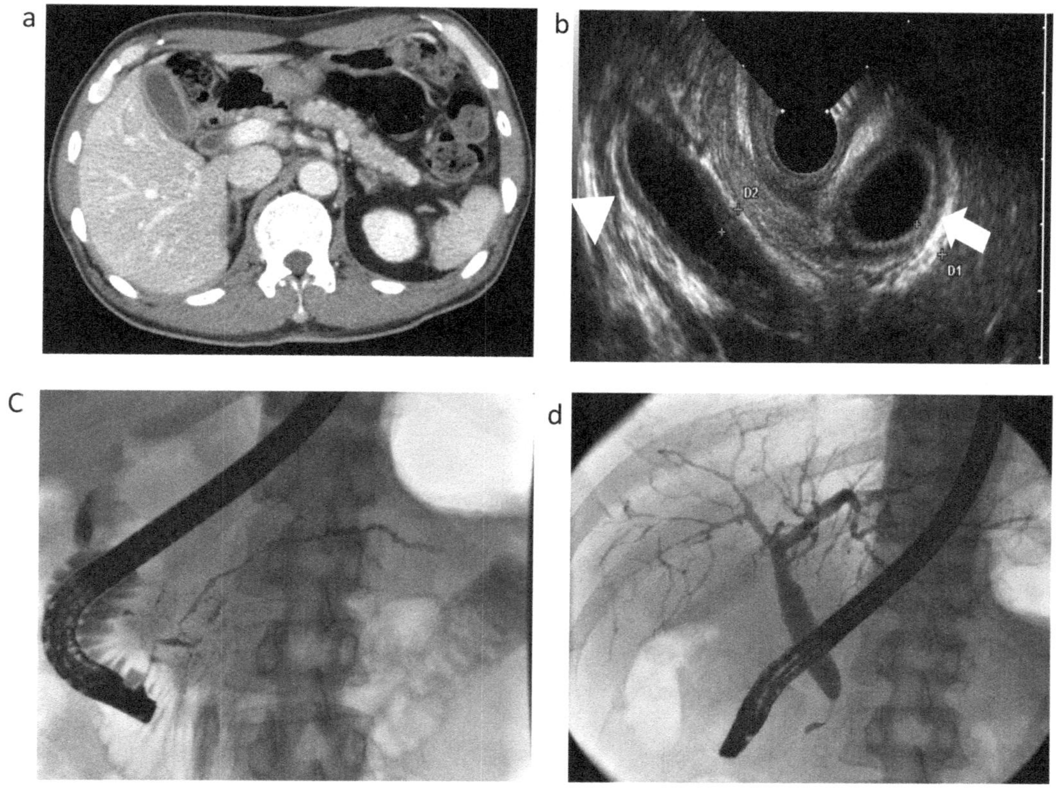

Fig. 1 A typical case of diffuse IgG4-related cholecystitis. **a** Abdominal CT showed diffuse pancreatic enlargement and diffuse thickness in the whole gall bladder. **b** EUS revealed thickening of the walls of the bile duct (4.5 mm, arrow head) and gall bladder (6.5 mm, arrow). **c** ERP showed diffuse narrowing of the main pancreatic duct. **d** ERC revealed diffuse narrowing of the intrahepatic and lower common bile ducts

Table 1 Summary of IgG4-related cholecystitis mimicking gallbladder cancer

	Author	Age	Sex	IgG4 (md/dl)	Location	Symptom	IgG4-SC	AIP	Diagnosis	Treatment
1	Gumbs [5]	68	F	NA	Funds	Abdominal pain	NA	+	ope	ope
2	Matsubayashi [7]	62	M	764	Diffuse	Jaundice	+	+	Imaging	PSL
3	Kawakami [8]	55	M	455	Fundus	NA	+	+	ope	ope
4	Lee [9]	59	M	75	Neck	Abdominal pain	+	–	Biospy	PSL
5	Shin [10]	58	M	NA	Body, Fundus	Abdominal pain	–	–	ope	ope
6	Feely [11]	61	F	17	Fundus	Jaundice	+	–	ope	ope
7	Feely [11]	71	F	NA	Fundus	Abdominal pain	NA	NA	ope	ope
8	Feely [11]	53	M	NA	Diffuse	Abdominal pain	NA	NA	ope	ope
9	Inoue [12]	60	F	813	Fundus	NA	–	+	ope	ope
10	Li [13]	61	M	175	Diffuse	Jaundice	+	+	ope	ope
11	Takahashi [14]	18	M	40	Neck	Jaundice	–	–	ope	ope
12	Yamaguchi [15]	50	M	NA	Body, Fundus	Abdominal pain	–	–	ope	ope
13	Ishigami [16]	82	M	943	Diffuse	NA	–	+	ope	ope
14	Ichinokawa [17]	56	M	721	Fundus	No	–	+	ope	ope
15	Our case (2018)	67	M	231	Body, Fundus	No	+	+	ope	ope

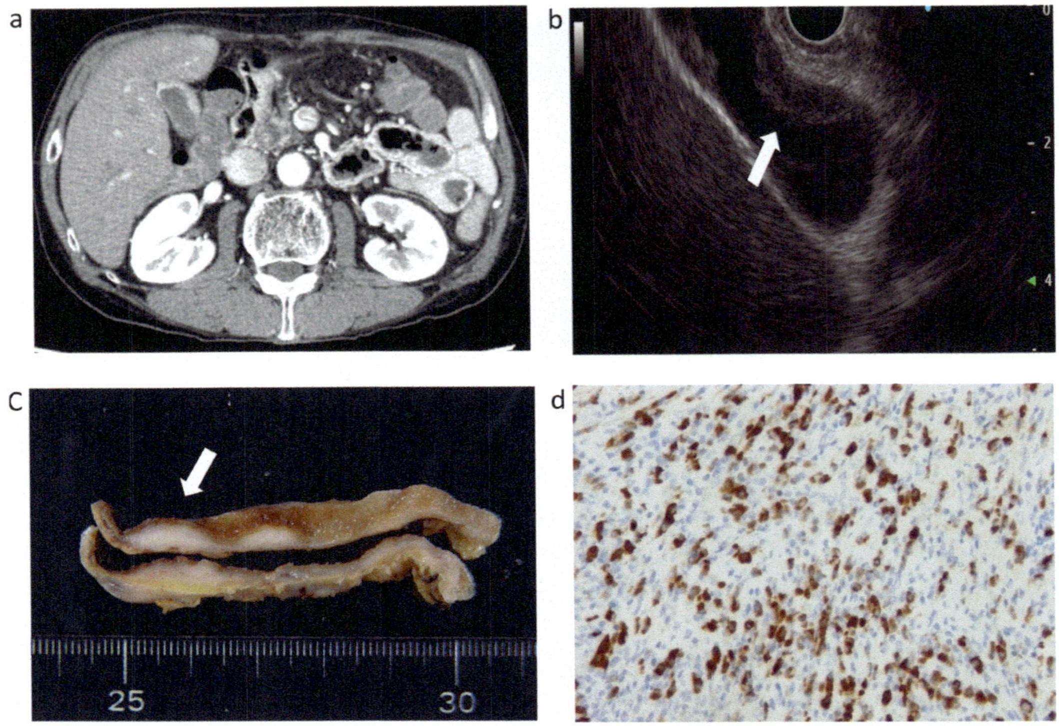

Fig. 2 A typical case of localized IgG4-related cholecystitis. **a** Abdominal CT showed pancreatic atrophy and localized thickness in the body of the gall bladder. **b** EUS revealed localized thickness measuring 6.1 mm in the body and fundus of gall bladder with smooth surface (arrow). **c** Analysis of the surgical specimen resulted in a white mass with normal epithelium of gall bladder wall (arrow). **d** Diffuse lymphoplasmacytic infiltration with affluent IgG4-positive plasma cells in the gall bladder was observed

IgG4-SC could be determined in 7 of the 15 cases, including 3 cases in which there was no association of both AIP and IgG4-SC. In that study, all patients with isolated IgG4-related cholecystitis were treated by surgical resection.

Pathology

Similar to diffuse IgG4-related cholecystitis, localized IgG4-related cholecystitis is characterized by transmural lymphoplasmacytic infiltration, storiform fibrosis, obliterative phlebitis, and abundant IgG4-positive plasma cells.

Rokitansky–Aschoff (RA) sinuses of adenomyomatosis are also frequently observed in localized IgG4-related cholecystitis. The gross findings of the surgical specimen are typically a localized tumor similar in appearance to adenomyomatosis [17], i.e., a yellow-white mass with multiple small cystic lesions [8, 12]. By contrast, the frequency of RA sinuses in diffuse IgG4-related cholecystitis is similar to that in chronic cholecystitis [3]. Xanthogranulomatous inflammation may also be observed [14].

A Typical Case of Localized IgG4-Related Cholecystitis

A 67-year-old male was referred to our hospital for further examination of new gallbladder lesion during the course of prednisolone treatment for IgG4-related cholangitis coexisting with AIP since 2 years ago. His serum IgG4 level was 231 mg/dl. Abdominal CT showed pancreatic atrophy and localized thickness in the body of the gallbladder (Fig. 2a). On MRCP, a diffuse dilatation of common bile duct without main pancreatic duct dilatation or stricture was observed, while EUS revealed localized thickness measuring 6.1 mm in the body and fundus of gallbladder with a smooth surface (Fig. 2b arrow). The localized mass maintained the normal epithelium of the gallbladder wall (Fig. 2b). Although the diagnosis was localized IgG4-related cholecystitis associated with AIP, the new appearance of gallbladder cancer could not be ruled out. The gallbladder was surgically resected because a restudy of the EUS images showed an irregularity of the localized mass. Analysis of the surgical specimen resulted in a white mass with normal epithelium of gallbladder wall (Fig. 2c arrow) and diffuse lymphoplasmacytic infiltration with affluent IgG4-positive plasma cells in the gallbladder (Fig. 2d).

A Case of Gallbladder Cancer Resembling Localized IgG4-Related Cholecystitis Associated with AIP

In the following, we report a case of gallbladder cancer similar to localized IgG4-related cholecystitis. The presence of AIP complicated the diagnosis.

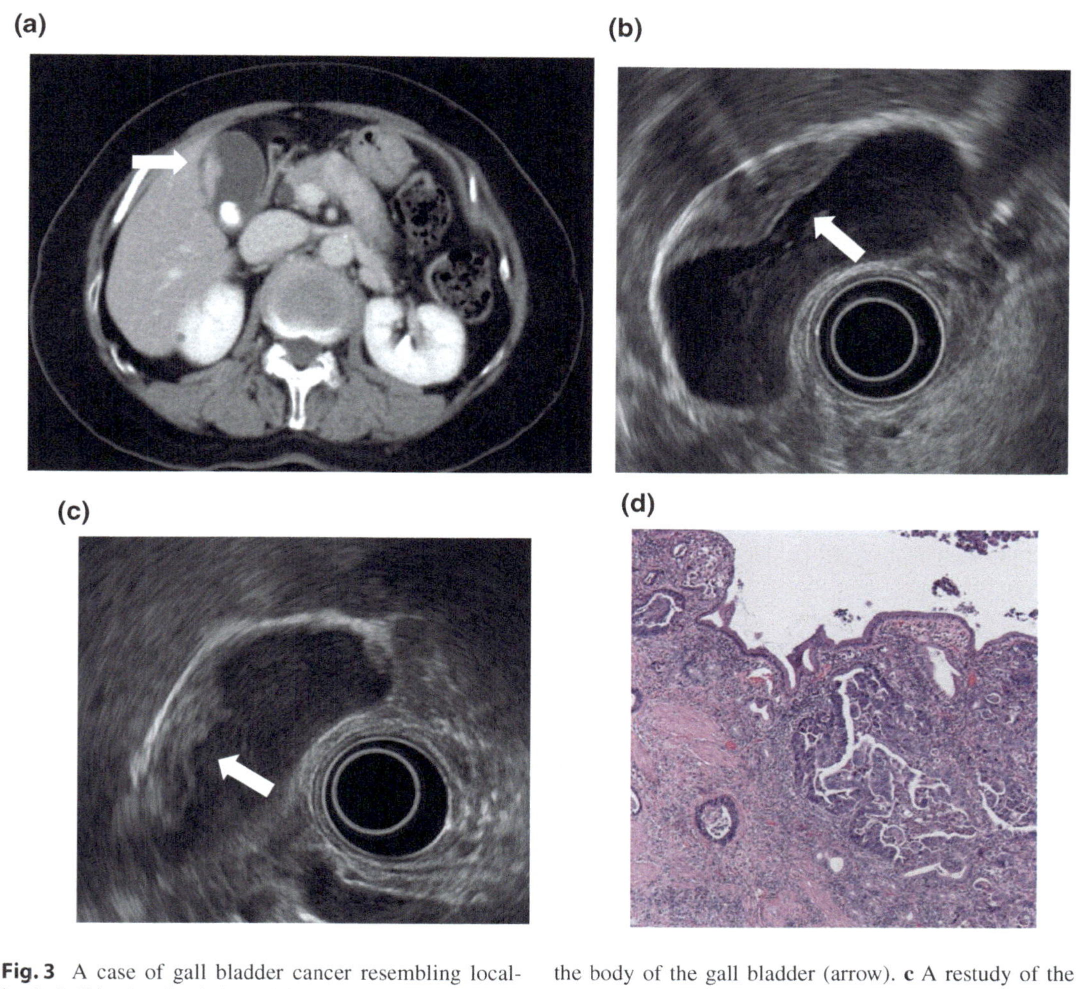

Fig. 3 A case of gall bladder cancer resembling localized IgG4-related cholecystitis associated with AIP. **a** Abdominal CT showed pancreatic enlargement and localized thickness in the body of the gall bladder (arrow). **b** EUS revealed a localized thickness in the body of the gall bladder (arrow). **c** A restudy of the EUS images showed an irregularity of the mass (arrow). **d** Analysis of the surgical specimen resulted in a diagnosis of moderately differentiated tubular adenocarcinoma of the gallbladder

A 75-year-old female was referred to our hospital for further examination of pancreatic enlargement. Her serum IgG4 level was 369 mg/dl. Abdominal CT showed pancreatic enlargement and localized thickness in the body of the gallbladder (Fig. 3a). On ERP, a diffuse narrowing of the main pancreatic duct was observed while EUS revealed a localized thickness in the body of the gallbladder (Fig. 3b). The localized mass maintained the normal epithelium of the gallbladder wall and featured RA sinuses mimicking adenomyomatosis (Fig. 3b). The diagnosis was localized IgG4-related cholecystitis associated with AIP. The patient was treated with steroids, which dramatically reduced the pancreatic enlargement. However, there was no change in the size of the localized mass in the gallbladder. The gallbladder was surgically resected because a restudy of the EUS images showed an irregularity of the mass (Fig. 3c). Analysis of the surgical specimen resulted in a diagnosis of moderately differentiated tubular adenocarcinoma of the gallbladder (Fig. 3d).

Conclusion

The characteristic findings of both diffuse and localized forms of IgG4-related cholecystitis have been described. Localized IgG4-related cholecystitis is difficult to diagnose; it must be distinguished from gallbladder cancer, which is still challenging.

References

1. Miyabe K, Zen Y, Cornell LD, Rajagopalan G, Chowdhary VR, Roberts LR, et al. Gastrointestinal and extra-intestinal manifestations of IgG4–related disease. Gastroenterology. 2018;155:990–1003.
2. Kamisawa T, Zen Y, Nakazawa T, Okazaki K. Advances in IgG4-related pancreatobiliary diseases. Lancet Gastroenterol Hepatol. 2018;3:575–85.
3. Abraham SC, Cruz-Correa M, Argani P, Furth EE, Hruban RH, Boitnott JK. Am J Surg Pathol. 2003;27:441–51.
4. Kamisawa T, Tu Y, Nakajima H, Egawa N, Tsuruta K, Okamoto A, et al. Sclerosing cholecystitis associated with autoimmune pancreatitis. World J Gastroenterol. 2006;12:3736–9.
5. Gumbs AA, Kim J, Kiehna E, Brink JA, Salem RR. Autoimmune pancreatitis presenting as simultaneous masses in the pancreatic head and gallbladder. JOP. 2005;6:455–9.
6. Kamisawa T, Takuma K, Anjiki H, Egawa N, Kurata M, Honda G, et al. Biliary lesions associated with autoimmune pancreatitis. Hepatogastroenterology. 2009;56:1190–3.
7. Matsubayashi H, Furukawa H, Uesaka K, Sasaki K, Ono H, Hruban RH. Autoimmune pancreatitis accompanied by cholecystitis, periaortitis and pseudotumors of the liver. Case Rep Gastroenterol. 2008;2:155–61.
8. Kawakami H, Eto K, Kuwatani M, Asaka M. Localized lymphoplasmacytic sclerosing cholecystitis in a patient with autoimmune pancreatitis. Int Med. 2010;49:2359–60 (Tokyo, Japan).
9. Lee YS, Lee SH, Lee MG, Lee SJ, Hwang JH, Shin E, et al. Immunoglobulin g4-related disease mimicking unresectable gallbladder cancer. Gut Liver. 2013;7:616–20.
10. Shin SW, Kim Y, Jeong WK, Kim J, Kim MY, Oh YH, et al. Isolated IgG4-related cholecystitis mimicking gallbladder cancer: a case report. Clin Imaging. 2013;37:969–71.
11. Feely MM, Gonzalo DH, Corbera M, Hughes SJ, Trevino JG, et al. IgG4-related cholecystitis presenting as biliary malignancy: report of three cases. J Gastrointest Surg. 2014;18:1710–5.
12. Inoue T, Okumura F, Mizushima T, Nishie H, Iwasaki H, Anbe K, et al. Localized IgG4-related cholecystitis mimicking gallbladder cancer. Int Med. 2015;54:1869–74 (Tokyo, Japan).
13. Li M, Zhou Q, Yang K, Brigstock D, Zang L, Xiu M, et al. Rare case of *Helicobacter pylori*-positive multiorgan IgG4-related disease and gastric cancer. World J Gastroenterol. 2015;21:3429–34.
14. Takahashi K, Ito H, Katsube T, Tsuboi A, Hashimoto M, Ota E, et al. Immunoglobulin G4-related sclerosing cholecystitis presenting as gallbladder cancer: a case report. Surg Case Rep. 2015;1:120.
15. Yamaguchi T, Kayahara M, Furukawa H, Satoh T, Oonishi I, Ooyama S, et al. A case of isolated IgG4-related cholecystitis mimicking gallbladder cancer. J Jpn Surg Assoc. 2015;76:3042–6 (in Japanese, Abstract in English).
16. Ishigami K, Shitani M, Kimura Y, Hasegawa T, Masaki Y, Ito A, et al. Ectopic relapse of IgG4-related disease presenting as IgG4-related sclerosing cholecystitis. Medicine. 2018;97:52.
17. Ichinokawa M, Matsumoto J, Kuraya T, Kuwabara S, Wada H, et al. A rare case of localized IgG4-related sclerosing cholecystitis mimicking gallbladder cancer. J Rural Med. 2019;14:138–42.

Gallbladder Lesions in Patients with Pancreaticobiliary Maljunction

Kensuke Yoshimoto, Terumi Kamisawa, Masataka Kikuyama, and Yoshinori Igarashi

Introduction

Pancreaticobiliary maljunction (PBM) is a congenital malformation in which the anatomical junction of the pancreatic and bile ducts occurs outside the duodenal wall. The diagnosis of PBM is made when direct cholangiography including endoscopic retrograde cholangiopancreatography (ERCP), or magnetic resonance cholangiopancreatography (MRCP), shows that the common channel is abnormally long and/or the pancreatic and bile ducts join abnormally. PBM has been classified into two types: PBM with biliary dilatation (congenital biliary dilatation) and PBM without biliary dilatation (Fig. 11.1) [1–3].

The sphincter of Oddi, which regulates the outflow of bile and pancreatic juice, is usually at the distal end of the pancreatic and bile ducts. However, in PBM, because of the excessive length of the common channel, the pancreaticobiliary junction is not directly affected by the sphincter. This then results in pancreatic juice and bile reflux, which can cause a variety of pathological biliary tract and pancreatic conditions [1, 3, 4].

Pathophysiology of the Biliary Tract in PBM

As noted above, the excessive length of the common channel in PBM causes the pancreaticobiliary junction to be unaffected by the action of the sphincter of Oddi. Since pancreatic duct hydropressure is normally higher than bile duct hydropressure, there is a frequent reflux of pancreatic juice into the biliary tract (pancreatobiliary reflux) in PBM. Persistent refluxed pancreatic juice damages the biliary tract epithelium, which promotes cancer development; thus, patients with PBM have higher rates of biliary tract cancers. On the other hand, there are also cases of bile reflux into the pancreatic duct (biliopancreatic reflux), which can cause pancreatitis (Fig. 11.2) [1, 3–6].

Pathological Findings in the Gallbladder of PBM Patients

On histopathological examination of the gallbladder in PBM, inflammation, hyperplasia, metaplasia, and dysplasia caused by stasis of

K. Yoshimoto · T. Kamisawa (✉) · M. Kikuyama
Department of Internal Medicine, Tokyo Metropolitan Komagome Hospital, 3-18-22 Honkomagome, Bunkyo-Ku, Tokyo 113-8677, Japan
e-mail: kamisawa@cick.jp

K. Yoshimoto · Y. Igarashi
Division of Gastroenterology and Hepatology, Omori Medical Center, Toho University School of Medicine, Tokyo, Japan

J. B. Chung and K. Okazaki (eds.), *Diseases of the Gallbladder*,
https://doi.org/10.1007/978-981-15-6010-1_11

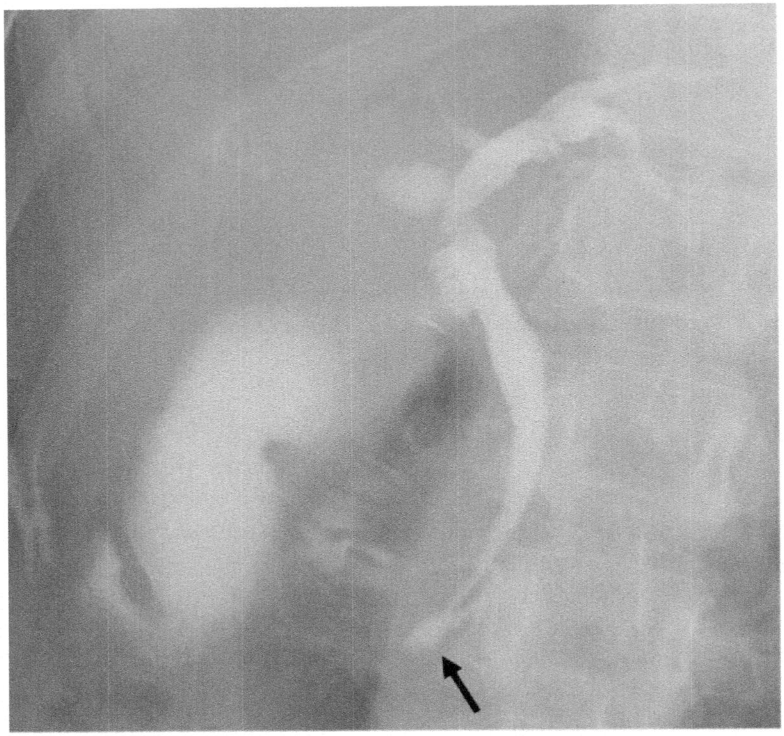

Fig. 11.1 Endoscopic cholangiopancreatogram of pancreaticobiliary maljunction without biliary dilatation associated with hyperplasia of gallbladder epithelium. Arrow: long common channel

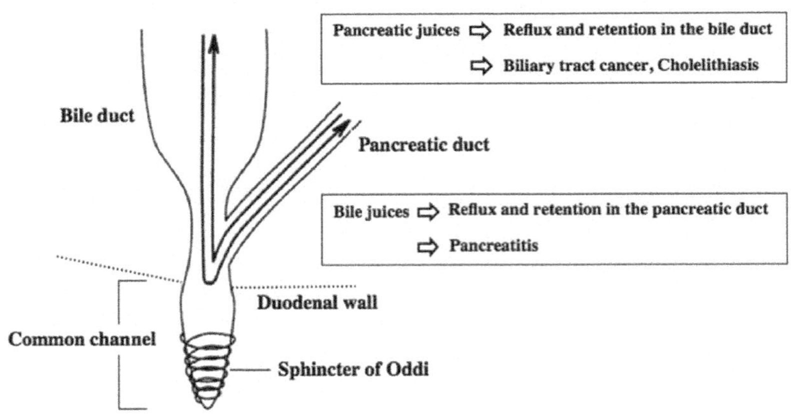

Fig. 11.2 Pathophysiology pf pancreaticobiliary maljunction (referred from Refs. [1, 6])

bile mixed with refluxed pancreatic juice can be seen. The characteristic finding is a hyperplastic change of the epithelium (Fig. 11.3) [5–14]. In our series, the gallbladder mucosa was significantly higher in PBM (6.3 mm) than in controls (3.2 mm, $p<0.01$), and epithelial hyperplasia of the gallbladder was significantly more frequent in PBM (73%) than in controls

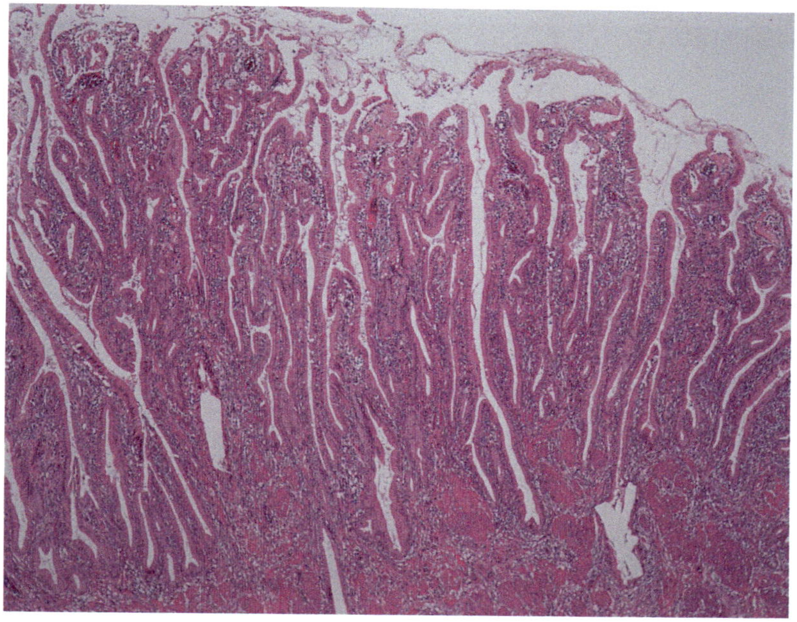

Fig. 11.3 Hyperplastic change of the epithelium in the gallbladder of a PBM patient (H&E staining)

(0%, $p<0.01$). In addition, the gallbladder epithelium of PBM patients showed a significantly higher Ki-67 labeling index, which is a marker of cell proliferative activity, than that of controls (8.1% vs. 1.4%, $p<0.01$) [4, 8, 9]. It has also been reported that the gallbladder epithelium showed the hyperplastic change in 39% [10]–91% [11] of PBM patients. Tokiwa et al. found gallbladder epithelial hyperplasia in 50% of 28 pediatric PBM patients [12]. In addition, there was a report of a hyperplastic polyp of the gallbladder in a 9-year-old girl with PBM [13], but high-grade hyperplasia has been reported to increase with age, and dysplasia or metaplasia of the gallbladder epithelium is rare in infancy, only being detected in adolescence and later [11, 14]. The mucosa around gallbladder cancer often shows dysplasia. Though hyperplastic epithelium can be seen at birth or from the early stages of infancy, dysplasia or metaplasia appears later. Given these findings, the carcinogenetic process in PBM appears to follow a sequence of hyperplasia–dysplasia–carcinoma [14, 15].

On imaging studies, hyperplastic change of the gallbladder epithelium presents as gallbladder wall thickening. In order to identify PBM without biliary dilatation early, PBM should be suspected in patients who show gallbladder wall thickening on screening ultrasound (US) (Fig. 11.4) and MRCP should be performed [16].

Biliary Tract Carcinogenesis in PBM

The carcinogenetic mechanism in PBM appears to involve the persistent refluxed pancreatic juice in the biliary tract. With an increased intraductal pressure of the common bile duct or bacterial infection, the refluxed proteolytic pancreatic enzymes and phospholipase A2 are easily activated in the biliary tract. Phospholipase A2 converts lecithin within the bile to lysolecithin, which causes extensive damage to the cell membrane [17]. Furthermore, secondary bile acids, especially taurodeoxycholic acid, have been found to be increased in the bile of PBM patients [18], and mutagenic substances that

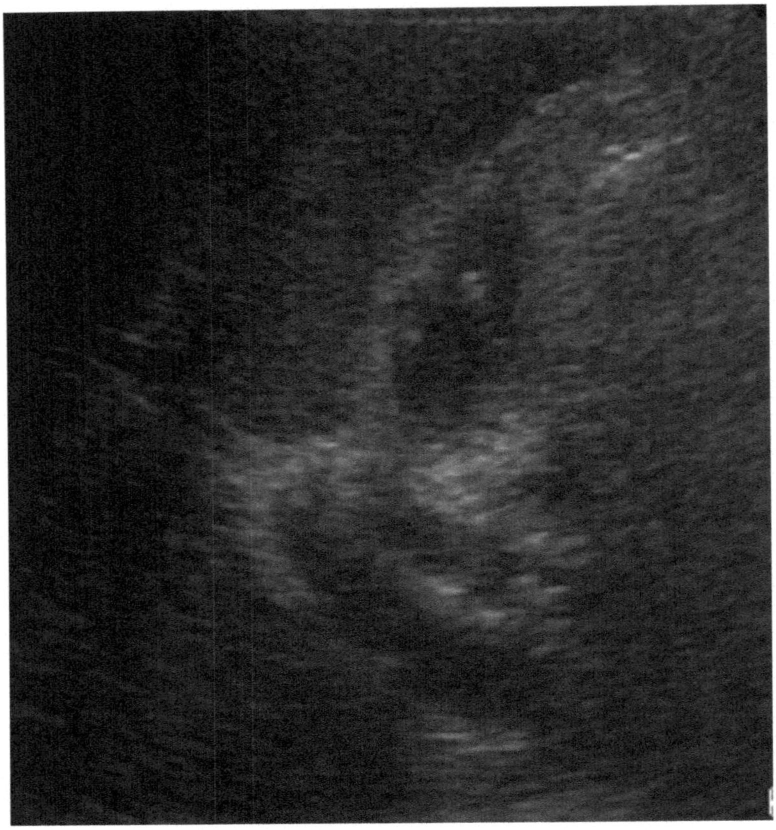

Fig. 11.4 Ultrasound showing thickening of the gallbladder wall in a PBM patient with the hyperplastic change of the gallbladder epithelium

damage DNA has been detected clinically in the bile of PBM patients as well as in experimental animal models [19, 20]. In the presence of such harmful substances, there is an acceleration of the cell cycle, various additional epithelial changes occur, and DNA is damaged.

There are frequent point mutations of K-ras oncogene in gallbladder and bile duct cancers. However, the noncancerous epithelium of the gallbladder and bile duct also shows K-ras mutation in PBM patients, as reported by Matsubara et al., who found K-ras mutation in the gallbladder and bile duct epithelium of PBM patients without biliary carcinoma in 33% and 40%, respectively [21], and Iwase et al., who found K-ras mutation in 36% of hyperplastic gallbladder lesions in PBM patients [22]. Aoki et al. reported K-ras mutation in 64% of gallbladder hyperplasia, 28% of metaplasia, and 17% of metaplasia cases in PBM patients [23]. In our series, 36% of PBM patients showed K-ras mutation in noncancerous gallbladder epithelium [4, 8]. Because the noncancerous epithelium and the epithelium of hyperplasia of the gallbladder show K-ras mutation, there appears to be a genetically precancerous state that represents an early event in multistep carcinogenesis in PBM patients.

Thus, in PBM patients, activated pancreatic enzymes, increased secondary bile acids, or other mutagens persistently attack biliary tract epithelial cells, resulting in hyperplastic change with an increase in cell proliferative activity. Then, oncogenes and/or tumor suppressor

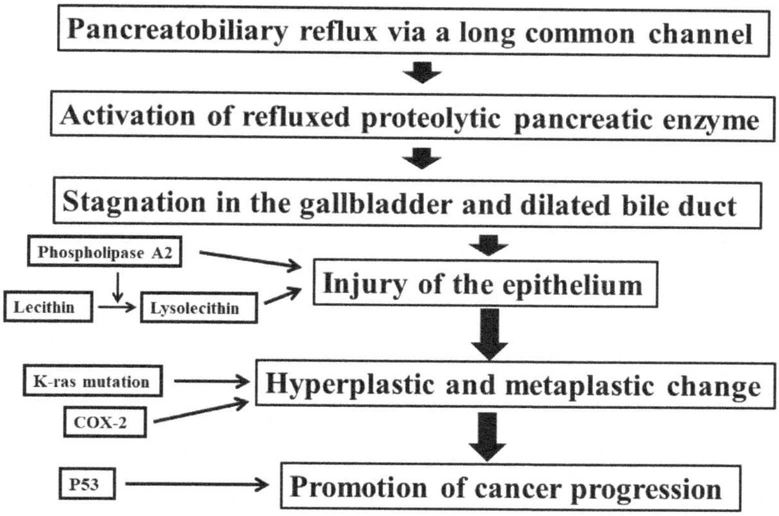

Fig. 11.5 Mechanism of biliary carcinogenesis in pancreaticobiliary maljunction (referred from Ref. [6])

genes in the epithelia mutate, leading to biliary tract cancer. Therefore, the biliary tract carcinogenesis in PBM patients appears to involve the hyperplasia–dysplasia–carcinoma sequence that occurs as a result of the chronic inflammation that pancreatic juice reflux into the biliary tract causes and this mechanism differs from the adenoma–carcinoma sequence or the de novo carcinogenesis of biliary tract cancers in persons without PBM (Fig. 11.5) [1, 6, 24].

Clinical Features of Biliary Cancer in PBM Patients

According to a nationwide survey in Japan ($n = 2561$) [25], 21.6% of adult patients with congenital biliary dilatation and 42.4% of PBM patients without biliary dilatation were found to have biliary cancer. In adult PBM patients with biliary cancers, 32.1% had bile duct cancer and 62.3% had gallbladder cancer among those with congenital biliary dilatation, whereas 7.3% had bile duct cancer and 88.1% had gallbladder cancer among those without biliary dilatation. In other words, in adult patients with congenital biliary dilatation, 6.9% had bile duct cancer and 13.4% had gallbladder cancer, whereas, in those without congenital biliary dilatation, 3.1% had bile duct cancer and 37.4% had gallbladder cancer. Only one pediatric patient with congenital biliary dilatation had an associated biliary cancer. The mean age when biliary cancer developed in PBM patients was 60.1 years for gallbladder cancer and 52.0 years for bile duct cancer in those with congenital biliary dilatation, and it was 58.6 years for gallbladder cancer in PBM patients without congenital biliary dilatation. Biliary cancers develop 15–20 years earlier in PBM patients than in those without PBM [26].

In our series of 129 PBM patients, 8 (11%) and 15 (21%) of 73 patients with congenital biliary dilatation had bile duct cancer and gallbladder cancer, respectively, compared to 2 (4%) and 43 (77%) of 56 patients with PBM without biliary dilatation. Metachronous ($n = 1$) and simultaneous ($n = 2$) multiple biliary cancers were included. It has been reported that concurrent PBM was seen in 19 (51%) of 37 patients with simultaneous double or multiple biliary cancers [27–31]. Among our 43 PBM patients without biliary dilatation who developed gallbladder cancer, gallstones were found in only 9%, significantly less than the 62% in patients without PBM who develop gallbladder cancer [32].

Conclusions

In PBM, the hyperplasia–dysplasia–carcinoma sequence triggered by the chronic inflammation caused by pancreatic juice reflux is thought to be involved in the development of biliary tract cancer. Gallbladder wall thickening is the imaging manifestation of hyperplastic change of the gallbladder epithelium. To detect PBM without biliary dilatation early, patients found to have gallbladder wall thickening on screening US, which is suspicious of PBM, should undergo MRCP.

Acknowledgements This work was supported by a grant from the Ministry of Health, Labor, and Welfare of Japan (19FC1008, Research on rare and intractable diseases, Health and Labor Sciences Research Grants).

References

1. Kamisawa T, Ando H, Suyama M, Shimada M, Morine Y, Shimada H, et al. Japanese clinical practice guidelines for pancreaticobiliary maljunction. J Gastroenterol. 2012;47:731–59.
2. Kamisawa T, Ando H, Hamada Y, Fujii H, Koshinaga T, Urushihara N, et al. Diagnostic criteria for pancreaticobiliary maljunction 2013. J Hepatobiliary Pancreat Sci. 2014;21:159–61.
3. Kamisawa T, Kaneko K, Itoi T, Ando H. Pancreaticobiliary maljunction and congenital biliary dilatation. Lancet Gastroenterol Hepatol. 2017;2:610–8.
4. Kamisawa T, Takuma K, Anjiki H, Egawa N, Kurata M, Honda G, et al. Pancreaticobiliary maljunction. Clin Gastroenterol Hepatol. 2009;7:S84–8.
5. Kamisawa T, Kuruma S, Tabata T, Chiba K, Iwasaki S, Koizumi S, et al. Pancreaticobiliary maljunction and biliary cancer. J Gastroenterol. 2015;50:273–9.
6. Kamisawa T, Kuruma S, Chiba K, Tabata T, Koizumi S, Kikuyama M. Biliary carcinogenesis in pancreaticobiliary maljunction. J Gastroenterol. 2017;52:158–63.
7. Hanada K, Itoh M, Fujii K, Tsuchida A, Hirata A, Ishimaru S, et al. Pathology and cellular kinetics of gallbladder with an anomalous junction of pancreaticobiliary duct. Am J Gastroenterol. 1996;91:1007–11.
8. Kamisawa T, Funata N, Hayashi Y, Egawa N, Nakajima H, Tsuruta K, et al. Pathologic changes in the non-carcinomatous epithelium of the gallbladder in patients with a relatively long common channel. Gastrointest Endosc. 2004;60:56–60.
9. Kamisawa T, Go K, Chen PY, Tu Y, Fujiwara T, Endoh J, et al. Lesions with a high risk of carcinogenesis in the gallbladder of patients with a long common channel. Dig Endosc. 2006;18:192–5.
10. Yamamoto M, Nakajo S, Tahara E, Ito M, Taniyama K, Shimamoto F, et al. Mucosal changes of the gallbladder in anomalous union with the pancreaticobiliary duct system. Pathol Res Pract. 1991;187:241–6.
11. Tanno S, Obara T, Fujii T, Mizukami Y, Shudo R, Nishino N, et al. Proliferative potential and K-ras mutation in epithelial hyperplasia of the gallbladder in patients with anomalous pancreaticobiliary ductal union. Cancer. 1998;83:267–75.
12. Tokiwa K, Iwai N. Early mucosal changes of the gallbladder in patients with anomalous arrangement of the pancreaticobiliary duct. Gastroenterology. 1996;110:1614–8.
13. Okada T, Sasaki F, Honda S, Matsuno Y, Kubota K, Todo S. Hyperplastic polyp of the gallbladder associated with pancreaticobiliary maljunction in a 9-year-old girl. Pediatr Surg Int. 2009;25:999–1002.
14. Tsuchida A, Itoi T. Carcinogenesis and chemoprevention of biliary tract cancer in pancreaticobiliary maljunction. World J Gastointest Oncol. 2010;2:130–5.
15. Funabiki T, Matsubara T, Miyakawa S, Ishihara S. Pancreaticobiliary maljunction and carcinogenesis to biliary and pancreatic malignancy. Langenbecks Arch Surg. 2009;394:159–69.
16. Takuma K, Kamisawa T, Tabata T, Hara S, Kuruma S, Inaba Y, et al. Importance of early diagnosis of pancreaticobiliary maljunction without biliary dilatation. World J Gastroenterol. 2012;18:3409–14.
17. Shimada K, Yanagisawa J, Nakayama F. Increased lysophosphatidylcholine and pancreatic enzyme content in bile of patients with anomalous pancreaticobiliary ductal junction. Hepatology. 1991;13:438–44.
18. Funabiki T, Sugiue K, Matsubara T, Amano H, Ochiai M. Bile acids and biliary carcinoma in pancreaticobiliary maljunction. Keio J Med. 1991;40:118–22.
19. Mizuno M, Kato T, Koyama K. An analysis of mutagens in the contents of the biliary tract in pancreaticobiliary maljunction. Surg Today. 1996;26:597–602.
20. Qian D, Kinouchi T, Kunitomo T, Kataoka K, Matin MA, Akimoto S, et al. Mutagenicity of the bile of dogs with an experimental model of an anomalous arrangement of the pancreaticobiliary duct. Carcinogenesis. 1993;14:743–7.
21. Matsubara T, Fakurai Y, Zhi LZ, Miura H, Ochiai M, Funabiki T. K-ras and p53 gene mutations in noncancerous biliary lesions of patients with pancreaticobiliary maljunction. J Hepatobiliary Pancreat Surg. 2002;9:312–21.
22. Iwase T, Nakazawa S, Yamao K, Yoshino J, Inui K, Yamachika H, et al. Ras gene point mutations in gallbladder lesions associated with anomalous connection of pancreatobiliary ducts. Hepatogastroenterology. 1997;44:1457–62.

23. Aoki T, Tsuchida A, Kasuya K, Aoki T, Saito H, Endo M, et al. Carcinogenesis in pancreaticobiliary maljunction. In: Aoki T, editor. KoyanagiY. Pancreaticobiliary maljunction. Tokyo: Igaku Tosho; 2002. p. 295–302.
24. Ishibashi H, Shimada M, Kamisawa T, Fujii H, Hamada Y, Kubota M, et al. Japanese clinical practice guidelines for congenital biliary dilatation. J Hepatobiliary Pancreat Sci. 2017;24:1–16.
25. Morine Y, Shiamda M, Takamatsu H, Araida T, Endo I, Kubota M, et al. Clinical Features of Pancreaticobiliary Maljunction: Update analysis of 2nd Japan-nationwide Survey. J Hepatobiliary Pancreat Surg. 2013;20:472–80.
26. Matsuda T, Marugame T, Kamo K, Katanoda K, Ajiki W, Sobue T, et al. Cancer incidence and incidence rates in Japan in 2003: based on data from 13 population-based cancer registries in the monitoring of cancer incidence in Japan (MCIJ) project. Jpn J Clin Oncol. 2009;39:850–8.
27. Ogawa A, Sugo H, Takamori S, Kojima K, Fukasawa M, Beppu T, et al. Double cancers in the common bile duct: molecular genetic findings with an analysis of LOH. J Hepatobiliary Pancreat Surg. 2001;8:374–8.
28. Okamoto A, Tsuruta K, Matsumoto G, Takahashi T, Kamisawa T, Egawa N, et al. Papillary carcinoma of the extrahepatic bile duct: characteristic features and implications in surgical treatment. J Am Coll Surg. 2003;196:394–401.
29. Fujii T, Kaneko T, Sugimoto H, Okochi O, Inoue S, Takeda S, et al. Metachronous double cancer of the gallbladder and common bile duct. J Hepatobiliary Pancreat Surg. 2004;11:280–5.
30. Hori H, Ajiki T, Fujita T, Okazaki T, Suzuki Y, Kuroda Y, et al. Double cancer of gall bladder and bile duct not associated with anomalous junction of the pancreaticobiliary duct system. Jpn J Clin Oncol. 2006;36:638–42.
31. Itoh T, Fuji N, Taniguchi H, Yasukawa S, Yasuda H, Wakabayashi N, et al. Double cancer of the cystic duct and gallbladder associated with low junction of the cystic duct. J Hepatobiliary Pancreat Surg. 2008;15:338–43.
32. Miyazaki M, Takada T, Miyakawa S, Tsukada K, Nagino M, Kondo S, et al. Risk factors for biliary tract and ampullary carcinomas and prophylactic surgery for these factors. J Hepatobiliary Pancreat Surg. 2008;15:15–24.

Dyskinesia of the Gallbladder

Seong Ji Choi and Chang Duck Kim

Introduction

In 1923, gallbladder dyskinesia was first described by Westphal as an autonomic nervous system dysfunction of the gallbladder [1]. Afterward, it has been described by different nomenclatures in the literature, including functional gallbladder disorder, chronic acalculous gallbladder dysfunction, chronic acalculous cholecystitis, biliary dysmotility, gallbladder spasm, and cystic duct syndrome [2]. Biliary dyskinesia is a functional gastrointestinal disorder that affects the gallbladder and sphincter of Oddi, called gallbladder dyskinesia and sphincter of Oddi dysfunction, respectively. Gallbladder dyskinesia is a motility disorder of the gallbladder characterized by biliary-type abdominal pain (biliary colic) and structurally normal gallbladder. True biliary colic consists of episodic, moderate to a severe, steady, right upper quadrant or epigastric pain, lasting for at least 30 minutes, plateauing in less than an hour, and subsiding in less than 6 hours; however, the pain is paradoxically not colicky but constant. The pain often radiates to the back and right infrascapular areas in combination with other symptoms, such as nausea, vomiting, and diaphoresis, and is typically worse postprandially, 1–2 hours after digestion of a fatty meal. One study suggested that biliary colic has a circadian rhythm, reporting that 38 of 50 patients (76%) had a 24-hour cycle of pain, with its peak at midnight, tending to occur at the same time of day [3]. Gallbladder dyskinesia is relatively rare, but its clinical manifestations are not easily distinguishable from those of high-prevalence diseases that can cause biliary pain, such as functional dyspepsia, gastroesophageal reflux disease, peptic ulcer disease, cholecystitis, and pancreatitis; the possibility of these diseases should be carefully reviewed before making a diagnosis. Therefore, understanding the nature of the disease is essential for both diagnosis and treatment.

Epidemiology

Dyskinesia of the gallbladder is a rare disease compared to other diseases of the gallbladder and functional gastrointestinal disorders. The true prevalence of gallbladder dyskinesia is unknown, but it has been estimated in a few studies based on the number of patients with biliary colic combined with normal gallbladder

S. J. Choi · C. D. Kim (✉)
Division of Gastroenterology and Hepatology, Department of Internal Medicine, Korea University College of Medicine, 73 Goryeodae-ro, 02841 Seoul, Republic of Korea
e-mail: kumcge@korea.ac.kr

S. J. Choi
e-mail: coolandy@korea.ac.kr

J. B. Chung and K. Okazaki (eds.), *Diseases of the Gallbladder*,
https://doi.org/10.1007/978-981-15-6010-1_12

structure. Large population-based studies in the late 1980s showed that 7.6% of men and 20.7% of women, or overall 2.4% of adults complained of biliary colic in 5 years without gallstones in abdominal ultrasound imaging [4–6]. A population study carried out from 2005 to 2013 estimated a rate of 3.3% of gallbladder dyskinesia and 63.7% of biliary colic among patients who underwent cholecystectomy, and other studies estimated the rates of gallbladder dyskinesia between 26 and 38% in adults and 13 and 63% in children who underwent cholecystectomy [7–9]. A recent cross-sectional, general population study reported 10 patients with functional gallbladder disorder among 5931 adults, comprising 0.2% of the adult population, while 2083 controls (35.1%) complained of functional gastrointestinal disorders [10]. Incidence trends have differed between studies, with an incidence reported from stable to increasing, and may be affected by the development and adoption of different diagnostic tools over the reporting periods [7, 11]. Because of diagnostic uncertainty, shifting of operation indication and other aforementioned factors that might influence the diagnosis, one study reported that the incidence of gallbladder dyskinesia in the United States was 85 cases per million, doubling from 1991 to 2001 and was two times higher than those of other countries [12]. Overall, due to its diagnostic uncertainty, the prevalence of the disease is not certain and varies between studies.

Pathophysiology

Gallbladder stores the bile produced in the liver and secrets the concentrated bile juice into the duodenum in response to certain signals. The complex mechanisms underlying gallbladder function are well studied, but the etiology of gallbladder dyskinesia, which may be the outcome of combinations of dysfunctions in these mechanisms, is poorly understood.

There are several hypotheses proposed to illuminate the etiology of gallbladder dyskinesia, which can be divided into two broad categories: one considers dyskinesia as a mechanical/metabolic disorder and the other as a neurohormonal disorder. Mechanical/metabolic causes of gallbladder dyskinesia are due to crystal formation in the bile or the gallbladder wall, resulting from many different proposed mechanisms, such as cholesterolosis, microlithiasis, biliary sludge, chronic cholecystitis, gallbladder dysmotility, uncoordinated contraction between the gallbladder and cystic duct, and non-occluding cystic duct narrowing. The crystals may have formed at different stages of these mechanisms [13–16]. Moreover, crystals may eventually develop into organic abnormalities, such as gallstones or cholecystitis, may increase gallbladder pressure and cause biliary colic at any point during these processes [17]. However, not all patients with biliary colic that was relieved after cholecystectomy had histologic changes in their removed gallbladders; changes were observable in 44–100% of gallbladders, and those changes may or may not have been the cause or the outcome of poor gallbladder motility [18–20].

Neurohormonal causes of gallbladder dyskinesia include abnormalities in neuronal or hormonal regulation of the gallbladder. Stimulations of the vagus and celiac plexus affect the contraction and relaxation of the gallbladder, respectively, and any disruption in this stimulation results in abnormal gallbladder function [21]. Cholecystokinin (CCK) is a hormone widely accepted to be associated with biliary colic, through its abnormal release, decreased sensitivity of the gallbladder to CCK, or increased sensitivity of the cystic duct receptor to CCK [22]. One of the causes included in the neurohormonal etiology is visceral hypersensitivity or visceral neuropathy, a multifactorial entity that is well described in irritable bowel syndrome [23, 24]. Visceral hypersensitivity is an exaggerated response to normal or even stopped irritation after prolonged stimuli have altered and sensitized the nociceptor and brain–gut axis. Gallbladder dyskinesia is often associated with irritable bowel syndrome, delayed gastric emptying, gastric paresis, and chronic constipation, suggesting that these alterations may result from abnormal neurohormonal signaling pathways and pointing to possible panenteric motility disorder [25]. Even slight changes in any of these factors can induce biliary pain and be a cause of gallbladder dyskinesia.

Diagnosis

The diagnosis of gallbladder dyskinesia is a diagnosis of exclusion in patients with typical biliary pain. More common diseases with biliary pain should be focused and thoroughly investigated and excluded before making a diagnosis of gallbladder dyskinesia. Symptom-based criteria called the Rome criteria have been developed over many years to assist and standardize the clinical diagnosis of gallbladder dyskinesia. The Rome II criteria identified gallbladder dysfunction as an episode of severe steady epigastric and right upper quadrant pain of minimum 30 minutes duration, one or more pain episodes within the previous 12 months, and abnormal gallbladder function [26]. The Rome III criteria specified gallbladder dyskinesia more accurately and more concretely, and abnormal gallbladder function became a supportive but not required criterion for diagnosis [27]. The Rome IV criteria introduced diagnostic criteria for biliary pain (Table 1) and proposed diagnostic criteria for gallbladder dyskinesia, which include the described biliary pain (Table 2) [28]. Compared to the Rome III criteria, there was a minor change in the proposed criteria, quantitating "not significantly" to mean less than 20% (Table 1). Thorough physical examination and history taking, including the nature of the pain and its aggravating and relieving factors, such as food intake, should be performed in patients with suspected biliary pain to identify those who fulfill the criteria and require further investigation. Once the patients meet the criteria, they are to undergo several diagnostic studies to evaluate whether they meet the criteria for gallbladder dyskinesia. Figure 1 shows the algorithm for the diagnosis and treatment of gallbladder dyskinesia. The following are different diagnostic modalities that can be used in the diagnostic process.

Table 2 Rome IV diagnostic criteria for gallbladder dyskinesia [28]

1. Biliary pain
2. No structural gallbladder abnormality
Supportive criteria
The pain may be presented with
1. Low ejection fraction of gallbladder on scintigraphy
2. Normal liver enzymes, conjugated bilirubin, and amylase/lipase

Laboratory Tests

Blood tests, including testing of liver biochemistry and levels of pancreatic enzymes, should be performed to identify possible structural abnormalities in the liver, biliary system, and pancreas that might cause biliary pain. These results should be normal in order to diagnose gallbladder dyskinesia; if any of these results are abnormal, other diagnoses should be considered.

Table 1 Rome IV diagnostic criteria for biliary pain [28]

Pain located in the epigastrium and/or right upper quadrant and all of the following:
1. Builds up to a steady level lasting 30 minutes or longer
2. Recurrent symptoms at different intervals (not daily)
3. Severe enough to interrupt daily activities or lead to an emergency department visit
4. Not significantly (<20%) related to bowel movements
5. Not significantly (<20%) relieved by postural change or acid suppression
Supportive criteria
The pain may be presented with
1. Nausea and vomiting
2. Radiation to the back and/or right infra-subscapular region
3. Waking during the sleep

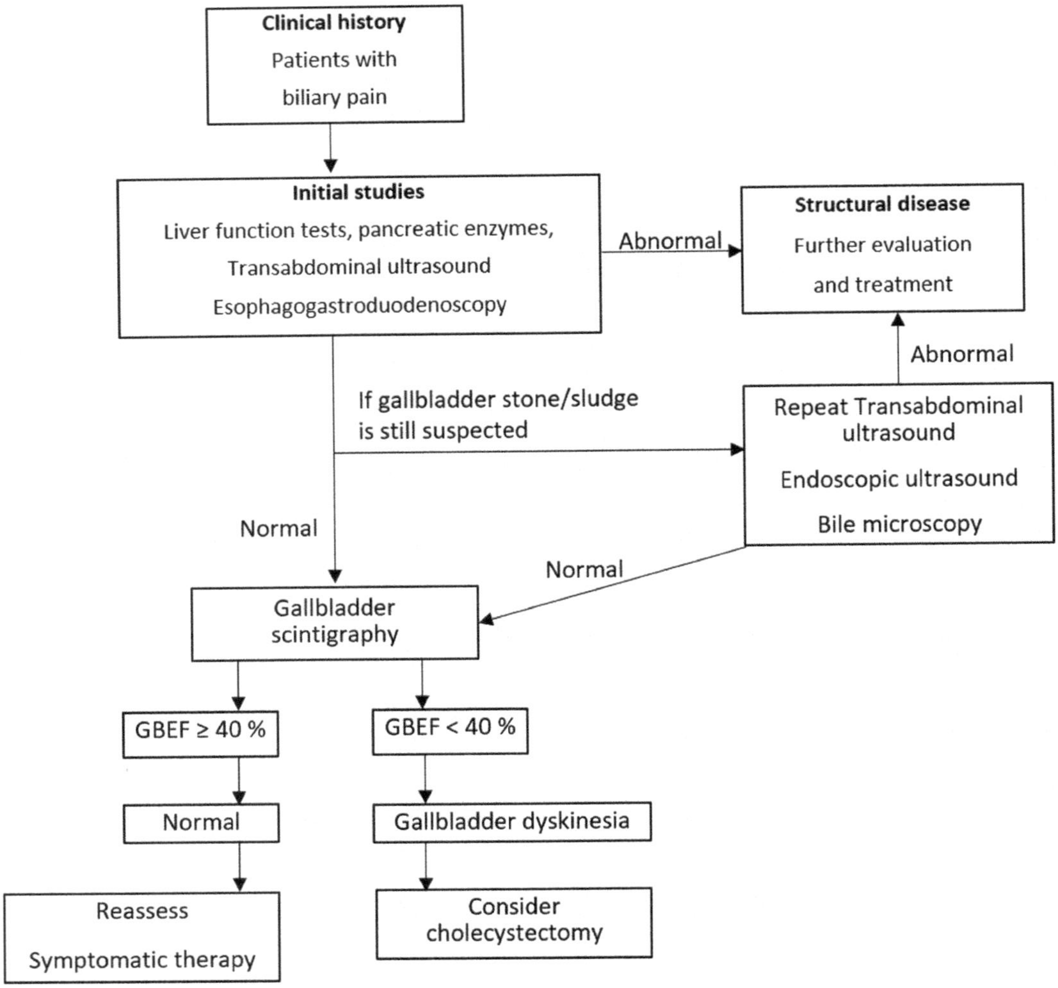

Fig. 1 Suggested algorithm for the diagnosis and treatment of gallbladder dyskinesia

Ultrasound

To evaluate potential structural abnormalities in the gallbladder, transabdominal ultrasound (TA-US) is recommended to rule out gallstones or gallbladder sludge. Even though there is inter-observer variability, TA-US remains the gold standard for detecting gallstones larger than 2 mm, with a sensitivity of>95% [29]. Gallstones can be easily detected by TA-US due to features such as echogenic focus, acoustic shadow, and gravitation dependence [30]. If gallstones or gallbladder sludge are suspected clinically but are not visualized in TA-US, the study can be repeated or endoscopic ultrasound (EUS) can be performed, which has shown better results in detecting gallbladder microlithiasis and can also screen for possible pancreatic lesions, such as chronic pancreatitis and tumors [31].

Endoscopy

The use of esophagogastroduodenoscopy is controversial, but can be a useful tool to rule out peptic ulcer disease and other structural abnormalities in the esophagus, stomach, and duodenum that could cause abdominal pain.

Microscopic Examination

Microscopic examination of gallbladder bile for microcrystal disease can also be performed to exclude microlithiasis and evaluate bile composition. Gallbladder bile can be collected directly during endoscopic retrograde cholangiopancreatography or from the duodenum following intravenous cholecystokinin (CCK) stimulation, and microscopic examination of the collected bile after immediate centrifugation can detect microlithiasis and cholesterol crystals. Cholesterol microcrystals are highly birefringent, with rhomboid shape under polarized light, and their presence strongly suggests microlithiasis. Calcium bilirubinate can be observed in the form of dark red-brown granules under light microscopy. However, the sensitivity and specificity of microscopic examination of duodenal bile are 67% and 91%, respectively, and the examination has not been widely accepted because of poor specificity and other technical issues [20, 31].

Assessment of Gallbladder Emptying

The quantity of gallbladder emptying can be measured as the gallbladder ejection fraction (GBEF), which is a percentage change calculated after a cholecystokinetic stimulus. The most prevalent method to estimate GBEF is CCK-stimulated cholescintigraphy (CCK-CS), which is a noninvasive, physiologic, and accurate assessment tool (Fig. 2). The role of CCK in gallbladder contraction and its clinical use was first reported in the mid-1900s, and Fink-Bennett et al. in 1985 combined CCK and nuclear imaging to measure GBEF [32]. Currently, sincalide™ (the 8 amino acid C-terminal fragment of cholecystokinin, CCK-8), which is a CCK analogue, is the only commercially available drug for CCK-CS. This test is performed after intravenous administration of ^{99m}technetium-labeled iminodiacetic acid (HIDA) analogue compounds, which have a high affinity for the liver and are excreted into the biliary tract, where they concentrate in the gallbladder. After either CCK administration or ingestion of fat-containing food, gallbladder emptying is stimulated and a net activity–time curve for the gallbladder can be calculated. Using a fatty meal for the stimulation of gallbladder contraction might be more physiologic and economical than using CCK, but the response to it may be variable and normal values have not been established in a protocol. Since there were wide variations in the methodologies of CCK-CS, an interdisciplinary panel recommended a protocol in 2011 [33]. The patient should be optimally prepared, with adequate fasting for at least 4 hours and adjustment of medications before the procedure, and intravenously injected HIDA radiotracer should fill the gallbladder within 60 minutes before sincalide infusion. A camera is placed in the left anterior oblique projection for adequate visualization of the gallbladder, duodenum, and small bowel, and 0.02 μg/kg of sincalide mixed with saline for a total 30–50 mL should be infused continuously for 60 minutes. At 60 minutes, GBEF is calculated as follows:

$$\text{GBEF}\ (\%) = \frac{\text{maximum counts} - \text{minimum counts}}{\text{maximum counts}}$$

Since studies with short CCK infusion duration resulted in varying GBEF values by stimulating CCK receptors in the cystic duct, infusion duration should be applied according to the protocol for reducing the variation of GBEF [22]. Cutoff values for abnormal GBEF vary from 35 to 50% and a value of 40% is the most widely accepted [34]. Figure 2 shows the examples of CCK-CS.

A low GBEF is not specific to or required for the diagnosis of gallbladder dyskinesia, but supports the diagnosis. The GBEF results values can change after a retest, and a low GBEF may also be observed in about 20% of healthy individuals or in patients with obesity, suffering from rapid weight loss, in a fasting state, with diabetes, celiac disease, steatohepatitis, liver cirrhosis, VIPoma, spinal cord injury, or irritable bowel syndrome, or having undergone prior foregut surgery [8, 35]. Medications, including

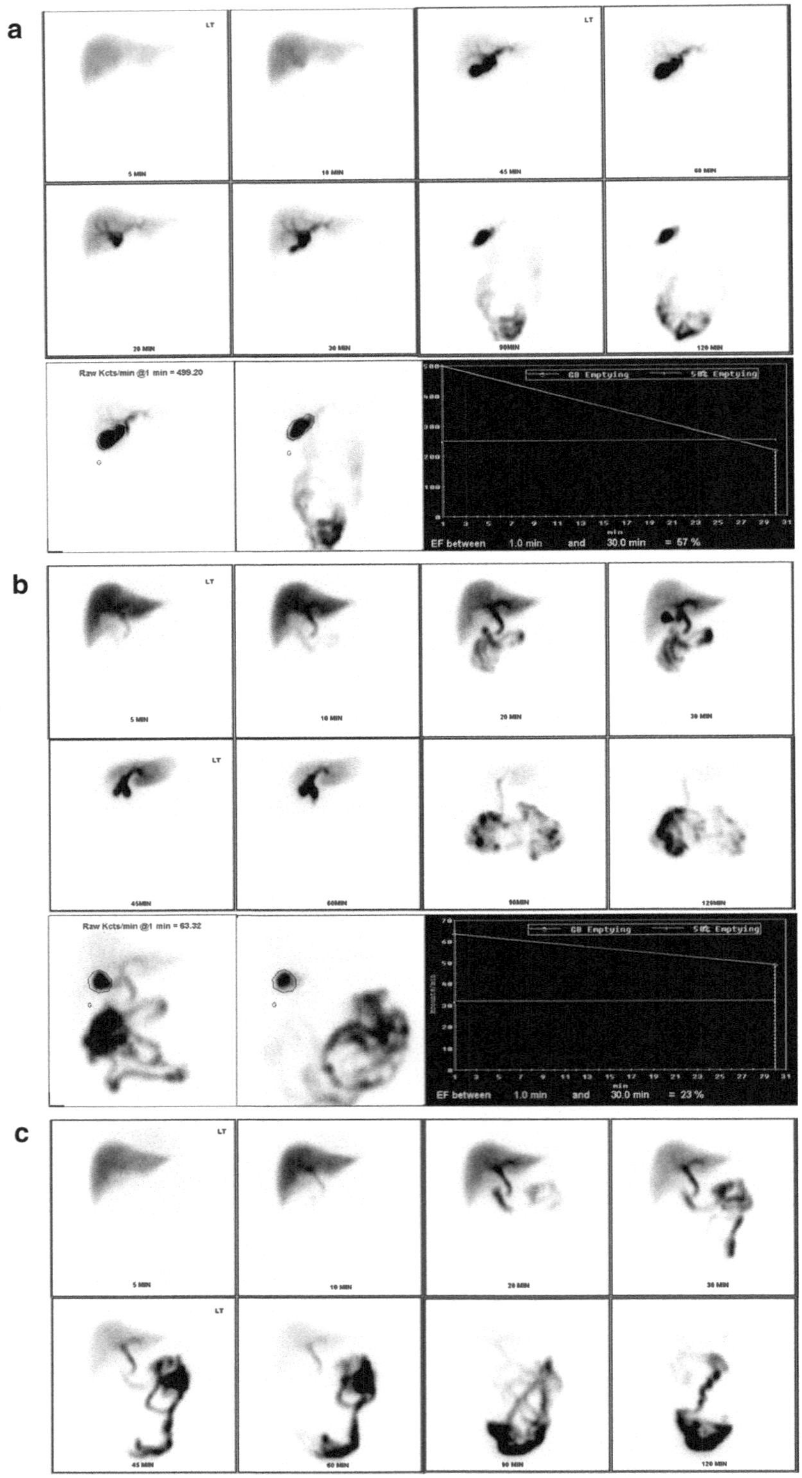

Fig. 2 A. Normal gallbladder emptying on gallbladder scintigraphy. After the injection of technetium 99-m-labeled mebrofenin, abdominal images are obtained at 10, 20, 30, 60, 90, and 120 minutes. The gallbladder is visualized 30 minutes after the injection of the radiopharmaceutical, and cholecystokinin is then infused after 60 minutes to evaluate gallbladder ejection function. The estimated ejection fraction is 57%. B. Decreased gallbladder emptying on gallbladder scintigraphy. The estimated ejection fraction is 23%. C. Gallbladder scintigraphy taken from patient B after cholecystectomy. No radiocontrast filling in previous gallbladder location

prokinetics, opiates, cholinomimetics, inhibitory hormones, nitric acid releasers, calcium channel blockers, and many other drugs can affect gallbladder contraction [36].

There is still controversy on performing cholecystectomy in patients with recurrent biliary pain with impaired gallbladder emptying without structural causes. Several studies support performing cholecystectomy in patients with biliary pain and reduced GBEF, and that 90–94% of those patients experience a significant improvement of pain [37, 38]. However, Singhal et al. reported that 43% of these patients still complained of persistent or recurrent symptoms in long-term follow-up, and a meta-analysis reported that patients with biliary pain and normal GBEF showed similar response rates to patients with biliary pain and abnormal GBEF [8, 39]. Because of these controversies surrounding the outcome of cholecystectomy, the surgery can be considered as a treatment option, but its use should be decided carefully.

There is a diagnostic dilemma for patients with typical biliary colic, normal laboratory findings, normal gallbladder structure, and normal gallbladder ejection fraction. These patients should be carefully followed with laboratory and imaging studies so as not to miss any diseases that show similar symptoms, and simultaneously treated with lifestyle modifications and symptomatic medical treatments. Cholecystectomy can be carefully considered if all follow-up studies show negative results and typical biliary colic continues.

Other Imaging Studies

Functional computed tomography and magnetic resonance (MR) cholangiography for diagnosing gallbladder dyskinesia are largely experimental, but they have shown to be applicable for calculating GBEF and detecting stones and other structural abnormalities [40, 41]. The recent development of hepatobiliary-specific gadolinium-based MR contrast agents, such as gadoxetic acid, made it possible to calculate GBEF accurately with MR cholangiography, and gadoxetic acid-contrasted MRI could be a potential alternative for CCK-CS in the near future [42]. Several studies have tried to measure GBEF using ultrasound with different techniques, but its applicability has not been established yet, and CCK-CS remains the standard diagnostic tool for GBEF [43, 44].

Pain Provocation Test

A pain provocation test using CCK in attempts to reproduce patients' symptoms has been used in supporting the diagnosis of gallbladder dyskinesia. Several studies advocate the use of the CCK provocation test as a tool for diagnosis of gallbladder dyskinesia and prediction of response to cholecystectomy [45, 46]. However, the sensitivity and specificity of the test in diagnosing gallbladder dyskinesia is low, considering that CCK can stimulate not only the gallbladder, but also other gastrointestinal organs, such as the duodenum and colon, and cause pain in these organs as well [47]. The false positive rate of CCK infusion is high, and even 15% of normal individuals showed positive results [1]. Moreover, abdominal cramping can be caused by bolus injections of CCK, and the subjective nature of pain makes it difficult to assess the effect of CCK on the gallbladder and predict the symptomatic relief by cholecystectomy in patients with gallbladder dyskinesia [16].

Differential Diagnosis

Gallbladder dyskinesia should be differentiated from organic disease and other common functional disorders. Any disease that could cause or whose effects can be mistaken as right upper quadrant abdominal pain should be considered in the diagnostic process. Diseases that should not be neglected include abdominal wall pain, bile duct obstruction, choledocholithiasis, cholelithiasis, functional sphincter of Oddi disorder, functional dyspepsia, gastritis, gastroesophageal reflux disease, gastroparesis, irritable bowel syndrome, pancreatitis, peptic ulcer disease, and pancreatobiliary malignancy.

Management

Medical Management

The medical management of gallbladder dyskinesia is at present poorly supported because of a lack of evidence. Medications recommended with limited evidence include tricyclic antidepressants, selective serotonin reuptake inhibitors, and gabapentin, which could be effective in some patients with functional gastrointestinal disorders accompanied by visceral hypersensitivity [48]. Prokinetics, bile acid composition modifiers, calcium channel blockers, and anti-inflammatory agents have also been suggested to be helpful, but their role and mechanisms of action are poorly understood [20]. Further studies are required to clarify their roles. Despite the lack of evidence for medical treatments, the diagnostic uncertainty of gallbladder dyskinesia and the comparative risks between medical and surgical management should be considered; medical treatment should be taken into account before cholecystectomy. Moreover, many studies have even reported that the symptoms of gallbladder dyskinesia improve significantly without any therapy [8].

Surgical Management

Cholecystectomy is considered as a standard treatment of gallbladder dyskinesia, recommended because of its effects on symptom resolution [1]. Gall and Chambers reported that 79% of patients with gallbladder dyskinesia experienced symptom relief after cholecystectomy, and Ozden and DiBaise reported 56% [49, 50]. In a retrospective study by Goncalves et al., patients with gallbladder dyskinesia who underwent cholecystectomy experienced symptom resolution in 80% of cases and symptom improvement in 20%, while 75% of patients who did not undergo cholecystectomy complained of persistent symptoms [51]. Several studies suggest that the response to cholecystectomy can be predicted by typical biliary colic symptom, low GBEF, or CCK provocation test, but this is still controversial [8]. Cholecystectomy may be considered in patients with normal GBEF after excluding other likely diagnoses that could produce similar symptoms and after medical treatment has failed. DiBaise and Oleynikov suggested in a systematic review that GBEF values did not predict a surgical outcome, and the symptoms of gallbladder dyskinesia improved significantly regardless of GBEF abnormalities [52]. A recent systematic review by Gudsoorkay et al. similarly suggests that there is no significant difference in relative risk between patients with normal and low GBEF, but patients with low GBEF show a significant improvement in symptoms with cholecystectomy compared to medical treatment, while patients with normal GBEF do not [53]. However, many of these studies were of the retrospective design, with small samples and a high risk of bias, so their results tend to be inconsistent and unreliable. There has been only one prospective, randomized, controlled trial that compared the efficacy of cholecystectomy to that of medical treatment in patients with decreased gallbladder ejection fraction; however, only 21 patients were enrolled in the study [54]. Prospective randomized clinical trials with sufficiently large patient cohorts and long follow-up periods are needed to establish well-accepted treatment guidelines for gallbladder dyskinesia.

References

1. Barnes SL, Clark DM, Schwartz RW. Biliary dyskinesia: a brief review. Curr Surg. 2004;61(5):428–34.
2. Goussous N, Kowdley GC, Sardana N, Spiegler E, Cunningham SC. Gallbladder dysfunction: how much longer will it be controversial? Digestion. 2014;90(3):147–54.
3. Rigas B, Torosis J, McDougall CJ, Vener KJ, Spiro HM. The circadian rhythm of biliary colic. J Clin Gastroenterol. 1990;12(4):409–14.

4. Rome Group for the Epidemiology and Prevention of Cholelithiasis (GREPCO). Prevalence of gallstone disease in an Italian adult female population. Am J Epidemiol. 1984;119(5):796–805.
5. The epidemiology of gallstone disease in Rome, Italy. Part I. Prevalence data in men. The Rome Group for Epidemiology and Prevention of Cholelithiasis (GREPCO). Hepatology. 1988;8(4):904–6.
6. Barbara L, Sama C, Morselli Labate AM, Taroni F, Rusticali AG, Festi D, et al. A population study on the prevalence of gallstone disease: the Sirmione Study. Hepatology. 1987;7(5):913–7.
7. Thiels CA, Hanson KT, Chawla KS, Topazian MD, Paley KH, Habermann EB, et al. Functional gallbladder disease: operative trends and short-term outcomes. Surgery. 2016;160(1):100–5.
8. Bielefeldt K, Saligram S, Zickmund SL, Dudekula A, Olyaee M, Yadav D. Cholecystectomy for biliary dyskinesia: how did we get there? Dig Dis Sci. 2014;59(12):2850–63.
9. Richmond BK. Response to: Laparoscopic cholecystectomy is safe and effective for the treatment of biliary dyskinesia in the pediatric population. Am Surg. 2010;76(12):1426.
10. Aziz I, Palsson OS, Tornblom H, Sperber AD, Whitehead WE, Simren M. The prevalence and impact of overlapping Rome IV-diagnosed functional gastrointestinal disorders on somatization, quality of life, and healthcare utilization: a cross-sectional general population study in three countries. Am J Gastroenterol. 2018;113(1):86–96.
11. Jones-Monahan K, Gruenberg JC. Chronic acalculous cholecystitis: changes in patient demographics and evaluation since the advent of laparoscopy. JSLS. 1999;3(3):221–4.
12. Preston JF, Diggs BS, Dolan JP, Gilbert EW, Schein M, Hunter JG. Biliary dyskinesia: a surgical disease rarely found outside the United States. Am J Surg. 2015;209(5):799–803; discussion.
13. Velanovich V. Biliary dyskinesia and biliary crystals: a prospective study. Am Surg. 1997;63(1):69–74.
14. Brugge WR, Brand DL, Atkins HL, Lane BP, Abel WG. Gallbladder dyskinesia in chronic acalculous cholecystitis. Dig Dis Sci. 1986;31(5):461–7.
15. Merg AR, Kalinowski SE, Hinkhouse MM, Mitros FA, Ephgrave KS, Cullen JJ. Mechanisms of impaired gallbladder contractile response in chronic acalculous cholecystitis. J Gastrointest Surg. 2002;6(3):432–7.
16. Amaral J, Xiao ZL, Chen Q, Yu P, Biancani P, Behar J. Gallbladder muscle dysfunction in patients with chronic acalculous disease. Gastroenterology. 2001;120(2):506–11.
17. Crowell MD, DiBaise JK, Lacy BE. Functional and motility disorders of the gastrointestinal tract: a case study approach. Chapter 13, Functional Gallbladder Disorder, pp. 153–160. Springer. 2015. https://doi.org/10.1007/978-1-4939-1498-2, ISBN 978-1-4939-1497-5.
18. Barron LG, Rubio PA. Importance of accurate preoperative diagnosis and role of advanced laparoscopic cholecystectomy in relieving chronic acalculous cholecystitis. J Laparoendosc Surg. 1995;5(6):357–61.
19. Patel NA, Lamb JJ, Hogle NJ, Fowler DL. Therapeutic efficacy of laparoscopic cholecystectomy in the treatment of biliary dyskinesia. Am J Surg. 2004;187(2):209–12.
20. Hansel SL, DiBaise JK. Functional gallbladder disorder: gallbladder dyskinesia. Gastroenterol Clin North Am. 2010;39(2):369–79, x.
21. Jones MW, Young M. Anatomy, abdomen and pelvis, gallbladder. Treasure Island (FL): StatPearls; 2019.
22. Francis G, Baillie J. Gallbladder dyskinesia: fact or fiction? Curr Gastroenterol Rep. 2011;13(2):188–92.
23. Farzaei MH, Bahramsoltani R, Abdollahi M, Rahimi R. The Role of Visceral Hypersensitivity in Irritable Bowel Syndrome: Pharmacological Targets and Novel Treatments. J Neurogastroenterol Motil. 2016;22(4):558–74.
24. Sood GK, Baijal SS, Lahoti D, Broor SL. Abnormal gallbladder function in patients with irritable bowel syndrome. Am J Gastroenterol. 1993;88(9):1387–90.
25. Penning C, Gielkens HA, Delemarre JB, Lamers CB, Masclee AA. Gall bladder emptying in severe idiopathic constipation. Gut. 1999;45(2):264–8.
26. Corazziari E, Shaffer EA, Hogan WJ, Sherman S, Toouli J. Functional disorders of the biliary tract and pancreas. Gut. 1999;45 Suppl 2:II48–54.
27. Behar J, Corazziari E, Guelrud M, Hogan W, Sherman S, Toouli J. Functional gallbladder and sphincter of oddi disorders. Gastroenterology. 2006;130(5):1498–509.
28. Cotton PB, Elta GH, Carter CR, Pasricha PJ, Corazziari ES. Rome IV. Gallbladder and sphincter of Oddi disorders. Gastroenterology. 2016;150(6):1420–1429.
29. Bortoff GA, Chen MY, Ott DJ, Wolfman NT, Routh WD. Gallbladder stones: imaging and intervention. Radiographics. 2000;20(3):751–66.
30. Gore RM, Thakrar KH, Newmark GM, Mehta UK, Berlin JW. Gallbladder imaging. Gastroenterol Clin North Am. 2010;39(2):265–87, ix.
31. Dahan P, Andant C, Levy P, Amouyal P, Amouyal G, Dumont M, et al. Prospective evaluation of endoscopic ultrasonography and microscopic examination of duodenal bile in the diagnosis of cholecystolithiasis in 45 patients with normal conventional ultrasonography. Gut. 1996;38(2):277–81.
32. Fink-Bennett D, DeRidder P, Kolozsi W, Gordon R, Rapp J. Cholecystokinin cholescintigraphic findings in the cystic duct syndrome. J Nucl Med. 1985;26(10):1123–8.
33. DiBaise JK, Richmond BK, Ziessman HH, Everson GT, Fanelli RD, Maurer A, et al. Cholecystokinin-cholescintigraphy in adults: consensus recommendations of an interdisciplinary panel. Clin Gastroenterol Hepatol. 2011;9(5):376–84.
34. Clark CJ. An Update on Biliary Dyskinesia. Surg Clin North Am. 2019;99(2):203–14.

35. Shaffer E. Acalculous biliary pain: new concepts for an old entity. Dig Liver Dis. 2003;35(Suppl 3): S20–5.
36. Jain AS, Simon S, Muthukrishnan I, Mohan AT, Balsubramaniam R. Standardization of "In-House fatty meal" methodology for cholescintigraphy. Indian J Nucl Med. 2015;30(4):303–8.
37. Khosla R, Singh A, Miedema BW, Marshall JB. Cholecystectomy alleviates acalculous biliary pain in patients with a reduced gallbladder ejection fraction. South Med J. 1997;90(11):1087–90.
38. Yost F, Margenthaler J, Presti M, Burton F, Murayama K. Cholecystectomy is an effective treatment for biliary dyskinesia. Am J Surg. 1999;178(6):462–5.
39. Singhal V, Szeto P, Norman H, Walsh N, Cagir B, VanderMeer TJ. Biliary dyskinesia: how effective is cholecystectomy? J Gastrointest Surg. 2012;16(1):135–40; discussion 40–1.
40. Vyas PK, Vesy TL, Konez O, Ciavellara DP, Hua K, Gaisie G. Estimation of gallbladder ejection fraction utilizing cholecystokinin-stimulated magnetic resonance cholangiography and comparison with hepatobiliary scintigraphy. J Magn Reson Imaging. 2002;15(1):75–81.
41. Inoue Y, Komatsu Y, Yoshikawa K, Akahane M, Isayama H, Ohtomo K, et al. Biliary motor function in gallstone patients evaluated by fatty-meal MR cholangiography. J Magn Reson Imaging. 2003;18(2):196–203.
42. Lee JK, Kim Y, Lee S, Park JE. Hepatobiliary phase of gadoxetic acid-enhanced MR in patients suspected of having gallbladder dyskinesia: comparison with hepatobiliary scintigraphy. Clin Imaging. 2015;39(1):66–71.
43. Donen A, Kantor R. Fatty meal ultrasonography in chronic acalculous cholecystitis. J Surg Case Rep. 2014;2014(11).
44. Irshad A, Ackerman SJ, Spicer K, Baker NL, Campbell A, Anis M, et al. Ultrasound evaluation of gallbladder dyskinesia: comparison of scintigraphy and dynamic 3D and 4D ultrasound techniques. AJR Am J Roentgenol. 2011;197(5):1103–10.
45. Rhodes M, Lennard TW, Farndon JR, Taylor RM. Cholecystokinin (CCK) provocation test: long-term follow-up after cholecystectomy. Br J Surg. 1988; 75(10):951–3.
46. Carr JA, Walls J, Bryan LJ, Snider DL. The treatment of gallbladder dyskinesia based upon symptoms: results of a 2-year, prospective, nonrandomized, concurrent cohort study. Surg Laparosc Endosc Percutan Tech. 2009;19(3):222–6.
47. Smythe A, Majeed AW, Fitzhenry M, Johnson AG. A requiem for the cholecystokinin provocation test? Gut. 1998;43(4):571–4.
48. Mapel DW. Functional disorders of the gastrointestinal tract: Cost effectiveness review. Best Pract Res Clin Gastroenterol. 2013;27(6):913–31.
49. Gall CA, Chambers KJ. Cholecystectomy for gall bladder dyskinesia: symptom resolution and satisfaction in a rural surgical practice. ANZ J Surg. 2002;72(10):731–4.
50. Ozden N, DiBaise JK. Gallbladder ejection fraction and symptom outcome in patients with acalculous biliary-like pain. Dig Dis Sci. 2003;48(5):890–7.
51. Goncalves RM, Harris JA, Rivera DE. Biliary dyskinesia: natural history and surgical results. Am Surg. 1998;64(6):493–7; discussion 7–8.
52. Delgado-Aros S, Cremonini F, Bredenoord AJ, Camilleri M. Systematic review and meta-analysis: does gall-bladder ejection fraction on cholecystokinin cholescintigraphy predict outcome after cholecystectomy in suspected functional biliary pain? Aliment Pharmacol Ther. 2003;18(2):167–74.
53. Gudsoorkar VS, Oglat A, Jain A, Raza A, Quigley EMM. Systematic review with meta-analysis: cholecystectomy for biliary dyskinesia-what can the gallbladder ejection fraction tell us? Aliment Pharmacol Ther. 2019;49(6):654–63.
54. Yap L, Wycherley AG, Morphett AD, Toouli J. Acalculous biliary pain: cholecystectomy alleviates symptoms in patients with abnormal cholescintigraphy. Gastroenterology. 1991;101(3):786–93.

Incidental Gallbladder Carcinoma

Jae Uk Chong, Jin Ho Lee, and Kuk Hwan Kwon

Introduction

According to global cancer statistics 2018, gallbladder cancer (GBC) accounts for 1.2% of all cancer diagnoses, but 1.7% of all cancer deaths [1]. GBC is a rare yet fatal disease with poor prognosis of reported less than 5% in 5-year survival [2, 3]. Such a poor prognosis results from discovery at late stages due to vague or absent symptoms. The absence of submucosa and serosa layers between the gallbladder and the liver may have a role in the early invasion of GBC into the liver [4]. SEER cancer statistics review shows that only one in five GBC cases is diagnosed at an early stage even in a highly advanced country such as the United States [5]. Occasionally, GBC is diagnosed during or following cholecystectomy for unsuspected benign disease of the gallbladder. These cases are termed as "incidental gallbladder cancer" and present several dilemmas for further management. With laparoscopic cholecystectomy as the current gold standard for treatment of cholecystolithiasis and the most frequently performed surgical procedure worldwide for benign gallbladder diseases, the incidence of incidental GBC has also increased with some reporting up to 3% [6]. Additionally, incidental GBC is reported to be associated with more favorable pathologic characteristics such as lower tumor grade and T-stage compared to non-incidental GBC, which usually presents with concerning signs of malignancy such as jaundice and weight loss [7]. When diagnosed with incidental GBC, the current guideline recommends re-resection for T1b, T2, and T3 disease unless contraindicated by advanced disease or poor performance status [8]. However, there are still controversies in the management of incidental GBC and risk factors have not yet been fully elaborated. In this chapter, we explored up-to-date knowledge for all aspects of incidental GBC.

Epidemiology

The widespread use of laparoscopic cholecystectomy has led to the discovery of incidental gallbladder cancer at an earlier stage. GBC is discovered incidentally during histopathology following 0.25–3.0% of laparoscopic cholecystectomies [9]. This constitutes a majority of GBC diagnoses (50–70%) [7, 10]. While GBC is rare, it is the most common malignant disease of the biliary tract [11]. Incidences have been reported to vary greatly by geographical regions and ethnicity. GBC commonly occurs in South America, in countries such as Chile, Bolivia,

J. U. Chong (✉) · J. H. Lee · K. H. Kwon
Department of Surgery, NHIS Ilsan Hospital, Yonsei University College of Medicine, Goyang-si, Gyeonggi-do, Korea
e-mail: jaeuk1216@nhimc.or.kr

J. B. Chung and K. Okazaki (eds.), *Diseases of the Gallbladder*,
https://doi.org/10.1007/978-981-15-6010-1_13

and Ecuador, and in Asia, in parts of India, Pakistan, Japan, and Korea [12, 13]. Mapuche Indians in Chile demonstrate the highest rate of GBC: 12.3/100,000 for males and 27.3/100,000 for females [14]. GBC is also found in high frequency in Eastern and Central Europe, but in low frequency in Western and Mediterranean Europe, and in the United States [4]. This variation may be a result of differences in both environmental and genetic factors. In regions with a high prevalence of GBC, surgeons should practice with more vigilance to discover incidental GBC during laparoscopic cholecystectomy for presumed benign gallbladder diseases.

Risk Factors

Currently known risk factors for GBC include advanced age, female sex, polyps greater than 1 cm, porcelain GB, anomalous pancreatobiliary ductal union, and gallstones. In terms of incidental GBC, results of the American College of Surgeons-National Surgical Quality Improvement Program (ACS-NSQIP) database showed that the conversion of laparoscopic cholecystectomy to open cholecystectomy, advanced age (≥65 years old), Asian or African-American race, an elevated alkaline phosphatase level (≥120units/L), and female sex were independent risk factors [15]. The combination of risk factors increased the risk of incidental GBC: 6.3-fold increase for one factor, 16.7-fold increase for two factors, 30.0-fold increase for three factors, and 47.4-fold increase in risk of incidental GBC for all four factors.

Recently, the risk score model to predict incidental GBC has also been proposed based on the data from the Swedish Registry of Gallstone Surgery and Endoscopic Retrograde Cholangiopancreatography (GallRiks) [16]. The model was based on five clinical variables including age, female gender, previous cholecystitis, bilirubin level, and the presence of acute cholecystitis. Risk scores were divided into low risk (<3.5 points), intermediate risk (3.5–8 points), and high risk (>8 points). Each clinical variables were given points as following: 0 for age<60 years, 3.5 for age 60–69 years, 6.5 for age 70–79 years, 16 for age ≥80 years, 3.5 for female gender, 1.5 for previous cholecystitis, 1.5 for normal bilirubin levels/acute cholecystitis, and 2.0 for elevated bilirubin levels/no acute cholecystitis. With reference to the low-risk group, the intermediate-risk group had 3.6 times increased risk and the high-risk group had 18 times more risk of GBC.

Under the circumstances of increased risk, as previously reported, surgeons should be more attentive and prepared to perform adequate R0 resection at initial operation when incidental GBC is discovered.

Tumor Markers

Currently, there are no biomarkers for incidental GBC as tumor markers are not routinely checked for benign gallbladder diseases. For GBC, carcinoembryonic antigen (CEA) and carbohydrate antigen (CA) 19–9 are most commonly utilized as tumor markers. CEA is a broad-spectrum tumor marker that is found in gastrointestinal cancer and in the normal embryonic gut, pancreas, and biliary tract. CEA level greater than 4 ng/mL is 93% specific for GBC but only 50% sensitive [17]. CA 19–9 greater than 20 IU/mL has 79% sensitivity and 79% specificity for GBC [17]. Wen et al. have shown that a combination of an elevated preoperative CEA and CA 19–9 was associated with a poor prognosis and values within normal range showed the best prognosis [18]. However, prognostic accuracy of both CEA and CA 19–9 is rather low and other markers such as CA 242 and thymidine kinase have been proposed in the past [19, 20]. Role of tumor markers and other biomarkers need to be evaluated and discovered in incidental GBC.

Diagnosis

Preoperative diagnosis of incidental GBC is difficult in clinical practice as there is no mass seen on preoperative imaging, and cholecystectomy is performed for presumed benign stone disease. Focal or diffuse wall thickening may be present due to chronic or acute cholecystitis. Since GBC may present with wall thickening in 20–30% of cases, the differential diagnosis should be more actively sought [21].

In a study comparing non-incidental GBC and incidental GBC, sonographic characteristics showed a significantly different width of gallbladder (41.6 mm vs. 32.3 mm, $p=0.009$, respectively) and gallbladder wall thickness (8.0 mm vs. 5.5 mm, $p=0.016$, respectively) [22]. Incidental GBC was found with less wall thickening and smaller gallbladder width with the common presence of cholelithiasis. Findings suggested that incidental GBC has only mildly thickened gallbladder wall with difficulty in distinguishing from the inflammatory thickening. Suspicious cases of the small gallbladder with wall thickening may require further radiological evaluation to differentiate incidental GBC.

Multi-detector computed tomography (MDCT) has also been used to distinguish between benign and malignant causes of gallbladder wall thickening according to gallbladder enhancement and have reported sensitivity and positive predictive values of 75.9–82.8% and 80.0–82.8%, respectively [23]. In the study, MDCT findings of "thick" one-layer pattern with heterogeneous enhancement and two-layer pattern with "thick" enhancing inner wall $\geq$2.6 mm and "thin" weakly or nonenhancing outer wall $\leq$3.4 mm indicated signs of malignant flat gallbladder wall thickening rather than benign disease. The diagnostic accuracy of these enhancing patterns as signs of malignancy was 87.6–89.1%.

Another emerging technique for differentiating the wall thickening includes real-time elastography using acoustic radiation force impulse (ARFI). High intensity-focused ultrasound is used to evaluate the tissue stiffness in the liver, breast, and other organs [24]. Benign and malignant nodules in various organs are differentiated by using much higher stiffness present in malignant tissues due to the increased cell density compared to tissues with chronic inflammation and fibrosis [25].

Kapoor et al. [26] showed that real-time elastography diagnosed GBC with a mean shear wave velocity of 3.41 m/s [95% CI: 3.1–3.7 m/s]. With a cutoff value of 2.7 m/s, elastography showed sensitivity and specificity of 100% and 91.3%, respectively for diagnosing GBC with an overall accuracy of 92.8%. A false positive rate of 8.5% occurring in acute cholecystitis was also reported.

For suspicious wall thickening of gallbladder, routine use of elastography during ultrasonography combined with MDCT may assist in the earlier discovery of incidental GBC.

Stage Distribution at Presentation

Systemic review and meta-analysis of 2145 incidental GBC patients [27] showed that nearly half were T2 stage with a pooled proportion of 47.0% (95% CI: 0.421–0.519) at presentation. T1 and T3 were discovered at similar rate with pooled proportion of 23.0% (95% CI: 0.178–0.291) for T1 and 25.1% (95% CI: 0.195–0.317) for T3. Pooled proportion of lymph node metastases was 14.2% (95% CI: 0.107–0.185). Results of a multicenter study on 724 GBC cases by the French Surgical Association showed that 85% of cases were identified as T3 or T4 [28]. While GBC is usually discovered at an advanced stage, incidental GBC is diagnosed at an earlier stage. With early diagnosis, prognosis is greatly influenced. The 5-year overall survival rate for T1a and T1b is over 95% [29] and for T2 is 70% [30]. In order to increase the survival of GBC, efforts to discover more incidental GBC may be essential.

Pathologic Examination and Staging

Pathologic examination is important for appropriate staging and further management. Yet, no consensus has been met on a uniform pathologic examination protocol for those with no clinical or imaging suspicion for GBC and no apparent abnormality on gross examination. Due to limited resources and low risk of cancer, some centers do not recommend a microscopic examination in these situations [31]. However, results from GallRiks data showed that routine pathologic examination rather than selective uncovers a higher proportion of incidental GBC [32]. The current guideline suggests a routine histopathological examination of gallbladder specimens including minimal microscopic evaluation of three sections and the cystic duct margin, particularly in areas of high incidence [8].

Once a diagnosis is confirmed as GBC, correct staging according to the depth of invasion is critical in establishing further treatment. (Table 1) Staging influences disease management and prognosis. Current AJCC 8th cancer staging manual [33] for gallbladder cancer contains several changes from the previous edition. First, the T2 category (stage II) was separated into T2a (stage IIA) and T2b (stage IIB), depending on the tumor location on peritoneal or hepatic side of the gallbladder, respectively. This change was based on results from a multi-institutional study showing worse survival after resection of T2 GBC on the hepatic side of the gallbladder [34]. Second, the N category has been changed from an anatomic location-based system to a number-based system. Regional metastatic lymph nodes along the cystic duct, common bile duct, hepatic artery, and/or portal vein are classified into N1 and N2 stages, depending on the involvement of 1–3 LNs and $\geq$4 LNs, respectively. Periaortic, pericaval, superior mesenteric artery, and/or celiac artery lymph nodes are now classified as distant metastasis. Finally, retrieval of at least six lymph nodes is recommended in patients with T1b or greater.

Restaging Prior to Re-Resection

After the diagnosis of GBC has been confirmed, appropriate staging workup should be undertaken to exclude disseminated disease or obvious early recurrence. Patients should undergo chest and abdominal CT as a minimum requirement for restaging and consider other imaging modalities such as MRI and PET for selected cases based on features on CT or MRI.

In a retrospective Surveillance, Epidemiology and End Results (SEER) database study, CT scan was the most utilized perioperative imaging modality [35]. MRI can also be used to detect vascular invasion, biliary tract involvement, liver

Table 1 TNM staging according to AJCC 8th edition

Stage group	T category	T-criteria	N category	M category
0	Tis	carcinoma in situ	N0	M0
I	T1a	Invades lamina propria	N0	M0
	T1b	Invades muscular layer	N0	M0
IIA	T2a	Invades the perimuscular connective tissue on the peritoneal side, without involvement of the serosa	N0	M0
IIB	T2b	Invades the perimuscular connective tissue on the hepatic side, with no extension into the liver	N0	M0
IIIA	T3	Tumor perforates the serosa or directly invades the liver or one other adjacent organ or structure, such as the stomach, duodenum, colon, pancreas, omentum or extrahepatic bile ducts	N0	M0
IIIB	T1-3		N1	M0
IVA	T4	Invades the main portal vein or hepatic artery or invades two or more extrahepatic organs or structures	N0-1	M0
IVB	Any T		N2	M0
	Any T		Any N	M1

*N1: 1–3 regional lymph node metastases, N2: 4 or more regional lymph node metastases

invasion, and lymph node involvement with reliable accuracy [36].

The role of PET-CT has not been sufficiently proven in a prospective fashion for patients with GBC; however, numerous retrospective studies have reported some utility. In a study from Memorial Sloan Kettering Cancer Center, PET results altered the management of 23% of GBC patients [37]. A study evaluating 108 patients undergoing PET before re-resection found that PET was useful in stratifying patients for effective treatment and significantly higher uptake was associated with residual disease [38]. PET was also reported useful in the assessment of local residual disease in T1b GBC [38]. If there is no uptake in PET for T1b, re-resection was not recommended due to the low risk of residual disease.

Surgical Strategy

Reoperation for incidental GBC should have two fundamental objectives: R0 resection and clearance of the locoregional lymph nodes.

For tumor contained within the mucosa (Tis or T1a), cholecystectomy alone is sufficient for complete R0 resection as the risk of lymph node dissemination is low. With negative resection margins, 5-year survival after simple cholecystectomy is reported between 99% and 100% with a less than 2% risk of lymph node involvement [39]. However, great care should be exercised to prevent bile spillage during operation. If the surgeon cannot guarantee an adequate resection without spillage during laparoscopy, open cholecystectomy should be considered.

For T1b GBC, current guidelines recommend extended resection with lymphadenectomy because of the possibility of nodal involvement in about 10% [39, 40]. However, there are controversies in the necessity of re-resection in T1b GBC. According to National Comprehensive Cancer Network Guidelines 2019, for T1b and greater, postoperative workup including CT and MRI along with consideration for staging laparoscopy are recommended. In cases of resectable state, hepatic resection and lymphadenectomy are recommended with bile duct resection when needed. For unresectable cases, chemotherapy, radiation therapy, and/or best supportive care are recommended [41]. While NCCN guidelines recommend a more radical approach to T1b, the results of a systemic review found no definite evidence that extended cholecystectomy provides a survival benefit over simple cholecystectomy in T1b GBC [39]. Nevertheless, since the lymph node metastasis is considerable (10%), regional lymphadenectomy should be performed for the treatment and staging of GBC.

T2 GBC is often diagnosed incidentally after laparoscopic cholecystectomy and it is well known that 5-year overall survival is superior when re-resection with extended cholecystectomy is performed (55–90% vs. 0–40%) [42, 43]. Extended cholecystectomy includes resection of the gallbladder bed and hepatectomy to achieve an R0 resection; a 2–3-cm margin is commonly used. The extent of liver resection ranges from partial hepatectomies (nonanatomical or anatomical resection of segments 4a and 5) to major extended hepatectomies. Anatomical resection of segments 4a and 5 is considered a good oncologic option for GBC because the cystic vein drains into segment 4a (37–90%) and segment 5 (52–90%) [44, 45]. A more radical method of routine right extended hepatectomy including caudate lobectomy has also been proposed. However, results have not shown improved survival for major resection over nonanatomical liver resection and increased morbidity has been associated with major resection [46, 47]. Consequently, complete R0 resection with limited liver resection is the recommended approach to GBC, as long as negative margins are achieved.

With the newly introduced subdivision of T2 based on the tumor location, there are recent debates on the necessity of extended cholecystectomy for all peritoneal side T2 GBC [48]. The presence of residual disease in incidental GBC has been reported to be 57–70% for T2 and 77–91% T3 [49, 50]. Residual disease has a profound impact on survival. Patients without residual disease after re-resection had a better

5-year survival than those with residual disease (84.8% vs. 36.9%, p=0.01) [50]. In order to better predict the risk of residual disease, Ethun et al. [51] proposed the gallbladder cancer predictive risk score (GBRS) based on T-stage, tumor differentiation, lymphovascular invasion (LVI), and perineural invasion (PNI). Each pathologic characteristic was assigned a following value: T1a-0, T1b-1, T2–2, T3/4–3, well-diff-1, mod-diff-2, poor-diff-3, LVI-negative-1, LVI-positive-2, PNI-negative-1, PNI-positive-2. The values were added and separated into three risk groups including low risk (3–4), intermediate risk (5–7), and high risk (8–10). In the high-risk group, chances of locoregional residual disease were estimated to be 61% and re-resection is necessary if possible. For intermediate-risk group, the risk of locoregional residual disease is estimated to be 24% and re-resection should be aggressively pursued. In the low-risk group, however, re-resection may not be necessary with low chances of residual disease. The approach to incidental GBC is still controversial because of the difficulty in comparing data derived from nonuniform case studies. Application of GBRS may be limited in the current form because of a limited number of patients evaluated for developing the scoring system. However, with further validation in a larger population, GBRS may prove to be a great tool in optimizing the treatment strategy.

Intraoperative Findings

Events during the operation may influence oncologic outcome and treatment strategy. In a result based on German registry, intraoperative gallbladder perforation resulted in significantly higher local recurrence rate (38.4% vs. 27.2%, p=0.047) [52]. Gallbladder perforation or bile spillage during operation has been associated with poor oncologic outcomes and increased risk of peritoneal carcinomatosis [53–57]. Ouchi et al. [54] reported that gallbladder perforation during laparoscopic cholecystectomy was found in 94 of 470 patients (20%). Risk factors associated with gallbladder perforation is not clear but increased T stage and severity of inflammation may cause greater difficulty during operation, leading to higher chances of intraoperative gallbladder perforation. In acute cholecystitis, severe gallbladder inflammation such as emphysematous and gangrenous cholecystitis is highly associated with gallbladder perforation [58]. While the association between intraoperative gallbladder perforation and inflammation in gallbladder cancer has not yet been found, preoperatively elevated neutrophil–lymphocyte ratio (NLR>5) [59] and presence of inflammation [60] were found to be associated with poor oncologic outcome after curative resection for GBC. Utmost care to prevent bile spillage and gallbladder perforation is indisputably necessary during operation.

Perioperative Therapy

Role of adjuvant chemotherapy in GBC has not yet been fully elucidated. The majority of recurrences after resection of GBC was found to be distant, emphasizing the systemic nature of GBC and the need for multimodal therapy [61]. In a series of incidental GBC, adjuvant chemotherapy has been shown to be associated with better survival [7]. A meta-analysis of 6712 patients also supported the use of adjuvant therapy after surgery for biliary tract cancers [62]. Until recently, a combination of cisplatin and gemcitabine has been preferred regimen based on the Advanced Biliary Cancer (ABC)-02 trial, which demonstrated in a randomized controlled trial of 410 patients with advanced biliary tract malignancies (149 patients with GBC) [63]. Results showed an overall survival of 11.7 months for cisplatin plus gemcitabine versus 8.1 months for gemcitabine alone. However, the overall application was less than 30% and treatment benefit was small [64]. A recent BILCAP (BILiary CAPecitabine) randomized controlled trial in 447 patients showed that 6 months of adjuvant capecitabine improved overall survival compared to placebo [65]. Thus, this regimen is currently recommended after the re-resection of incidental GBC [66]. Current guidelines and consensus statements recommend adjuvant chemotherapy for any T2 disease and above with N1 disease, given the high risk of recurrence and nodal involvement [8, 67].

In terms of radiotherapy, the utility in adjuvant setting has not been proven. There are no randomized trials for radiotherapy and is only performed in some centers. Currently, chemoradiation is recommended only in microscopically positive surgical resection margin (R1 resection) [66]. There is no evidence for the use of neoadjuvant therapy prior to re-resection.

Conclusion

GBC is a rare yet fatal disease. Most cases are discovered incidentally while treating a benign disease, indicating the importance of surveillance during laparoscopic cholecystectomy. Incidental GBC is generally diagnosed at an earlier stage and carries a better prognosis than nonincidental GBC. Therapy can be multimodal yet surgical intervention is the mainstay of GBC treatment. A simple cholecystectomy is adequate for GBC contained within mucosa (Tis, T1a). For T1b and above, reoperation for incidental GBC should have two fundamental objectives: R0 resection and clearance of the locoregional lymph nodes. The role of adjuvant therapy needs further investigation in better detail and for subgroups. Until then, adjuvant capecitabine seems to improve oncologic outcomes. Due to the rarity of the disease, efforts to recruit patients into ongoing multicenter clinical trials and further prospective studies are warranted for a better understanding of incidental GBC.

References

1. Bray F, Ferlay J, Soerjomataram I, Siegel RL, Torre LA, Jemal A. Global cancer statistics 2018: GLOBOCAN estimates of incidence and mortality worldwide for 36 cancers in 185 countries. CA Cancer J Clin. 2018;68:394–424.
2. Batra Y, Pal S, Dutta U, Desai P, Garg PK, Makharia G, et al. Gallbladder cancer in India: a dismal picture. J Gastroenterol Hepatol. 2005:20:309–14.
3. Cubertafond P, Mathonnet M, Gainant A, Launois B. Radical surgery for gallbladder cancer. Results of the French surgical association survey. Hepatogastroenterology. 1999;46:1567–71.
4. Levy AD, Murakata LA, Rohrmann CA Jr. Gallbladder carcinoma: radiologic-pathologic correlation. Radiographics. 2001;21:295–314.
5. Howlader N, Noone A, Krapcho M, Miller D, Bishop K, Kosary C, et al. SEER cancer statistics review, 1975-2014. Bethesda, MD: National Cancer Institute; 2017. https://seer.cancer.gov/csr/1975_2014/.
6. Toyonaga T, Chijiiwa K, Nakano K, Noshiro H, Yamaguchi K, Sada M, et al. Completion radical surgery after cholecystectomy for accidentally undiagnosed gallbladder carcinoma. World J Surg. 2003;27:266–71.
7. Ethun CG, Le N, Lopez-Aguiar AG, Pawlik TM, Poultsides G, Tran T, et al. Pathologic and prognostic implications of incidental versus nonincidental gallbladder cancer: a 10-institution study from the United States extrahepatic biliary malignancy consortium. Am Surg. 2017;83:679–86.
8. Aloia TA, Jarufe N, Javle M, Maithel SK, Roa JC, Adsay V, et al. Gallbladder cancer: expert consensus statement. HPB (Oxford). 2015;17:681–90.
9. Cavallaro A, Piccolo G, Di Vita M, Zanghì A, Cardì F, Di Mattia P, et al. Managing the incidentally detected gallbladder cancer: algorithms and controversies. Int J Surg. 2014;12:S108–19.
10. Butte JM, Matsuo K, Gönen M, D'Angelica MI, Waugh E, Allen PJ, et al. Gallbladder cancer: differences in presentation, surgical treatment, and survival in patients treated at centers in three countries. J Am Coll Surg. 2011;212:50–61.
11. Lazcano-Ponce EC, Miquel J, Muñoz N, Herrero R, Ferrecio C, Wistuba II, et al. Epidemiology and molecular pathology of gallbladder cancer. CA Cancer J Clin. 2001;51:349–64.
12. Randi G, Franceschi S, La Vecchia C. Gallbladder cancer worldwide: geographical distribution and risk factors. Int J Cancer. 2006;118:1591–602.
13. Strom BL, Soloway RD, Rios-Dalenz JL, Rodriguez-Martinez HA, West SL, Kinman JL, et al. Risk factors for gallbladder cancer. An international collaborative case–control study. Cancer. 1995;76:1747–56.
14. Hundal R, Shaffer EA. Gallbladder cancer: epidemiology and outcome. Clin Epidemiol. 2014;6:99–109.
15. Pitt SC, Jin LX, Hall BL, Strasberg SM, Pitt HA. Incidental gallbladder cancer at cholecystectomy: when should the surgeon be suspicious? Ann Surg. 2014;260:128–33.
16. Muszynska C, Nilsson J, Lundgren L, Lindell G, Andersson R, Sandström P, et al. A risk score model to predict incidental gallbladder cancer in patients scheduled for cholecystectomy. Am J Surg. 2020. https://doi.org/10.1016/j.amjsurg.2020.01.039.
17. Strom BL, Maislin G, West SL, Atkinson B, Herlyn M, Saul S, et al. Serum CEA and CA 19-9: potential

future diagnostic or screening tests for gallbladder cancer? Int J Cancer. 1990;45:821–4.
18. Wen Z, Si A, Yang J, Yang P, Yang X, Liu H, et al. Elevation of CA19-9 and CEA is associated with a poor prognosis in patients with resectable gallbladder carcinoma. HPB (Oxford). 2017;19:951–6.
19. Liska V, Treska V, Skalicky T, Fichtl J, Bruha J, Vycital O, et al. Evaluation of tumor markers and their impact on prognosis in gallbladder, bile duct and cholangiocellular carcinomas–a pilot study. Anticancer Res. 2017;37:2003–9.
20. Rana S, Dutta U, Kochhar R, Rana SV, Gupta R, Pal R, et al. Evaluation of CA 242 as a tumor marker in gallbladder cancer. J Gastrointest Cancer. 2012;43:267–71.
21. Vijayakumar A, Vijayakumar A, Patil V, Mallikarjuna M, Shivaswamy B. Early diagnosis of gallbladder carcinoma: an algorithm approach. ISRN Radiol. 2012;2013. https://doi.org/10.5402/2013/239424.
22. Wang J-H, Liu B-J, Xu H-X, Sun L-P, Li D-D, Guo L-H, et al. Clinical, pathological and sonographic characteristics of unexpected gallbladder carcinoma. Int J Clin Exp Med. 2015;8:11109–16.
23. Kim SJ, Lee JM, Lee JY, Kim SH, Han JK, Choi BI, et al. Analysis of enhancement pattern of flat gallbladder wall thickening on MDCT to differentiate gallbladder cancer from cholecystitis. AJR Am J Roentgenol. 2008;191:765–71.
24. Fahey B, Nelson R, Bradway D, Hsu S, Dumont D, Trahey G. In vivo visualization of abdominal malignancies with acoustic radiation force elastography. Phys Med Biol. 2007;53:279–93.
25. Cho SH, Lee JY, Han JK, Choi BI. Acoustic radiation force impulse elastography for the evaluation of focal solid hepatic lesions: preliminary findings. Ultrasound Med Biol. 2010;36:202–8.
26. Kapoor A, Kapoor A, Mahajan G. Differentiating malignant from benign thickening of the gallbladder wall by the use of acoustic radiation force impulse elastography. J Ultrasound Med. 2011;30:1499–507.
27. Choi KS, Choi SB, Park P, Kim WB, Choi SY. Clinical characteristics of incidental or unsuspected gallbladder cancers diagnosed during or after cholecystectomy: a systematic review and meta-analysis. World J Gastroenterol. 2015;21:1315–23.
28. Cubertafond P, Gainant A, Cucchiaro G. Surgical treatment of 724 carcinomas of the gallbladder. Results of the French Surgical Association Survey. Ann Surg. 1994;219:275–80.
29. Jang J-Y, Heo JS, Han Y, Chang J, Kim JR, Kim H, et al. Impact of type of surgery on survival outcome in patients with early gallbladder cancer in the era of minimally invasive surgery: oncologic safety of laparoscopic surgery. Medicine. 2016;95:e3675.
30. Jung W, Jang J-Y, Kang MJ, Chang YR, Shin YC, Chang J, et al. Effects of surgical methods and tumor location on survival and recurrence patterns after curative resection in patients with T2 gallbladder cancer. Gut Liver. 2016;10:140–6.
31. Renshaw AA, Gould EW. Submitting the entire gallbladder in cases of dysplasia is not justified. Am J Clin Pathol. 2012;138:374–6.
32. Lundgren L, Muszynska C, Ros A, Persson G, Gimm O, Valter L, et al. Are incidental gallbladder cancers missed with a selective approach of gallbladder histology at cholecystectomy? World J Surg. 2018;42:1092–9.
33. Edge SB, Byrd DR, Compton CC, Fritz AG, Greene FL, Trotti A, et al. AJCC Cancer Staging Manual. 8th ed. New York: Springer; 2017.
34. Shindoh J, de Aretxabala X, Aloia TA, Roa JC, Zimmitti G, Javle M, et al. Tumor location is a strong predictor of tumor progression and survival in T2 gallbladder cancer: an international multicenter study. Ann Surg. 2015;261:733–9.
35. Mayo SC, Shore AD, Nathan H, Edil B, Wolfgang CL, Hirose K, et al. National trends in the management and survival of surgically managed gallbladder adenocarcinoma over 15 years: a population-based analysis. J Gastrointest Surg. 2010;14:1578–91.
36. Miller G, Jarnagin W. Gallbladder carcinoma. Eur J Surg Oncol. 2008;34:306–12.
37. Corvera CU, Blumgart LH, Akhurst T, DeMatteo RP, D'Angelica M, Fong Y, et al. 18F-fluorodeoxyglucose positron emission tomography influences management decisions in patients with biliary cancer. J Am Coll Surg. 2008;206:57–65.
38. Goel M, Tamhankar A, Rangarajan V, Patkar S, Ramadwar M, Shrikhande SV. Role of PET CT scan in redefining treatment of incidental gall bladder carcinoma. J Surg Oncol. 2016;113:652–8.
39. Lee SE, Jang JY, Lim CS, Kang MJ, Kim SW. Systematic review on the surgical treatment for T1 gallbladder cancer. World J Gastroenterol. 2011;17:174–80.
40. Lee SE, Jang JY, Kim SW, Han HS, Kim HJ, Yun SS, et al. Surgical strategy for T1 gallbladder cancer: a nationwide multicenter survey in South Korea. Ann Surg Oncol. 2014;21:3654–60.
41. National Comprehensive Cancer Network. NCCN Guidelines for Hepatobiliary Cancers [Internet]. Philadelphia: c2020 [accessed on 2020 Feb 11]. Avaliable at: https://www.nccn.org/about/news/ebulletin/ebulletindetail.aspx?ebulletinid=3679.
42. Goetze TO, Paolucci V. Benefits of reoperation of T2 and more advanced incidental gallbladder carcinoma: analysis of the German registry. Ann Surg. 2008;247:104–8.
43. Shirai Y, Yoshida K, Tsukada K, Muto T. Inapparent carcinoma of the gallbladder. An appraisal of a radical second operation after simple cholecystectomy. Ann Surg. 1992;215:326–31.
44. Yoshimitsu K, Honda H, Kaneko K, Kuroiwa T, Irie H, Chijiiwa K, et al. Anatomy and clinical importance of cholecystic venous drainage: helical CT observations during injection of contrast medium into the cholecystic artery. AJR Am J Roentgenol. 1997;169:505–10.

45. Suzuki M, Yamamoto K, Unno M, Katayose Y, Endo K, Oikawa M, et al. Detection of perfusion areas of the gallbladder vein on computed tomography during arterial portography (CTAP)–the background for dual S4a. S5 hepatic subsegmentectomy in advanced gallbladder carcinoma. Hepatogastroenterology. 2000;47:631–5.
46. Shirai Y, Wakai T, Sakata J, Hatakeyama K. Regional lymphadenectomy for gallbladder cancer: rational extent, technical details, and patient outcomes. World J Gastroenterol. 2012;18:2775–83.
47. Horiguchi A, Miyakawa S, Ishihara S, Miyazaki M, Ohtsuka M, Shimizu H, et al. Gallbladder bed resection or hepatectomy of segments 4a and 5 for pT2 gallbladder carcinoma: analysis of Japanese registration cases by the study group for biliary surgery of the Japanese Society of Hepato-Biliary-Pancreatic Surgery. J Hepatobiliary Pancreat Sci. 2013;20:518–24.
48. Lee H, Choi DW, Park JY, Youn S, Kwon W, Heo JS, et al. Surgical strategy for T2 gallbladder cancer according to tumor location. Ann Surg Oncol. 2015;22:2779–86.
49. Isambert M, Leux C, Métairie S, Paineau J. Incidentally-discovered gallbladder cancer: when, why and which reoperation? J Visc Surg. 2011;148:e77–84.
50. Pawlik TM, Gleisner AL, Vigano L, Kooby DA, Bauer TW, Frilling A, et al. Incidence of finding residual disease for incidental gallbladder carcinoma: implications for re-resection. J Gastrointest Surg. 2007;11:1478–87.
51. Ethun CG, Postlewait LM, Le N, Pawlik TM, Buettner S, Poultsides G, et al. A novel pathology-based preoperative risk score to predict locoregional residual and distant disease and survival for incidental gallbladder cancer: a 10-institution study from the US extrahepatic biliary malignancy consortium. Ann Surg Oncol. 2017;24:1343–50.
52. Goetze TO, Paolucci V. Use of retrieval bags in incidental gallbladder cancer cases. World J Surg. 2009;33:2161–5.
53. Suzuki K, Kimura T, Ogawa H. Is laparoscopic cholecystectomy hazardous for gallbladder cancer? Surgery. 1998;123:311–4.
54. Ouchi K, Mikuni J, Kakugawa Y. Organizing Committee ttACotJSoBS. Laparoscopic cholecystectomy for gallbladder carcinoma: results of a Japanese survey of 498 patients. J Hepatobiliary Pancreat Surg. 2002;9:256–60.
55. Yamaguchi K, Chijiiwa K, Ichimiya H, Sada M, Kawakami K, Nishikata F, et al. Gallbladder carcinoma in the era of laparoscopic cholecystectomy. Arch Surg. 1996;131:981–4.
56. Tian Y-H, Ji X, Liu B, Yang G-Y, Meng X-F, Xia H-T, et al. Surgical treatment of incidental gallbladder cancer discovered during or following laparoscopic cholecystectomy. World J Surg. 2015;39:746–52.
57. Goussous N, Maqsood H, Patel K, Ferdosi H, Muhammad N, Sill AM, et al. Clues to predict incidental gallbladder cancer. Hepatobiliary Pancreat Dis Int. 2018;17:149–54.
58. Jansen S, Stodolski M, Zirngibl H, Gödde D, Ambe PC. Advanced gallbladder inflammation is a risk factor for gallbladder perforation in patients with acute cholecystitis. World J Emerg Surg. 2018;13:9. https://doi.org/10.1186/s13017-018-0169-2.
59. Beal EW, Wei L, Ethun CG, Black SM, Dillhoff M, Salem A, et al. Elevated NLR in gallbladder cancer and cholangiocarcinoma–making bad cancers even worse: results from the US extrahepatic biliary malignancy consortium. HPB (Oxford). 2016;18:950–7.
60. Han HS, Cho JY, Yoon YS, Ahn K, Kim H. Preoperative inflammation is a prognostic factor for gallbladder carcinoma. Br J Surg. 2011;98:111–6.
61. Patkar S, Ostwal V, Ramaswamy A, Engineer R, Chopra S, Shetty N, et al. Emerging role of multimodality treatment in gall bladder cancer: Outcomes following 510 consecutive resections in a tertiary referral center. J Surg Oncol. 2018;117:372–9.
62. Horgan AM, Amir E, Walter T, Knox JJ. Adjuvant therapy in the treatment of biliary tract cancer: a systematic review and meta-analysis. J Clin Oncol. 2012;30:1934–40.
63. Valle J, Wasan H, Palmer DH, Cunningham D, Anthoney A, Maraveyas A, et al. Cisplatin plus gemcitabine versus gemcitabine for biliary tract cancer. New Engl J Med. 2010;362:1273–81.
64. Mantripragada KC, Hamid F, Shafqat H, Olszewski AJ. Adjuvant therapy for resected gallbladder cancer: analysis of the National Cancer Data Base. J Natl Cancer Inst. 2017;109:djw202.
65. Primrose JN, Fox RP, Palmer DH, Malik HZ, Prasad R, Mirza D, et al. Capecitabine compared with observation in resected biliary tract cancer (BILCAP): a randomised, controlled, multicentre, phase 3 study. Lancet Oncol. 2019;20:663–73.
66. Shroff RT, Kennedy EB, Bachini M, Bekaii-Saab T, Crane C, Edeline J, et al. Adjuvant therapy for resected biliary tract cancer: ASCO clinical practice guideline. J Clin Oncol. 2019;37:1015–27.
67. Valle JW, Borbath I, Khan SA, Huguet F, Gruenberger T, Arnold D. Biliary cancer: ESMO clinical practice guidelines for diagnosis, treatment and follow-up. Ann Oncol. 2016;27:v28–37.

Gallbladder Cancer

Epidemiology

Jin Heon Lee

Introduction

The gallbladder (GB) is a small pear-shaped hollow organ, which stores and concentrates bile before it is released into small intestine. In humans, the gallbladder lies beneath the liver and can be subjected to gallstone, which is a strong risk factor for gallbladder cancer (GBC). In most cases, histology of GBC is adenocarcinomas, which arise from the secretory cells of GB mucosa. Infrequent form of GBC, papillary adenocarcinoma arises from papillary cells of mucosal layer and has a better prognosis than adenocarcinoma [1, 2]. The characteristics of GB anatomy are attributable to difficulty in early diagnosis at initial stage of GBC without routine medical checkup.

Among 33 leading diseases of cancer registered in GLOBOCAN 2018 over the past five years, the estimated number of prevalent cases of breast cancer (6,875,099 cases) is the highest and colorectal cancer (4,789,635 cases), prostate cancer (3,724,658 cases), lung cancer (2,129,964 cases), and thyroid cancer (1,997,846 cases) follow in order. GBC is ranked 26th, with 233,820 cases, followed by Hodgkin Lymphoma [3] (Fig. 1).

J. H. Lee (✉)
Department of Internal Medicine, Gangdong Sacred Heart Hospital, Hallym University College of Medicine, Gangdong-Gu #445, Seoul, Korea
e-mail: john114d@daum.net

Global Incidence and Mortality

GBC is an uncommon digestive tract cancer with the incidence rate of 2–3 cases per 100,000 people [4–7]. This contributes 1.2% of all cancer incidences and 1.7% of all global cancer deaths. GBC occurs mainly after the age of 60's in both sexes [1, 8, 9]. The number of GBC is rising steadily similar to other malignant tumors, mainly due to global population growth. According to the recent GLOBOCAN 2018 report, data from Global Cancer Observatory (GCO) (https://gco.iarc.fr), an interactive web-based platform presenting global cancer statistics for cancer control and research, the annual incidence of gallbladder cancer, however, is ranked as 20th frequent tumor (219,420 cases) and 17th deadly cancer (165,087 cases) [3].

With a mortality rate of 75.2%, gallbladder cancer is the 7th poor prognostic tumor among 33 cancer disease entities. According to world statistics in 2018, gallbladder cancer age-standardized mortality rates for both sexes (per 100,000) were 1.7 with the highest rate reported in Bolivia (10.6). The subsequent eight countries were as following; Thailand (6.7), Chile (5.4), Nepal (4.5), Republic of Korea (4.1), Bangladesh (3.5), Japan (3.3), Slovakia (3.2), and Peru (3.1).

GBC occurs in the body of gallbladder in about one-thirds of the cases. As the surface of the gallbladder wall attaches to the liver with

J. B. Chung and K. Okazaki (eds.), *Diseases of the Gallbladder*,
https://doi.org/10.1007/978-981-15-6010-1_14

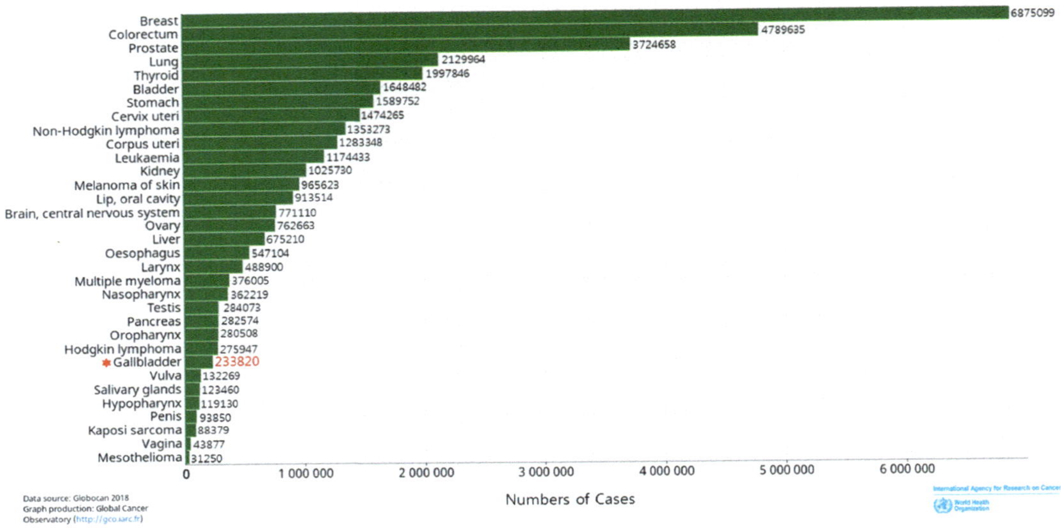

Fig. 1 Estimated number of 33 prevalent cancer cases (5-year) worldwide, both sexes, all ages. *Source* data from GLOBOCAN 2018, obtained from Global Cancer Observatory (GCO) (https://gco.iarc.fr)

no serosal layer, hepatic invasions commonly occur without any symptoms. More than 50% of GBC patients who undergo surgery already have lymph node metastasis and only 10% can be completely resected. Adenocarcinoma is the most frequent histologic type, accounting for 98% of all gallbladder tumors; two-thirds of these are moderately or poorly differentiated. In fact, even in a highly developed country like the United States, only about 1 in 5 gallbladder cancers are diagnosed at early stages, which explains GBC's poor prognosis. Such poor prognostic tumor diseases include pancreatic cancer, hepatoma, esophageal cancer, lung cancer, mesothelioma, and brain tumor (Fig. 2) [3, 6, 10, 11].

Worldwide Distribution Pattern of Gallbladder Cancer

The global distribution of GBC is not uniform, and its frequency varies greatly from region to region [1, 2, 4, 12]. The estimated number of prevalence cases in the last 5 years, in proportion per 100,000 people, is higher in Southeastern Asia, Central Europe, North Africa, and especially in Latin America (Fig. 3). However, the global maps of the estimated crude incidence rates in 2018 show that Japan, Republic of Korea, Europe, Canada, Australia, and Thailand tend to be higher, when compared to their prevalence rate. Considering the fact that GBC has been described as the "rich and old people's disease", the possible explanation of this phenomenon may be the increase of obese and old-age population in Eastern Asia, Europe, and Canada. For the Latin America area, especially Andes region, environmental exposures to various chemicals, lifestyle, ethnicity, regional intrinsic risk factors that predispose to carcinogenesis and specific dietary habits may be the answer to this situation (Fig. 4).

In 2018, in terms of total estimated number of GBC patients according to nationality, China (54,131 cases) was ranked comes first with India (25,999 cases) ranking as the second country with the most cases, due to their large population. Japan ranked third position with 24,823 cases and United States (11,496 cases) followed (Fig. 5). But the estimated crude incidence rate was the highest in Japan with 19.5 cases per 100,000 people. Subsequent countries with high rates included Chile (14.8), Republic of Korea (14.1), and Bolivia (13.4) (Fig. 6).

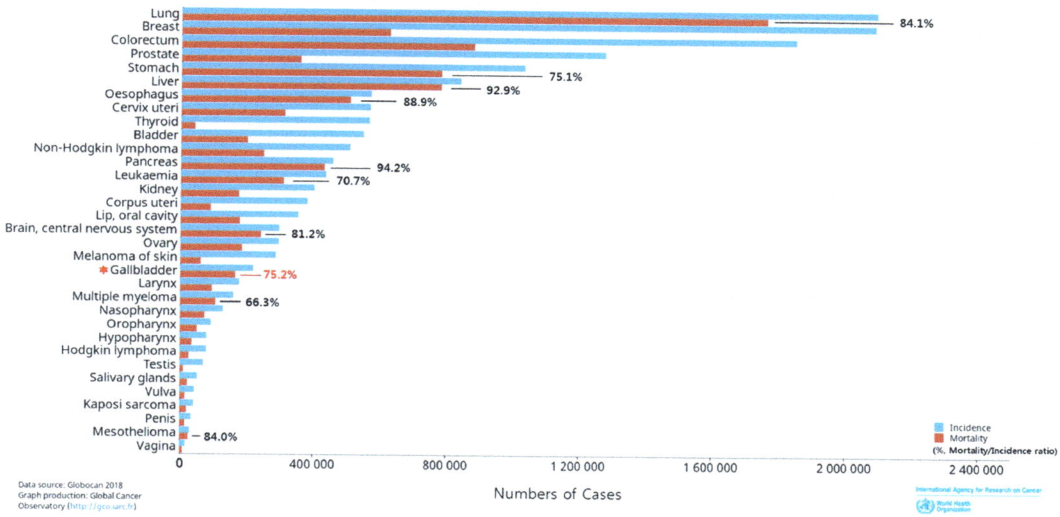

Fig. 2 Estimated number of 33 incident cancer cases and deaths worldwide, both sexes, all ages. The top 10 cancer diseases with the highest mortality/incidence ratio (%) are marked. *Source* data from GLOBOCAN 2018, obtained from Global Cancer Observatory (GCO) (https://gco.iarc.fr)

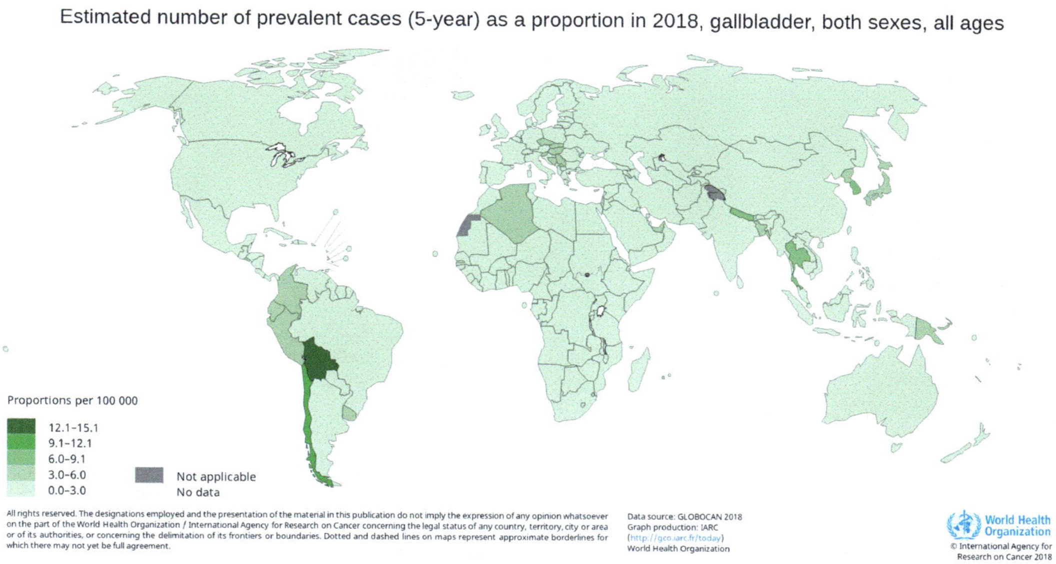

Fig. 3 Estimated number of prevalent cases (5-yr) as a proportion in 2018, gallbladder cancer, both sexes, all ages worldwide. *Source* data from GLOBOCAN 2018, obtained from Global Cancer Observatory (GCO) (https://gco.iarc.fr)

Considering the fact that GBC increases with age, like many other cancer diseases, one of the reasons for this phenomenon may be due to Japan and Republic of Korea's increasing proportion of aged population.

In order to emphasize ethnicity and to remove the bias of different demographic features of each country, age-standardized incidence rates can be calculated, with Bolivia taking the lead with 14.0 cases per 100,000

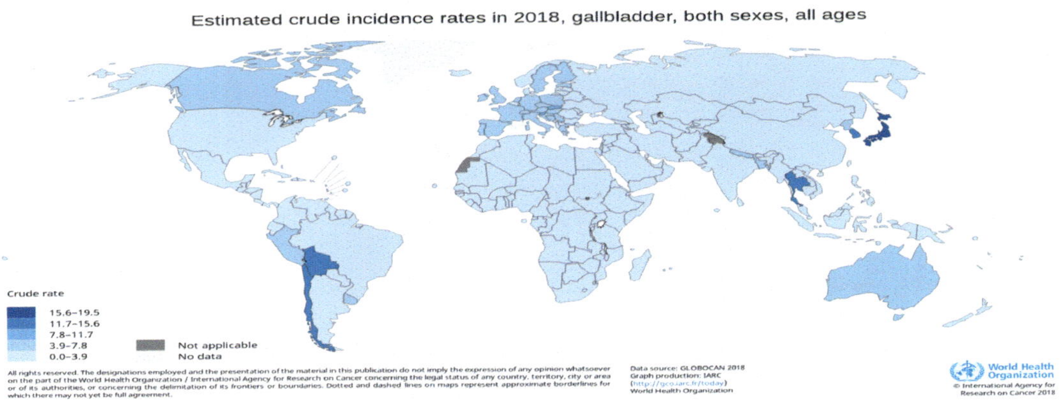

Fig. 4 Estimated crude incidence rates in 2018, gallbladder cancer, both sexes, all ages worldwide *Source* data from GLOBOCAN 2018, obtained from Global Cancer Observatory (GCO) (https://gco.iarc.fr)

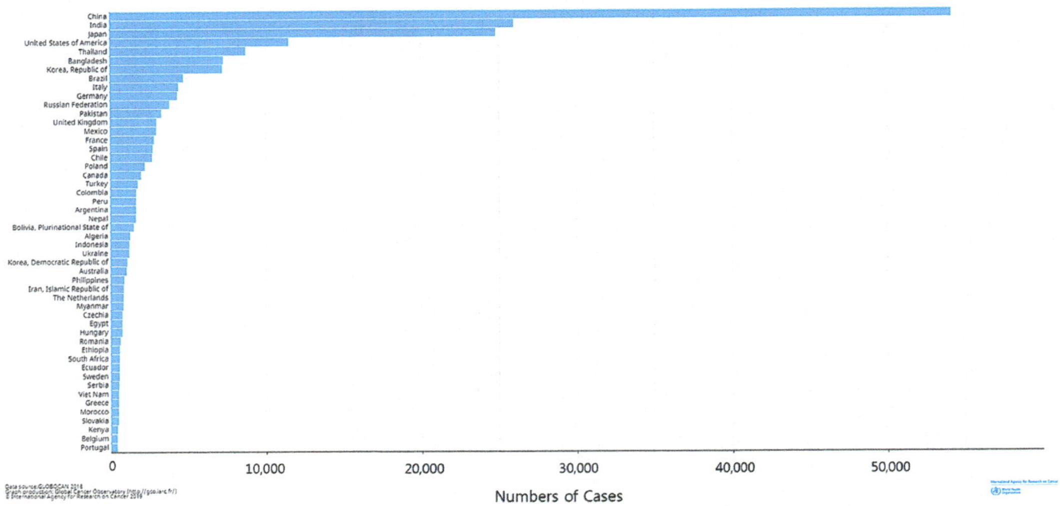

Fig. 5 Estimated number of incident cases of gallbladder cancer, according to nationality, both sexes, all ages. *Source* data from GLOBOCAN 2018, obtained from Global Cancer Observatory (GCO) (https://gco.iarc.fr)

people. The next six countries are as following; Chile (9.3), Thailand (7.4), Republic of Korea (6.8), Nepal (5.1), Peru (4.8), and Japan (4.5) (Fig. 7). This result is consistent with the known facts of high incidence of GBC in Mapuche Indians and American Indians when ethnicity is taken into consideration and when analyzed geographically. The Andes area in Latin America and some far Eastern and Southeastern Asia also show high incidences [1, 2, 13–16]. In addition, these areas have close relationship with relatively high frequency of gallbladder stones (female Mapuche and American Indian, 49% and 64–73%, respectively) (Fig. 8) and salmonella infection, both of which are known risk factors for gallbladder cancer [13, 17–20]. Gallbladder stones particularly are closely related to GBC as they are observed in about 85% of gallbladder cancer patients. The relatively high incidence rate

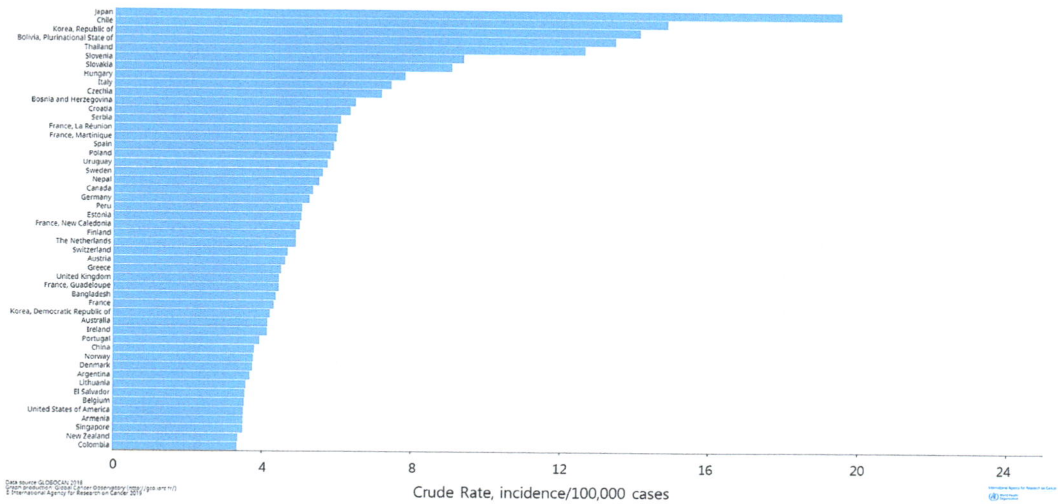

Fig. 6 Estimated crude incidence rates in 2018, gallbladder cancer, according to nationality, both sexes, all ages. *Source* data from GLOBOCAN 2018, obtained from Global Cancer Observatory (GCO) (https://gco.iarc.fr)

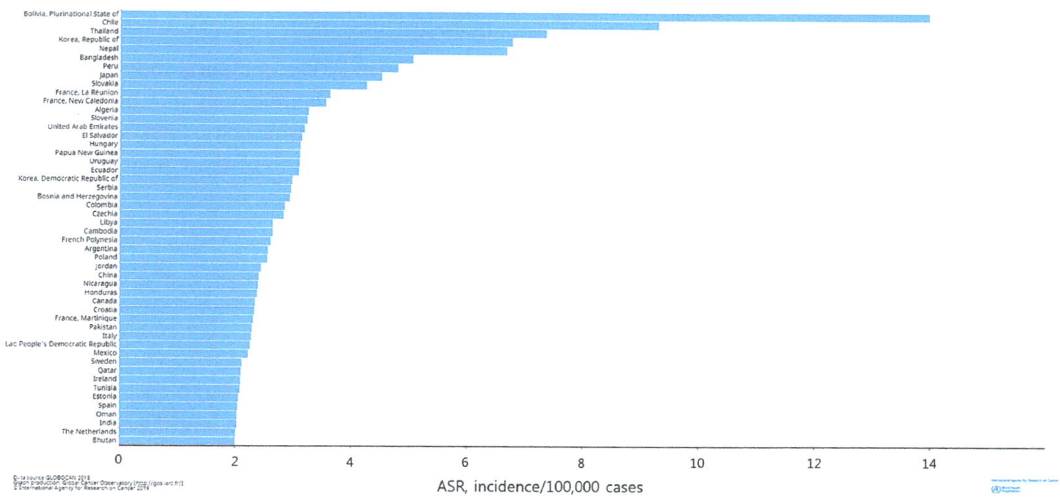

Fig. 7 Estimated age-standardized incidence rates in 2018, gallbladder cancer, according to nationality, both sexes, all ages. *Source* data from GLOBOCAN 2018, obtained from Global Cancer Observatory (GCO) (https://gco.iarc.fr)

in Southeast Asia and Thailand seems related to the regions' improved economic status. In addition, in cases of far eastern Asian countries such as Republic of Korea and Japan, rapidly increasing proportion of aged people probably contributes to GBC incidences in the region.

Sex Ratio and Socioeconomic Status

GBC is the only digestive organ cancer that is more common among women than men. While crude incident rate of GBC was known to be two times higher in women when compared to

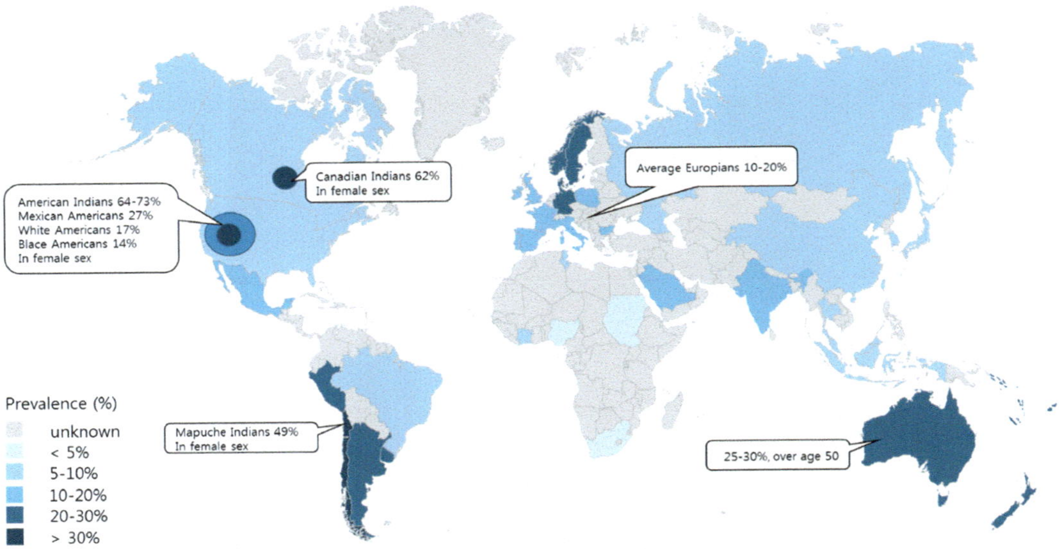

Fig. 8 Worldwide prevalence of gallstone. Prevalence is inordinately high in north American Indians, western Andes Indians and Northern Europeans; somewhat lower in European and American whites; intermediate in Asians and black Americans, and quite low in black Africans. (adopted from ref. 10)

men, the number of estimated incidence was 97,396 for men and 122,024 for women (Male: Female = 1: 1.25) in GLOBOCAN 2018 report. Possible explanation for this feature is women's tendency to live longer. However, estimated age-standardized incidence rate of GBC shows little difference around the world with the sex ratio of 2.4: 2.2 (Female: Male) [1, 3]. Furthermore, the incidence rate in men is 1.5 times higher than women in Melanesian in the South Pacific region. Similar trends are observed in Eastern Asia, Southern Europe, Southeastern Asia, Western Europe and North America (Fig. 9).

If the entire world's population is classified according to income status and/or Human Development Index (HDI), there is a high estimated age-standardized incidence rate of GBC in the upper class. Eating relatively more fatty meals, higher Body Mass Index (BMI), and easier access to health care may also contribute to increasing consequences (Fig. 10). While GBC tends to occur in higher rates in the upper socioeconomic class, mortality rate is slightly lower compared to mid-class patients, probably due to early diagnosis and proper management such as surgery. As mentioned above, in GBC, early diagnosis and treatment is crucial for the patients [21, 22]. Additionally, GBC is known to occur more in Caucasians than Africans, which may not be attributable to genetic differences, but rather due to better overall socioeconomic status in Caucasians. Figure 4 shows ethnically randomized distribution.

Global Trends and Future Expectation of Gallbladder Cancer Incidence

Estimated age-standardized incidence rate of GBC has slightly decreased or has been similar over the past decades. Utilizing the past data, future occurrence model of GBC cases was predicted (Fig. 11). Marked increment in number of GBC cases in Asia is probably due to the fast population growth. The world's population is projected to grow from 7.7 billion in 2019 to 8.5 billion in 2030 (10% increase), and further to 9.7 billion in 2050 (26% increase) and to 10.9 billion in 2100 (42% increase). India, especially, is expected to add nearly 273 million people between 2019 and 2050 and surpass China

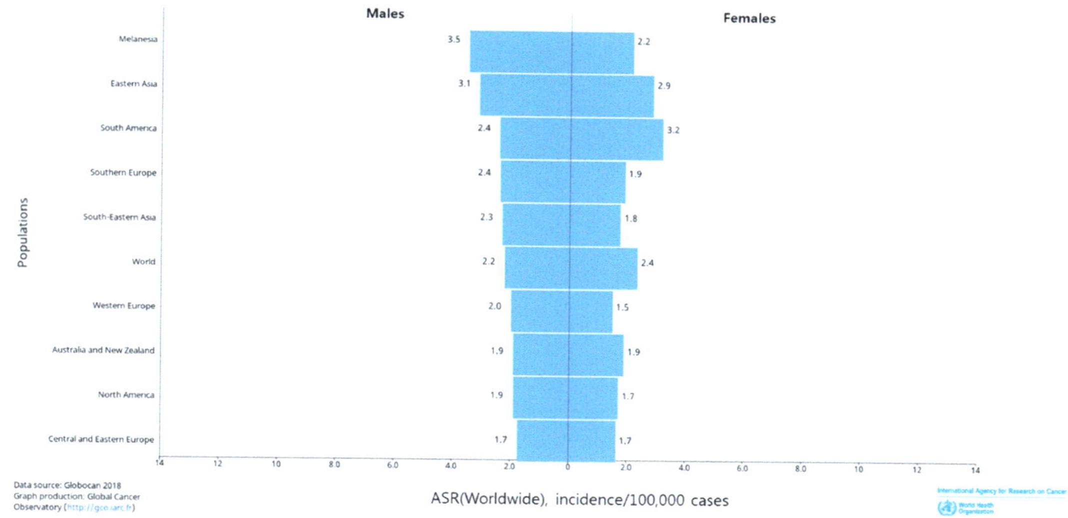

Fig. 9 Estimated age-standardized incidence rates according to sex, 2018, gallbladder cancer, all ages. *Source* data from GLOBOCAN 2018, obtained from Global Cancer Observatory (GCO) (https://gco.iarc.fr)

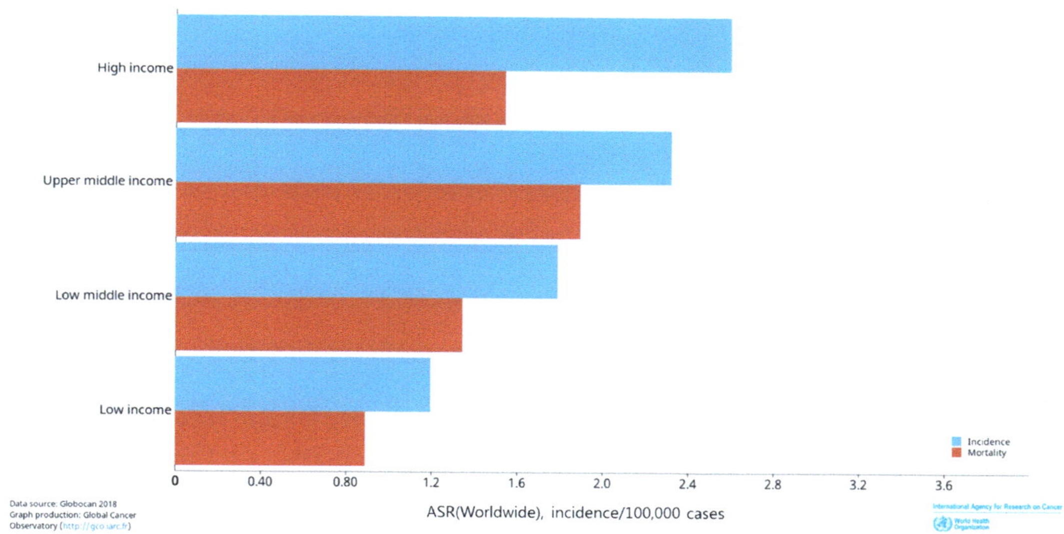

Fig. 10 Estimated age-standardized incidence rates in 2018, according to income level, gallbladder cancer, both sexes, all ages. *Source* data from GLOBOCAN 2018, obtained from Global Cancer Observatory (GCO) (https://gco.iarc.fr)

as the world's most populous country around 2027. Another reason for increment of GBC cases in Asia is socioeconomic development of China and the increasing aging status of the general population in Republic of Korea and Japan [1, 8, 23, 24].

Although GBC mortality has decreased remarkably over the past several decades in majority of countries, no further improvement was shown after 2000s in many countries, probably due to increasing prevalence of the obesity, but the mechanism is not fully understood. In

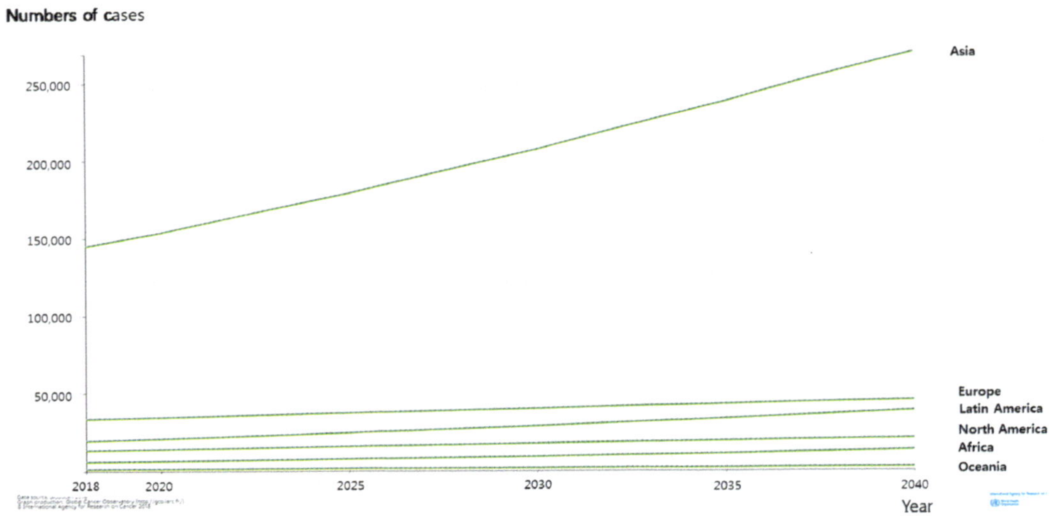

Fig. 11 Estimated expectation number of incident cases of gallbladder cancer from 2018 to 2040, both sexes, all ages. *Source* data from GLOBOCAN 2018, obtained from Global Cancer Observatory (GCO) (https://gco.iarc.fr)

histological point of view, incidence of papillary adenocarcinoma tends to be increasing recently, or even higher than adenocarcinoma in some countries like United States, further data is required for the assessment of global incidence rate [1, 9, 25].

Conclusion

Although estimated age-standardized incidence rate of GBC has slightly decreased or has been similar over the past decades, the number of GBC cases is expected to increase worldwide by 2050, especially in Asia. The high incidence rate of GBC is observed in the areas with a high proportion of old-aged people, high HDI, high BMI, and high GB stone prevalence. In the ethnical point of view, high incidence rate of GBC is noted in Indians in America and Andes region, especially in Mapuche Indians. The female sex was slightly dominant in terms of the estimated age-standardized incidence rate (Male: Female = 1: 1.09). The GBC mortality rate has decreased remarkably over the past several decades in majority of countries, but no more improvement was shown after 2000s in many countries.

References

1. Prashanth R, Tagore S, Krishna CT, Adam B. Epidemiology of gallbladder cancer. Clin Exp Hepatol. 2019;5(2):93–102.
2. Rajveer H, Eldon AS. Gallbladder cancer: epidemiology and outcome. Clin Epidemiol. 2014;6(1): 99–109.
3. Bray F, Ferlay J, Soerjomataram I, Siegel RL, Torre LA, Jemal A. Global cancer statistics 2018: GLOBOCAN estimates of incidence and mortality worldwide for 36 cancers in 185 countries. CA Cancer J Clin. 2018;68:394–424.
4. Randi G, Franceschi S, Vecchia C. Gallbladder cancer worldwide: geographical distribution and risk factors. Int J Cancer. 2006;118:1591–602.
5. Hueman MT, Vollmer CM, Pawlik TM. Evolving treatment strategies for gallbladder cancer. Ann Surg Oncol. 2009;16:2101–15.
6. Siegel RL, Miller KD, Jemal A, Mahdavifar N, Pakzad R, Ghoncheh M, et al. Epidemiology, incidence, and mortality of gallbladder cancer and its relation with development in the world. Ann Trop Med Public Health. 2017;10:563–70.
7. Lazcano-Ponce EC, Miquel JF, Munoz N, Herrero R, Ferrecio C, Wistuba II, et al. Epidemiology and molecular pathology of gallbladder cancer. CA Cancer J Clin. 2001;51:349–64.
8. Kim BW, Oh CM, Choi HY, Park JW, Cho HS, Ki MR. Incidence and overall survival of biliary tract cancers in South Korea from 2006 to 2015: using the national health information database. Gut and Liver. 2019;13(1):104–13.

9. Wi YJ, Woo HT, Won YJ, Jang JY, Shin AS. Trends in gallbladder cancer incidence and survival in Korea. Cancer Res Treat. 2018;50(4):1444–51.
10. Siegel RL, Miller KD, Jemal A. Cancer statistics, 2019. CA Cancer J Clin. 2019;69(1):7–34.
11. Miller G, Jarnagin WR. Gallbladder carcinoma. Eur J Surg Oncol. 2008;34(3):306–12.
12. Misra S, Chaturvedi A, Misra NC, Sharma ID. Carcinoma of the gallbladder. Lancet Oncol. 2003;4:167–76.
13. Stinton LM, Shaffer EA. Epidemiology of gallbladder disease: cholelithiasis and cancer. Gut Liver. 2012;6(2):172–87.
14. Paltoo DN, Chu KC. Patterns in cancer incidence among American Indians/Alaska Natives, United States, 1992–1999. Public Health Rep. 2004;19:443–51.
15. Kapoor VK, McMichael AJ. Gallbladder cancer: an 'Indian' disease. Natl Med J India. 2003;16:209–13.
16. Nervi F, Duarte I, Gomez G, Rodriguez G, Del Pino G, Ferrerio O, et al. Frequency of gallbladder cancer in chile, a high-risk area. Int J Cancer. 1988;41:657–60.
17. Strom BL, Soloway RD, Rios-Dalenz JL, Rodriguez-Martinez HA, West SL, Kinman JL, et al. Risk factors for gallbladder cancer. Int Collaborative Case-Control Study. Cancer. 1995;76:1747–56.
18. Csendes A, Becerra M, Rojas J, Medina E. Number and size of stones in patients with asymptomatic and symptomatic gallstones and gallbladder carcinoma: a prospective study of 592 cases. J Gastrointest Surg. 2000;4:481–5.
19. Dutta U, Garg PK, Kumar R, Tandon RK. Typhoid carriers among patients with gallstones are at increased risk for carcinoma of the gallbladder. Am J Gastroenterol. 2000;95:784–7.
20. Nagaraja V, Eslick GD. Systematic review with meta-analysis: the relationship between chronic Salmonella typhi carrier status and gall-bladder cancer. Aliment Pharmacol Ther. 2014;39(8):745–50.
21. Li ZM, Wu ZX, Han B, Mao YQ, Chen HL, Han SF, et al. The association between BMI and gallbladder cancer risk: a meta-analysis. Oncotarget. 2016;7:43669–79.
22. Weiderpass E, Pukkala E. Time trends in socioeconomic differences in incidence rates of cancers of gastro-intestinal tract in Finland. BMC Gastroenterol. 2006;6:41–58.
23. Goding Sauer A, Siegel RL, Jemal A, Fedewa SA. Current prevalence of major cancer risk factors and screening test use in the United States: disparities by education and race/ethnicity. Cancer Epidemiol Biomarkers Prev. 2019;284:629–42.
24. Boutros C, Gary M, Baldwin K, Somasundar P. Gallbladder cancer: past, present and an uncertain future. Surg Oncol. 2012;21:183–91.
25. Henley SJ, Weir HK, Jim MA, Watson M, Richardson LC. Gallbladder cancer incidence and mortality, United States 1999-2011. Cancer Epidemiol Biomarkers Prev. 2015;24:1319–26.

Risk Factors

Jeong Hun Seo

Introduction

While generally considered rare, gallbladder cancer is the most common malignant tumor of the biliary tract worldwide. It is an extremely lethal disease, with an overall mean survival of six months [1]. The reason for poor prognosis is partly due to its aggressive biologic behavior and a *lack* of sensitive screening tests for early detection. Epidemiological studies have shown a wide range of geographical and ethnic variations, with higher rates in certain areas and remarkable rarity in others [2]. This difference suggests that the combination of local environmental factors and genetic predisposition is associated with its carcinogenesis. This review provides a comprehensive overview of risk factors associated with the development of gallbladder cancer.

Risk Factors

Multifactorial factors contribute to the development of gallbladder cancer. The risk factors for gallbladder cancer can be divided into three broad categories as follows.

(1) Demographic factors

① Age
② Female sex and parity
③ Obesity
④ Geography and ethnicity
⑤ Genetic factors and family history

(2) Diseases of the gallbladder and bile duct

① Gallstones
② Gallbladder polyps
③ Gallbladder adenomyomatosis
④ Xanthogranulomatous cholecystitis
⑤ Porcelain gallbladder
⑥ Pancreaticobiliary maljunction
⑦ Primary sclerosing cholangitis

(3) Environmental/lifestyle factors

① Chronic infection: *Salmonella, Helicobactor*
② Exposures and medications
③ Lifestyle factors

Demographic Factors

Age

The incidence of gallbladder cancer tends to increase continuously with age. More than two-thirds of patients diagnosed with gallbladder cancer are older than 65 years, and the average age at diagnosis in the US is

J. H. Seo (✉)
Division of Gastroenterology, Department of Internal Medicine, National Health Insurance Service Ilsan Hospital, Yonsei University College of Medicine, Goyang-si, Gyeonggi-do, Korea
e-mail: jhsuh@nhimc.or.kr

J. B. Chung and K. Okazaki (eds.), *Diseases of the Gallbladder*,
https://doi.org/10.1007/978-981-15-6010-1_15

72 years. According to US data from 2015, the age-adjusted incidence rates (per 100,000 people) increased from 0.2 among those 20–49 years of age to 1.6 in those 50–64 years of age, to 4.3 among those 65–74 years of age, and to 8.1 for individuals over the age of 75 years [3].

Female Sex and Parity

Gallbladder cancer occurs two to six times more often in women than men in most countries [4]; therefore, sex is a recognized risk factor for gallbladder cancer. The female predominance of gallbladder cancer suggests a role of female sex hormones. Estrogen increases biliary cholesterol saturation and decreases bile salt secretion, while progesterone impairs gallbladder emptying to promote the development of gallstones, which is the most important risk factor for gallbladder cancer. Prolonged lifetime estrogen exposure is associated with an increased risk of gallbladder cancer through early menarches, late menopause, multiple pregnancies, and estrogen replacement therapy. Serum estrogen levels rise about 100-fold during pregnancy; thus, higher parity is associated with increased lifetime exposure to estrogen. The female-to-male ratio of gallbladder cancer is above 2 in most countries but is only about 1.3 in Korea and Japan [5]. One possible explanation for the relatively high incidence of gallbladder cancer in men than women in these countries may be the difference in the prevalence of *Clonorchis sinensis*.

Obesity

Obese individuals have an increased risk of developing gallbladder cancer. Overweight and obesity were associated with 14 and 56% higher risk of gallbladder cancer, respectively. For each five-point increase in Body Mass Index (BMI), the Relative Risks (RRs) of developing gallbladder cancer increase by 1.59 for women and 1.09 for men [6]. The association between obesity and risk of gallbladder cancer is stronger in women than in men, and overweight is only associated with gallbladder cancer in women [7]. Other anthropometric factors such as waist circumference, hip circumference, and waist-to-hip ratio were all associated with gallbladder cancer. Diabetes mellitus is a risk factor for gallstone disease and gallbladder cancer. In a meta-analysis of 20 studies, diabetic individuals had a 1.56-fold increased risk of gallbladder cancer compared to that in nondiabetics [8]. Patients with diabetes have an increased risk of developing gallbladder cancer even in the absence of gallstones [9]. It is not clear whether obesity plays an important mediating role in the association between diabetes and gallbladder cancer.

The potential biological mechanisms for the carcinogenesis of gallbladder associated with obesity include increased concentrations of hormones such as insulin or estrogen, which increase the formation of gallstones. Obesity-related mediators such as Insulin-like Growth Factor (IGF)-1, adipokines, inflammatory factors, and pro-inflammatory cytokines may contribute to cancer-related processes. Leptin and adiponectin secreted by adipose tissue are also involved in carcinogenesis [6].

In conclusion, adiposity is associated with an increased risk of gallbladder cancer, suggesting that weight management can help to minimize the risk of gallbladder cancer [10].

Geography and Ethnicity

The incidence of gallbladder cancer shows marked geographical variability. The rates are highest in Chile (27/100,000), India (21.5/100,000), Poland (14/100,000), south Pakistan (11.3/100,000), and Japan (7/100,000) [11]. The incidence in Korea from 1999 to 2013 was 2.96–3.12 per 100,000 in men and 2.79–3.03 in women [12]. In contrast, gallbladder cancer is rare in the western world including the US, UK, and Canada. Gallbladder cancer tends to particularly afflict indigenous populations, and ethnic rates can prevail even in different geographic locations. This suggests that gallbladder cancer may result from interactions between innate genetic predisposition and exposure to environmental risk factors.

Genetic Factors and Family History

A family history of gallbladder cancer can slightly increase the risk of gallbladder cancer [13]. A Swedish family-cancer database was the first to report the familial clustering of gallbladder cancer, in which the risk of gallbladder cancer was increased in female immigrants from Chile and the Indian subcontinent while some Northern European immigrants showed decreased risks compared to native Swedes [14]. Therefore, some persistent damage was inflicted before emigration, and racial factors were more important than environmental factors. A study from the Utah Cancer Registry estimated that 26% of all gallbladder cancers are familial [15].

Gallbladder cancer has also been associated with multiple familial polyposis/Gardner syndrome and Peutz–Jeghers syndrome. Multiple genetic mutations are likely involved in the pathogenesis of gallbladder cancer. The early molecular changes may include p53 mutation, cyclooxygenase-2 overexpression, mitochondrial DNA mutations, and abnormal hypermethylation of various tumor suppressor gene promoters [16].

Diseases of the Gallbladder and Bile Duct

Gallstones

Gallstones are the most important risk factor for the development of gallbladder cancer, with a Relative Risk (RR) of 4.9 [5]. Among patients with gallbladder cancer, 70–90% have a history of gallstones. Furthermore, the incidence of gallbladder cancers is well correlated with the prevalence of gallstone disease. However, compared to the high prevalence of gallstones, gallbladder cancer occurs in less than 1% of patients with gallstones; therefore, gallstones alone cannot be considered a single cause of gallbladder cancer [17]. The reasons why some individuals with gallstone disease develop cancer while most do not remain unknown.

Gallstone characteristics influence the risk of gallbladder cancer. Increasing gallstone size is associated with a greater risk of gallbladder cancer. The risk of developing gallbladder cancer increases by 10.1-fold and 2.4-fold for gallstones larger than 3 and 2.0–2.9 cm in diameter, respectively, compared to stones less than 1 cm [18]. In addition to size, gallstone weight and volume are also associated with gallbladder cancer. Average volumes of 6, 8, and 10 mL have relative cancer risks of 5, 7, and 11-fold, respectively [19]. As the duration of gallstone increases, so does the RR of gallbladder cancer, with an RR of 4.9 for gallstones with duration of 5–19 years and 6.2 for durations exceeding 20 years [20] American Indians who have a high incidence of gallbladder cancer also have a high prevalence of cholesterol gallstones, suggesting that those with cholesterol stones are at a higher risk than those with pigment stone [21, 22].

The exact mechanism by which gallstones predisposes individuals to gallbladder cancer remains debatable. During the secretion of cholesterol from the liver to gallbladder in gallstone formation, other toxic substances may be released simultaneously and cause malignant changes in the gallbladder. Two candidates are orphan nuclear receptors and the adenosine triphosphate-binding cassette transporter family, which may increase gallbladder epithelium exposure to carcinogenic compounds [23]. Chronic irritation due to gallstones and the local production of carcinogens such as secondary bile acid promote progressive morphological damage through a metaplasia–dysplasia–carcinoma sequence [24]. A Danish study reported that it takes approximately 15 years to progress from dysplasia to advanced cancer [21].

Although gallstones are an associated risk factor and there is an inverse correlation between cholecystectomy for gallstone and gallbladder cancer rate [25], studies of their natural history and decision analysis do not favor prophylactic cholecystectomy for clinically silent gallstones [26, 27]. Screening for gallbladder cancer in patients with gallstones is not currently recommended.

Gallbladder Polyps

Gallbladder polyps are incidentally found on Ultrasound (US) and appear as fixed, echogenic masses protruding into the gallbladder lumen without an acoustic shadow [28]. Gallbladder polyps are relatively common, with a prevalence of 3–7% in abdominal US and 2–12% in cholecystectomy specimens. The majority are pseudotumors with no neoplastic potential, including cholesterol polyps (60%), adenomyomatosis (25%), or inflammatory polyps (10%). The most common benign neoplastic lesion is adenoma. Benign adenomas, accounting for approximately 4% of all gallbladder polyps, have malignant potential, although the role of adenomas in the pathogenesis of carcinoma is controversial. Adenomas may play a role in some cases of gallbladder cancer; however, the absence of adenoma remnants in mucosa adjacent to adenocarcinoma suggests that these tumors may not universally play a role in carcinogenesis [1]. In the carcinogenesis of gallbladder cancer, the dysplasia-carcinoma sequence is considered the predominant mechanism over the adenoma-carcinoma sequence because malignant transformation of adenoma or concomitant presence of adenoma and carcinoma are not common findings [29, 30].

Although most gallbladder polyps are benign, malignant polyps are present in some cases. Polyp size is the most important risk factor for malignancy, with gallbladder polyps larger than 10 mm significant predictors of malignancy, while most polyps less than 10 mm are benign and remain static for long periods [31]. Other factors predicting malignancy include solitary sessile polyps, presence of gallstones, patient age over 50 years, and, most importantly, rapid polyp growth [32].

The management of incidentally detected gallbladder polyp is controversial. Cholecystectomy is recommended for gallbladder polyps $\geq$ 10 mm or symptomatic polyps irrespective of size. If the patient has risk factors for gallbladder malignancy and a polyp measuring 6–9 mm, cholecystectomy is suggested if the patient is fit and accepts surgery [33]. However, these suggestions are not firm evidence-based consensus guidelines.

Gallbladder polyps should be followed by serial US; however, there is no consensus regarding screening interval. Practical recommendations advise an initial review within 6 months and then annual follow-up or every 6 months for at least 2 years until stability is documented [34]. The most recent European Society of Gastrointestinal and Abdominal Radiology (ESGAR) guidelines recommended follow-up US of the gallbladder at 6 months and 1 year and then yearly up to 5 years in polyps measuring 6–9 mm. In polyps under 6 mm, follow-up is advised at 1, 3, and 5 years; however, patients with risk factors for malignancy should receive the more extensive follow-up recommended for polyps of 6–9 mm without risk factors [33]. The duration of follow-up in patients with apparently stable gallbladder polyps has not been established. Wiles et al. demonstrated that gallbladder polyps that do grow appear to do so slowly and concluded that a 5-year follow-up should be advised [28]. Another study suggested that a follow-up of at least 10 years were necessary [35] because it took about 7 years for the development of neoplasia in gallbladder polyps [36]. The decision to terminate follow-up is dependent on the judgment of the clinician, and it may be more efficient to develop flexible and tailored follow-up plans rather than follow fixed or inflexible guidelines.

Alternative imaging modalities may provide additional information for the diagnosis of gallbladder polyps. Compared to conventional US, Endoscopic Ultrasound (EUS) showed a greater accuracy to predict neoplastic gallbladder polyps by analyzing EUS features and scoring systems [37]. Utilization of other imaging modalities such as ContrastEnhanced Ultrasound (CEUS) and Contrast-Enhanced Harmonic EUS (CEH-EUS) increased the diagnostic accuracy for gallbladder polyps. CEUS features highly suggestive of malignancy include the destruction of the gallbladder wall, heterogeneously enhancing patterns, and rapid contrast washout [38]. The presence of irregular intratumoral vessels or perfusion defects on CEH-EUS may be sensitive and accurate predictors of malignant polyps [39].

As a new technique, real-time elastography showed that all benign gallbladder polyps appeared to have a high-strain elastographic pattern, which may be useful in the characterization of gallbladder polyps but should be used as an auxiliary means of diagnosis [40].

Gallbladder Adenomyomatosis

Gallbladder Adenomyomatosis (GBA) is characterized by epithelial proliferation and hypertrophy of the muscles of the gallbladder wall with the outpouching of the mucosa into the thickened muscular layer, known as Rokitansky-Aschoff sinuses (RAS). GBA is frequently observed in cholecystectomy specimens, with a prevalence of 1–9% [41]. GBA has three morphological types—fundal (localized), segmental, and diffuse—according to the localization in the gallbladder wall. The fundal type is the most common pattern and is characterized by a local wall thickening on the gallbladder fundus. The segmental type, located in the gallbladder body, is annular and separates the gallbladder into two communicating compartments. The diffuse type includes thickening of the entire GB wall [42]. Gallstones are present in more than 50% of patients with GBA and up to 90% with segmental type [43]. Most patients with GBA are asymptomatic but, if present, the symptoms may result from the presence of gallstones. US is the imaging modality of choice for GBA diagnosis. The features on US are focal or diffuse gallbladder wall thickening with small anechoic cystic spaces and/or echogenic foci and comet-tail artifacts. Small anechoic cystic spaces (1–10 mm) representing clear bile-filled RAS are pathognomonic for GBA.

GBA is a benign lesion as the hyperplastic epithelium of GBA has no higher neoplastic potential than that of a normal gallbladder. Some studies have reported an increased prevalence of gallbladder cancer in patients with segmental-type GBA (6.6%) compared to that in patients without GBA or with other GBA patterns (4.3%), with more marked differences in patients over 60 years of age [43, 44]. However, these results may have been influenced by the higher prevalence of gallstones in patients with segmental-type GBA, which is a well-known risk factor for gallbladder cancer. Thus, GBA itself is not a precancerous lesion but gallstones secondary to GBA may lead to dysplastic changes and cancer. GBA may increase in size over time; however, this change alone is not considered an index of malignancy [41, 45]. Although GBA is not generally considered a premalignant lesion, GBA-positive gallbladder cancer is more often diagnosed in advanced stages because preceding GBA may interfere with early gallbladder cancer detection [46, 47].

There are no universally accepted guidelines for GBA management. Given the lack of malignancy potential, asymptomatic GBA theoretically requires no specific treatment when imaging provides a definite diagnosis. Cholecystectomy is usually indicated for symptomatic patients or in cases with inconclusive imaging findings. However, some doctors may prefer surgical options in patients with segmental-type GBA, given its higher association with gallbladder cancer, and in patients with diffuse-type GBA given the possible difficulties in identifying coexisting malignancies [42, 48].

New methods have been proposed to improve diagnostic accuracy. CEUS can be performed if RAS cannot be clearly identified in baseline US. RAS appear avascular in every phase of the dynamic study in CEUS, independently from their content. Magnetic Resonance Imaging (MRI) should be reserved for cases that are unclear on US and CEUS. At MRI, RAS can be identified with extremely high sensitivity by visualizing intramural cystic images in a "pearl necklace" configuration, which is pathognomonic of GBA [41].

Xanthogranulomatous Cholecystitis

Xanthogranulomatous Cholecystitis (XGC) is an uncommon form of chronic cholecystitis characterized by abnormal wall thickening and severe proliferative fibrosis with multiple yellow-brown intramural nodules. The incidence of XGC was 1.3–5.2% in resected gallbladder specimens [49]. XGC is frequently misdiagnosed as gallbladder cancer because its clinical and radiological features often mimic those of gallbladder cancer. The ultrasonographic characteristics of XGC include moderate-to-marked thickening of the gallbladder wall with oval hypoechoic nodules. As the frequency of coexisting XGC and gallbladder cancer is nearly 10% [49], XGC association with cancer is controversial. One study suggests the malignant potential of XGC for its upregulated oncogenes (BCL-2, c-Myc) [50], while another suggests the inflammatory nature of XGC through the expression of p53, proliferating cell nuclear antigen (PCNA), and beta-catenin [51]. Although XGC itself may not be the direct cause of gallbladder cancer, knowledge of clinicopathological features would help clinicians to manage gallbladder lesions associated with XCG because the association of XGC with gallbladder cancer makes treatment decisions difficult.

Porcelain Gallbladder

Porcelain Gallbladder (PGB) refers to gallbladder wall calcification. When calcium deposits become extensive, the gallbladder is called "porcelain" due to its bluish color and fragile, even brittle, consistency. The pathogenesis is associated with chronic gallbladder inflammation, and approximately 90% of patients have associated gallstones. PGB occurs in 0.8% of all cholecystectomies [22]. It has a female preponderance (5:1) and is usually diagnosed in the sixth decade. Patients are usually asymptomatic and PGB is found incidentally on plain abdominal radiographs, US, or Computed Tomography (CT) images showing the characteristic calcification of the gallbladder wall. In general, US findings are classified into three types based on the extent and pattern of wall calcification: type I is characterized by a hyperechoic semilunar structure with posterior acoustic shadowing; type II displays a curvilinear echogenic structure with acoustic shadowing; and type III is characterized by irregular clumps of echoes with posterior acoustic shadowing [22]. While type I corresponds to complete intramural calcification, types II and III reflect changes in selective mucosal calcification.

There is no definite consensus on the incidence rate of gallbladder cancer from PGB. Previous studies reported concomitant incidence of gallbladder cancer ranging from 12.5 to 61% [52, 53]. A recent systematic review of 340 patients with gallbladder calcifications reported an incidence of gallbladder malignancy of 21%. However, when studies with obvious selection bias were excluded, the rate of gallbladder malignancy fell to 6% in patients with gallbladder calcification compared to 1% in a matched cohort of patients without gallbladder calcification [54]. Khan et al. reported incidence of gallbladder cancer in PGB patients as low as 2–3% [55]. Stephen et al. found that the incidence of gallbladder cancer was related to the calcification pattern, with selective mucosal calcification causing a significant cancer risk compared to diffuse intramural calcification, which was less likely to develop malignancy [52]. Hence, gallbladders with partial, stippled, or multiple punctate calcifications in the mucosa may benefit from prophylactic cholecystectomy while an observational approach may be appropriate for those with a continuous band of calcification in the muscular layer [54, 56].

The management of PGB has been controversial for decades. Due to the high incidence of cancer in early studies, prophylactic cholecystectomy was previously routinely recommended. However, based on recent evidence suggesting a much lower incidence of cancer, prophylactic cholecystectomy appears appropriate for healthy patients, whereas a nonoperative approach should be considered in patients with significant comorbidities. Patients who are managed conservatively may need close follow-up to detect malignancy.

Pancreaticobiliary Maljunction

Pancreaticobiliary Maljunction (PBM), also known as anomalous pancreaticobiliary ductal junction or anomalous pancreaticobiliary ductal union, is an established risk factor for gallbladder cancer especially in relatively young female patients without gallbladder stones. PBM is particularly common in the Asian population and may explain the high incidence of gallbladder cancer in East Asia [57]. Approximately 10% of patients with gallbladder cancer have this junction anomaly [1]. PBM is a congenital malformation in which the junction of the pancreatic and bile ducts is located outside the duodenal wall. PBM can be divided into two types: with biliary dilatation (congenital biliary dilatation) and without biliary dilatation. Most PBM cases detected in childhood are associated with biliary dilatation; however, one-third of PBM detected in adults do not show biliary dilatation. PBM patients with biliary dilatation often present symptoms of pancreatitis or cholangitis in childhood, whereas those without biliary dilatation rarely have symptoms and most patients are not diagnosed until the onset of advanced-stage gallbladder cancer [58]. PBM is diagnosed when an abnormally long common channel and/or an abnormal union between the pancreatic and bile ducts is evident on direct cholangiography such as Endoscopic Retrograde Cholangiopancreatography (ERCP) or Magnetic Resonance Cholangiopancreatography (MRCP).

The sphincter of Oddi, which is normally located at the distal end of the pancreatic and bile ducts, regulates the outflow of the pancreatic juice and bile. Because of the markedly long common channel in PBM, sphincter activity does not affect the pancreaticobiliary junction, which allows reciprocal reflux of pancreatic juice or bile. As the hydropressure in the pancreatic duct is usually greater than that in the bile duct, reflux of pancreatic juice into the biliary tract is frequent in PBM, which explains the higher rates of carcinogenesis of the biliary tract in patients with PBM [57, 59]. Carcinogenesis in PBM appears to be related to the stagnation of the pancreatic juice refluxed into the biliary tract. Refluxed proteolytic pancreatic enzymes and phospholipase A2 activation in the biliary tract produce strong cytotoxic substances such as lysolecithin. Exposure to harmful substances induces epithelial hyperplasia with increased cell proliferation. This leads to *K-ras* oncogene and/or *p53* tumor suppressor gene mutations in the epithelium and subsequent cancer development and progression. The reported incidence of epithelial hyperplasia of the gallbladder of PBM patients without biliary dilatation was 72–91% [58]. The Ki-67 labeling index, a marker of cell proliferation activity, was significantly higher in the gallbladder epithelium of PBM patients than in that of controls (8.1 vs. 1.4%) [60]. The predominant mechanism responsible for the development of biliary tract cancer in patients with PBM appears to be the hyperplasia-dysplasia-carcinoma sequence resulting from chronic inflammation induced by refluxed pancreatic juice, which is different from the adenoma-carcinoma sequence or de novo carcinogenesis seen in patients without PBM [57, 61].

A nationwide survey in Japan [62] reported prevalences of biliary tract cancers in adult PBM patients with and without biliary dilatation of 21.6 and 42.4%, respectively. Among PBM patients with biliary tract cancers, bile duct and gallbladder cancers were present in 32.1 and 62.3% of patients with biliary dilatation and 7.3 and 88.1% of those without biliary dilatation. Thus, bile duct and gallbladder cancer occurred in 6.9 and 13.4% of patients with congenital biliary dilatation and 3.1 and 37.4% of patients without biliary dilatation. Furthermore, biliary tract cancers developed at an early age in PBM patients (mean 50–60 years), about 15–20 years earlier than those without PBM [57].

Once PBM is diagnosed, prophylactic biliary surgery is recommended before the onset of malignant changes. Cholecystectomy and resection of the extrahepatic bile duct is an established standard for the surgical treatment in PBM patients with congenital biliary dilatation [63]. However, the treatment of PBM without biliary dilatation remains controversial. Only prophylactic cholecystectomy is performed in many institutes because most biliary cancers in PBM patients without biliary dilatation are gallbladder cancer [64]. However, some surgeons suggest excision of the extrahepatic bile duct with the gallbladder in PBM patients without biliary dilatation because such patients have a higher risk of bile duct cancer than the general population [65].

Compared to congenital biliary dilatation, PBM without biliary dilatation is difficult to diagnose early because they rarely evoke symptoms. In PBM without biliary dilatation, epithelial hyperplasia of the gallbladder induced by long-standing continuous stasis of the bile intermingled with refluxed pancreatic juice is a characteristic pathological change [66]. To achieve early detection of PBM without biliary dilatation, MRCP is recommended for patients with gallbladder wall thickening on screening ultrasonography under suspicion of PBM [58, 61].

Primary Sclerosing Cholangitis

Primary Sclerosing Cholangitis (PSC) is a chronic liver disease characterized by chronic inflammation and fibrosis of the intra- and extrahepatic bile ducts. Patients with PSC have a significantly increased risk of cholangiocarcinoma, gallbladder cancer, and colorectal cancer. The risk of gallbladder cancer increases via a metaplasia-dysplasia-carcinoma sequence [22], and the lifetime incidence of gallbladder cancer in patients with PSC is estimated to be 3–14% [67]. On imaging, gallbladder cancer can manifest a mass (45–60%), thickened gallbladder wall (20–30%), or polypoid lesion (15–25%) [68]. The European Association for the Study of the Liver (EASL) reported that adenocarcinoma is found in more than 50% of patients of PSC with gallbladder mass lesions regardless of their size [69]. Therefore, cholecystectomy should be considered in all patients with PSC for gallbladder masses of any size or gallbladder polyps greater than 8 mm in size, while polyps less than 8 mm may be closely monitored because of the high surgical risk of PSC patients and the unlikelihood to be malignant [69–71]. The American Association for the Study of Liver Diseases (AASLD) recommends annual surveillance of gallbladder cancer with US screening to detect mass lesions in the gallbladder [72].

Environmental/Lifestyle Factors

Chronic Infection

Chronic infection by *Salmonella* (*S. typhi* and *S. paratyphi*) or *Helicobacter (H. pylori and H. bilis)* may predispose individuals to gallbladder cancer [73, 74]. Approximately 2–5% of patients with acute *S. Typhi* infection become chronic asymptomatic carriers, with the gallbladder being a site of persistence [75]. Chronic infection with *S. typhi* has been associated with an increased risk of gallbladder cancer, although the mechanism underlying this association is unknown. Epidemiological studies have shown that chronic *S. typhi* carriers have an 8.47-fold increased risk of gallbladder cancer compared to non-carriers [76]. In a meta-analysis of studies from South Asia, Nagaraja et al. reported a 4.28-fold increased risk of gallbladder cancer in chronic typhoid carriers [77]. Latin American countries such as Chile and Bolivia, where typhoid fever is endemic, have the highest rates of gallbladder cancer worldwide, with summary RRs of 4.6 and 4.7 for studies using Vi antibody serology and culture techniques, respectively [78]. Due to the risk of gallbladder cancer, management options for chronic typhoid carriers should include either elective cholecystectomy or careful monitoring by US [77].

Several *Helicobacter* species can colonize the hepatobiliary tract in humans, where they cause chronic inflammation. A study of Japanese and Thai populations found that the Odds Ratios (ORs) for bile duct or gallbladder cancer with *H. bilis* compared to gallstone and/or cholecystitis were 6.50 in Japanese and 5.86 in Thai patients [79]. *H. pylori* was detected in the bile 9.9 times more frequently in patients with biliary tract cancer compared to patients in the control group [80]. However, other studies failed to demonstrate an increased risk of gallbladder cancer in the presence of *H. bilis* [81] or *H. pylori* [82]. Therefore, the possible role of *Helicobacter* species in the development of gallbladder cancer requires verification. Other chronic infections with liver flukes, including *Clonorchis sinensis* and *Opisthorchis viverrini,* are highly associated with cholangiocarcinoma but have not been evaluated for the risk of gallbladder cancer.

Chronic gallbladder infection may predispose individuals to gallbladder cancer through several mechanisms. Beta-glucuronidase excreted by bacteria may deconjugate bile acids and metabolites, rendering them highly active intermediates that bind to DNA [83]. Long-term chronic inflammation results in the sustained release of inflammatory mediators such as cytokines, chemokines, reactive oxygen species, and prostaglandins into the tissue microenvironment. Inflammation by cytokines induces oncogene activation and tumor suppressor gene inactivation, leading to cell transformation, mutated cell proliferation, and apoptosis inhibition, eventually leading to gallbladder cancer [84].

Exposures and Medications

Occupational and environmental exposures to carcinogens may increase the risk of gallbladder cancer. The presumed mechanism by which toxic substances contribute to gallbladder carcinogenesis is chronic exposure of the gallbladder epithelium to carcinogenic metabolites of toxins excreted from the liver into bile [85]. Prolonged exposure to some heavy metals may result in gallbladder cancer. Patients with gallbladder cancer have significantly lower levels of selenium and zinc and higher levels of copper, lead, cadmium, chromium, and nickel in serum and bile. These findings indicate that deficiencies in trace elements such as selenium and zinc may lead to a loss of their protective roles against cancer and that the remaining heavy metals have carcinogenic properties [86, 87]. Workers in rubber plants or textile factories or those exposed to nitrosamines have increased risks of gallbladder cancer [88]. An increased risk was also reported among miners exposed to radon [1]. Those living in the Gangetic belt in India, an industrial region with high levels of pollutants in untreated domestic sewage, industrial, and agricultural effluents containing aromatic hydrocarbons, nitrosamines, and chemicals such as nitrates and nitrites, have a nearly 10-fold increased risk of developing gallbladder cancer [89]. Fungal aflatoxin, ochratoxin A, and arsenic exposure may also be associated with increased risks of gallbladder cancer [90–92].

Increased risk of gallbladder cancer has also been associated with some medications. Hormone Replacement Therapy (HRT) and use of oral contraceptives have different impacts on the risk of gallbladder cancer. Postmenopausal women undergoing oral estrogen or estrogen-progesterone therapy are at increased risks of gallstones and gallbladder cancer [93]; however, the risk associated with oral contraceptive use remains controversial [94]. Large prospective cohort studies have suggested that HRT increases the risk of gallbladder disease in postmenopausal women, and transdermal estrogen replacement therapy has a lower risk for gallbladder disease than oral therapy (RR 1.17 *vs.* 1.74) [95]. Transdermal estrogens are absorbed through the skin and enter the systemic circulation directly, bypassing first-pass metabolism by the liver. Therefore, the concentrations of estrogens and their metabolites in the bile are low, which explains the lower risk of gallbladder disease. Drugs including methyldopa and isoniazid may increase the risk of gallbladder cancer; however, the associations are weak [96, 97].

Lifestyle Factors

Although the association between dietary intake and gallbladder cancer is unclear, dietary factors may influence the production of gallbladder cancer through potential effects on gallstone formation [31]. Higher intakes of energy and carbohydrate can increase the risk of gallbladder cancer because obesity plays an important role in the development of gallbladder cancer. However, adequate intake of fruits and vegetables may have a preventive effect against gallbladder cancer, which could be attributed to their high levels of vitamins, carotenes, and fiber [98]. High consumption of fish may also play an important role in gallbladder cancer prevention by increasing the inhibitory effect of biliary linolenic acid on mutagens in gallbladder bile [99]. A recent prospective cohort study of Swedish adults showed an association between coffee consumption and a reduced risk of gallbladder cancer. The protective effect of coffee consumption may be mediated via reduced gallstone formation. Coffee consumption stimulates cholecystokinin release, enhances gallbladder contraction, and decreases cholesterol crystallization in the bile [100]. Tea consumption also reduced the risk of gallbladder cancer in women but not in men [101].

Cigarettes can damage DNA and cause genetic mutations, which may increase the risk of gallbladder cancer. A recent study reported a 19% increased RR among current smokers and a dose-response relationship between smoking and gallbladder cancer [102]. The association between alcohol consumption and the risk of gallbladder cancer was also dose-dependent. A meta-analysis by Bagnardi et al. of eight studies showed that heavy drinking (>50 g of alcohol/day), but not moderate and light drinking, was associated with an RR of 2.64 for gallbladder cancer [103].

Conclusion

Gallbladder cancer is a deadly, aggressive, and multifactorial disease with complex interplays between genetic and environmental risk factors. In the carcinogenesis of gallbladder cancer, the dysplasia-carcinoma and metaplasia-dysplasia-carcinoma sequences induced by chronic inflammation are considered more important models than the adenoma-carcinoma sequence. In countries with high rates of cholecystectomy, the incidence of gallbladder cancer has decreased following the recommendation for prophylactic cholecystectomy in patients with risk factors. Therefore, investigation of risk factors is important. While gallstones are the most common risk factor for gallbladder cancer, less than 1% of patients with gallstones develop gallbladder cancer; thus, prophylactic cholecystectomy or screening for gallbladder cancer is not necessary. Patients with gallbladder polyps>10 mm have increased malignant potential and prophylactic cholecystectomy is recommended. However, for small gallbladder polyps, less concern seems appropriate since most do not become gallbladder cancer. Based on recent evidence suggesting a much lower incidence of cancer in patients with PGB, cholecystectomy is not routinely recommended for all patients and is limited to healthy patients. PBM, which is more common in young Asian women without gallstones, should be kept in mind as these patients may have a high risk of gallbladder cancer. Once PBM is diagnosed, prophylactic biliary surgery is recommended. Patients with PSC would benefit from annual surveillance of gallbladder cancer with US screening to detect mass lesions in the gallbladder. For the primary prevention of gallbladder cancer, further research is needed to identify the complex relationship between environmental and genetic risks and elucidate the multifactorial pathophysiology of gallbladder cancer. Cancer genomics and new molecular biology techniques may be helpful to reveal the overall molecular pathogenesis of gallbladder cancer, which will guide strategies for prevention and modern therapeutic approaches.

References

1. Hundal R, Shaffer EA. Gallbladder cancer: epidemiology and outcome. Clin Epidemiol. 2014;6:99–109.
2. Roa I, de Aretxabala X. Gallbladder cancer in chile: what have we learned? Curr Opin Gastroenterol. 2015;31:269–75.
3. Surveillance, Epidemiology, and End Results Program. SEER*Explorer: An interactive website for SEER cancer statistics. 2019; 2020.
4. Duffy A, Capanu M, Abou-Alfa GK, Huitzil D, Jarnagin W, Fong Y, et al. Gallbladder cancer (GBC): 10-year experience at memorial sloan-kettering cancer centre (MSKCC). J Surg Oncol. 2008;98:485–9.
5. Randi G, Franceschi S, La Vecchia C. Gallbladder cancer worldwide: Geographical distribution and risk factors. Int J Cancer. 2006;118:1591–602.
6. Vucenik I, Stains JP. Obesity and cancer risk: evidence, mechanisms, and recommendations. Ann N Y Acad Sci. 2012;1271:37–43.
7. Tan W, Gao M, Liu N, Zhang G, Xu T, Cui W. Body mass index and risk of gallbladder cancer: systematic review and meta-analysis of observational studies. Nutrients. 2015;7:8321–34.
8. Gu J, Yan S, Wang B, Shen F, Cao H, Fan J, et al. Type 2 diabetes mellitus and risk of gallbladder cancer: a systematic review and meta-analysis of observational studies. Diabetes Metab Res Rev. 2016;32:63–72.
9. Lai H, Chang S, Lin C, Chen C, Chou J, Peng C, et al. Does diabetes mellitus with or without gallstones increase the risk of gallbladder cancer? results from a population-based cohort study. J Gastroenterol. 2013;48:856–65.
10. Jackson SS, Van Dyke AL, Zhu B, Pfeiffer RM, Petrick JL, Adami H, et al. Anthropometric risk

factors for cancers of the biliary tract in the biliary tract cancers pooling project. Cancer Res. 2019;79:3973–82.
11. Bray F, Ferlay J, Soerjomataram I, Siegel RL, Torre LA, Jemal A. Global cancer statistics 2018: GLOBOCAN estimates of incidence and mortality worldwide for 36 cancers in 185 countries. CA Cancer J Clin. 2018;68:394–424.
12. Wi Y, Woo H, Won Y, Jang J, Shin A. Trends in gallbladder cancer incidence and survival in Korea. Cancer Res Treat. 2018;50:1444–51.
13. Hemminki K, Li X. Familial liver and gallbladder cancer: a nationwide epidemiological study from sweden. Gut. 2003;52:592–6.
14. Hemminki K, Mousavi SM, Brandt A, Ji J, Sundquist J. Liver and gallbladder cancer in immigrants to sweden. Eur J Cancer. 2010;46:926–31.
15. Srivastava K, Srivastava A, Sharma KL, Mittal B. Candidate gene studies in gallbladder cancer: a systematic review and meta-analysis. Mutat Res. 2011;728:67–79.
16. Roa JC, Vo Q, Araya JC, Villaseca M, Guzmán P, Ibacache GS, et al. [Inactivation of CDKN2A gene (p 16) in gallbladder carcinoma]. Rev Med Chil. 2004; 132:1369–76.
17. Henley SJ, Weir HK, Jim MA, Watson M, Richardson LC. Gallbladder cancer incidence and mortality, united states 1999-2011. Cancer Epidemiol Biomarkers Prev. 2015;24:1319–26.
18. Boutros C, Gary M, Baldwin K, Somasundar P. Gallbladder cancer: past, present and an uncertain future. Surg Oncol. 2012;21:183–91.
19. Roa I, de Aretxabala X, Araya JC, Roa J. Preneoplastic lesions in gallbladder cancer. J Surg Oncol. 2006;93:615–23.
20. Zatonski WA, Lowenfels AB, Boyle P, Maisonneuve P, Bueno de Mesquita HB, Ghadirian P, et al. Epidemiologic aspects of gallbladder cancer: a case-control study of the SEARCH program of the international agency for research on cancer. J Natl Cancer Inst. 1997; 89:1132–8.
21. Stinton LM, Shaffer EA. Epidemiology of gallbladder disease: cholelithiasis and cancer. Gut Liver. 2012;6:172–87.
22. Goetze TO. Gallbladder carcinoma: prognostic factors and therapeutic options. World J Gastroenterol. 2015;21:12211–7.
23. Pilgrim CHC, Groeschl RT, Christians KK, Gamblin TC. Modern perspectives on factors predisposing to the development of gallbladder cancer. HPB (Oxford). 2013;15:839–44.
24. Jain K, Mohapatra T, Das P, Misra MC, Gupta SD, Ghosh M, et al. Sequential occurrence of preneoplastic lesions and accumulation of loss of heterozygosity in patients with gallbladder stones suggest causal association with gallbladder cancer. Ann Surg. 2014;260:1073–80.
25. Shaffer EA. Gallbladder cancer: the basics. Gastroenterol Hepatol (NY). 2008;4:737–41.
26. Tewari M. Contribution of silent gallstones in gallbladder cancer. J Surg Oncol. 2006;93:629–32.
27. Williams CI, Shaffer EA. Gallstone disease: Current therapeutic practice. Curr Treat Options Gastroenterol. 2008;11:71–7.
28. Wiles R, Varadpande M, Muly S, Webb J. Growth rate and malignant potential of small gallbladder polyps–systematic review of evidence. Surgeon. 2014;12:221–6.
29. Trivedi V, Gumaste VV, Liu S, Baum J. Gallbladder cancer: adenoma-carcinoma or dysplasia-carcinoma sequence? Gastroenterol Hepatol (NY). 2008;4:735–7.
30. Goldin RD, Roa JC. Gallbladder cancer: A morphological and molecular update. Histopathology. 2009;55:218–29.
31. Lazcano-Ponce EC, Miquel JF, Muñoz N, Herrero R, Ferrecio C, Wistuba II, et al. Epidemiology and molecular pathology of gallbladder cancer. CA Cancer J Clin. 2001;51:349–64.
32. Myers RP, Shaffer EA, Beck PL. Gallbladder polyps: epidemiology, natural history and management. Can J Gastroenterol. 2002;16:187–94.
33. Wiles R, Thoeni RF, Barbu ST, Vashist YK, Rafaelsen SR, Dewhurst C, et al. Management and follow-up of gallbladder polyps: Joint guidelines between the european society of gastrointestinal and abdominal radiology (ESGAR), european association for endoscopic surgery and other interventional techniques (EAES), international society of digestive surgery—European federation (EFISDS) and european society of gastrointestinal endoscopy (ESGE). Eur Radiol. 2017;27:3856–66.
34. Bhatt NR, Gillis A, Smoothey CO, Awan FN, Ridgway PF. Evidence based management of polyps of the gall bladder: a systematic review of the risk factors of malignancy. Surgeon. 2016;14:278–86.
35. Gallahan WC, Conway JD. Diagnosis and management of gallbladder polyps. Gastroenterol Clin North Am. 2010;39:359–67.
36. Park JY, Hong SP, Kim YJ, Kim HJ, Kim HM, Cho JH, et al. Long-term follow up of gallbladder polyps. J Gastroenterol Hepatol. 2009;24:219–22.
37. Cho JH, Park JY, Kim YJ, Kim HM, Kim HJ, Hong SP, et al. Hypoechoic foci on EUS are simple and strong predictive factors for neoplastic gallbladder polyps. Gastrointest Endosc. 2009;69:1244–50.
38. Liu L, Xu H, Lu M, Xie X, Wang W, Hu B, et al. Contrast-enhanced ultrasound in the diagnosis of gallbladder diseases: a multi-center experience. PLoS ONE. 2012;7:e48371.
39. Choi J, Seo D, Choi JH, Park DH, Lee SS, Lee SK, et al. Utility of contrast-enhanced harmonic EUS in the diagnosis of malignant gallbladder polyps (with videos). Gastrointest Endosc. 2013;78:484–93.
40. Teber MA, Tan S, Dönmez U, İpek A, Uçar AE, Yıldırım H, et al. The use of real-time elastography in the assessment of gallbladder polyps: preliminary observations. Med Ultrason. 2014;16:304–8.

41. Bonatti M, Vezzali N, Lombardo F, Ferro F, Zamboni G, Tauber M, et al. Gallbladder adenomyomatosis: imaging findings, tricks and pitfalls. Insights Imaging. 2017;8:243–53.
42. Golse N, Lewin M, Rode A, Sebagh M, Mabrut JY. Gallbladder adenomyomatosis: diagnosis and management. J Visc Surg. 2017;154:345–53.
43. Nishimura A, Shirai Y, Hatakeyama K. Segmental adenomyomatosis of the gallbladder predisposes to cholecystolithiasis. J Hepatobiliary Pancreat Surg. 2004;11:342–7.
44. Nabatame N, Shirai Y, Nishimura A, Yokoyama N, Wakai T, Hatakeyama K. High risk of gallbladder carcinoma in elderly patients with segmental adenomyomatosis of the gallbladder. J Exp Clin Cancer Res. 2004;23:593–8.
45. Agrawal S, Khurana J, Daruwala C. Gallbladder adenomyomatosis: a malignant masquerader. Dig Liver Dis. 2012;44:e23.
46. Kai K, Irie H, Ide T, Masuda M, Kitahara K, Miyoshi A, et al. Actual status of clinical diagnosis in patients with primary gallbladder cancer associated with adenomyomatosis. Indian J Gastroenterol. 2013;32:386–91.
47. Kai K, Ide T, Masuda M, Kitahara K, Miyoshi A, Miyazaki K, et al. Clinicopathologic features of advanced gallbladder cancer associated with adenomyomatosis. Virchows Arch. 2011;459:573–80.
48. Pellino G, Sciaudone G, Candilio G, Perna G, Santoriello A, Canonico S, et al. Stepwise approach and surgery for gallbladder adenomyomatosis: a mini-review. HBPD INT. 2013;12:136–42.
49. Suzuki H, Wada S, Araki K, Kubo N, Watanabe A, Tsukagoshi M, et al. Xanthogranulomatous cholecystitis: difficulty in differentiating from gallbladder cancer. World J Gastroenterol. 2015;21:10166–73.
50. Zhuang PY, Zhu MJ, Wang JD, Zhou XP, Quan ZW, Shen J. Xanthogranulomatous cholecystitis: a clinicopathological study of its association with gallbladder carcinoma. J Dig Dis. 2013;14:45–50.
51. Ghosh M, Sakhuja P, Agarwal AK. Xanthogranulomatous cholecystitis: a premalignant condition? HBPD INT. 2011;10:179–84.
52. Stephen AE, Berger DL. Carcinoma in the porcelain gallbladder: a relationship revisited. Surgery. 2001;129:699–703.
53. Cunningham SC, Alexander HR. Porcelain gallbladder and cancer: ethnicity explains a discrepant literature? Am J Med. 2007;120:17–8.
54. Schnelldorfer T. Porcelain gallbladder: a benign process or concern for malignancy? J Gastrointest Surg. 2013;17:1161–8.
55. Khan ZS, Livingston EH, Huerta S. Reassessing the need for prophylactic surgery in patients with porcelain gallbladder: case series and systematic review of the literature. Arch Surg. 2011;146:1143–7.
56. DesJardins H, Duy L, Scheirey C, Schnelldorfer T. Porcelain gallbladder: is observation a safe option in select populations? J Am Coll Surg. 2018;226:1064–9.
57. Kamisawa T, Ando H, Suyama M, Shimada M, Morine Y, Shimada H. Japanese clinical practice guidelines for pancreaticobiliary maljunction. J Gastroenterol. 2012;47:731–59.
58. Takuma K, Kamisawa T, Tabata T, Hara S, Kuruma S, Inaba Y, et al. Importance of early diagnosis of pancreaticobiliary maljunction without biliary dilatation. World J Gastroenterol. 2012;18:3409–14.
59. Kamisawa T, Ando H, Hamada Y, Fujii H, Koshinaga T, Urushihara N, et al. Diagnostic criteria for pancreaticobiliary maljunction 2013. J Hepatobiliary Pancreat Sci. 2014;21:159–61.
60. Kamisawa T, Takuma K, Anjiki H, Egawa N, Kurata M, Honda G, et al. Pancreaticobiliary maljunction. Clin Gastroenterol Hepatol. 2009;7:84–8.
61. Kamisawa T, Kuruma S, Chiba K, Tabata T, Koizumi S, Kikuyama M. Biliary carcinogenesis in pancreaticobiliary maljunction. J Gastroenterol. 2017;52:158–63.
62. Morine Y, Shimada M, Takamatsu H, Araida T, Endo I, Kubota M, et al. Clinical features of pancreaticobiliary maljunction: Update analysis of 2nd japan-nationwide survey. J Hepatobiliary Pancreat Sci. 2013;20:472–80.
63. Kamisawa T, Ando H, Shimada M, Hamada Y, Itoi T, Takayashiki T, et al. Recent advances and problems in the management of pancreaticobiliary maljunction: feedback from the guidelines committee. J Hepatobiliary Pancreat Sci. 2014;21:87–92.
64. Tashiro S, Imaizumi T, Ohkawa H, Okada A, Katoh T, Kawaharada Y, et al. Pancreaticobiliary maljunction: retrospective and nationwide survey in japan. J Hepatobiliary Pancreat Surg. 2003;10:345–51.
65. Funabiki T, Matsubara T, Miyakawa S, Ishihara S. Pancreaticobiliary maljunction and carcinogenesis to biliary and pancreatic malignancy. Langenbecks Arch Surg. 2009;394:159–69.
66. Tsuchida A, Itoi T, Endo M, Kitamura K, Mukaide M, Itokawa F, et al. Pathological features and surgical outcome of pancreaticobiliary maljunction without dilatation of the extrahepatic bile duct. Oncol Rep. 2004;11:269–76.
67. Razumilava N, Gores GJ, Lindor KD. Cancer surveillance in patients with primary sclerosing cholangitis. Hepatology. 2011;54:1842–52.
68. Sandrasegaran K, Menias CO. Imaging and screening of cancer of the gallbladder and bile ducts. Radiol Clin North Am. 2017;55:1211–22.
69. European Association for the Study of the Liver. EASL clinical practice guidelines: management of cholestatic liver diseases. J Hepatol. 2009;51:237–67.
70. Lindor KD, Kowdley KV, Harrison ME. ACG clinical guideline: primary sclerosing cholangitis. Am J Gastroenterol. 2015;110:646–59.
71. Eaton JE, Thackeray EW, Lindor KD. Likelihood of malignancy in gallbladder polyps and outcomes following cholecystectomy in primary sclerosing cholangitis. Am J Gastroenterol. 2012;107:431–9.

72. Chapman R, Fevery J, Kalloo A, Nagorney DM, Boberg KM, Shneider B, et al. Diagnosis and management of primary sclerosing cholangitis. Hepatology. 2010;51:660–78.
73. Kumar S, Kumar S, Kumar S. Infection as a risk factor for gallbladder cancer. J Surg Oncol. 2006;93:633–9.
74. Gonzalez-Escobedo G, Marshall JM, Gunn JS. Chronic and acute infection of the gallbladder by salmonella typhi: Understanding the carrier state. Nat Rev Microbiol. 2011;9:9–14.
75. Levine MM, Black RE, Lanata C. Precise estimation of the numbers of chronic carriers of salmonella typhi in santiago, chile, an endemic area. J Infect Dis. 1982;146:724–6.
76. Samaras V, Rafailidis PI, Mourtzoukou EG, Peppas G, Falagas ME. Chronic bacterial and parasitic infections and cancer: a review. J Infect Dev Ctries. 2010;4:267–81.
77. Nagaraja V, Eslick GD. Systematic review with meta-analysis: the relationship between chronic salmonella typhi carrier status and gallbladder cancer. Aliment Pharmacol Ther. 2014;39:745–50.
78. Koshiol J, Wozniak A, Cook P, Adaniel C, Acevedo J, Azócar L, et al. Salmonella enterica serovar typhi and gallbladder cancer: a case-control study and meta-analysis. Cancer Med. 2016;5:3310–235.
79. Matsukura N, Yokomuro S, Yamada S, Tajiri T, Sundo T, Hadama T, et al. Association between Helicobacter bilis in bile and biliary tract malignancies: H. bilis in bile from japanese and thai patients with benign and malignant diseases in the biliary tract. Jpn J Cancer Res. 2002; 93:842–7.
80. Bulajic M, Maisonneuve P, Schneider-Brachert W, Müller P, Reischl U, Stimec B, et al. Helicobacter pylori and the risk of benign and malignant biliary tract disease. Cancer. 2002;95:1946–53.
81. Pandey M, Mishra RR, Dixit R, Jaiswal R, Shukla M, Nath G. Helicobacter bilis in human gallbladder cancer: results of a case-control study and a meta-analysis. Asian Pac J Cancer Prev. 2010;11:343–7.
82. Mishra RR, Tewari M, Shukla HS. Helicobacter pylori and pathogenesis of gallbladder cancer. J Gastroenterol Hepatol. 2011;26:260–6.
83. Hill MJ. Chronic bacterial infection and subsequent human carcinogenesis. Eur J Cancer Prev. 1995;4:127–8.
84. Li Y Zhang, Ma H. Chronic inflammation and gallbladder cancer. Cancer Lett. 2014; 345:242–8.
85. Tsuchiya Y, Terao M, Okano K, Nakamura K, Oyama M, Ikegami K, et al. Mutagenicity and mutagens of the red chili pepper as gallbladder cancer risk factor in chilean women. Asian Pac J Cancer Prev. 2011;12:471–6.
86. Rustagi T, Dasanu CA. Risk factors for gallbladder cancer and cholangiocarcinoma: similarities, differences and updates. J Gastrointest Cancer. 2012;43:137–47.
87. Basu S, Singh MK, Singh TB, Bhartiya SK, Singh SP, Shukla VK. Heavy and trace metals in carcinoma of the gallbladder. World J Surg. 2013;37:2641–6.
88. Rawla P, Sunkara T, Thandra KC, Barsouk A. Epidemiology of gallbladder cancer. Clin Exp Hepatol. 2019;5:93–102.
89. Dixit R, Shukla V. Why is gallbladder cancer common in the gangetic belt? In: Sudhakaran PR, editors. Perspectives in cancer prevention-translational cancer research. 1st ed. Springer; 2013. p. 145–51.
90. Koshiol J, Gao Y, Dean M, Egner P, Nepal C, Jones K, et al. Association of aflatoxin and gallbladder cancer. Gastroenterology. 2017;153:488–94.
91. Ikoma T, Tsuchiya Y, Asai T, Okano K, Ito N, Endoh K, et al. Ochratoxin A contamination of red chili peppers from chile, bolivia and peru, countries with a high incidence of gallbladder cancer. Asian Pac J Cancer Prev. 2015;16:5987–91.
92. Ganesan N, Bambino K, Boffetta P, Labgaa I. Exploring the potential carcinogenic role of arsenic in gallbladder cancer. Eur J Cancer Prev. 2020;29:100–9.
93. Cirillo DJ, Wallace RB, Rodabough RJ, Greenland P, LaCroix AZ, Limacher MC, et al. Effect of estrogen therapy on gallbladder disease. JAMA. 2005;293:330–9.
94. Shaffer EA. Gallstone disease: epidemiology of gallbladder stone disease. Best Pract Res Clin Gastroenterol. 2006;20:981–96.
95. Liu B, Beral V, Balkwill A, Green J, Sweetland S, Reeves G. Gallbladder disease and use of transdermal versus oral hormone replacement therapy in postmenopausal women: prospective cohort study. BMJ. 2008;337:280–3.
96. Brodén G, Bengtsson L. Biliary carcinoma associated with methyldopa therapy. Acta Chir Scand Suppl. 1980;500:7–12.
97. Lowenfels AB, Norman J. Isoniazid and bile duct cancer. JAMA. 1978;240:434–5.
98. Rai A, Mohapatra SC, Shukla HS. A review of association of dietary factors in gallbladder cancer. Indian J Cancer. 2004;41:147–51.
99. Serra I, Tsuchiya Y, Hori Y, Villegas R, Oyama M, Makiguchi T, et al. Effect of dietary intake on the levels of biliary unsaturated free fatty acids having inhibitory activity on mutagens. Asian Pac J Cancer Prev. 2009;10:899–902.
100. Larsson SC, Giovannucci EL, Wolk A. Coffee consumption and risk of gallbladder cancer in a prospective study. J Natl Cancer Inst. 2017;109:1–3.
101. Zhu G, Hua J, Wang Z, She F, Chen Y. Tea consumption and risk of gallbladder cancer: a meta-analysis of epidemiological studies. Mol Clin Oncol. 2015;3:613–8.
102. Aune D, Vatten LJ, Boffetta P. Tobacco smoking and the risk of gallbladder disease. Eur J Epidemiol. 2016;31:643–53.
103. Bagnardi V, Rota M, Botteri E, Tramacere I, Islami F, Fedirko V, et al. Alcohol consumption and site-specific cancer risk: A comprehensive dose-response meta-analysis. Br J Cancer. 2015;112:580–93.

Gene Mutations and Its Clinical Significance

Sang Hoon Lee and Seung Woo Park

Introduction

Gallbladder cancer (GBC) is a rare malignancy of biliary tract cancer (BTC), characterized by late presentation and poor prognosis. There is a significant difference in its incidence with respect to geography and ethnic background. The highest incidence has been observed in parts of South America, East and South Asia, and in Native American and Asian population in North America (see Chap. "Epidemiology") [1, 2]. These differences in incidence rates in GBC could be interpreted as the difference in environmental exposure and genetic aberrations. Epidemiologic risk factors for GBC include age, female gender, family history, obesity, cholelithiasis, chronic cholecystitis, porcelain gallbladder, polyps, chronic infection by Salmonella species, and exposure to certain chemicals and heavy metals, accompanied with various genetic factors (see Chap. "Risk Factors") [3].

The recent advance of genomic sequencing has led to a better understanding of carcinogenesis in several cancers, including GBC. Earlier, traditional candidate gene studies with low throughput approaches, like Polymerase Chain Reaction (PCR), restriction fragment length polymorphism (RFLP), PCR-single stranded conformation polymorphism (SSCP), and direct sequencing, were used to detect mutations in cancers. Recently, Next-generation sequencing (NGS) has been introduced. NGS focuses on the sequencing of whole exons (exome sequencing). NGS technique can provide increased sequence coverage of a particular region of interest at high throughput with lower cost when compared to conventional gene sequencing. With the advent of high-throughput approaches, large-scale genome-wide association studies (GWAS) have made it possible to explore the entire genome for the GBC specific susceptibility genomic loci.

This chapter unravels the genetic landscape of GBC based on different approaches including candidate gene approach, GWAS, and other high-throughput sequencing methods. Furthermore, identification of the contribution of both germline and somatic mutations in the carcinogenesis would be further helpful not only in better understanding of this malignancy but also in disease management and targeted therapy.

Germline Mutations

Candidate Gene Approach

A large number of researches have reported the susceptibility loci for GBC. Almost available literature had evaluated the role of gene alterations

S. H. Lee · S. W. Park (✉)
Department of Internal Medicine, Yonsei University College of Medicine, Seoul, Korea
e-mail: swoopark@yuhs.ac

S. H. Lee
e-mail: lshjjang_2000@yuhs.ac

J. B. Chung and K. Okazaki (eds.), *Diseases of the Gallbladder*,
https://doi.org/10.1007/978-981-15-6010-1_16

in GBC risk in several genes of hormone pathway [4], inflammatory pathway [5–11], DNA-repair pathway [12–15], drug metabolism pathway [16–20], hedgehog pathway [21], apoptosis pathway [22, 23], and Wnt signaling pathway [24]. However, these studies were limited to small sample size. In fact, further multigene and meta-analysis studies were demonstrated to exclude the association of most single nucleotide polymorphism(s) (SNPs) on GBC susceptibility [25–27]. Therefore, further evaluation through large sample sized studies in different populations is required to provide the definitive conclusion of association of a particular candidate gene in conferring GBC risk.

GWAS-Based Approach

To date, only two GWAS are reported in GBC. The first GWAS in GBC was from Japan, which included 41 patients and 866 controls with a replication cohort consisting of 30 cases and 898 controls. It revealed that the SNP rs7504990 in the *DCC* gene was found to associate with an increased risk of GBC [28]. Also, two new SNPs (rs2229080 and rs714) in the same gene were replicated in a larger sized study in Indian population [29]. These results implied that *DCC* variants are a useful marker for GBC susceptibility.

In a recent large-scale GWAS study in Indian population, the discovery cohort consisted of 1042 GBC cases and 1709 controls and replication cohort contained 428 GBC cases and 420 non-cancer controls from another cohort from North India. Significant association of 19 markers (15 intronic SNPs, 1 synonymous SNP, and 3 ANPs in the 5' upstream region) in the chromosomal region 7q21.12, localizing to the *ABCB4* genes, was observed with the most notable SNPs after replication and meta-analysis being rs1558375, rs17209837, and rs4148808. Furthermore, GWAS heritability test also suggested that the common variants are associated with substantial variation in GBC risk (sibling relative risk 3.15, 95% CI 1.80-5.49) [30]. The function of *ABCB4* gene is one of the hepatobiliary phospholipid transporters that translocate the phosphatidylcholine from the inner leaflet of the canalicular membrane of the hepatocyte. In vitro animal study showed the knockout of the *ABCB4* gene results in hepatic inflammation and its deficiency increases reactive oxygen species accumulation, lipid peroxidation, and DNA damage [31]. Therefore, it is plausible that genetic variants in *ABCB4* gene modify transport process and might be responsible in GBC carcinogenesis.

Somatic Mutation

Low Throughput Approaches

Several studies have shown the effect of somatic mutation in GBC carcinogenesis and disease prognosis, with low throughout approaches such as PCR-RFLP, PCR-SSCP, and direct sequencing. Most extensively evaluated oncogenes in GBC are *K-ras* and *p53* gene.

K-ras mutation is mostly detected at codon 12 in *K-ras* gene with high prevalence (33 ~ 59%) in GBC patients [32–35]. Also, the sites of *p53* mutation were well known to be located in exon 5 to 8 and this prevalence was ranged from 31 to 50% [35, 36]. However, these studies were limited to evaluate the influence of single or few mutations in signaling pathway and so, the role of each gene will be summarized in the following section.

High-Throughput Approaches

With advent of high throughout approaches like mass Sequenom array, whole exome or genome sequencing (WES/WGS), detection of somatic mutations in multiple genes has become quite easy. The somatic mutation and the type of mutations prevalent in human cancer, globally, have been collected in the Catalogue of Somatic Mutations in Cancer (COSMIC) online database (www.cancer.sanger.ac.uk). Based on the COSMIC database, the top 20 most mutated genes in GBC tissue are delineated in Fig. 1.

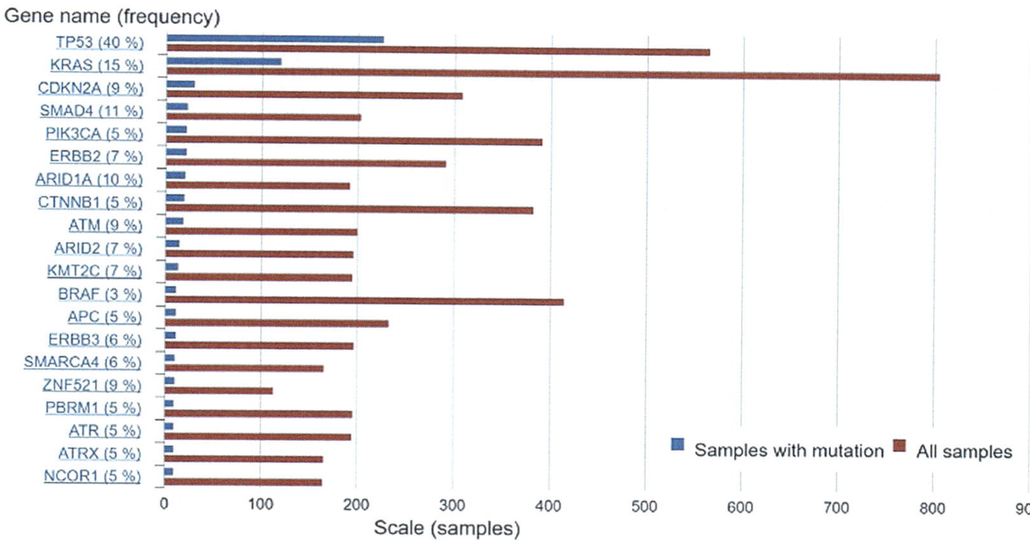

Fig. 1 Illustration of top 20 somatic mutations in gallbladder cancer (GBC) retrieved from COSMIC database (www.cancer.snager.ac.uk/cosmic)

The list of the most prevalent mutations in GBC is as follows: TP53, KRAS, PI3K/AKT/mTOR pathway, chromatin-remodeling pathway, and ErbB pathway. We will discuss the role of somatic mutations in GBC carcinogenesis and its clinical significance.

Tp53

The somatic mutation of tumor suppression gene *p53* has been found in approximately above half of GBC patients (45 ~ 64%) [37–43]. Furthermore, it was regarded as one of the earliest change in the development of GBC, being detected in one-third of normal and dysplastic epithelia acquired from gallbladders with gallstone but without cancer [44]. Additionally, the excessive accumulation of p53 protein in gallbladder dysplasia (0 ~ 32%) and carcinoma in situ lesion (45 ~ 86%) also supported that TP53 abnormality is an early event in GBC carcinogenesis [45–48].

Kras

K-ras mutation is detected in about 15% of GBC patients in high throughout evaluation (8 ~ 19%) [38–43] with significant predictor for poor survival [49]. One study in Japan represented that *K-ras* mutation is more frequently detected in GBC patients having anomalous junction of the pancreaticobiliary tract [35, 50]. By contrast, at least in Chilean patients with cholelithiasis and chronic cholecystitis, *K-ras* mutations were rare, while *p53* mutation arises early during multistage pathogenesis [47, 51]. Although some authors maintained that two distinct pathogenetic pathways had histologic and molecular differences in GBCs associated with anomalous pancreaticobiliary duct junction and those associated with gallstones [52, 53], its clinical role in GBC carcinogenesis was under debate and needed to validate through large-scale sophisticated method.

PI3K/AKT/MTOR Pathway

Deshpande et al. demonstrated the presence of activating mutations in *PIK3CA* (12.5%) gene notably in GBC, as compared to other BTCs [54]. In the study which identified 14 and 26 hotspot mutations through mass spectroscopy-based profiling in 57 cases and NGS in 15 cases among resected GBC cases, PI3 kinase pathway (*STK11, RICTOR, TSC2*) mutations happened commonly(49). Another multigene NGS studies showed that mTOR pathway genes, *PIK3CA* (7 ~ 22%), *PTEN* (3.8 ~ 7%), and *TSC1* (7%), were also mutated [37, 38, 40, 41, 55]. Furthermore, one laboratory finding demonstrated that knockdown *TROP2* gene resulted in smaller xenograft tumors from GBC cell lines in vivo by regulating PI3K/AKT pathway [56]. Conclusively, PI3K/AKT/mTOR pathway could be a potential therapeutic target for GBC management.

Chromatin-Remodeling Pathway

Through WES of 32 intrahepatic cholangiocarcinomas and 8 GBCs, chromatin-remodeling genes including *BAP1, ARID1A, and PBRM1* frequently harbored inactivating mutations in almost half of intrahepatic cholangiocarcinomas; however, *PBRM1* and another chromatin-remodeling gene *KMT2C (MLL3)* were identified in GBC cases, but no mutations in *BAP1* and *ARIDA1A* were screened in GBC patients [37]. Recent large-scale multigene NGS study including total 153 BTCs with 26 GBCs revealed the somatic mutations of chromatin-remodeling genes in GBC—*ARIDA1A* (11.5%), *BAP1* (3.8%), *PBRM1* (7.7%) and *SMARCB1* (7.7%) [41]. Another large-scale study of 260 BTCs (including 28 GBCs) uncovered the distinct mutational pattern of GBC in chromatin-remodeling genes—*ARID2* (18%), *PBRM1* (7%), *MLL2* (11%), *MLL3* (11%), *KDM4A* (7%), and *TET1 ~ 3* (11%), which differ from those of other BTCs [55]. These genetic alterations in chromatin-remodeling pathway can affect the epigenetic instability and are potentially targeted as anti-cancer drugs such as Histone deacetylase (HDAC) inhibitor or DNA-demethylating agents.

ErbB Pathway

One study on 57 tumor-normal pairs reported high portion of mutations in *ERBB3* (11.8%), along with *P53* (47.1%) and *K-ras* (7.8%) gene mutations. The authors further represented ErbB signaling pathway (including *EGFR*, *ERBB2*, *ERBB3*, *ERBB4*, and their downstream gene) to be the most extensively mutated pathway, affecting 36.8% (21/57) of the GBC samples [39]. Several studies have shown *EGFR* or *ERBB3* mutations predominant in GBC tissue samples [40, 55, 57]. An expression study in ErbB2 and its functional ligand, Muc4 in BK5.erbB2 transgenic mice in GBC reported that Muc4 is upregulated during GBC growth by potentiating ErbB2 signaling [58], thereby highlighting the key role of the ErbB signaling pathway in GBC pathogenesis.

Others

CDKN2

CDKN2 gene, also known as *MTS1* or *p16*$^{\mathrm{INK4}}$, is a well-known tumor suppressor gene and considered as one of the most frequently altered somatic mutation in GBC (7 ~ 19%) [40, 42], but clinical meaning is indeterminate in GBC.

Microsatellite Instability

Mismatch repair (MMR) gene mutations and the resultant microsatellite instability (MSI) are infrequently detected in GBC [59, 61]. Although MSI was identified in a minority of GBC cases, these unique cases were correlated with favorable prognosis and degree of global DNA hypermethylation [60, 61]. In particular, unresectable or metastatic GBC patients with MSI-high/deficient MMR tumors are associated with high-prevalent mutations, and thus may benefit from immune checkpoint inhibitor such as pembrolizumab [62, 63].

Miscellaneous

Some studies contained Japanese GBC patients identified SMAD4 mutation [42, 43, 57], but its clinical significance remains still unknown in GBC carcinogenesis.

One study also showed that *TERT* promoter mutations and APOBEC-mediated somatic mutational signature, which was associated with *APOBEC3B* expression and a high number of mutation number, preferentially contributed to GBC rather than cholangiocarcinoma. Furthermore, they also demonstrated that hypermutated cases were significantly enriched in the

BTC subgroup with the poorest prognosis, which had characteristic elevation in the expression of immune checkpoint molecules [55]. Accordingly, immune-modulating treatments might be potentially promising options for these patients.

Summary

GBC is enriched with multiple mutations, from germline mutations such as genetic susceptibility of *DCC* and *ABCB4* variants to somatic mutations including TP53, KRAS, PI3K/AKT/mTOR pathway, chromatin-remodeling pathway, and ErbB pathway genes in GBC tissues. The further understanding of gene polymorphisms in GBC carcinogenesis will be available to targeted therapy-based approaches for better clinical recommendations in the future.

References

1. Jemal A, Bray F, Center MM, Ferlay J, Ward E, Forman D. Global cancer statistics. CA Cancer J Clin. 2011;61(2):69–90.
2. Patel T. Worldwide trends in mortality from biliary tract malignancies. BMC Cancer. 2002;2:10.
3. Duffy A, Capanu M, Abou-Alfa GK, Huitzil D, Jarnagin W, Fong Y, et al. Gallbladder cancer (GBC): 10-year experience at Memorial Sloan-Kettering Cancer Centre (MSKCC). J Surg Oncol. 2008;98(7):485–9.
4. Srivastava A, Sharma KL, Srivastava N, Misra S, Mittal B. Significant role of estrogen and progesterone receptor sequence variants in gallbladder cancer predisposition: a multi-analytical strategy. PLoS ONE. 2012;7(7):e40162.
5. Srivastava K, Srivastava A, Pandey SN, Kumar A, Mittal B. Functional polymorphisms of the cyclooxygenase (PTGS2) gene and risk for gallbladder cancer in a North Indian population. J Gastroenterol. 2009;44(7):774–80.
6. Sakoda LC, Gao YT, Chen BE, Chen J, Rosenberg PS, Rashid A, et al. Prostaglandin-endoperoxide synthase 2 (PTGS2) gene polymorphisms and risk of biliary tract cancer and gallstones: a population-based study in Shanghai. China. Carcinogenesis. 2006;27(6):1251–6.
7. Hsing AW, Sakoda LC, Rashid A, Andreotti G, Chen J, Wang BS, et al. Variants in inflammation genes and the risk of biliary tract cancers and stones: a population-based study in China. Cancer Res. 2008;68(15):6442–52.
8. Vishnoi M, Pandey SN, Choudhuri G, Mittal B. IL-1 gene polymorphisms and genetic susceptibility of gallbladder cancer in a north Indian population. Cancer Genet Cytogenet. 2008;186(2):63–8.
9. Srivastava A, Pandey SN, Choudhuri G, Mittal B. CCR5 Delta32 polymorphism: associated with gallbladder cancer susceptibility. Scand J Immunol. 2008;67(5):516–22.
10. Srivastava K, Srivastava A, Kumar A, Mittal B. Significant association between toll-like receptor gene polymorphisms and gallbladder cancer. Liver Int. 2010;30(7):1067–72.
11. Sharma KL, Misra S, Kumar A, Mittal B. Higher risk of matrix metalloproteinase (MMP-2, 7, 9) and tissue inhibitor of metalloproteinase (TIMP-2) genetic variants to gallbladder cancer. Liver Int. 2012;32(8):1278–86.
12. Srivastava K, Srivastava A, Mittal B. Polymorphisms in ERCC2, MSH2, and OGG1 DNA repair genes and gallbladder cancer risk in a population of Northern India. Cancer. 2010;116(13):3160–9.
13. Srivastava A, Srivastava K, Pandey SN, Choudhuri G, Mittal B. Single-nucleotide polymorphisms of DNA repair genes OGG1 and XRCC1: association with gallbladder cancer in North Indian population. Ann Surg Oncol. 2009;16(6):1695–703.
14. Zhang M, Huang WY, Andreotti G, Gao YT, Rashid A, Chen J, et al. Variants of DNA repair genes and the risk of biliary tract cancers and stones: a population-based study in China. Cancer Epidemiol Biomarkers Prev. 2008;17(8):2123–7.
15. Jiao X, Wu Y, Zhou L, He J, Yang C, Zhang P, et al. Variants and haplotypes in Flap endonuclease 1 and risk of gallbladder cancer and gallstones: a population-based study in China. Sci Rep. 2015;5:18160.
16. Sakai K, Loza E, Roig GV, Nozaki R, Asai T, Ikoma T, et al. CYP1A1, GSTM1, GSTT1 and TP53 polymorphisms and risk of gallbladder cancer in bolivians. Asian Pac J Cancer Prev. 2016;17(2):781–4.
17. Tsuchiya Y, Kiyohara C, Sato T, Nakamura K, Kimura A, Yamamoto M. Polymorphisms of cytochrome P450 1A1, glutathione S-transferase class mu, and tumour protein p53 genes and the risk of developing gallbladder cancer in Japanese. Clin Biochem. 2007;40(12):881–6.
18. Xu HL, Cheng JR, Andreotti G, Gao YT, Rashid A, Wang BS, et al. Cholesterol metabolism gene polymorphisms and the risk of biliary tract cancers and stones: a population-based case-control study in Shanghai, China. Carcinogenesis. 2011;32(1):58–62.
19. Gong Y, Zhang L, Bie P, Wang H. Roles of ApoB-100 gene polymorphisms and the risks of gallstones and gallbladder cancer: a meta-analysis. PLoS ONE. 2013;8(4):e61456.
20. Rai R, Sharma KL, Misra S, Kumar A, Mittal B. CYP17 polymorphism (rs743572) is associated with increased risk of gallbladder cancer in tobacco users. Tumour Biol. 2014;35(7):6531–7.

21. Dixit R, Pandey M, Tripathi SK, Dwivedi AN, Shukla VK. Comparative Analysis of Mutational Profile of Sonic hedgehog Gene in Gallbladder Cancer. Dig Dis Sci. 2017;62(3):708–14.
22. Rai R, Sharma KL, Sharma S, Misra S, Kumar A, Mittal B. Death receptor (DR4) haplotypes are associated with increased susceptibility of gallbladder carcinoma in north Indian population. PLoS ONE. 2014;9(2):e90264.
23. Srivastava K, Srivastava A, Mittal B. Caspase-8 polymorphisms and risk of gallbladder cancer in a northern Indian population. Mol Carcinog. 2010;49(7):684–92.
24. Yadav A, Gupta A, Yadav S, Rastogi N, Agrawal S, Kumar A, et al. Association of Wnt signaling pathway genetic variants in gallbladder cancer susceptibility and survival. Tumour Biol. 2016;37(6):8083–95.
25. Srivastava K, Srivastava A, Kumar A, Mittal B. Gallbladder cancer predisposition: a multigenic approach to DNA-repair, apoptotic and inflammatory pathway genes. PLoS ONE. 2011;6(1):e16449.
26. Sharma KL, Rai R, Srivastava A, Sharma A, Misra S, Kumar A, et al. A multigenic approach to evaluate genetic variants of PLCE1, LXRs, MMPs, TIMP, and CYP genes in gallbladder cancer predisposition. Tumour Biol. 2014;35(9):8597–606.
27. Rai R, Kim JJ, Misra S, Kumar A, Mittal B. A multiple interaction analysis reveals ADRB3 as a potential candidate for gallbladder cancer predisposition via a complex interaction with other candidate gene variations. Int J Mol Sci. 2015;16(12):28038–49.
28. Cha PC, Zembutsu H, Takahashi A, Kubo M, Kamatani N, Nakamura Y. A genome-wide association study identifies SNP in DCC is associated with gallbladder cancer in the Japanese population. J Hum Genet. 2012;57(4):235–7.
29. Rai R, Sharma KL, Tiwari S, Misra S, Kumar A, Mittal B. DCC (deleted in colorectal carcinoma) gene variants confer increased susceptibility to gallbladder cancer (Ref. No.: Gene-D-12-01446). Gene. 2013; 518(2):303-9.
30. Mhatre S, Wang ZM, Nagrani R, Badwe R, Chiplunkar S, Mittal B, et al. Common genetic variation and risk of gallbladder cancer in India: a case-control genome-wide association study. Lancet Oncology. 2017;18(4):535–44.
31. Tebbi A, Levillayer F, Jouvion G, Fiette L, Soubigou G, Varet H, et al. Deficiency of multidrug resistance 2 contributes to cell transformation through oxidative stress. Carcinogenesis. 2016;37(1):39–48.
32. Ajiki T, Fujimori T, Onoyama H, Yamamoto M, Kitazawa S, Maeda S, et al. K-ras gene mutation in gall bladder carcinomas and dysplasia. Gut. 1996;38(3):426–9.
33. Roa JC, Anabalon L, Tapia O, Melo A, de Aretxabala X, Roa I. Frequency of K-ras mutation in biliary and pancreatic tumors. Rev Med Chile. 2005;133(12):1434–40.
34. Singh MK, Chetri K, Pandey UB, Kapoor VK, Mittal B, Choudhuri G. Mutational spectrum of K-ras oncogene among Indian patients with gallbladder cancer. J Gastroen Hepatol. 2004;19(8):916–21.
35. Hanada K, Tsuchida A, Iwao T, Eguchi N, Sasaki T, Morinaka K, et al. Gene mutations of K-ras in gallbladder mucosae and gallbladder carcinoma with an anomalous junction of the pancreaticobiliary duct. Am J Gastroenterol. 1999;94(6):1638–42.
36. Takagi S, Naito E, Yamanouchi H, Ohtsuka H, Kominami R, Yamamoto M. Mutation of the P53 gene in gallbladder cancer. Tohoku J Exp Med. 1994;172(3):283–9.
37. Jiao Y, Pawlik TM, Anders RA, Selaru FM, Streppel MM, Lucas DJ, et al. Exome sequencing identifies frequent inactivating mutations in BAP1, ARID1A and PBRM1 in intrahepatic cholangiocarcinomas. Nat Genet. 2013;45(12):1470–3.
38. Kumari N, Corless CL, Warrick A, Beadling C, Nelson D, Neff T, et al. Mutation profiling in gallbladder cancer in Indian population. Indian J Pathol Microbiol. 2014;57(1):9–12.
39. Li M, Zhang Z, Li X, Ye J, Wu X, Tan Z, et al. Whole-exome and targeted gene sequencing of gallbladder carcinoma identifies recurrent mutations in the ErbB pathway. Nat Genet. 2014;46(8):872–6.
40. Javle M, Bekaii-Saab T, Jain A, Wang Y, Kelley RK, Wang K, et al. Biliary cancer: utility of next-generation sequencing for clinical management. Cancer. 2016;122(24):3838–47.
41. Simbolo M, Fassan M, Ruzzenente A, Mafficini A, Wood LD, Corbo V, et al. Multigene mutational profiling of cholangiocarcinomas identifies actionable molecular subgroups. Oncotarget. 2014;5(9):2839–52.
42. Noguchi R, Yamaguchi K, Ikenoue T, Terakado Y, Ohta Y, Yamashita N, et al. Genetic alterations in Japanese extrahepatic biliary tract cancer. Oncol Lett. 2017;14(1):877–84.
43. Wardell CP, Fujita M, Yamada T, Simbolo M, Fassan M, Karlic R, et al. Genomic characterization of biliary tract cancers identifies driver genes and predisposing mutations. J Hepatol. 2018;68(5):959–69.
44. Moreno M, Pimentel F, Gazdar AF, Wistuba II, Miquel JF. TP53 abnormalities are frequent and early events in the sequential pathogenesis of gallbladder carcinoma. Ann Hepatol. 2005;4(3):192–9.
45. Kamel D, Paakko P, Nuorva K, Vahakangas K, Soini Y. p53 and c-erbB-2 protein expression in adenocarcinomas and epithelial dysplasias of the gall bladder. J Pathol. 1993;170(1):67–72.
46. Wee A, Teh M, Raju GC. Clinical importance of p53 protein in gall bladder carcinoma and its precursor lesions. J Clin Pathol. 1994;47(5):453–6.
47. Wistuba II, Gazdar AF, Roa I, Albores-Saavedra J. p53 protein overexpression in gallbladder carcinoma and its precursor lesions: an immunohistochemical study. Hum Pathol. 1996;27(4):360–5.

48. Ajiki T, Onoyama H, Yamamoto M, Asaka K, Fujimori T, Maeda S, et al. p53 protein expression and prognosis in gallbladder carcinoma and premalignant lesions. Hepatogastroenterology. 1996;43(9):521–6.
49. Javle M, Rashid A, Churi C, Kar S, Zuo MX, Eterovic AK, et al. Molecular characterization of gallbladder cancer using somatic mutation profiling. Hum Pathol. 2014;45(4):701–8.
50. Matsubara T, Sakurai Y, Sasayama Y, Hori H, Ochiai M, Funabiki T, et al. K-ras point mutations in cancerous and noncancerous biliary epithelium in patients with pancreaticobiliary maljunction. Cancer. 1996;77(8 Suppl):1752–7.
51. Wistuba II, Sugio K, Hung J, Kishimoto Y, Virmani AK, Roa I, et al. Allele-specific mutations involved in the pathogenesis of endemic gallbladder carcinoma in Chile. Cancer Res. 1995;55(12):2511–5.
52. Sasatomi E, Tokunaga O, Miyazaki K. Precancerous conditions of gallbladder carcinoma: overview of histopathologic characteristics and molecular genetic findings. J Hepatobiliary Pancreat Surg. 2000;7(6):556–67.
53. Itoi T, Watanabe H, Ajioka Y, Oohashi Y, Takel K, Nishikura K, et al. APC, K-ras codon 12 mutations and p53 gene expression in carcinoma and adenoma of the gall-bladder suggest two genetic pathways in gall-bladder carcinogenesis. Pathol Int. 1996;46(5):333–40.
54. Deshpande V, Nduaguba A, Zimmerman SM, Kehoe SM, Macconaill LE, Lauwers GY, et al. Mutational profiling reveals PIK3CA mutations in gallbladder carcinoma. BMC Cancer. 2011;11:60.
55. Nakamura H, Arai Y, Totoki Y, Shirota T, Elzawahry A, Kato M, et al. Genomic spectra of biliary tract cancer. Nat Genet. 2015;47(9):1003–10.
56. Li X, Teng S, Zhang Y, Zhang W, Zhang X, Xu K, et al. TROP2 promotes proliferation, migration and metastasis of gallbladder cancer cells by regulating PI3K/AKT pathway and inducing EMT. Oncotarget. 2017;8(29):47052–63.
57. Neyaz A, Husain N, Gupta S, Kumari S, Arora A, Awasthi NP, et al. Investigation of targetable predictive and prognostic markers in gallbladder carcinoma. J Gastrointest Oncol. 2018;9(1):111–25.
58. Miyahara N, Shoda J, Kawamoto T, Ishida H, Ueda T, Akimoto Y, et al. Interaction of Muc4 and ErbB2 in a transgenic mouse model of gallbladder carcinoma: potential pathobiological implications. Oncol Rep. 2014;32(5):1796–802.
59. Mishra PK, Raghuram GV, Jatawa SK, Bhargava A, Varshney S. Frequency of genetic alterations observed in cell cycle regulatory proteins and microsatellite instability in gallbladder adenocarcinoma: a translational perspective. Asian Pac J Cancer Prev. 2011;12(2):573–4.
60. Moy AP, Shahid M, Ferrone CR, Borger DR, Zhu AX, Ting D, et al. Microsatellite instability in gallbladder carcinoma. Virchows Arch. 2015;466(4):393–402.
61. Matsuda Y. Microsatellite instability meets gallbladder cancer. J Gastroenterol. 2000;35(10):798–9.
62. Le DT, Durham JN, Smith KN, Wang H, Bartlett BR, Aulakh LK, et al. Mismatch repair deficiency predicts response of solid tumors to PD-1 blockade. Science. 2017;357(6349):409–13.
63. Le DT, Uram JN, Wang H, Bartlett BR, Kemberling H, Eyring AD, et al. PD-1 blockade in tumors with mismatch-repair deficiency. N Engl J Med. 2015;372(26):2509–20.

Staging by Radiological Imaging

Kengo Yoshimitsu

Introduction

Because the gallbladder is a small organ, high spatial resolution images are mandatory for accurate staging assessment of gallbladder carcinoma (GBC), and therefore, CT and MRI are the two major modalities commonly used in clinical practice for this purpose. In this chapter, the staging system of GBC is based on the Union for International Cancer Control (UICC) classification 8th edition [1] (Tables 1 and 2).

Scanning Techniques of CT and MRI

CT

An example of CT protocol is shown in Table 3. Multidetector-row CT with 64 or more rows is preferable. Contrast medium injection and scanning phases are similar to those of liver protocol, but slice thickness should be thinner, namely, 1–2 mm [2]. Usually, four phases are obtained: precontrast scan is used for assessing the presence of calcification or stones, arterial phase is useful to assess the arterial anatomy and the neovascularity of GBC, portal phase best provides the anatomical details of GBC, venous anatomy, and the presence of liver metastasis, and the equilibrium phase is important to visualize the desmoplastic characteristic of GBC. Particularly, the assessment of subserosal delayed enhancement is important for the assessment of T2 or more advanced lesions [3], and therefore, the equilibrium phase should also be obtained with a thin slice at the adequate delay time (240 s) [4].

MR Imaging

A 1.5-T or 3.0-T magnet is preferable. A dynamic scan using 3D T1-weighted images is the main sequence for evaluation, the concept of which is similar to that of CT, as mentioned earlier, but MRI is superior to CT in terms of contrast resolution. T2- and diffusion-weighted images (DWI) are used to characterize the lesion, but may sometimes serve for invasion depth assessment. Out-of-phase T1-weighted image is useful to separate GBC and adjacent organ by demonstrating the preserved fatty plane as shown as a layer of signal reduction [2].

MR cholangiopancreatography (MRCP) is obtained at the same time as conventional MR imaging, or as a separate examination, which is excellent for the assessment of the whole image of the biliary duct system. Usually, an oral contrast medium (OCM) is given before the MRCP

K. Yoshimitsu (✉)
Faculty of Medicine, Department of Radiology, Fukuoka University, Fukuoka, Japan
e-mail: kegno@fukuoka-u.ac.jp

J. B. Chung and K. Okazaki (eds.), *Diseases of the Gallbladder*,
https://doi.org/10.1007/978-981-15-6010-1_17

Table 1 UICC staging 8th edition [1]

	M0			M1
	N0	N1	N2	Any N
T1	Satge I	Stage IIIB	Stage IVB	Stage IVB
T2a	Stage IIA			
T2b	Stage IIB			
T3	Stage IIIA			
T4	Stage IVA	Stage IVB		

examination to suppress the signal from gastrointestinal fluid, but care should be taken as to the timing of OCM administration. Because OCM has T1 shortening property in addition to T2 shortening effect, OCM in bowel may cause artifacts due to peristalsis, which would degrade the image quality of the dynamic study, if OCM is given beforehand. Furthermore, it is possible that OCM regurgitates into the biliary tree and obscure the visualization of the lower bile duct, particularly in those with Odd's sphincter dysfunction, for example, those after any intervention to the papilla, or those with juxta-papillary diverticula [5]. In our institute, therefore, OCM is given only when gastrointestinal fluid hampers the quality of MRCP, at the end of the examination after dynamic study [2]. An example of MR protocol is shown in Table 4.

Diagnostic Performance of CT and MRI for Each Factor Staging

T Factor Assessment

Because T factor or local spread of GBC directly affects the therapeutic approach and patient prognosis, correct preoperative assessment of T factor is of great importance, particularly differentiation of T1 versus T2, and T2 versus more advanced lesions [6]. As for T2 lesions, it has been shown that those on the hepatic side are more likely to

Table 2 T factor definition according to UICC 8th edition [1]

	Definition
T1	Invades lamina propria (1a) or muscular layer (1b)
T2a	Invades PMFT (subserosal layer) on the peritoneal side
T2b	Invades PMFT on the liver side
T3	Invades through serosa, or directly into one nearby organ (liver, stomach, duodenum, pancreas, extrahepatic bile duct)
T4	Invades into PV or HA, or two or more nearby organs except for the liver

PMFT: perimuscular fibrous tissue, PV: portal vein, HA: hepatic artery

Table 3 Example of CT protocol (64-row MDCT)

	120 kVp, auto mAs
Detector configuration	0.5 mm × 64, or 1 mm × 32
Table speed	26.5 mm/rotation
Slice thickness	0.5 mm or 1 mm collimation, 1 mm or 2 mm reconstruction
Phase scanning	Precontrast Arterial phase: 20 s after the triggering (150 HU at the abdominal aorta), Portal venous phase: 60 s Equilibrium phase: 240 s
Iodine contrast medium	300–370 mgI/mL, total volume 600 mgI/kg Injection duration 30 s, 20-G needle

Table 4 Example of MRI protocol

Name	Sequence	TR/TE etc.	Slice thk/gap	Other information
2D MRCP (oblique coronal)	BH FS-FSE	∞/800 (ETL 256)	4–8 cm	3–5 directions to cover the liver and pancreas
T1/T2 coronal	BH balanced sequence	3.5/1.8 ms	4–5/0 mm	Optional
T2WI axial	BH FSE	∞/120 (ETL 80)	4–5/0 mm	To cover liver through papilla
T1WI axial	BH dual-echo 2DGRE	150/2.3&4.2 ms FA 70–90°	4–5/0 mm	To cover liver through papilla
DWI axial	FB FS2DEPI	5000/65 (b = 0 & 800–1000)	4–5/0 mm	To cover liver through papilla
Dynamic study axial	BH FS3DGRE	4.3/2.1 ms FA 15–30°	3/0 mm or 4/-2 mm	Precontrast, arterial phase by bolus tracking, portal venous, and equilibrium phase
Oral contrast medium administration, if needed				
3D MRCP with navigation	FS 3DFSE	∞/87 (ETL 124)	2/-1 mm	

BH: breath-hold, FS: fat suppression, FSE: fast spin-echo, ETL: echo-train length, GRE: gradient-echo, FA: flip angle, DWI: diffusion-weighted image, EPI: echo-planar, b: b factor [mm2/sec], MRCP: magnetic resonance cholangiopancreatography

be associated with neural or lymphatic invasion, and resultantly worse prognosis than those on the peritoneal side [7]. Recently, the importance of T1a versus T1b differentiation has also been emphasized, as the number of GBC incidentally found at laparoscopic cholecystectomy increases; T1a lesion has little chance to be associated with nodal metastasis and therefore does not require additional treatment, but T1b lesion does [8]. In the assessment of direct invasion to the liver parenchyma (T3 or T4), care should be taken that early enhancement around the gallbladder fossa does not indicate a positive sign of direct invasion in most of the cases because increased cholecystic venous drainage to the liver parenchyma (segments IV and V) due to the presence of GBC is often observed as such [9]. Representative cases are shown in Figs. 1, 2, 3, 4, 5 and 6.

CT

The criteria for the assessment of each T factor are proposed for CT [6] and summarized in Table 5. The reported diagnostic accuracies using single helical CT with 3-mm collimation were 86, 71, 81, and 94% for T1, T2, T3, and T4 lesions, respectively [10], and those for MDCT with 0.75–2.5-mm collimation were 94.7, 89.8, and 100% for T1 versus ≧T2, ≦T2 versus ≧T3, and ≦T3 versus T4 lesions, respectively [6]. Care should be taken that these results are based on the previous UICC systems, not on the latest version. However, the overall diagnostic performance of CT using the current technique can be considered relatively satisfactory in terms of diagnostic accuracy.

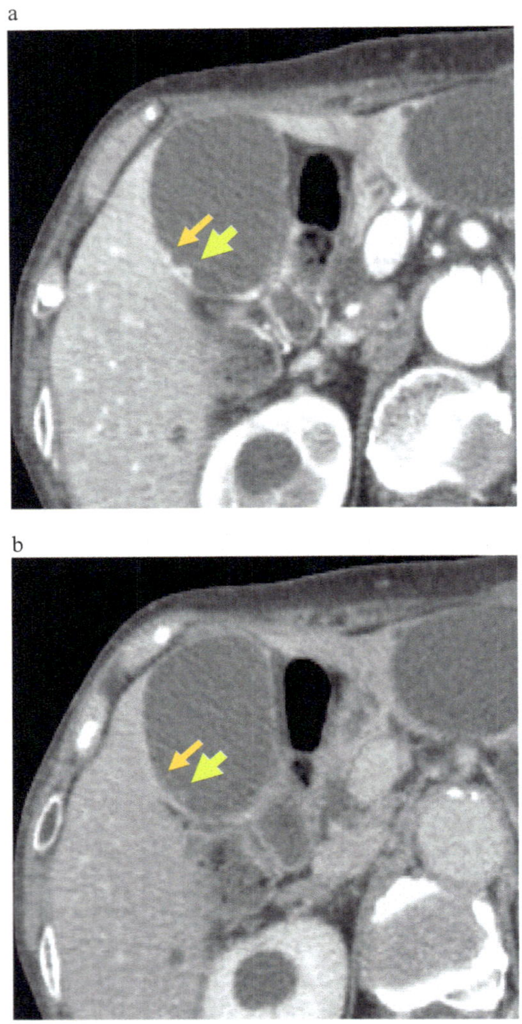

Fig. 1 T1a lesion in a 74-year-old woman. At the body of the gallbladder, small polypoid lesions were found. 1a Arterial phase CT The lesions show apparent enhancement (arrows). 1b Equilibrium phase CT. Lesions show apparent washout (arrows). Note contiguously preserved gallbladder wall. By referring to the MR criteria (Table 2), the lesion can be diagnosed as T1a gallbladder carcinoma

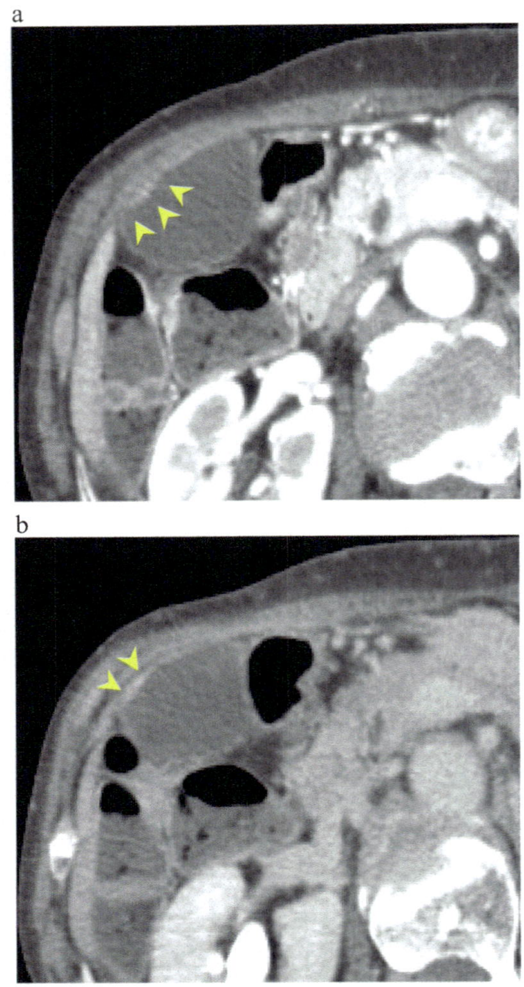

Fig. 2 T2a lesion in the same patient as Fig. 1. At the fundal side of the organ, a flat wall thickening lesion was present 2a Arterial phase CT. The mucosal aspect of the lesion show enhancement (arrows). 2b Equilibrium phase CT. Delayed or prolonged enhancement of the serosal aspect is apparent (arrows)

MRI

The criteria for the assessment of each T factor are proposed for MRI [8] and summarized in Table 6. There are few reports describing the diagnostic performance of MRI in the stage assessment of GBC, but according to Kim et al. [8], diagnostic accuracies were 95.4 and 93.0%, 90.7 and 87.2%, 88.4 and 80.3%, and 100 and 96.5%, for T1a versus ≧T1b, T1 versus ≧T2, ≦T2 versus ≧T3, and ≦T3 versus T4 lesions, respectively, by two independent readers. Again, it should be noted that these results are based on the previous UICC systems, not on the latest version.

a

b

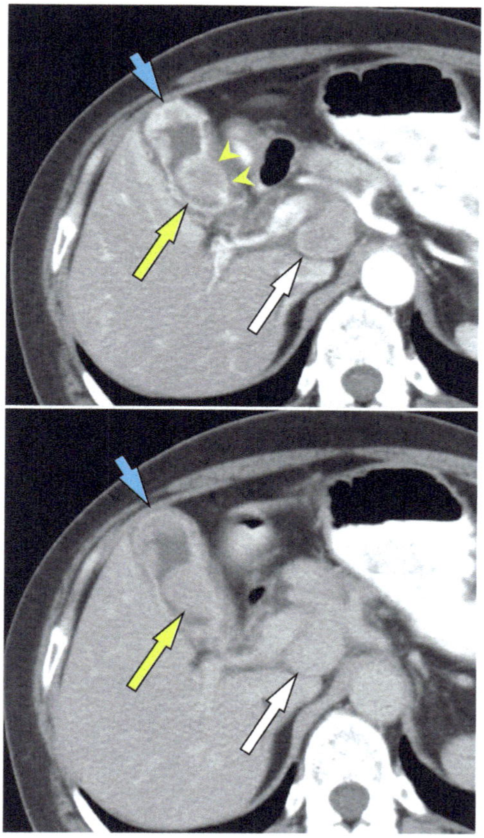

Fig. 3 T1 and T2 lesions with nodal metastasis (N1) in a 67-year-old woman 3a Arterial phase CT. Flat elevated lesion at the fundus shows apparent enhancement [blue arrow], but a nodular lesion at the body (yellow arrow) appears relatively hypovascular as compared to the fundal lesion, which shows bulging towards the serosal aspect (arrowheads). The former turned out to be T1 (predominantly T1a but partially T1b), and the latter T2a lesion. 3b Equilibrium phase CT. The fundal lesion shows apparent washout with preserved gallbladder wall (blue arrow), whereas the one at the body shows slightly prolonged enhancement (yellow arrow). Note 2 cm enlarged lymph node at the portocaval region (white arrow), showing similar enhancement pattern as the body lesion, rather than the fundal lesion. At laparotomy, the gallbladder was successfully resected, but the metastatic node was found inseparable from the portal vein and common hepatic artery possibly due to invasion, and therefore left behind

Although there is no direct comparative study between CT and MRI, the diagnostic performance of MRI appears at least comparable to that of MDCT in the assessment of T factor of GBC.

N Factor Assessment

N factor is also an important prognostic factor in patients with GBC. UICC definition for N factor is as follows: N0: no nodal metastasis, N1: 3 or less metastasized nodes, N2: 4 or more metastasized nodes [1]. Metastatic nodes are diagnosed usually based on the size or heterogeneous enhancement for both CT and MRI. Various size criteria have been proposed, depending upon the literature, but 1 cm or larger is a generally accepted criterion. Other criteria reported include larger than 5 mm in the shortest axis, lobulated or speculated margin, or internal necrosis [11, 12]. A recent meta-analysis [13] suggested a significant uncertainty regarding the optimal imaging strategy for the pre-operative detection of metastatic nodes in GBC patients, reporting varying sensitivity, and unreliability for the detection of metastatic nodes less than 1 cm in size. Of note, paraaortic nodal metastasis is considered distant metastasis (M factor). Representative cases are shown in Figs. 3 and 6.

CT

Reported sensitivities of CT in diagnosing metastatic lymph nodes ranges from 59 to 92%, with a median of 51%, based on four previously published literatures [13–17]. In contrast, specificity was available only in one study [15], reporting 100%.

MRI

Reported sensitivities of MRI in diagnosing metastatic lymph nodes ranges from 25 to 93%,

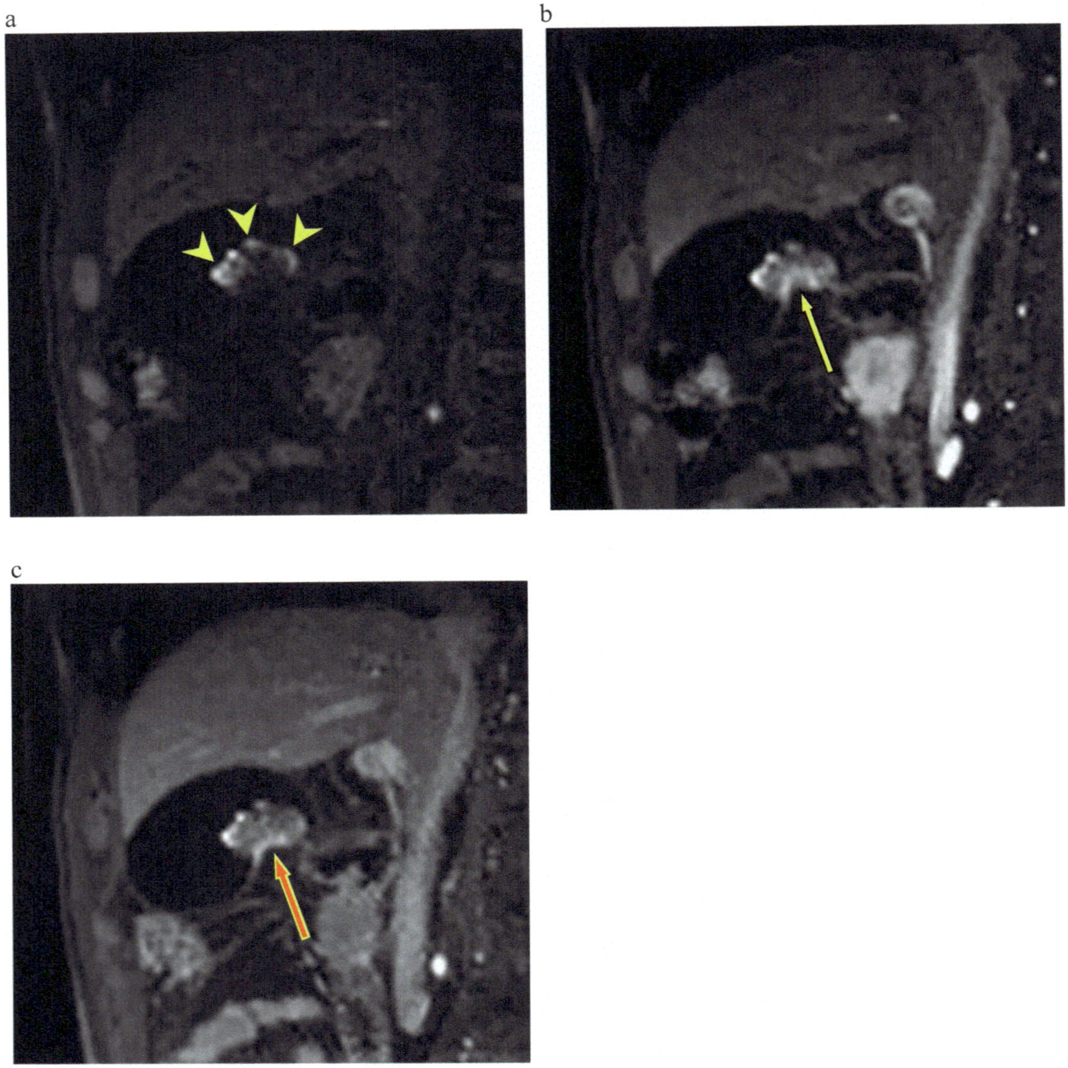

Fig. 4 T2a lesion showing subserosal delayed enhancement at the base of the polypoid lesion 4a Precontrast sagittal T1-weighted image for dynamic study. High signal along the cephalad aspect of the lesion (arrowhead s) represents coagulated bile juice attached to the lesion. 4b Arterial phase. The lesion shows apparent enhancement. The arc-shaped enhancement at the base of the lesion is considered to represent venous drainage from the tumor. 4c Equilibrium phase. The lesion shows slight prolong enhancement. Note curvilinear enhancement at the base of the lesion, representing fibrous tissue due to the desmoplastic reaction caused by tumor infiltration. Although the arc-shaped enhancement in 4B and this curvilinear enhancement look similar in appearance, but should clearly be differentiated from each other because these two represent two different phenomena: the former represents enhancement due to venous return from the tumor, and the latter contrast medium retention in the fibrous tissue at the base, suggesting a subserosal invasion of the tumor [3]

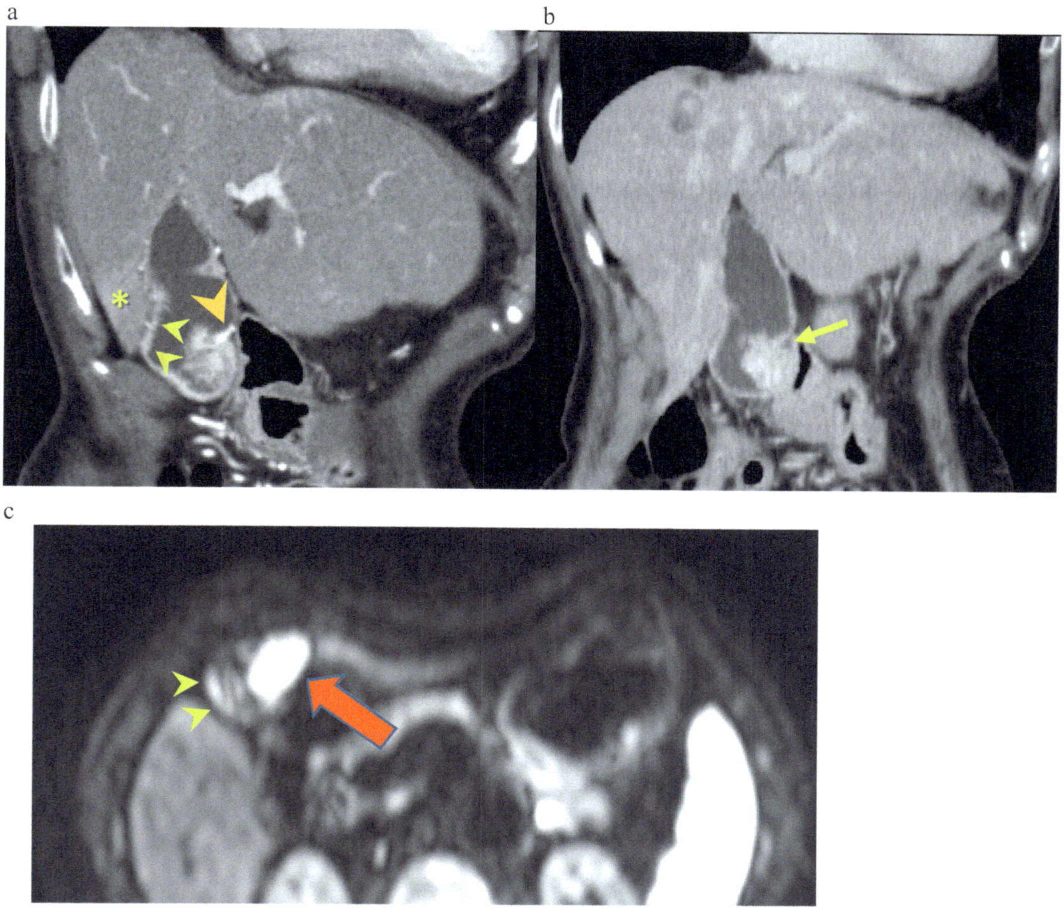

Fig. 5 T1b lesion in a 65-year-old woman. A large polypoid lesion was found at the fundus 5a Oblique coronal CT, arterial phase. The lesion shows heterogeneity. Note strong linear enhancement at the base (large arrowhead), representing venous drainage via a thin stalk. Irregular mucosal enhancement along the hepatic side of the organ (small arrowheads) turned out to be mucosal cancerous tissue (T1a). Note the faint enhancement of adjacent liver tissue (*) represents increased cholecystic venous drainage due to the presence of cancer, not a sign of direct invasion [9]. 5b Oblique coronal CT, equilibrium phase. The major part of the lesion shows washout but also shows prolonged enhancement in part. Note there is no prolonged or delayed enhancement at all at the base, suggesting that the tumor is not invading the subserosal layer. An arrow indicates "dimpling". 5c Transaxial diffusion-weighted image ($b = 800$ s/mm^2). The lesion exhibits strong high intensity (arrow). The faint curvilinear signal at the hepatic side indicates mucosal cancerous tissue, as mentioned in 5a

with a median of 72%, based on five previously published literatures [8, 18–21]. Reported specificities ranged from 26 to 71% with a median of 56%, based on four previously published literatures [8, 19–21].

Other Approaches

According to Ramos-Font et al. [22], the accuracy of fluorodeoxyglucose (FDG) positron emission tomography (PET) in diagnosing nodal metastasis

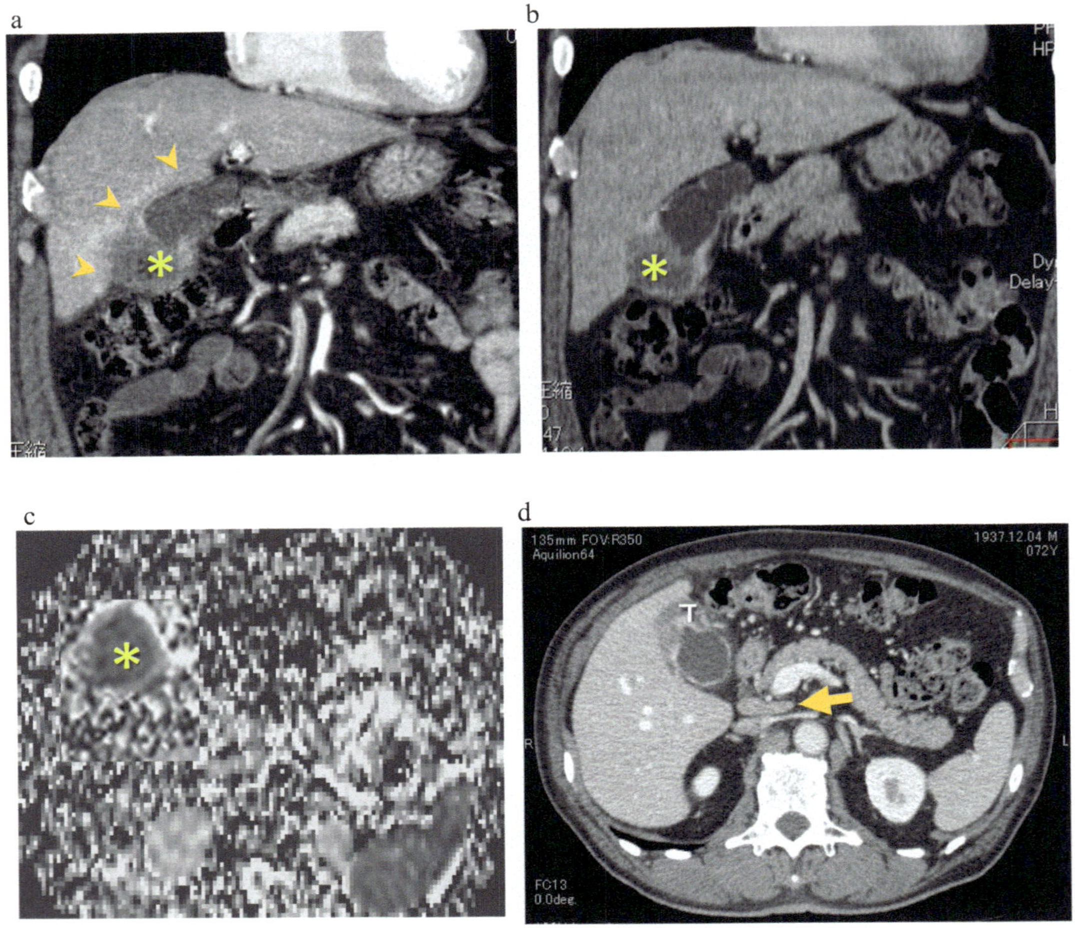

Fig. 6 T4 lesion in a 74-year-old man 6a Coronal CT, arterial phase. A 3 cm mass (*) at the fundus apparently invades both liver and hepatic flexure of the colon. Note faint enhancement in the liver along the gallbladder bed indicates increased cholecystic venous drainage due to the presence of cancer, not a sign of direct invasion [9]. 6b Coronal CT, equilibrium phase. The lesion shows faint heterogeneous enhancement (*). 6c Apparent diffusion coefficient (ADC) map. The lesion shows restricted diffusion, with an ADC value of 0.91×10^{-3} mm^2/s (*). 6d Axial CT, portal venous phase. Note enlarged nodes at the portocaval region (arrow). There were enlarged nodes at the paraaortic regions as well (not shown), all of which showed apparent FDG uptake at PET scan. The patient was clinically diagnosed as T4N2M1 and underwent chemotherapy. T indicates the primary gallbladder cancer

in GBC patients was 87.5%. PET was also reported to be useful to confirm nodal metastasis which was suspicious on CT with an odd's ratio of 7.1 [23].

Morine et al. have reported that apparent diffusion coefficient (ADC) values obtained from DWI of MRI less than 1.8×10^{-3} mm^2/s provided the sensitivity 75% and positive predictive value of 82% in diagnosing nodal metastasis, along with size criteria of maximum diameter larger than 8 mm and long-to-short axis ration less than 2 providing 81% sensitivity and 45% positive predictive value [24].

M Factor Assessment

M factors are defined as follows: M0: no distant metastasis, M1: metastasis to distant organs,

Table 5 CT criteria [6]

UICC staging	CT criteria
T1	Polypoid lesions without focal thickening of the gallbladder wall, or Nodular or flat lesions with mucosal enhancement or Focal thickening of the inner enhancing layer of the gallbladder wall with a clear, low-attenuated outer wall
T2a T2b	Nodular or sessile lesions associated with focal thickening of the gallbladder wall at what was considered to be attachment sites and with the presence of an apparently smooth fat plane separating the adjacent organs, or Diffuse wall thickening with heterogeneous enhancement, or Diffuse wall thickening with strong, thick inner wall enhancement and weak enhancement of the outer layer (two-layered pattern), with the presence of an apparently smooth fat plane separating the adjacent organs
T3	Lesions showing loss of a fat plane separating the lesions from a single adjacent organ, indicating tumor involvement ($\leq$2 cm into the liver), or Apparent nodularity on the serosal aspect, indicating serosal exposure of the tumor Tumor perforates the serosa (visceral peritoneum) and directly invades the liver or one other adjacent organ or structure (such as the stomach; duodenum; colon; or pancreas, omentum, or extrahepatic bile ducts)
T4	Tumor invades main portal vein or hepatic artery or invades multiple extrahepatic organs or structures

Table 6 MR criteria [8]

UICC staging	MRI criteria
T1	T1a: Gross morphology: Polypoid lesions without focal thickening of the GB wall T2WI: Intact low SI of the muscle layer HAP: even, thin mucosal enhancement without thickening
	T1b: Gross morphology: Polypoid/nodular lesions with focal thickening of the GB wall * Retraction of the GB wall at the tumor base (dimpling) can be found at this stage because of the muscle layer involvement T2WI: loss of low SI at the base of the tumor
T2a T2b	Gross morphology: apparent nodularity with a smooth and clear margin on the serosal aspect T1-opposed phase: external nodular bulging without disruption of the outer low SI And with the presence of a smooth fat plane separating the adjacent organs PVP: full-thickness, homogeneous or heterogeneous enhancement of the thickened wall Delayed phase: delayed subserosal enhancement suggesting subserosal involvement at the tumor base
T3	Gross morphology: apparent nodularity or irregular margin on the serosal aspect, indicating serosal exposure of the tumor T1-opposed phase: disruption of the outer low SI rim (fat plane between the gallbladder and adjacent organs), suggesting a direct invasion of the liver and/or one other adjacent organ or structure such as the stomach, duodenum, colon, pancreas, omentum, or extrahepatic bile duct
T4	Tumor invades the main portal vein or hepatic artery or invades two or more extrahepatic organs or structures

GB: gallbladder, T2WI: T2-weighted image, SI: signal intensity, HAP: hepatic arterial phase, PVP: portal venous phase

including liver, peritoneal cavity, and lung. There have been little investigations describing the diagnostic performance of radiological modalities focusing on the detection of GBC distant metastasis. Karla N et al. reported that five out of seven (71.4%) GBC patients with distant metastasis were correctly called on preoperative MDCT [15]. Ramos-Font C described the accuracy of PET in detecting overall distant metastasis is 95.9% [22].

As for liver metastasis in general, gadoxetate-enhanced MRI has higher diagnostic performance than CT or PET [25]. It would be useful to keep in mind for radiologists that early-stage liver metastasis from GBC is conveyed via cholecystic venous blood [26], and therefore it would almost always be observed around gallbladder fossa, rather than at the sites far away from the gallbladder. As for peritoneal implants, CT or PET may be the modalities of choice for diagnosis. For lung metastasis, CT is usually chosen as a diagnostic tool.

Other Radiological Approaches in Gallbladder Cancer Staging and Prognosis Prediction

Recently, Min et al. reported that ADC value of the main tumor (GBC) was significantly correlated to histological grades and UICC staging, and furthermore, it was the only factor to be related to disease-free survival rate for GBC patients, whereas histological grades and UICC staging were not [27]. SUV max at PET has also been reported to be a possible biomarker to predict the prognosis of GBC patients along with the UICC staging, nodal metastasis status, and curative versus non-curative treatment [28, 29].

Summary

State-of-the-art CT and MRI can provide fairly good accuracy in staging GBC, particularly for T factor. Adding PET or ADC information may not only enhance the diagnosis when CT or MRI findings are equivocal, particularly for N and M factors but also be independent biomarkers to predict the prognosis of GBC patients.

References

1. Gallbladder cancer stages. American Cancer Society. https://www.cancer.org/cancer/gallbladder-cancer/detection-diagnosis-staging/staging.html.
2. Standard imaging technique in gastrointestinal organs. Chapter 5, gastrointensitnal tract. In: Japanese Radiological society ed. The Japanese Imaging Guideline 2016. Tokyo: Kanehara; 2016. P268–272, *in Japanese.*
3. Yoshimitsu K, Nishihara Y, Okamoto D, Ushijima Y, Nishie A, Yamaguchi K, et al. Magnetic resonance differentiation between T2 and T1 gallbladder carcinoma: significance of subserosal enhancement on the delayed phase dynamic study. Magn Reson Imaging. 2012;30:854–9.
4. Shinagawa Y, Sakamoto K, Sato K, Ito E, Urakawa H, Yoshimitsu K. Usefulness of new subtraction algorithm in estimating degree of liver fibrosis by calculating extracellular volume fraction obtained from routine liver CT protocol equilibrium phase data: Preliminary experience. Eur J Radiol. 2018 Jun;103:99–104.
5. Sakamoto K, Shinagawa Y, Inoue K, Morita A, Urakawa H, Fujimitsu R, et al. Obliteration of the biliary system after administration of an oral contrast medium is probably due to regurgitation: a pitfall on MRCP. Magn Reson Med Sci. 2016;15(1):137–43.
6. Kim SJ, Lee JM, Lee JY, Kim SH, Han JK, Choi BI, et al. Analysis of enhancement pattern of flat gallbladder wall thickening on MDCT to differentiate gallbladder cancer from cholecystitis. AJR Am J Roentgenol. 2008 Sep;191(3):765-71.
7. Shindo J, de Aretxabala X, Aloia TA, Roa JC, Roa I, Zimmitti G, et al. Tumor location is a strong predictor of tumor progression and survival in T2 gallbladder cancer. Ann Surg. 2015;261:733–9.
8. Kim SJ, Lee JM, Lee ES, Han JK, Choi BI. Preoperative staging of gallbladder carcinoma using biliary MR imaging. J Magn Reson Imaging. 2015 Feb;41(2):314-21.
9. Yoshimitsu K, Honda H, Kaneko K, Kuroiwa T, Irie H, Chijiiwa K, et al. Anatomy and clinical importance of cholecystic venous drainage: helical CT observations during injection of contrast medium into the cholecystic artery. AJR Am J Roentgenol. 1997 Aug;169(2):505-10.
10. Yoshimitsu K, Honda H, Shinozaki K, Aibe H, Kuroiwa T, Irie H, et al. Helical CT of the local spread of carcinoma of the gallbladder: evaluation according to the TNM system in patients who underwent surgical resection. AJR Am J Roentgenol. 2002 Aug;179(2):423-8.
11. Weber SM, DeMatteo RP, Fong Y, Blumgart LH, Jarnagin WR. Staging laparoscopy in patients with extrahepatic biliary carcinoma. Ann Surg. 2002;235:392–9.
12. Jarnagin WR, Bodniewicz J, Dougherty E, Conlon K, Blumgart LH, Fong Y. A prospective analysis of staging laparoscopy in patients with primary and secondary hepatobiliary malignancies. J Gastrointest Surg. 2000;4:34–43.
13. de Savornin Lohman EAJ, de Bitter TJJ, van Laarhoven CJHM, Hermans JJ, de Haas RJ, de Reuver PR. The diagnostic accuracy of CT and MRI for the detection of lymph node metastases in gallbladder

cancer: A systematic review and meta-analysis. Eur J Radiol. 2019 Jan;110:156-62.
14. Engels JT, Balfe DM, Lee JK. Biliary carcinoma: CT evaluation of extrahepatic spread. Radiology. 1989;172(1):35–40.
15. Kalra N, Suri S, Gupta R, Natarajan SK, Khandelwal N, Wig JD. MDCT in the staging of gallbladder carcinoma. AJR Am J Roentgenol. 2006;186(3):758–62.
16. Ohtani T, Shirai Y, Tsukada K, Muto T, Hatakeyama K. Spread of gallbladder carcinoma: CT evaluation with pathologic correlation. Abdom Imaging. 1996;21(3):195–201.
17. Oikarinen H, Päivänsalo M, Lähde S, Tikkakoski T, Suramo I. Radiological findings in cases of gallbladder carcinoma. Eur J Radiol. 1993;17(3):179–83.
18. Kim JH, Kim TK, Eun HW, Kim BS, Lee MG, Kim PN, et al. Preoperative evaluation of gallbladder carcinoma: efficacy of combined use of MR imaging, MR cholangiography, and contrast-enhanced dual-phase three-dimensional MR angiography. J Magn Reson Imaging. 2002;16(6):676–84.
19. Schwartz LH, Black J, Fong Y, Jarnagin W, Blumgart L, Gruen D, et al. Gallbladder carcinoma: findings at MR imaging with MR cholangiopancreatography. J Comput Assist Tomogr. 2002;26(3):405–10.
20. Tseng JH, Wan YL, Hung CF, Ng KK, Pan KT, Chou AS, et al. Diagnosis and staging of gallbladder carcinoma. Evaluation with dynamic MR imaging. Clin Imaging. 2002;26(3):177–82.
21. Kaza RK, Gulati M, Wig JD, Chawla YK. Evaluation of gall bladder carcinoma with dynamic magnetic resonance imaging and magnetic resonance cholangiopancreatography. Australas Radiol. 2006;50(3):212–7.
22. Ramos-Font C, Gómez-Rio M, Rodríguez-Fernández A, Jiménez-Heffernan A, Sánchez Sánchez R, Llamas-Elvira JM. Ability of FDG-PET/CT in the detection of gallbladder cancer. J Surg Oncol. 2014 Mar;109(3):218-24.
23. Leung U, Pandit-Taskar N, Corvera CU, D'Angelica MI, Allen PJ, Kingham TP, et al. Impact of pre-operative positron emission tomography in gallbladder cancer. HPB (Oxford). 2014 Nov;16(11):1023-30.
24. Morine Y, Shimada M, Imura S, Ikemoto T, Hanaoka J, Kanamoto M, et al. Detection of Lymph Nodes Metastasis in Biliary Carcinomas: Morphological Criteria by MDCT and the Clinical Impact of DWI-MRI. Hepatogastroenterology. 2015 Jun;62(140):777-81.
25. Standard imaging technique in gastrointestinal organs. Chapter 5, gastrointensitnal tract. In: Japanese Radiological society ed. The Japanese Imaging Guideline 2016. Tokyo: Kanehara; 2016. p. 307–10, *in Japanese*.
26. Yoshimitsu K, Honda H, Kuroiwa T, Irie H, Aibe H, Tajima T, et al. Liver metastasis from gallbladder carcinoma: anatomic correlation with cholecystic venous drainage demonstrated by helical computed tomography during injection of contrast medium in the cholecystic artery. Cancer. 2001 Jul 15;92(2):340-8.
27. Min JH, Kang TW, Cha DI, Kim SH, Shin KS, Lee JE, et al. Apprarent diffusion coefficient as a potential marker for tumour differentiation, staging and long-term clinical outcomes in gallbladder cancer. Eur Radiol. 2019 Jan;29(1):411-21.
28. Hwang JP, Lim I, Na II, Cho EH, Kim BI, Choi CW, et al. Prognostic value of SUVmax measured by fluorine-18 fluorodeoxyglucose positron emission tomography with computed tomography in patients with gallbladder cancer. Nucl Med Mol Imaging. 2014 Jun;48(2):114-20.
29. Lee JY, Kim HJ, Yim SH, Shin DS, Yu JH, Ju DY, et al. Primary tumor maximum standardized uptake value measured on 18F-fluorodeoxyglucose positron emission tomography-computed tomography is a prognostic value for survival in bile duct and gallbladder cancer. Korean J Gastroenterol. 2013 Oct;62(4):227-33.

Roles of PET/CT in Evaluating Gallbladder and Hepatobiliary Tumors

Motoki Nishimura, Nagara Tamaki, Shigenori Matsushima, and Kei Yamada

Introduction

Gallbladder carcinoma is a common carcinoma in the biliary cells and in the gastroenteric system as well [1]. An early diagnosis seems to be difficult due to its anatomical location, lack of typical symptoms, and aggressive biologic characteristics. In addition, gallbladder carcinoma is a highly aggressive malignancy. The 5-year survival rate of gallbladder cancer is reported at less than 15% [2]. In a recent study, 80% of the patients had metastatic disease and only 20% had potentially resectable disease at the time of diagnosis [3]. Thus, accurate evaluation and staging are important to provide a suitable indication of surgery [4].

Several diagnostic tools have been used in this setting, including ultrasonography (US), computed tomography (CT), magnetic resonance (MR), endoscopic retrograde cholangiopancreatography (ERCP), and percutaneous transhepatic cholangiography (PTC). This chapter introduces a new and elegant molecular imaging technique using positron emission tomography (PET).

Value of FDG-PET for Oncological Cases

Fluorine-18-fluorodeoxyglucose (FDG) and PET/CT have been proposed as a noninvasive imaging method to assess the disease extent in patients with various cancer.

Since most of the malignant lesion use glucose as an energy source, FDG as a marker of exogenous glucose utilization has been used for detecting and characterizing malignant lesions using whole-body PET imaging. FDG PET has been proposed for diagnosis, staging, the effectiveness of treatment and the prediction of long-term survival in different malignancies [5–8]. Hybrid PET/CT device permits enhanced detection and characterization of neoplastic lesions, by a combination of the functional data obtained by PET with morphological data obtained by CT.

M. Nishimura · N. Tamaki (✉) · S. Matsushima · K. Yamada
Department of Radiology, Kyoto Prefectural University of Medicine, 465 Kajii-Cho, Kawaramachi-Hirokoji, Kamigyoku-Ku, Kyoto 602-8566, Japan
e-mail: natamaki@koto.kpu-m.ac.jp

M. Nishimura
e-mail: mnsmr@koto.kpu-m.ac.jp

S. Matsushima
e-mail: matsu@koto.kpu-m.ac.jp

K. Yamada
e-mail: kyamada@koto.kpu-m.ac.jp

J. B. Chung and K. Okazaki (eds.), *Diseases of the Gallbladder*,
https://doi.org/10.1007/978-981-15-6010-1_18

Clinical Applications of FDG-PET for Gallbladder Cancer

The typical example of FDG PET-CT in a patient with gallbladder cancer is shown in Fig. 1. A high FDG uptake is well observed in an area of gallbladder cancer.

There are a number of reports showing different values of sensitivity and specificity for diagnostic accuracy of FDG PET or PET/CT [1, 4, 9–25]. In addition, a systematically reviewed and meta-analyzed report has also indicated the value and limitation for the diagnostic value of FDG PET for diagnosing gallbladder carcinoma [26]. Their pooled results of the meta-analysis indicate that FDG PET studies showed good sensitivity (87%) and specificity (78%) in the evaluation of primary tumors with a high value of the AUC (0.88) in patients with gallbladder carcinoma. Possible sources of false positive results are inflammatory diseases of the gallbladder (Fig. 2). On the other hand, possible false negative results are small size and/or low-grade tumors (Fig. 3). Regarding the diagnostic work-up of patients with gallbladder carcinoma, FDG PET and PET/CT may have little diagnostic advantage over traditional imaging modalities in detecting primary gallbladder carcinoma [4].

FDG PET and PET/CT may have important roles complementary to US, MR, CT, PTC, and ERCP in staging gallbladder carcinoma patients. Since FDG PET is a whole-body scanning technique, it allows the detection of unsuspected metastatic lymph nodes or distant spread that may lead to major changes in the surgical management of patients with biliary tract cancer [24] (Fig. 4). Since incidental diagnosis of gallbladder carcinoma is increasing, the role of PET/CT for an effective treatment has been discussed [27]. The pT1b patients on PET/CT may be observed as the chance of relapse is low. On the other hand, chemotherapy may be needed for all pT2 patients due to the high incidence

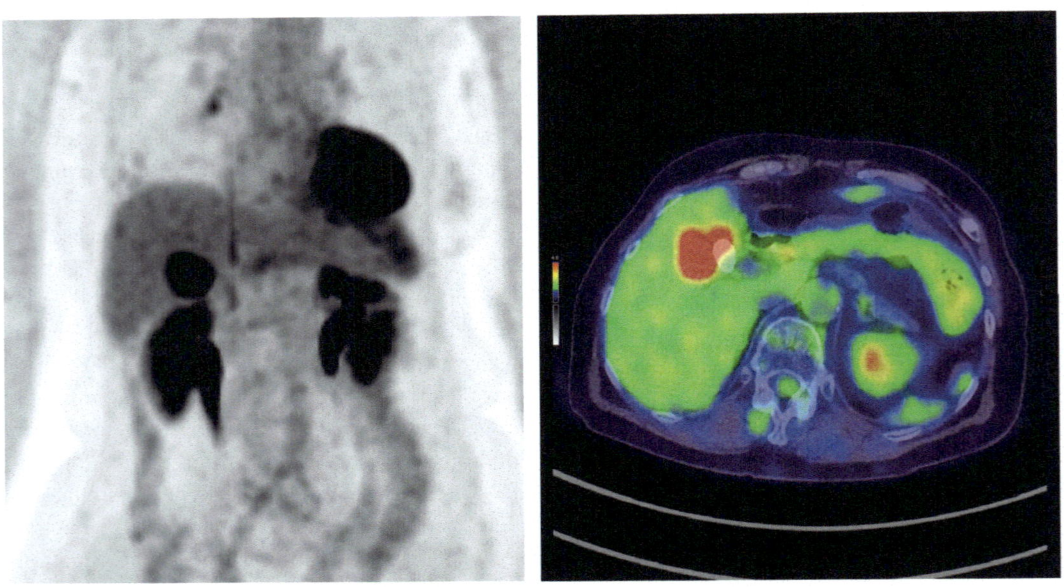

Fig. 1 FDG PET maximum intensity projection (MIP) image (left) and PET/CT fusion image (right) of a 76-year-old female patient with advanced gallbladder cancer MIP image shows focal area of high FDG uptake in the right upper abdomen. Fusion image reveals a calcified gallstone in the gallbladder and high uptake (SUV max 12.7) in wall thickening of the gallbladder body. High uptake area spread to segment 5 of the liver, suggested intrahepatic invasion. Two months later, she underwent surgery and adenocarcinoma of gallbladder was proved by pathological examination

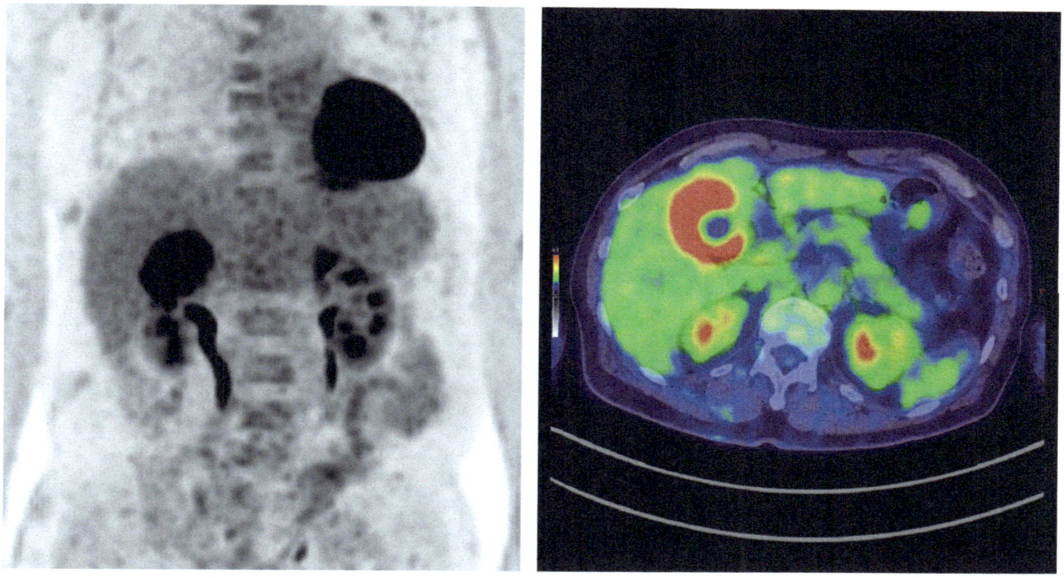

Fig. 2 FDG PET MIP image (left) and PET/CT fusion image (right) of a 65-year-old male patient with xanthogranulomatous cholecystitis (XGC). MIP image shows focal area of high FDG uptake in the right upper abdomen Fusion image reveals high uptake (SUV max 16.5) as along wall thickening from fundus to body of the gallbladder. Two months later, he underwent surgery and xanthogranulomatous cholecystitis was proved by pathological examination

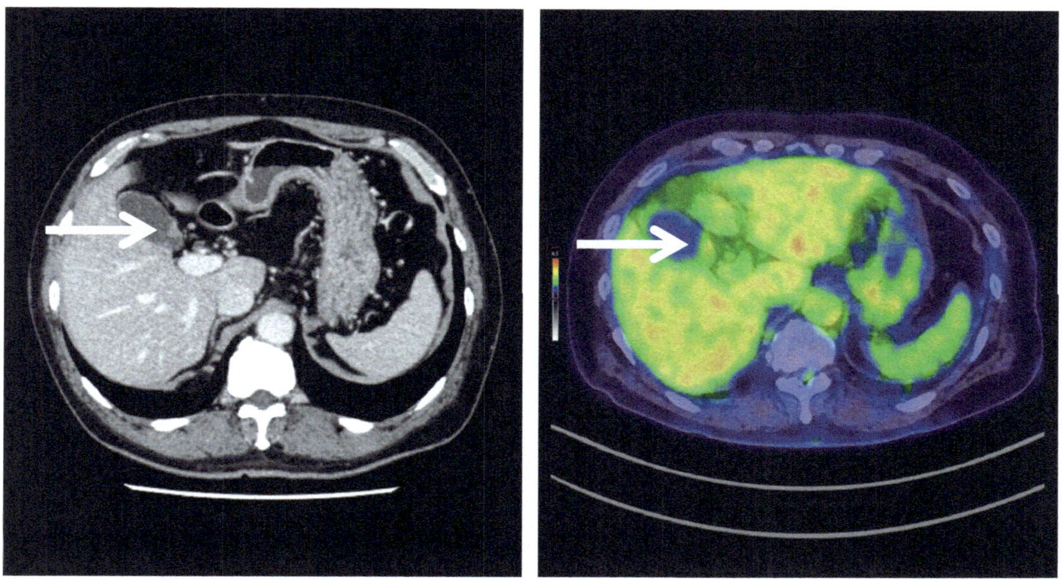

Fig. 3 Contrast-enhanced CT image (left) and FDG PET/CT fusion image (right) of a 68-year-old male patient with early gallbladder cancer Contrast-enhanced CT image shows focal wall thickening of the gallbladder neck. Fusion image reveals slightly high uptake (SUV max 3.0) in the gallbladder neck (white arrow). Two months later, he underwent surgery and adenocarcinoma (tub1 > tub2) of gallbladder was proved by pathological examination

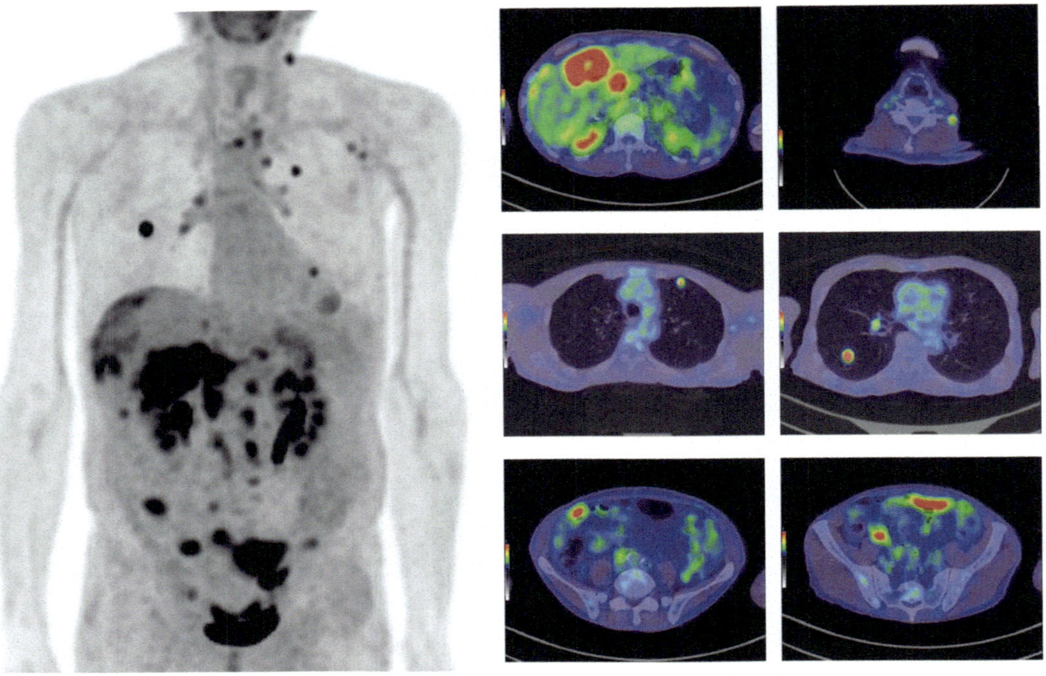

Fig. 4 FDG PET MIP image (left) and PET/CT fusion images (right) of a 75-year-old male patient with gallbladder cancer and systemic metastasis MIP image shows multiple focal high FDG uptakes in the abdomen, left supraclavicular fossa, chest, and pelvis. Fusion images reveal high uptake in the gallbladder tumor, left supraclavicular lymph node metastasis, pulmonary metastases, and peritoneal dissemination

of recurrence and nodal metastasis [27]. Since PET/CT was in good agreement with the final outcome compared to CT, PET/CT tended to show a better prediction on resectability than CT, especially due to unexpected distant metastasis [28]. There are a number of recent papers indicating diagnostic as well as prognostic values of PET/CT for patients with gallbladder carcinoma [29, 30].

Since most patients with gallbladder carcinoma are diagnosed incidentally after cholecystectomy, FDG PET is not commonly used for evaluating gallbladder carcinoma. On the other hand, FDG PET is typically used for initiating staging after cholecystectomy or restaging when recurrence is suspected [31, 32]. An increase in FDG uptake is well demonstrated in gallbladder carcinoma and has been helpful in identifying recurrence in the areas of incision when CT cannot differentiate scar tissue from tumor recurrence [26, 33]. While FDG PET may accumulate in both gallbladder carcinoma and inflammation, the addition of delayed imaging may improve differentiating between two lesions [13].

Clinical Applications of FDG-PET for Hepatobiliary Cancer

FDG PET/CT has also been used for assessing hepatobiliary carcinoma with reported sensitivity varied from 61 to 90% [10, 34, 35]. The diagnostic value may be highly dependent on the tumor form. FDG PET was more helpful in patients with nodular cholangiocarcinoma than those with the infiltrating variety (Fig. 5). Infiltrating cholangiocarcinoma may not have a sufficient cellular mass density due to the limited value of spatial resolution of PET (usually 4–7 mm in FWHM in recent high-performance PET camera). In addition, false positive findings may often be seen in patients with a biliary stent, probably

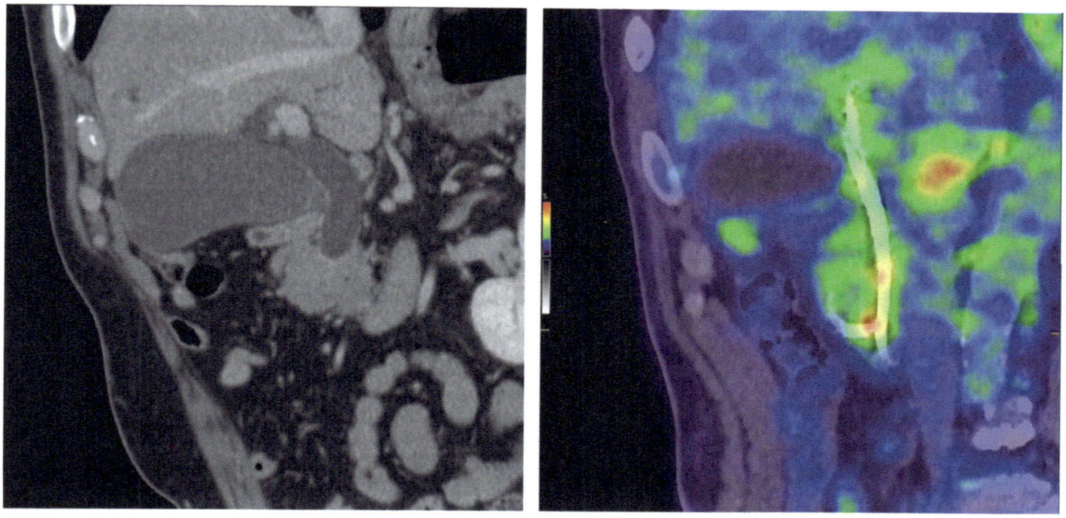

Fig. 5 Contrast-enhanced CT image (left) and FDG PET/CT fusion image (right) of a 67-year-old male patient with extrahepatic bile duct cancer Contrast-enhanced CT oblique-coronal plane image shows occlusion of distal common bile duct and dilatation of proximal common bile duct. Fusion image reveals high uptake in the distal common bile duct. High uptake in the lymph node in the hepatoduodenal ligament suggested lymph node metastasis. Two months later, he underwent pancreaticoduodenectomy. Adenocarcinoma (tub1 >por2, with sarcomatoid change) of distal bile duct and lymph node metastasis was proved by pathological examination

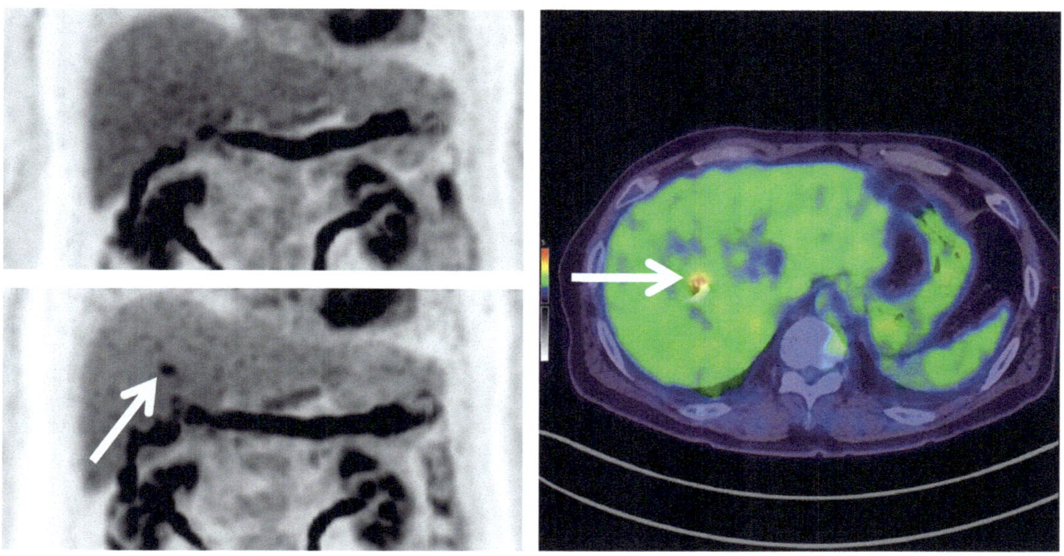

Fig. 6 FDG PET MIP images (left) and PET/CT fusion image (right) of a 67-year-old male patient with intrahepatic cholangiocellular carcinoma On 60-min MIP image (left top), no abnormal FDG uptake can be identified in the liver. On the other hand, 110-min MIP image (left bottom) and fusion image (right) reveal focal high uptake in the right hepatic duct (white arrow). Two months later, he underwent extended right hepatectomy and adenocarcinoma (tub1 > tub2 > por2) of right hepatic duct and bile duct was proved by pathological examination

due to inflammatory changes and also in patients with acute cholangitis where high FDG uptake may be seen. FDG PET has an important role in patient management since the metastatic diseases were unsuspected on the conventional imaging modalities. FDG PET findings may often show falsely negative for metastatic disease, but such lesions were detected during surgery. One of the limited sensitivities for detecting lesions may be due to the relatively high background activity of the FDG uptake in the liver. But a better contrast of the lesion may be seen by the delayed FDG imaging (90–120 min after injection) as compared to the conventional 60-min imaging after injection (Fig. 6) [13, 36, 37]. All extra-abdominal metastatic lesions were correctly detected by FDG PET [35].

Patients with primary sclerosing cholangitis may often develop cholangiocarcinoma. Therefore, a noninvasive method to detect cholangiocarcinoma small enough to allow for intended curative surgery is needed. CT and US have a poor sensitivity for the detection of such early cholangiocarcinoma. Dynamic FDG PET may hold a promise to detect cholangiocarcinoma and differentiates it from nonmalignant tissue [38].

Conclusions

We conclude that FDG PET may have an important role for evaluating biliary malignant tumors by detecting unsuspected distant metastasis, and thus, providing suitable patient management. However, FDG PET has high false negative rate for infiltrating cholangiocarcinoma, and also high false positive rate for acute inflammation. A wise use of FDG PET is required in a variety of clinical settings considering such values and limitations of FDG PET.

References

1. Ramos-Font C, Gómez-Rio M, Rodríguez-Fernández A, Jiménez-Heffernan A, Sánchez Sánchez R, Llamas-Elvira JM. Ability of FDG-PET/CT in the detection of gallbladder cancer. J Surg Oncol. 2014; 109:218–24.
2. Donohue JH. Present status of the diagnosis and treatment of gallbladder carcinoma. J Hepatobiliary Pancreat Surg. 2001;8:530–4. https://doi.org/10.1007/s005340100021.
3. Butte JM, Redondo F, Waugh E, Meneses M, Pruzzo R, Parada H, et al. The role of PET-CT in patients with incidental gallbladder cancer. HPB (Oxford). 2009;11:585–91. https://doi.org/10.1111/j.1477-2574.2009.00104.x.
4. Albazaz R, Patel CN, Chowdhury FU, Scarsbrook AF. Clinical impact of FDG PET-CT on management decisions for patients with primary biliary tumours. Insights Imaging. 2013;4:691–700.
5. Maldonado A, Gonzalez-Alenda FJ, Alonso M, Sierra JM. PET-CT in clinical oncology. Clin Transl Oncol. 2007;9:494–505. https://doi.org/10.1007/s12094-007-0093-5.
6. Higashi K, Ueda Y, Arisaka Y, Sakuma T, Nambu Y, Oquchi M, et al. 18 F-FDG uptake as a biologic prognostic factor for recurrence in patients with surgically resected non-small-cell lung cancer. J Nucl Med. 2002;43:39–45.
7. Kim JH, Yoo SW, Kang SR, Cho SG, Oh JR, Chong A, et al. Prognostic significance of metabolic tumor volume measured by 18 F-FDG PET/CT in operable primary breast cancer. Nucl Med Mol Imaging. 2012;46:278–85. https://doi.org/10.1007/s13139-012-0161-9.
8. Kim SH, Won KS, Choi BW, Jo I, Zeon SK, Chung WJ, et al. Usefulness of F-18 FDG PET/CT in the evaluation of early treatment response after interventional therapy for hepatocellular carcinoma. Nucl Med Mol Imaging. 2012;46:102–10. https://doi.org/10.1007/s13139-012-0138-8.
9. Koh T, Taniguchi H, Yamaguchi A, Kunishima S, Yamagishi H. Differential diagnosis of gallbladder cancer using positron emission tomography with fluorine-18-labeled fluoro-deoxyglucose (FDG-PET) J Surg Oncol. 2003;84:74–81.
10. Anderson CD, Rice MH, Pinson CW, Chapman WC, Chari RS, Delbeke D. Fluorodeoxyglucose PET imaging in the evaluation of gallbladder carcinoma and cholangiocarcinoma. J Gastrointest Surg. 2004;8:90–7.
11. Rodríguez-Fernández A, Gómez-Río M, Llamas-Elvira JM, Ortega-Lozano S, Ferrón-Orihuela JA, Ramia-Angel JM, Mansilla-Roselló A, Martínez-del-Valle MD, Ramos-Font C. Positron-emission tomography with fluorine-18-fluoro-2-deoxy-D-glucose for gallbladder cancer diagnosis. Am J Surg. 2004;188:171–5.
12. Wakabayashi H, Akamoto S, Yachida S, Okano K, Izuishi K, Nishiyama Y, et al. Significance of fluorodeoxyglucose PET imaging in the diagnosis of malignancies in patients with biliary stricture. Eur J Surg Oncol. 2005;31:1175–9.
13. Nishiyama Y, Yamamoto Y, Fukunaga K, Kimura N, Miki A, Sasakawa Y, et al. Dual-time-point FDG PET for the evaluation of gallbladder carcinoma. J Nucl Med. 2006;47:633–8.

14. Oe A, Kawabe J, Torii K, Kawamura E, Higashiyama S, Kotani J, et al. Distinguishing benign from malignant gallbladder wall thickening using FDG-PET. Ann Nucl Med. 2006;20:699–703.
15. Petrowsky H, Wildbrett P, Husarik DB, Hany TF, Tam S, Jochum W, et al. Impact of integrated positron emission tomography and computed tomography on staging and management of gallbladder cancer and cholangiocarcinoma. J Hepatol. 2006;45:43–50.
16. Shukla PJ, Barreto SG, Arya S, Shrikhande SV, Hawaldar R, Purandare N, et al. Does PET-CT scan have a role prior to radical re-resection for incidental gallbladder cancer? HPB (Oxford). 2008;10:439–45.
17. Corvera CU, Blumgart LH, Akhurst T, DeMatteo RP, D'Angelica M, Fong Y, et al. 18F-fluorodeoxyglucose positron emission tomography influences management decisions in patients with biliary cancer. J Am Coll Surg. 2008;206: 57–65.
18. Furukawa H, Ikuma H, Asakura-Yokoe K, Uesaka K. Preoperative staging of biliary carcinoma using 18F-fluorodeoxyglucose PET: prospective comparison with PET+CT. MDCT and histopathology. Eur Radiol. 2008;18:2841–7.
19. Furukawa H, Ikuma H, Asakura K, Uesaka K. Prognostic importance of standardized uptake value on F-18 fluorodeoxyglucose-positron emission tomography in biliary tract carcinoma. J Surg Oncol. 2009;100:494–9.
20. Lee SW, Kim HJ, Park JH, Park DI, Cho YK, Sohn CI, et al. Clinical usefulness of FDG PET-CT for patients with gallbladder cancer and cholangiocarcinoma. J Gastroenterol. 2010;45:560–6.
21. Zhu AX, Meyerhardt JA, Blaszkowsky LS, Kambadakone AR, Muzikansky A, Zheng H, et al. Efficacy and safety of gemcitabine, oxaliplatin, and bevacizumab in advanced biliary-tract cancers and correlation of changes in 18-fluorodeoxyglucose PET with clinical outcome: a phase 2 study. Lancet Oncol. 2010;11:48–54.
22. Lee J, Yun M, Kim KS, Lee JD, Kim CK. Risk stratification of gallbladder polyps (1-2 cm) for surgical intervention with FDG PET/CT. J Nucl Med. 2012;53:353–8.
23. Kumar R, Sharma P, Kumari A, Halanaik D, Malhotra A. Role of FDG PET/CT in detecting recurrent gallbladder carcinoma. Clin Nucl Med. 2012;37:431–5.
24. Yamada I, Ajiki T, Ueno K, Sawa H, Otsubo I, Yoshida Y, et al. Feasibility of (18) F-fluorodeoxyglucose positron-emission tomography for preoperative evaluation of biliary tract cancer. Anticancer Res. 2012;32:5105–10.
25. Lee JY, Kim HJ, Yim SH, Shin DS, Yu JH, Ju DY, et al. Primary tumor maximum standardized uptake value measured on 18F-fluorodeoxyglucose positron emission tomography-computed tomography is a prognostic value for survival in bile duct and gallbladder cancer. Korean J Gastroenterol. 2013;62:227–33.
26. Annunziata S, Pizzuto DA, Caldarella C, Galiandro F, Sadeghi R, Treglia G. Diagnostic accuracy of fluorine-18-fluorodeoxyglucose positron emission tomography in gallbladder cancer: a meta-analysis. World J Gastroenterol. 2015;21(40):11481–8.
27. Goel M, Tamhankar A, Rangarajan V, Patkar S, Ramadwar M, Shrikhande SV. Role of PET CT scan in redefining treatment of incidental gall bladder carcinoma. J Surg Oncol. 2016;113(6):652–8. https://doi.org/10.1002/jso.24198.
28. Kim J, Ryu JK, Kim C, Paeng JC, Kim YT. Is there any role of positron emission tomography computed tomography for predicting resectability of gallbladder cancer? J Korean Med Sci. 2014;29(5):680–4.
29. Lee JY, Kim HJ, Yim SH, Shin DS, Yu JH, Ju DY, et al. Primary tumor maximum standardized uptake value measured on ^{18}F-fluorodeoxyglucose positron emission tomography-computed tomography is a prognostic value for survival in bile duct and gallbladder cancer. Korean J Gastroenterol. 2013 Oct;62(4):227-33.
30. Ma KW, Cheung TT, She WH, Chok KSH, Chan ACY, Dai WC, et al. Diagnostic and prognostic role of 18-FDG PET/CT in the management of resectable biliary tract cancer. World J Surg. 2018;42(3):823–34.
31. Drouart E, Delamarre J, Capron JP. Cutaneous seeding of gallbladder cancer after laparoscopic cholecystectomy. N Eng J Med. 1991;325(18):1316.
32. Hoh CK, Hawkins RA, Glaspy JA, et al. Cancer detection with whole-body PEY using ^{18}F-fluoro-2-deoxy-D-glucose. J Comput Assisted Tomogr. 1993;40:244–6.
33. Lomis KD, Vitola JV, Delbeke D, et al. Recurrent gallbladder carcinoma at laparotomy port sites diagnosed by PET scan: implications for primary and radical second operations. Am Surg. 1997;63:341–5.
34. Keiding S, Hasen SB, Rasmussen HH, Gee A, Kruse A, Roelsgaard K, et al. Detection of cholangiocarcinoma in primary sclerosing cholangitis by positron emission tomography. Hepatology. 1998;28:700–6.
35. Kluge R, Schmidt F, Caca K, et al. Positron emission tomography with ^{18}F-fluoro-2-deoxy-D-glucose for diagnosis and staging of bile duct cancer. Hepatology. 2001;33:1029–35.
36. Dong A, Dong H, Zhang L, Zuo C. F-18 FDG uptake in borderline intraduactal papillary neoplasms of the bile duct. Ann Nucl Med. 2012;26(7):594–8.
37. Schillaci O. Use of dual-point fluorodeoxyglucose imaging to enhance sensitivity and specificity. Semin Nucl Med. 2012;42(4):267–80.
38. Prytz H, Keiding S, Bjornsson E, et al. Dynamic FDG-PET is useful for detection of cholangiocarcinoma in patients with PSC listed for liver transplantation. Hepatology. 2007;44(6):1572–80.

Diagnostic Strategies for Early Diagnosis

Yoshiki Hirooka, Senju Hashimoto, and Ryoji Miyahara

Introduction

The poor prognosis of advanced gallbladder cancer has been described previously in this specialized book. The main purpose of this chapter is how to diagnose early gallbladder cancer.

The "Clinical practice guidelines for the management of biliary tract cancers 2015" [1] published in 2015 was updated to the third edition in 2019. Figure 1 shows the algorithm for diagnosing gallbladder cancer in the "Clinical practice guidelines for management of biliary tract cancers: the 3rd edition."

According to this algorithm, a diagnosis using a blood test abnormality or TUS (transabdominal ultrasonography) from cohorts having high risks and some clinical symptoms is considered to be the first step to diagnosis.

In this section, we first describe what high-risk groups and clinical symptoms are. Next, we will discuss abnormal blood tests and some TUS findings.

According to the algorithm, EUS (endoscopic ultrasonography) has the third step and is positioned as a close examination for staging. EUS also contributes to the early diagnosis of gallbladder cancer, but this time, details will be given to the EUS chapter.

We will also discuss the Japanese approach or Japanese basic policy to cytology and biopsy, and lastly, we refer to tumor markers for early diagnosis of gallbladder cancer.

High-Risk Groups

Considering the following conditions as risk factors for gallbladder cancer and conducting first step tests such as TUS contributes to early diagnosis of gallbladder cancer.

Pancreaticobiliary Maljunction (PBM)

PBM is known to cause a high incidence of gallbladder cancer in both dilated and non-dilated bile ducts types [2, 3]. When PBM is diagnosed, prophylactic cholecystectomy is recommended. It is often experienced that advanced gallbladder cancer is found prior to the identification of PBM. Diagnosing PBM using TUS is directly linked to the early diagnosis of gallbladder cancer.

Y. Hirooka (✉) · S. Hashimoto · R. Miyahara
Department of Gastroenterology and Gastroenterological Oncology, Fujita Health University School of Medicine, 1-98, Dengakugakubo, Kutsutake-Cho, Toyoake, Aichi 470-1192, Japan
e-mail: yoshiki.hirooka@fujita-hu.ac.jp

S. Hashimoto
e-mail: hsenju@fujita-hu.ac.jp

R. Miyahara
e-mail: ryoji.miyahara@fujita-hu.ac.jp

J. B. Chung and K. Okazaki (eds.), *Diseases of the Gallbladder*,
https://doi.org/10.1007/978-981-15-6010-1_19

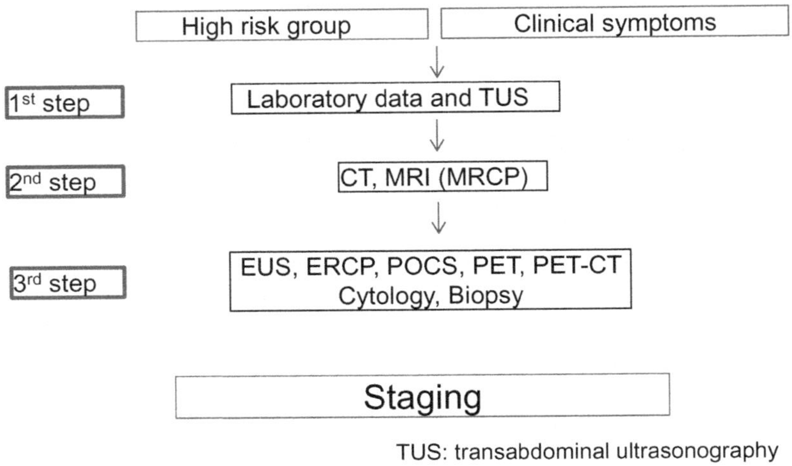

Fig. 1 Diagnostic algorithm for gallbladder cancer. Japanese Society of Hepato-Biliary-Pancreatic Surgery updated "Clinical practice guidelines for the management of biliary tract cancers 2015: the 2nd English edition" to the 3rd Japanese edition (English edition is now under revision). This algorithm for gallbladder cancer was created based on the Japanese 3rd edition

Gallbladder Stone

Many epidemiological studies have reported that gallbladder stones are a risk factor for gallbladder cancer. Risk factors for gallbladder cancer include stones with a diameter of 3 cm or more, symptomatic cases, and a long period of diseases [4–6]. It is thought that chronic inflammation associated with gallstones promotes dysplasia and canceration. However, long-term follow-up of subclinical gallbladder stones has a very low incidence of gallbladder cancer and no clear evidence of a causal relationship between gallstones and cancer is found [7].

Porcelain Gallbladder

Porcelain gallbladder has been associated with a high incidence of gallbladder cancer, but according to a systematic review by Schnelldorfer, only 6% of gallbladder cancer in 124 cases of Porcelain gallbladder excluding selection bias, with a background-matched control. It is concluded that there is a significant difference compared with the group, but it is not the risk factor as previously pointed out [8].

Infection

The association between Salmonella infection and gallbladder cancer is known, and it is thought that chronic inflammation due to infection plays a role in the process of carcinogenesis. Meta-analysis reports that Salmonella infection is significantly more at risk for gallbladder cancer than control gallstone disease [9].

Adenomyomatosis

Segmental adenomyomatosis of the gallbladder is believed to cause cholestasis at the base of the constricted gall bladder, leading to stone formation and cancer, but there is no clear evidence [10, 11].

Clinical Symptoms

Initial symptoms of gallbladder cancer have been reported as upper right abdominal pain (50–80%), jaundice (10–44%), nausea and vomiting (15–68%), and weight loss (10–72%) [12, 13]. Jaundice (extrahepatic bile duct infiltration) requires extended resection and therefore has a high mortality rate of 7–11%, and the median survival time after resection is poor at 14–18 months. Non-jaundice cases are accidentally found by TUS (transabdominal ultrasonography) at screening and cholecystectomy for cholelithiasis.

For early diagnosis of gallbladder cancer, it is necessary to consider a strategy for diagnosing in some way before the above-mentioned symptoms appear.

Abnormal Blood Tests

Biliary tract enzymes are mainly elevated due to bile duct obstruction, and it has been reported that ALP and γ-GTP are elevated in about 70% of patients with early bile duct cancer [14, 15]. Prolonged bile duct obstruction may also increase AST and ALT due to hepatocellular injury. However, it is poor in specificity and needs to be distinguished from liver disease due to viral, alcoholic, etc.

Abnormal blood tests do not always contribute to early detection of gallbladder cancer.

TUS (Transabdominal Ultrasonography) Findings

TUS, which is minimally invasive and can be performed at the bedside and has a high diagnostic ability, is essential for the first step diagnostic imaging. The ability of TUS to depict gallbladder tumors is extremely high, and the accuracy rate of gallbladder cancer among gallbladder tumors is as high as 70–90% [16]. It has been reported that the accuracy rate can be further increased by using high-resolution ultrasound [17], ultrasound Doppler method [18], and ultrasound contrast agents [16, 19].

Polypoid Lesions

Gallbladder cancer should be suspected if the size is 10 mm or more, and regardless of the size, when there is a broad basis or a tendency to increase on the image, and when the target is diagnosed malignant, it should be performed closer examination using TUS.

Figure 2 shows the algorithm for the diagnosis of depth invasion of gallbladder cancer [20].

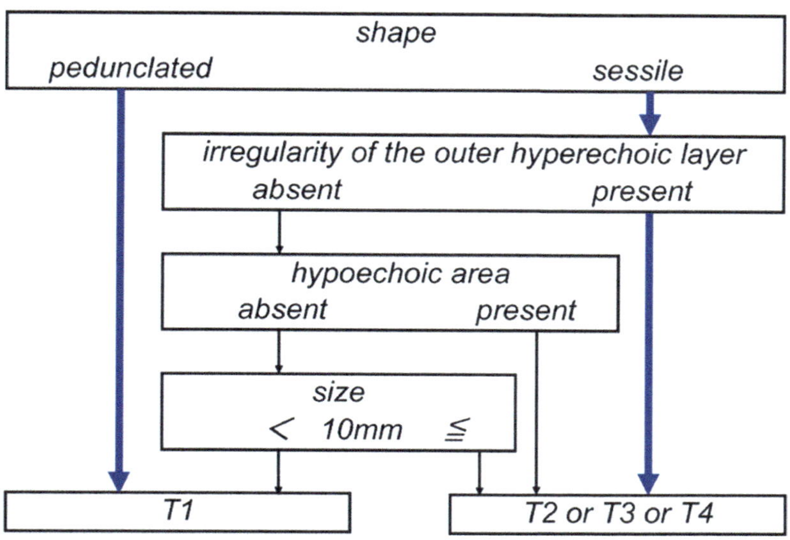

Fig. 2 Algorithm for the diagnosis of depth invasion of GBC (gallbladder cancer). A consensus has already built for both shape and irregularity of the outer hyperechoic layer. Hypoechoic area and size of GBC may be helpful for differentiation

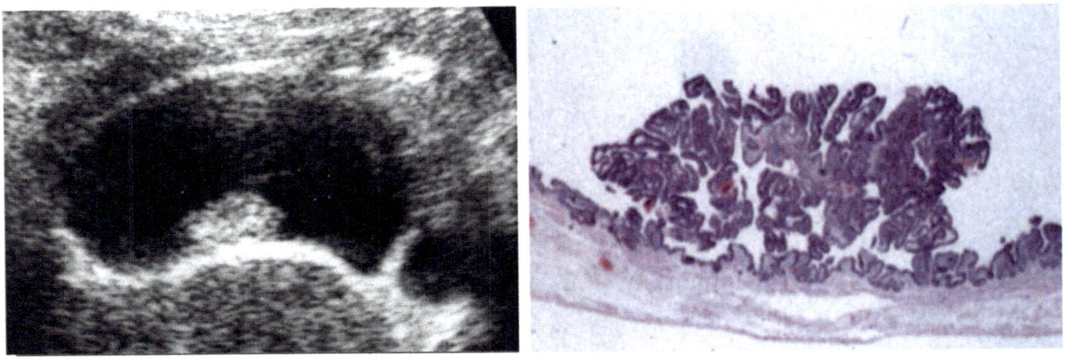

Fig. 3 Gallbladder cancer (depth invasion: M). **a** The tumor was depicted as having sessile base with the size around 10 mm. **b** Surgical treatment revealed the tumor invasion limited to the mucosa

Figure 3 indicates the early stage of gallbladder cancer. The tumor was depicted as having a sessile base with the size around 10 mm. Surgical treatment revealed the tumor invasion limited to the mucosa.

Diagnosis of PBM Without Biliary Dilatation

B-Mode Imaging

PBM cases without bile duct dilatation are risk factors for gallbladder cancer but are difficult to detect because they do not involve bile duct dilatation. Among the cases with a uniform smooth thickness of the gallbladder wall, there are cases of PBM [21]. Finding such cases may contribute to early diagnosis of gallbladder cancer. Figure 4 demonstrates the uniform smooth thickness of the gallbladder wall. Figure 5 shows the PBM without biliary dilatation. In some cases, PBM may be visualized on B-mode images from characteristic gallbladder wall thickening.

Color Doppler Flow Imaging

A differential diagnosis was made in 1996 by assessing hemodynamics within gallbladder elevated lesions [18].

Then, the differential diagnosis of gallbladder lesions and the assessment of PBM by evaluating the blood flow velocity of the gallbladder wall blood flow (branch of cystic artery) became possible [22, 23]. Figure 6 shows the distribution of the measured gallbladder blood wall flow. Setting 30 cm/sec as the cut-off value allowed all cancer cases to be picked up. When 25 cm/sec was set at as the cut-off value for differentiation between lesions with PBM and without PBM, sensitivity and specificity for diagnosing PBM were 88.2% and 89.2%, respectively [23]. Figure 7 shows the uniform gallbladder wall thickness and color flow signals were observed along with the gallbladder wall. The measured value of gallbladder blood flow velocity was about 26 cm/sec, leading to suspicion of PBM case. Figure 8 demonstrates this case was diagnosed as hyperplasia without cancerous change.

Cytology and Biopsy

Cytology and biopsy for gallbladder cancer differ depending on whether the subject is operable or inoperable.

Operable Cases

Pretreatment biopsy and cytology for gallbladder cancer are different from those for bile duct cancer in the following two points.

First, if gallbladder carcinoma does not involve bile duct invasion, ERCP or PTBD as a treatment for reducing jaundice is not essential.

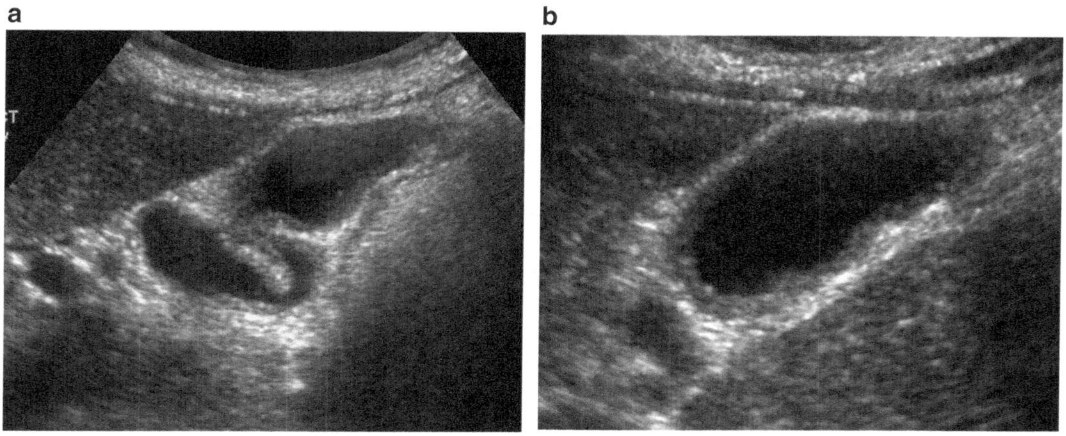

Fig. 4 Uniform smooth thickness of the gallbladder wall. The gall bladder wall thickened from neck and body (**a**) to fundus (**b**) without disruption of wall layer structure

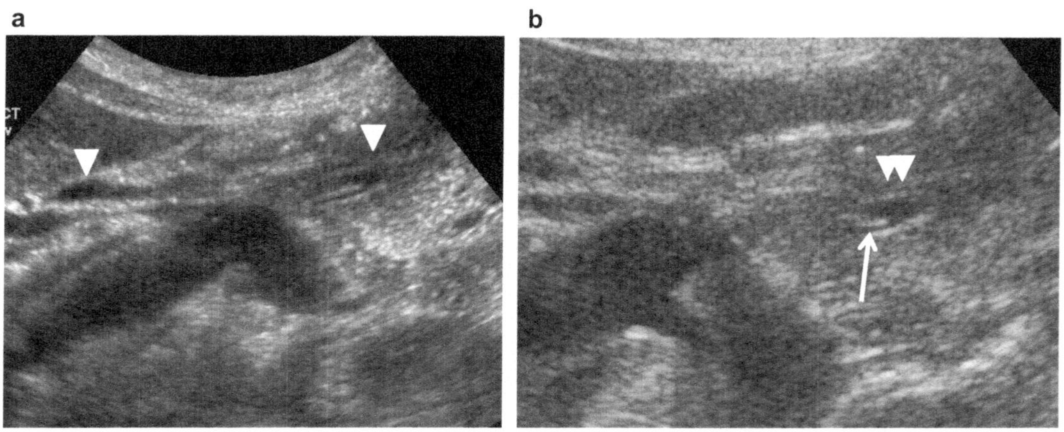

Fig. 5 Pancreaticobiliary maljunction without biliary dilatation. **a** Bile duct (arrow head) without dilatation was observed from the hilum to the place nearby duodenal major papilla. **b** Bile duct (arrow head) and main pancreatic duct (arrow) communicated inside the pancreas

Pre-biopsy/cytology is the only procedure for that purpose.

Second, the resection methods vary from cholecystectomy to extended cholecystectomy, extended hepatic lobectomy and pancreaticoduodenectomy. If T1 gallbladder cancer is suspected (depth is less than the muscularis muscularis), cholecystectomy is indicated because of excisional biopsy, so pretreatment biopsy and cytology are not necessarily required. When the lesion is estimated gallbladder cancer deeper than T2, it is necessary to have a preoperative biopsy or cytology, since the operation is more than an extended cholecystectomy. It has been reported that nasal gallbladder drainage and gallbladder bile cytology are useful for transpapillary pretreatment biopsy and cytology [24]. However, technically feasible facilities are still limited and can only be presented in the recommendation. A high accuracy rate of EUS-FNA for gallbladder lesions has also been reported (80–100%) [25–27], but due to complications of bile peritonitis [28], the possibility of dissemination cannot be ruled out.

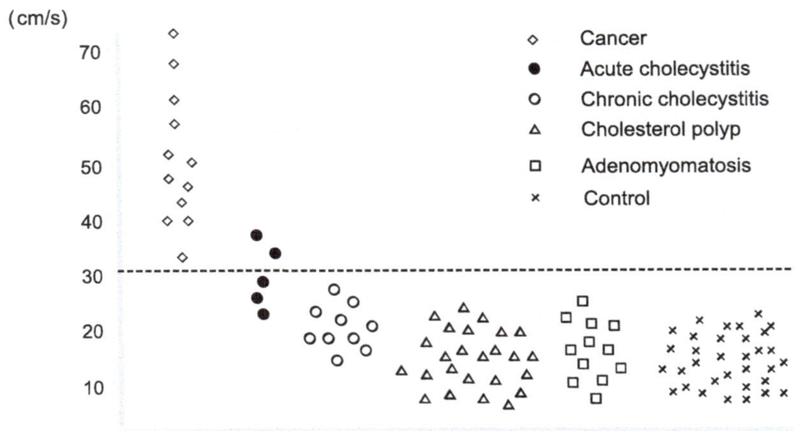

Fig. 6 Distribution of gallbladder wall blood flow. Setting 30 cm/s as the cut-off value allowed all cancer cases to be picked up

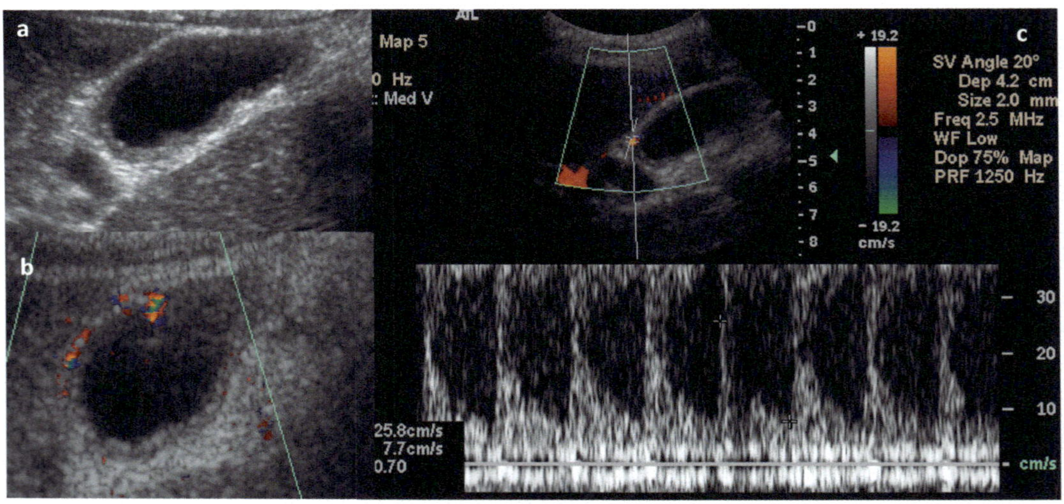

Fig. 7 Case with pancreaticobiliary maljunction. **a** showed the uniform gallbladder wall thickness and color flow signals were observed along with the gallbladder wall (**b**). Measured value of gallbladder blood flow velocity was about 26 cm/s, leading to suspicion of PBM case (**c**)

Inoperable Cases

If resection is not indicated, a percutaneous approach or high sensitivity to determine treatment is the same as for cholangiocarcinoma. We recommend pre-treatment biopsy or cytology with EUS-FNA (96% sensitivity). However, punctures must be kept in the gallbladder wall to avoid risk and should be performed at a facility that is skilled in the procedure.

Tumor Markers for Early Diagnosis of Gallbladder Cancer

Till date, there is no reliable tumor marker developed which can be employed in the diagnosis of gallbladder cancer [29]. The only two markers, i.e., carcinoembryonic antigen (CEA) and carbohydrate antigen 19-9 are most often elevated in advanced stages with low specificity. So, most often, they are not used in the

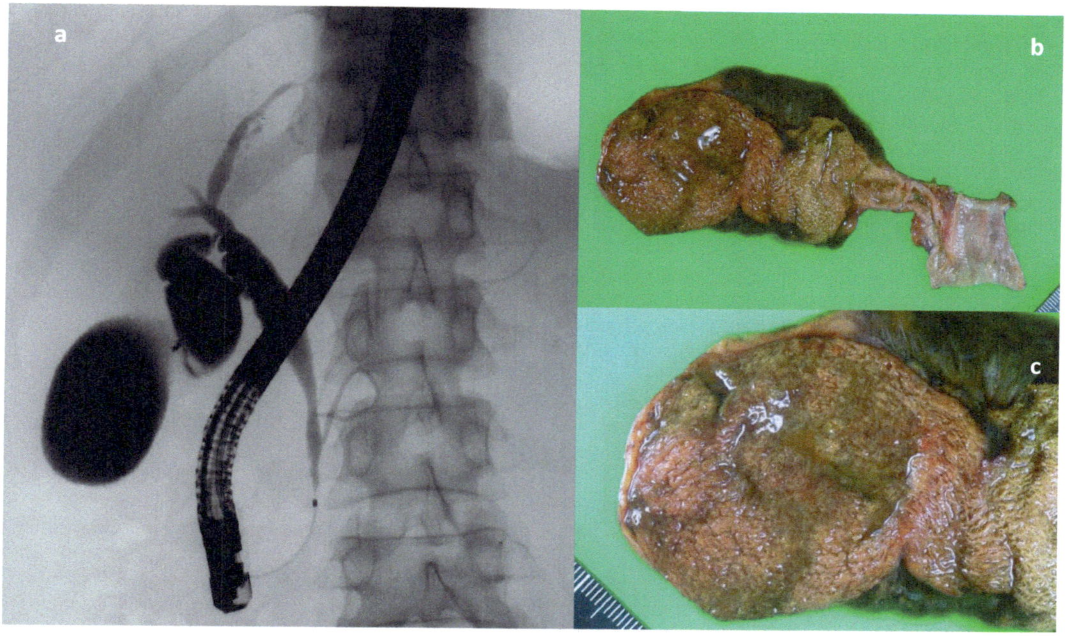

Fig. 8 Case with pancreaticobiliary maljunction (Fig. 7 and this figure are the same case). **a** ERCP showed the pancreaticobiliary maljunction. **b**, **c** Resected specimens. Despite severe wall thickening around the fundus of the gallbladder, there were no malignant findings in the area, with only hyperplastic mucosa

standalone diagnosis of gallbladder cancer [30]. However, there are other tumor markers like CA125, CA19-9, CEA (carcinoembryonic antigen), cancer antigens (CA), and CA242, which are for diagnosis of different other types of cancer (e.g., gastric, liver, pancreatic), have also been researched in the diagnosis of gallbladder cancer but the obtained results are highly inconsistent [31, 32]. In addition, some previous reports have shown CA 242, RCAS1 (receptor-binding cancer antigen expressed on SiSo cells), CA15-3, Mac-2BP (macrophage galactose-specific lectin-2-binding protein), Fragments of cytokeratin-19 (CYFRA 21-1) are frequently present in the blood of cancer patients and shown to be associated with gallbladder cancer with variable sensitivity and specificity.

The tumor markers available for diagnosis gallbladder cancer have also not of very high specificity and not discovered until an advanced stage of the disease leading to the complexity of the treatment. Exome sequencing of gallbladder cancer tissue has found ERBB pathway as the most dysregulated pathway in this disease. Although the studies have been published in highly distinguished journals, they need to be validated before clinical implication.

Conclusion

Transabdominal ultrasonography plays an important role in the detection of early gallbladder cancer and an appearance of useful biomarkers for early detection of gallbladder cancer is eagerly awaited.

References

1. Miyazaki M, Yoshitomi H, Miyakawa S, Uesaka K, Unno M, Endo I, et al. Clinical practice guidelines for the management of biliary tract cancers 2015: the 2nd English edition. J Hepatobiliary Pancreat Sci. 2015;22:249–73.
2. Morine Y, Shimada M, Takamatsu H, Araida T, Endo I, Kubota M, et al. Clinical features of pancreaticobiliary maljunction: update analysis of 2nd Japan-nationwide survey. J Hepatobiliary Pancreat Sci. 2013;20:472–80.

3. Kamisawa T, Kuruma S, Chiba K, Tabata T, Koizumi S, Kikuyama M. Pancreaticobiliary maljunction and biliary cancer. J Gastroenterol. 2015;50:273–9.
4. Diehl AK. Gallstone size and the risk of gallbladder cancer. JAMA. 1983;250:2323–6.
5. Scott TE, Carroll M, Cogliano FD, Smith BF, Lamorte WW. A case-control assessment of risk factors for gallbladder carcinoma. Dig Dis Sci. 1999;44:1619–25.
6. Serra I, Yamamoto M, Calvo A, Cavada G, Báez S, Endoh K, et al. Association of chili pepper consumption, low socioeconomic status and longstanding gallstones with gallbladder cancer in a Chilean population. Int J Cancer. 2002;102:407–11.
7. Sheth S, Bedford A, Chopra S. Primary gallbladder cancer: recognition of risk factors and the role of prophylactic cholecystectomy. Am J Gastroenterol. 2000;95:1402–10.
8. Schnelldorfer T. Porcelain gallbladder: a benign process or concern for malignancy? J Gastrointest Surg. 2013;17:1161–8.
9. Nagaraja V, Eslick GD. Systematic review with meta-analysis: the relationship between chronic Salmonella typhi carrier status and gall-bladder cancer. Aliment Pharmacol Ther. 2014;39:745–50.
10. Ootani T, Shirai Y, Tsukada K, Muto T. Relationship between gallbladder carcinoma and the segmental type of adenomyomatosis of the gallbladder. Cancer. 1992;69:2647–52.
11. Nabatame N, Shirai Y, Nishimura A, Yokoyama N, Wakai T, Hatakeyama K. High risk of gallbladder carcinoma in elderly patients with segmental adenomyomatosis of the gallbladder. J Exp Clin Cancer Res. 2004;23:593–8.
12. Cubertafond P, Gainant A, Cucchiaro G. Surgical treatment of 724 carcinomas of the gallbladder. Results of the French Surgical Association Survey. Ann Surg. 1994;219:275–80.
13. Misra S, Chaturvedi A, Misra NC, Sharma ID. Carcinoma of the gallbladder. Lancet Oncol. 2003;4:167–76.
14. Cha JM, Kim MH, Lee SK, Seo DW, Lee SS, Lee JH, et al. Clinicopathological review of 61 patients with early bile duct cancer. Clin Oncol (R Coll Radiol). 2006;18:669–77.
15. Stepien M, Fedirko V, Duarte-Salles T, Ferrari P, Freisling H, Trepo E, et al. Prospective association of liver function biomarkers with development of hepatobiliary cancers. Cancer Epidemiol. 2016;40:179–87.
16. Inui K, Yoshino J, Miyoshi H. Diagnosis of gallbladder tumors. Intern Med. 2011;50:1133–6.
17. Kim JH, Lee JY, Baek JH, Eun HW, Kim YJ, Han JK, et al. High-resolution sonography for distinguishing neoplastic gallbladder polyps and staging gallbladder cancer. Am J Roentgenol. 2015;204:W150–9.
18. Hirooka Y, Naitoh Y, Goto H, Furukawa T, Ito A, Hayakawa T. Differential diagnosis of gall-bladder masses using colour Doppler ultrasonography. J Gastroenterol Hepatol. 1996;11:840–6.
19. Wang W, Fei Y, Wang F. Meta-analysis of contrast-enhanced ultrasonography for the detection of gallbladder carcinoma. Med Ultrason. 2016;18:281–5.
20. Okaniwa S. Role of conventional ultrasonography in the diagnosis of gallbladder polypoid lesions. J Med Ultrason. 2019. https://doi.org/10.1007/s10396-019-00989-5.
21. Takuma K, Kamisawa T, Tabata T, Hara S, Kuruma S, Inaba Y, et al. Importance of early diagnosis of pancreaticobiliary maljunction without biliary dilatation. World J Gastroenterol. 2012;18:3409–14.
22. Hayakawa S, Goto H, Hirooka Y, Itoh A, Taki T, Watanabe Y, et al. Colour Doppler-guided spectral analysis of gall-bladder wall flow. J Gastroenterol Hepatol. 1998;13:181–5.
23. Kawashima H, Hirooka Y, Itoh A, Hashimoto S, Itoh T, Hara K, et al. Use of color Doppler ultrasonography in the diagnosis of anomalous connection in pancreatobiliary disease. World J Gastroenterol. 2005;11:1018–22.
24. Itoi T, Sofuni A, Itokawa F, Kurihara T, Tsuchiya T, Moriyasu F, et al. Preoperative diagnosis and management of thick-walled gallbladder based on bile cytology obtained by endoscopic transpapillary gallbladder drainage tube. Gastrointest Endosc. 2006;64:512–9.
25. Hijioka S, Mekky MA, Bhatia V, Sawaki A, Mizuno N, Hara K, et al. Can EUS-guided FNA distinguish between gallbladder cancer and xanthogranulomatous cholecystitis? Gastrointest Endosc. 2010;72:622–7.
26. Jacobson BC, Pitman MB, Brugge WR. EUS-guided FNA for the diagnosis of gallbladder masses. Gastrointest Endosc. 2003;57:251–4.
27. Varadarajulu S, Eloubeidi MA. Endoscopic ultrasound-guided fine-needle aspiration in the evaluation of gallbladder masses. Endoscopy. 2005;37:751–4.
28. Jacobson BC, Waxman I, Parmar K, Kauffman JM, Clarke GA, Van Dam J. Endoscopic ultrasound-guided gallbladder bile aspiration in idiopathic pancreatitis carries a significant risk of bile peritonitis. Pancreatology. 2002;2:26–9.
29. Sharma A, Sharma KL, Gupta A, Yadav A, Kumar A. Gallbladder cancer epidemiology, pathogenesis and molecular genetics: Recent update. World J Gastroenterol. 2017;23:3978–98.
30. Srivastava K, Srivastava A, Mittal B. Potential biomarkers in gallbladder cancer: present status and future directions. Biomarkers. 2013;18:1–9.
31. He CZ, Zhang KH, Li Q, Liu XH, Hong Y, Lv NH. Combined use of AFP, CEA, CA125 and CAl9-9 improves the sensitivity for the diagnosis of gastric cancer. BMC Gastroenterol. 2013;13:87. https://doi.org/10.1186/1471-230X-13-87.
32. Zhang D, Yu M, Xu T, Xiong B. Predictive value of serum CEA, CA19-9 and CA125 in diagnosis of colorectal liver metastasis in Chinese population. Hepatogastroenterology. 2013;60:1297–301.

Recent Advances of Surgical Treatment for Gallbladder Carcinoma

Michiaki Unno

Introduction

Surgery for gallbladder carcinoma is much better than other treatments, so that it is necessary to determine whether resection is possible or not. If there are no unresectable factors, surgical resection is recommended in principle. The surgical procedure for gallbladder carcinoma greatly differs depending on the depth of invasion, for example, laparoscopic cholecystectomy (LC) to hepatopancreaticoduodenectomy (HPD). However, it is quite difficult to diagnose the precise extent of gallbladder carcinoma preoperatively even with extracorporeal ultrasonography (US), CT, and endoscopic ultrasonography (EUS). Therefore, the surgery must be considered with inaccuracy in preoperative diagnosis.

In 2017, Japan Biliary Association started the prospective observational study, named "GALLOP study". The aim of this study is to diagnose and register the differential diagnosis between benign and malignant and the depth of gallbladder carcinoma before the operation and clarify the accuracy, sensitivity, and specificity of preoperative staging. Moreover, we believe that surgical outcome according to preoperative diagnosis will be clear. From October 2017 to September 2019, we have enrolled 359 cases of suspected gallbladder carcinoma. Final analysis, including surgical outcomes, is scheduled for fall 2021.

T1 Gallbladder Carcinoma

Gallbladder carcinoma in intramucosal ('m' cancer: T1a) and muscularis propria ('mp' cancer: T1b) basically have a good prognoses even in simple cholecystectomy, because there is theoretically no lymph node metastasis and distant metastasis in pT1a and pT1b gallbladder carcinoma. Therefore, it is essential to perform a meticulous microscopic investigation of the surgical specimen, with special attention given to the depth of invasion.

Now laparoscopic cholecystectomy (LC) is widely accepted for cholecystolithiasis or benign gallbladder polyp. However, the Japanese guidelines do not recommend LC for gallbladder carcinoma [1], because LC may increase the risk of peritoneal dissemination and port site recurrence due to bile leakage from gallbladder injury [2, 3].

In recent years, laparoscopic instruments and surgical techniques have been developed, so that LC has been gradually performed on T1 gallbladder carcinoma. However, LC or laparoscopic-expanded cholecystectomy for gallbladder carcinoma has been a challenge and

M. Unno (✉)
Department of Surgery, Tohoku University Graduate School of Medicine, 1-1, Seiryo-Machi, Aoba-Ku, Sendai, Miyagi 980-8574, Japan
e-mail: m_unno@surg.med.tohoku.ac.jp

J. B. Chung and K. Okazaki (eds.), *Diseases of the Gallbladder*,
https://doi.org/10.1007/978-981-15-6010-1_20

should be performed as a clinical study with sufficient informed consent. Recetly, some reports indicate that the prognosis of patients with incidental gallbladder carcinoma is almost the same between by open cholecystectomy and by LC [4–7]. Since there is no bile leakage if performed by the expert surgeon, it is possible that the indication of LC for gallbladder carcinoma may be expanded in the future.

T2, T3, and T4 Gallbladder Carcinoma

If the gallbladder carcinoma is deeper than muscularis propria, direct liver invasion and lymph node metastasis might occur. Therefore, cholecystectomy with liver resection and lymph node dissection is necessary. There were some arguments in the extent of hepatectomy that perform a subsegmental hepatectomy (Segment 4b + Segment 5) to ensure a sufficient surgical margin or an extended cholecystectomy with minimal liver resection in T2 gallbladder carcinoma. In the Japanese national survey, there is no prognostic difference between patients with subsegmental hepatectomy and minimal hepatectomy in T2 carcinoma [8]. Therefore, the Japanese guidelines recommends the extended cholecystectomy with minimal hepatectomy and lymph node dissection in hepato-duodenal ligament and around the hepatic artery in T2 gallbladder carcinoma [1].

In addition, if cystic duct margin and lymph nodes in hepatoduodenal ligament are negative, prophylactic extrahepatic bile duct resection for lymph node dissection is not recommended in the Japanese guidelines. There is no evidence that shows that combined extrahepatic bile duct resection improves the surgical outcomes [8]. However, the extrahepatic bile duct resection could be acceptable in patients with advanced lymph node metastasis or with cancer invading the neck of the gallbladder.

Moreover, to consider the inaccuracy in preoperative diagnosis, it might be appropriate to perform subsegmental hepatectomy and/or combined extrahepatic bile duct resection for patients with strongly suspected hepatic invasion or bile duct invasion and/or lymph node metastasis.

However, for patients with advanced gallbladder carcinoma in which there is massive invasion to the hepatoduodenal ligament, hepatic artery, and/or portal vein, or for advanced gallbladder carcinoma with metastasis of the posterior lymph nodes of the pancreas, HPD could be necessary for curative resection. However, HPD is not recommended for highly advanced gallbladder carcinoma, because an acceptable prognosis cannot be expected even if such a highly invasive resection (HPD) is performed [9].

Incidental Gallbladder Carcinoma

The incidental gallbladder carcinoma that is found by postoperative pathological examination is not rare. The incidence is 0.3–1.0% in gallbladder resected for cholecystolithiasis [10–12]. In patients with carcinoma invasion limited to the mucosa or muscularis propria, additional resection is not necessary. On the other hand, in patients with subserosa invasion or deeper, an additional resection with liver resection and lymph node dissection should be considered, because some reports showed an additional resection improved the prognosis [13, 14]. In addition, there is no prognostic difference between patients with incidental gallbladder carcinoma who underwent a two-stage operation and simultaneously one-stage resection [15]. Therefore, the Japanese guidelines strongly proposed that the simultaneous or sequential additional resection should be considered [1].

Conclusion

The surgical procedure for gallbladder carcinoma depends on the depth of invasion. The curative resection is most important for surgical treatment of gallbladder carcinoma.

References

1. Miyazaki M, Yoshitomi H, Miyakawa S, Uesaka K, Unno M, Endo I, et al. Clinical practice guidelines for the management of biliary tract cancers 2015: the 2nd English edition. J Hepatobiliary Pancreat Sci. 2015;22(4):249–73.
2. Reddy YP, Sheridan WG. Port-site metastasis following laparoscopic cholecystectomy: a review of the literature and a case report. Eur J Surg Oncol. 2000;26(1):95–8.
3. Wullstein C, Woeste G, Barkhausen S, Gross E, Hopt UT. Do complications related to laparoscopic cholecystectomy influence the prognosis of gallbladder cancer? Surg Endosc. 2002;16(5):828–32.
4. Yoshida T, Matsumoto T, Sasaki A, Morii Y, Ishio T, Bandoh T, et al. Laparoscopic cholecystectomy in the treatment of patients with gall bladder cancer. ACS. 2000;191(2):158–63.
5. Whalen GF, Bird I, Tanski W, Russell JC, Clive J. Laparoscopic cholecystectomy does not demonstrably decrease survival of patients with serendipitously treated gallbladder cancer. J Am Coll Surg. 192(2):189–95.
6. Sarli L, Contini S, Sansebastiano G, Gobbi S, Costi R, Roncoroni L. Does laparoscopic cholecystectomy worsen the prognosis of unsuspected gallbladder cancer? Arch Surg. 2000;135(11):1340–4.
7. de Aretxabala XA, Roa IS, Mora JP, Orellana JJ, Riedeman JP, Burgos LA, et al. Laparoscopic Cholecystectomy: Its Effect on the Prognosis of Patients with Gallbladder Cancer. World J Surg. 2004;28(6):544–7.
8. Horiguchi A, Miyakawa S, Ishihara S, Miyazaki M, Ohtsuka M, Shimizu H, et al. Gallbladder bed resection or hepatectomy of segments 4a and 5 for pT2 gallbladder carcinoma: analysis of Japanese registration cases by the study group for biliary surgery of the Japanese Society of Hepato-Biliary-Pancreatic Surgery. J Hepatobiliary Pancreat Sci. 2013;20(5):518–24.
9. Yamamoto Y, Sugiura T, Okamura Y, Ito T, Ashida R, Uemura S, et al. Is combined pancreatoduodenectomy for advanced gallbladder cancer justified? Surgery. 2016;159(3):810–20.
10. Varshney S, Buttirini G, Gupta R. Incidental carcinoma of the gallbladder. Eur J Surg Oncol (EJSO). 2002;28(1):4–10.
11. Yamamoto H, Hayakawa N, Kitagawa Y, Katohno Y, Sasaya T, Takara D, et al. Unsuspected gallbladder carcinoma after laparoscopic cholecystectomy. J Hepatobiliary Pancreat Surg. 2005;12(5):391–8.
12. Choi SB, Han HJ, Kim CY, Kim WB, Song T-J, Suh SO, et al. Incidental gallbladder cancer diagnosed following laparoscopic cholecystectomy. World J Surg. 2009;33(12):2657–63.
13. Wakai T, Shirai Y, Hatakeyama K. Radical Second Resection Provides Survival Benefit for Patients with T2 Gallbladder Carcinoma First Discovered after Laparoscopic Cholecystectomy. World J Surg. 2002;26(7):867–71.
14. Goetze TO, Paolucci V. Prognosis of incidental gallbladder carcinoma is not influenced by the primary access technique: analysis of 837 incidental gallbladder carcinomas in the German Registry. Surg Endosc. 2013;27(8):2821–8.
15. Ouchi K, Mikuni J, Kakugawa Y, Organizing Committee, The 30th Annual Congress of the Japanese Society of Biliary Surgery. Laparoscopic cholecystectomy for gallbladder carcinoma: results of a Japanese survey of 498 patients. J Hepatobiliary Pancreat Surg. 2002;9(2):256–60.

Neoadjuvant and Adjuvant Chemotherapy

Seungmin Bang

Introduction

To date, surgical resection including adequate lymph node dissection remains the gold standard curative therapy for gallbladder cancer. However, prognosis after curative surgery is still poor with a 5-year survival rate less than 5% and recurrence rate ranging from 30 to 70% [1–3]. Adjuvant therapy or neoadjuvant therapy for solid tumors including gallbladder cancer is aimed to decrease the risk of eradication of pre-existing microscopic metastatic disease as well as inadequate surgery. Guidelines from the National Comprehensive Cancer Network (NCCN) and the European Society of Medical Oncology (ESMO) consider multiple neoadjuvant and adjuvant therapy options [4, 5]. However, the concrete evidence of neoadjuvant and adjuvant therapy for gallbladder cancer is not yet defined. In this chapter, the current status of neoadjuvant and adjuvant therapy for gallbladder cancer will be addressed by focusing on chemotherapy.

S. Bang (✉)
Division of Gastroenterology, Department of Internal Medicine, Yonsei University College of Medicine, Seoul, South Korea
e-mail: bang7028@yuhs.ac

Neoadjuvant Chemotherapy for Gallbladder Cancer

The main aims of neoadjuvant chemotherapy for gallbladder cancer is to exclude rapid progression and avoid futile surgery. However, it has several concerns with regards to delay in surgery and disease progression due to ineffective chemotherapy. Currently, neoadjuvant chemotherapy for gallbladder cancer is recommended when there is evidence of locoregionally advanced diseases including large mass invading liver and/or nodal disease [4]. However, there is no data from large-scaled prospective, randomized clinical trials supporting the notion of neoadjuvant chemotherapy for gallbladder cancer. Rather than, only very limited data were available from relatively small-scaled retrospective cohort studies.

As the clinical guideline of gallbladder cancer, currently available data for neoadjuvant chemotherapy are only focused on locally advanced cases with or without lymph node metastasis [4, 5]. In most studies, lymph node involvement was defined as radiologically enlarged or biopsy-proven cases (Table 1) [6–9]. So, in terms of indication of neoadjuvant therapy, more studies should be more evaluated even for earlier staged gallbladder cancer.

As for the regimen of neoadjuvant chemotherapy for gallbladder cancer, the current data is also still scanty (Table 1). Gemcitabine

J. B. Chung and K. Okazaki (eds.), *Diseases of the Gallbladder*,
https://doi.org/10.1007/978-981-15-6010-1_21

Table 1 Summary of neoadjuvant chemotherapy for gallbladder cancer

Reference	No of patients	Regimen	ORR (%)*	DCR (%)**	Resection rate (%)	R0 resection rate (%)
Chaudhari et al. [6]	160	GEMCIS*** or GEMOX****	52.5	74.1	58.0	98.4
Creasy et al. [7]	74	Gemcitabine (n = 68) and Gemcitabine + Platinum-based (n = 42)	25.7	77.0	13.5	100
Gangopadhyay et al. [8]	121	GEMCIS***		48.8	48.8	88.1
Selvakumar et al. [9]	21	FOLFOX*****	100	100	100	66.7

*ORR; Overall response rate, **DCR; Disease control rate, ***GEMCIS; Gemcitabine + cisplatin, ****GEMOX; Gemcitabine + oxaliplatin, *****FOLFOX; 5-Fluorouracil + leucovorin + oxaliplatin

monotherapy or gemcitabine combination therapies were the most common regimens. The overall response rate (complete remission + partial response) of neoadjuvant chemotherapy was 25 ~ 100% [6–9]. The wide range of overall response rate may be due to the limitations of available studies which have a relatively small number of patients and retrospectively analyzed. The resection rate and rate of complete resection (R0 resection) after neoadjuvant therapy are the most important treatment outcomes. As like overall response rate of chemotherapy, resection rate also showed a wide range from 12 to 100% [6–9]. However, R0 resection rate was relatively high enough to 80% [6–9]. Considering most of cases were locoregionally advanced diseases, the rate of R0 resection gives an important clue for the logicality of neoadjuvant chemotherapy.

Adjuvant Chemotherapy

Chemotherapy for biliary tract cancer including gallbladder cancer is the main treatment option because most of cases are diagnosed at an advanced stage [1]. However, most of the currently available regimen for gallbladder cancer was extrapolated from the experience with pancreatic cancer. In 2010, the Advanced Biliary Cancer-02 trial (ABC-02) was published [10]. This trial was a randomized phase III trial conducted comparison gemcitabine plus cisplatin versus gemcitabine alone for metastatic biliary tract cancer. 36.3% of all participants were gallbladder cancer patients. This study proved the superiority of gemcitabine plus cisplatin in terms of survival gain. This benefit was also confirmed in gallbladder cancer with subgroup analysis. With this study, gemcitabine plus cisplatin is the standard chemotherapy for metastatic gallbladder cancer now.

Even after surgical resection, the overall survival is poor with a high risk of recurrence. It is suggestive of the role for adjuvant chemotherapy in treatment of gallbladder cancer [1–3]. However, chemotherapy in the adjuvant setting for gallbladder cancer is still controversial (Table 2) [11–15]. The main reason is that most of the studies were retrospective manner and included all cases of biliary tract cancer (heterogeneity of the cases). Kayahara et al. analyzed the data of 4,770 patients of gallbladder cancer collected from 1988 to 1997 [11]. They reported patient outcomes were affected by age and sex. However, adjuvant chemotherapy did not provide a survival benefit. In 2018, Bergguist et al. reported a retrospective analysis using the National Cancer Database 2004–2012 cohort [12]. In their analysis, adjuvant chemotherapy showed survival benefit only in T2 or greater staged with node-positive gallbladder cancer. For the prospective clinical trial

Table 2 Summary of adjuvant chemotherapy for gallbladder cancer

References	Study type	Study arms	Regimen	OS or survival
Kayahara et al. [11]	Retrospective	Chemotherapy vs. Observation	NR*	5-year survival rate 33% versus 45% (p<0.05)
Bergquist et al. [12]	Retrospective	Chemotherapy versus Observation	NR*	In T2, 25 months versus 28 months (p=0.44) In T3, 11 months versus 8 months (p<0.01)
Takada et al. [13]	Prospective	Chemotherapy versus Observation	5-FU/Mitomycin	5-year survival rate 27% versus 14% (p=0.04)
Edeline et al. [14]	Prospective	Chemotherapy versus Observation	Gemcitabine/Oxaliplatin	76 months versus 51 months (p=0.74)
Primrose et al. [15]	Prospective	Chemotherapy versus Observation	Capecitabine	53 months versus 36 months (p=0.03)

*NR, Not reported

for gallbladder cancer, 3 reports are available [13–15]. In 2002, Takada et al. reported a phase III prospective clinical trial which included 112 patients of gallbladder cancer [13]. They conducted comparison adjuvant chemotherapy with 5-FU plus mitomycin C (MF) versus surgery alone. Interestingly, gallbladder cancer was the only one that showed significant clinical benefit for adjuvant chemotherapy. The 5-year survival rate of the MF group was 26.0% and the observation group was 14.4% (p=0.0367). In 2019, Primrose et al. reported a phase III prospective clinical trial with 447 patients of biliary tract cancer [14]. In this study, 78 patients of gallbladder cancer were enrolled. They conducted a comparison between adjuvant chemotherapy with oral capecitabine and observation. The overall survival was 51.1 months in the capecitabine group compared with 36.4 months in the observation group (adjusted hazard ration [HR] 0.81) in intention-to-treat analysis. And gallbladder cancer also showed benefit with adjuvant therapy with capecitabine (HR 0.84, 95% CI 0.43–1.63). Even these two relatively large prospective studies showed the benefit of adjuvant chemotherapy for gallbladder cancer, Edeline et al. reported a negative outcome with adjuvant chemotherapy [15]. They performed the PRODIGE 12-ACCORD 18-UNICANCER GI phase III trial with biliary tract cancer. They conducted a comparison between gemcitabine plus oxaliplatin (GEMOX) and observation. 38 (19.6%) patients of gallbladder cancer were enrolled. In the final analysis, this study did not show any benefit of GEMOX in overall survival and recurrence free survival. Furthermore, the subgroup analysis showed gallbladder cancer became worse with GEMOX (HR 2.559, 95% CI 1.037–6.318). They explain the reason for this result with difference in tumor biology and sensitivity to GEMOX.

With regard to the controversial data of the prospective study, there are two available meta-analyses. In 2012, Horgan et al. reported the first meta-analysis of adjuvant therapy for cholangiocarcinoma mostly with non-randomized studies [16]. They evaluated 20 studies from 1960 to 2010. Even though they fail to show the benefit of adjuvant therapy in both cholangiocarcinoma and gallbladder cancer, there was a significant benefit of adjuvant therapy with chemotherapy or chemoradiotherapy in margin-positive and/or node-positive diseases. In 2019, Karan et al. evaluated the benefit of adjuvant chemotherapy for cholangiocarcinomas including gallbladder cancer [17]. Thirty-five studies involving 42,917 patients were recruited for the analysis. For gallbladder cancer, 9 studies were included in the analysis. Compared with surgery only group, overall survival with any adjuvant chemotherapy showed significant improvement (HR 0.74, 95% CI 0.67–0.83). There were significant benefit in those with margin-positive surgeries (HR 0.83, 95% CI

0.77–0.91) and node-positive diseases (HR 0.82, 95% CI 0.76–0.89). And gallbladder cancer also showed the benefit of adjuvant chemotherapy (HR 0.78, 95% CI 0.66–0.92).

Conclusion

Neoadjuvant chemotherapy can be applied in the situation of locoregionally advanced gallbladder cancer. However, it is required to be more validated in terms of indications and the appropriate combination of drug. And furthermore, it should be evaluated what is the most appropriate therapeutic modality among chemotherapy, chemoradiation, and radiation therapy alone.

Adjuvant chemotherapy for gallbladder cancer seems to be beneficial, especially in case of node-positive and/or resection margin-positive diseases. And gemcitabine or oral 5-FU like capecitabine can be considered as the chemotherapeutic agent for adjuvant chemotherapy. However, it should be more validated in terms of the most effective regimen and chemotherapy itself as the adjuvant treatment for gallbladder cancer.

References

1. Duffy A, Capanu M, Abou-Alfa GK, Huitzil D, Jarnagin W, Fong Y, et al. Gallbladder cancer (GBC): 10-year experience at memorial Sloan-Kettering cancer Centre (MSKCC). J Surg Oncol. 2008;98(7):485–9.
2. Park JS, Yoon DS, Kim KS, Choi JS, Lee WJ, Chi HS, et al. Actual recurrence patterns and risk factors influencing recurrence after curative resection with stage II gallbladder carcinoma. J Gastrointest Surg. 2007;11:631–7.
3. Jarnagin WR, Ruo L, Little SA, Klimstra D, D'Angelica M, DeMatteo RP, et al. Patterns of initial disease recurrence after resection of gallbladder carcinoma and hilar cholangiocarcinoma: implications for adjuvant therapeutic strategies. Cancer. 2003;98:1689–700.
4. Network NCCN. NCCN clinical practice guidelines in oncology. Hepatobiliary cancers version 3.2019.
5. Valle JW, Borbath I, Khan SA, Huguet F, Gruenberger T, Arnold D. Biliary cancer: ESMO clinical practice guidelines for diagnosis, treatment and followup. Ann Oncol. 2016;5:28–37.
6. Chaudhari VA, Ostwal V, Patkar S, Sahu A, Toshniwal A, Ramaswamy A, et al. Outcome of neoadjuvant chemotherapy in "locally advanced/borderline resectable" gallbladder cancer: the need to define indications. HPB (Oxford). 2018;20(9):841–7.
7. Creasy JM, Goldman DA, Dudeja V, Lowery MA, Cercek A, Balachandran VP, et al. Systemic chemotherapy combined with resection for locally advanced gallbladder carcinoma: surgical and survival outcomes. J Am Coll Surg. 2017;224:906–16.
8. Gangopadhyay A, Nath P, Biswas J. Reduced dose intensity of chemotherapy may not lead to inferior palliation in locally advanced carcinoma of the gallbladder: an experience from a regional cancer centre in eastern India. J Gastrointest Can. 2015;46:297–300.
9. Selvakumar VP, Zaidi S, Pande P, Goel A, Kumar K. Resection after neoadjuvant chemotherapy in advanced carcinoma of the gallbladder: a retrospective study. Indian J Surg Oncol. 2015;6:16–9.
10. Valle J, Wasan H, Palmer DH, Cunningham D, Anthoney A, Maraveyas A, et al. Cisplatin plus gemcitabine versus gemcitabine for biliary tract cancer. N Engl J Med. 2010;362:1273–81.
11. Kayahara M, Nagakawa T. Recent trends of gallbladder cancer in Japan: an analysis of 4,770 patients. Cancer. 2007;110:572–80.
12. Bergquist JR, Shah HN, Habermann EB, Hernandez MC, Ivanics T, Kendrick ML, et al. Adjuvant systemic therapy after resection of node positive gallbladder cancer: time for a well-designed trial? (Results of a US-national retrospective cohort study). Int J Surg. 2018;52:171–9.
13. Takada T, Amano H, Yasuda H, Nimura Y, Matsushiro T, Kato H, et al. Study group of surgical adjuvant therapy for carcinomas of the pancreas and biliary tract. Is postoperative adjuvant chemotherapy useful for gallbladder carcinoma? A phase III multicenter prospective randomized controlled trial in patients with resected pancreaticobiliary carcinoma. Cancer. 2002;95(8):1685–95.
14. Primrose JN, Fox RP, Palmer DH, Malik HZ, Prasad R, Mirza D, et al. Capecitabine compared with observation in resected biliary tract cancer (BILCAP): a randomised, controlled, multicentre, phase 3 study. Lancet Oncol. 2019 May;20(5):663–73.
15. Edeline J, Benabdelghani M, Bertaut A, Watelet J, Hammel P, Joly JP, et al. Gemcitabine and oxaliplatin chemotherapy or surveillance in resected biliary tract cancer (PRODIGE 12-ACCORD 18-UNICANCER GI): a randomized phase III study. J Clin Oncol. 2019 Mar 10;37(8):658–67.
16. Horgan AM, Amir E, Walter T, Knox JJ. Adjuvant therapy in the treatment of biliary tract cancer: a systematic review and meta-analysis. J Clin Oncol. 2012;30:1934–40.
17. Rangarajan K, Simmins G, Manas D, Malik H. Systemic adjuvant chemotherapy for cholangiocarcinoma surgery: a systemic review and meta-analysis. Eur J Sur Oncol 2019; Epub ahead of print.

Role of Radiation Therapy

Keiko Shibuya

Introduction

Radiation therapy (RT) is a cancer treatment that can be used for almost all organ-derived cancers. RT has some outstanding features, one of which is the less invasive nature of the procedure. Thus, RT is often indicated as a curative treatment in elderly patients or patients with contraindications for surgery because of other illnesses or conditions.

RT technology has significantly progressed over the past decade. The most innovative advance was the transition from a two-dimensional to a three-dimensional (3D) treatment planning that was based on computed tomography (CT) images. This enabled us to understand the positional relationship among the tumors and normal organs within three dimensions. In addition, adoption of a multi-leaf collimator (MLC) has proved useful in making radiation fields fit the shape of the tumors, thereby leading to a significant reduction in the radiation dose to the normal tissues. Using these techniques, RT methods, which are referred to as 3D conformal radiation therapy (3D-CRT), were developed and widely used, thus becoming one of the most popular RT systems. With 3D-CRT, patients can be more safely treated at higher doses as compared to previous treatments, with the RT outcomes showing improvement in several types of cancer.

Moreover, in 2000, a new technology called high-precision radiotherapy, which includes stereotactic radiosurgery (SRS), stereotactic body radiotherapy (SBRT), intensity-modulated radiotherapy (IMRT) and image-guided radiotherapy (IGRT), was developed. Using these techniques, tumors can be irradiated more precisely and selectively with higher doses without increasing adverse events.

Currently, however, it is well known that surgery is the first and only curative treatment choice for gallbladder cancer (GBC). Even so, at the time of diagnosis, this cancer is often unresectable and even if it is resected, local recurrence without distant metastasis is frequent and local lesions are the most influential factors for prognosis [1]. In addition, even if the tumor is not resectable, the rate of distant metastasis at diagnosis has not been found to be that high [1]. Considering these together, adding RT as a modality of local therapy for GBC seems a reasonable strategy. Results of a retrospective analysis of queried information (2004–2013, n = 1,199) from the National Cancer Database (NCDB) on patients who had received chemotherapy or chemoradiotherapy for GBC without distant metastasis in the past showed that the

K. Shibuya (✉)
Department of Radiation Oncology, Osaka City University, Graduate School of Medicine, Osaka, Japan
e-mail: shibuya.keiko@med.osaka-cu.ac.jp

J. B. Chung and K. Okazaki (eds.), *Diseases of the Gallbladder*,
https://doi.org/10.1007/978-981-15-6010-1_22

median overall survival (OS) in the respective cohorts was 8.8 months (95% CI, 7.1–8.5) in the chemotherapy group and 12.9 months (95% CI, 11.0–14.7) in the chemoradiotherapy group ($p = 0.001$) [2]. In the univariate and multivariate Cox proportional hazards model for OS, the addition of RT to the CT was shown to be independently associated with a higher OS. Although, this retrospective data may carry a selection bias, that said, the data did suggest that the addition of local therapy may have improved the survival of patients with unresectable locally advanced GBC.

However, when using RT for GBC, it remains unknown whether the introduction of new treatment techniques results in a sufficient advancement in the treatments. This is because the incidence of GBC is low and these radiotherapy or chemoradiation treatment regimens have yet to be definitively established. More importantly, the gallbladder and surrounding organs are constantly moving with respiratory motion, which presents a specific barrier when trying to adopt high-precision radiotherapy, such as SBRT or IMRT.

Recently, there has been some initial research and development into the use of four-dimensional radiotherapy, which is currently examining a new approach for solving the problems caused by movements of the target organs.

The current status and issues associated with RT for GBC, along with the development of new irradiation techniques, and new approaches are outlined in the text that follows.

High-Precision Radiotherapy

Stereotactic Body Radiotherapy (SBRT)

Stereotactic irradiation is a technique that irradiates a target three-dimensionally from multiple directions with millimeter precision. It was originally developed as a dedicated machine with cobalt-60 radioactive sources designed for gamma ray irradiation for intracranial diseases. However, SBRT using X-rays with a linear accelerator has recently been widely put into practice. The use of SBRT makes it possible to safely treat patients with very high doses exceeding 10 Gy per fraction, that we would normally expect to have a higher cytotoxic effect than conventional fractionated radiation therapy. In addition, we also expect this technique would be of greater benefit to patients, as reducing the number of treatments can lead to a reduction in the amount of time that the patients have to spend in the hospital.

Intensity-Modulated Radiotherapy (IMRT)

IMRT is a new technology of radiotherapy that allows the radiation dose intensity of a beam to be intentionally non-uniform by using a moving MLC with changing the shape of the radiation field very quickly over time during the irradiation. One of the applied types of IMRT is volumetric-modulated arc therapy (VMAT) that can create a more conformal dose distribution by using a gantry that rotates once or twice when emitting the beam, along with changing the rotation speed, dose rate, and shape of the radiation field. It is likely that the VMAT procedure will soon become mainstream, and help to make daily treatment times shorter than those now seen with IMRT.

With the adoption of IMRT or VMAT, it becomes possible to increase the dose gradually within the target volume or selectively increase the dose only to the tumor without increasing the dose to the normal organs that are located close to the tumor (Fig. 1).

Image-Guided Radiotherapy (IGRT)

IGRT is a treatment that uses collation technology that measures and corrects the displacement of the patient's position three-dimensionally and then reproduces the set-up position as determined in the treatment plan as much as possible over the entire course of the RT [3].

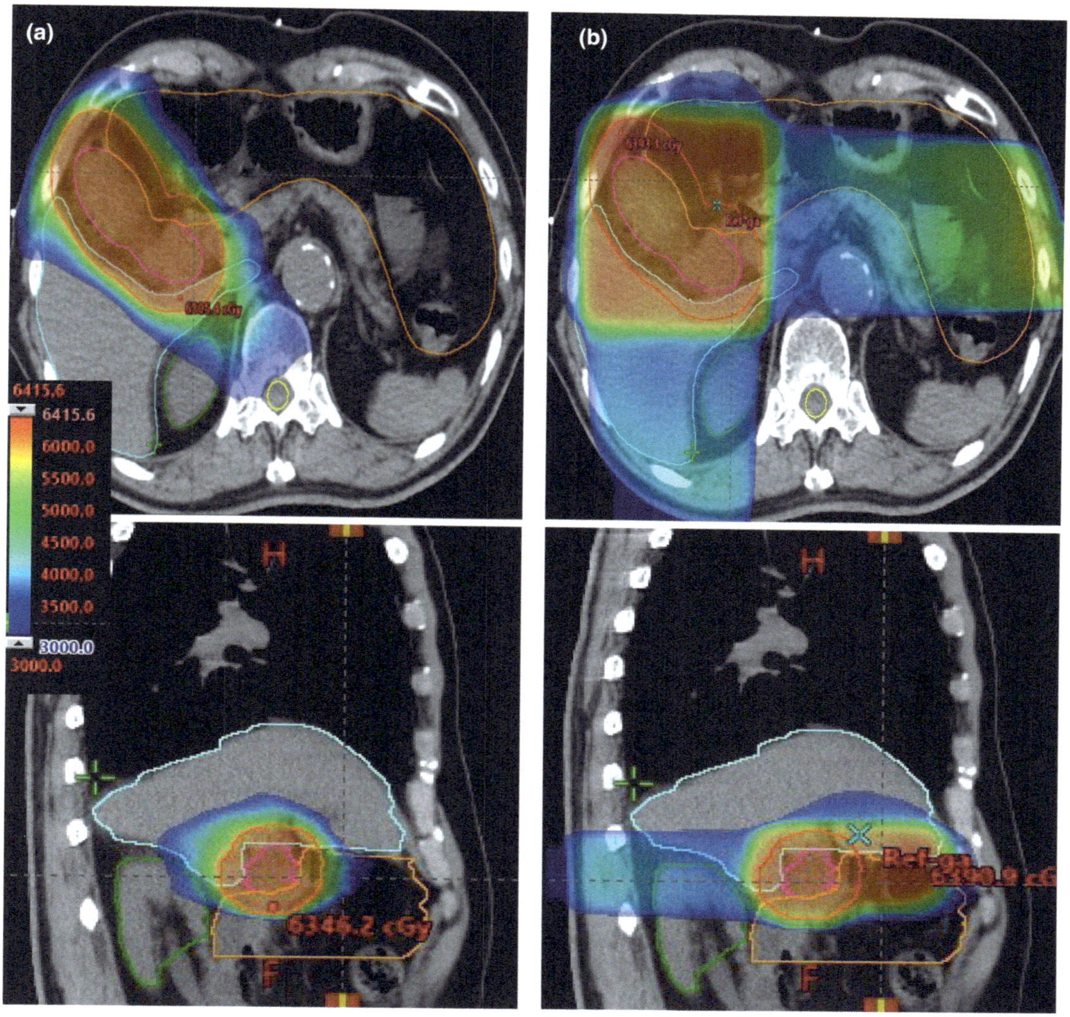

Fig. 1 Differences in dose distribution between IMRT (**a**) and 3D-CRT (**b**) in the treatment of gallbladder cancer: the irradiated volume of the liver and intestinal tract is much smaller in IMRT, as compared with 3D-CRT planning

One of the most basic and standard systems that has recently been installed on most linear accelerators in use is a system that acquires an image using a kV-based X-ray radiography device that is mounted on a treatment delivery apparatus and performs two-dimensional guidance in accordance with the bone structure. In addition, linear accelerators that have been equipped with imaging systems that can acquire CT images (cone beam computed tomography: CBCT) while rotating kV (or MV) X-ray tubes and detectors have quickly become the standard RT equipment. By using these systems, it becomes possible to determine the 3D position of the soft tissues (tumors and organs at risk) and then precisely collate them with the position originally observed on the planning CT imaging after the patient has once again been placed on the treatment table. Furthermore, there are other systems that have been developed and which are being used clinically that can track the position of the markers placed close to the tumor.

These dedicated devices for IGRT make it possible to pursue highly conformal dose distributions with higher dose prescriptions.

Significance of Intervention of RT in GBC

Role of RT for Unresectable GBC

Currently, there are no established standard treatments that can be used for unresectable GBC. In general, chemoradiotherapy is an option, just as it has been used for bile duct cancer. However, because of the very small number of patients with GBC, there have yet to be any large studies that have reported on the optimal radiation doses or chemoradiation regimens [4, 5]. At the present time, conventionally fractionated radiotherapy (50.4 Gy in 28 fractions to 60 Gy in 30 fractions) combined with concurrent 5-fluorouracil (5-FU)-based chemotherapy is suggested based on the data and results collected during the treatment of bile duct cancer. However, it was reported in a retrospective review of 52 patients with unresectable biliary cancer treated with definitive chemoradiotherapy [6] that the first site of disease progression was local in 72% with an actuarial local progression rate at 12 months of 59%. The median time to radiographic local progression was 9, 11, and 15 months in 27 patients who received a total dose of 30 Gy, 14 patients who received 36–50.4 Gy, and in 11 patients who received 54–85 Gy, respectively. These results suggest that higher doses of RT may improve local control, although the statistical power of this study was limited due to the small number of patients. GBC is particularly difficult to detect early, and at the time of diagnosis, it usually has invaded the liver and often has a considerable tumor diameter. As the tumor size increases, radiosensitivity tends to decrease. Thus, the notion that higher doses for locally advanced GBC are needed is easily supported by these observations.

In recent years, there have been attempts to deliver large ablative doses with hypofractionation using SBRT or IMRT. In 2015, a retrospective dose response analysis of 79 patients with inoperable intrahepatic cholangiocarcinoma who were treated with definitive RT between 2002 and 2014 was undertaken [7]. In this report, the 3-year OS rate for patients receiving ablative doses (67.5 Gy in 15 fractions or 75 Gy in 25 fractions) was 73% versus 38% as compared to those receiving lower doses (50.4 Gy in 28 fractions, 58.05 Gy in 15 fractions, or 60 Gy in 30 fractions) ($p = 0.017$).

However, the gallbladder is in close proximity to radiation-sensitive organs that are at high risk, such as the intestinal tract and, in some cases, the right kidney. In addition, the position of these organs is constantly changing due to respiration and/or bowel peristalsis. In order to ensure not only the accuracy of the treatment but also the reduction of the treatment-related adverse events, it is strongly recommended that the exact position of the tumors in each treatment be known, that is, using IGRT. Moreover, for liver tumors, it is always necessary to be careful with regard to the liver function. For example, in SBRT, the dose constraints for an average dose in a normal liver (non-tumor part) are recommended to be limited to 13–15 Gy (less than 6 Gy in patients with Child–Pugh B), while a normal liver with a critical volume ≥ 700 ml should be irradiated less than 15 Gy [8]. The safety of SBRT for Child–Pugh C patients has yet to be established.

Role of Adjuvant Radiation Therapy After Resection

Since many of the recurrences after resection occur locally, a number of studies have examined whether radiation and/or chemoradiation therapy after resection can reduce the relapse rate or prolong survival. However, to date, the effects of adjuvant RT with or without chemotherapy have not been clarified. Even if it is beneficial under certain conditions, it has yet to be established as to which patients would be potential candidates for adjuvant radiotherapy/chemoradiotherapy.

A retrospective review of a prospective database of 157 patients who underwent resection for biliary tract cancer, which included 63 GBC patients, demonstrated that neither neoadjuvant nor adjuvant therapy significantly prolonged the survival [9]. In this study, early surgical resection with more than 1 cm tumor-free margins was associated with improved probability of survival, which indicates that adjuvant local therapies are not always necessary in certain clinical conditions. Park et al. retrospectively evaluated the outcome of adjuvant therapy in 61 patients with stage II GBC, in which 28 patients received chemotherapy, 7 received RT, 8 received concurrent chemoradiotherapy, and 18 received surgery alone. Results showed that there was no evidence that adjuvant therapy was an effective treatment option [10].

On the other hand, several retrospective studies have suggested that adjuvant chemoradiation therapy might be associated with improved survival of GBC patients (Table 1) [11–14]. When using a multi-institutional national database in the US to evaluate the role of adjuvant therapies and subsequent outcomes in 291 patients undergoing curative-intent surgical resection, except for those with metastasis or an R2 margin, results showed there was significant improvement in 61 patients who received chemotherapy and in 44 who received chemoradiotherapy [12]. To minimize the confounding error due to the indication for treatments, multivariable and propensity-matched analyses were performed. These results showed that the adjuvant therapies remained independently associated with improved long-term outcomes, especially among patients with high-risk features including T3/T4 tumors and N1 disease. The hazard ratio (HR) of the OS was 0.38 and 0.26 ($p < 0.001$) for the chemotherapy and chemoradiotherapy, respectively. Similar results were observed for the disease-free survival (DFS) (chemotherapy HR 0.61 and chemoradiation therapy HR 0.43, $p < 0.05$), when compared with surgery alone. In the latest analyses of the NCDB that were conducted between 2004 and 2011, the outcome of 4775 patients with T2-3 or node-positive, nonmetastatic GBC, resected with grossly negative margins were evaluated [13]. The results for the inverse probability of treatment weighting analysis that was performed in order to minimize the treatment-related bias showed that adjuvant concurrent chemoradiation for T3 or node-positive disease had a modest early survival advantage, with an absolute difference at 2 years of 6.8% ($p = 0.009$). In 2018, a meta-analysis was performed to clarify the role of adjuvant radiotherapy [15]. This study examined 14 retrospective studies that included 9364 patients who met the criteria, although most of these had some risk of participant selection bias. Results showed that the RT group had a tendency to have more patients with unfavorable characteristics than the surgery alone group. Nevertheless, the findings of this study showed that RT significantly reduced the risk of death (HR 0.54; 95% CI 0.44–0.67; $p < 0.01$) and recurrence (HR 0.61; 95% CI 0.38–0.98; $p = 0.04$) compared with surgery alone. Furthermore, exploratory analyses demonstrated a survival benefit from RT for high-risk patients with lymph node-positive diseases (HR 0.61; $p < 0.001$) and R1 resections (HR 0.55; $p < 0.001$).

Although there are few prospective studies that have been conducted, a phase II trial [11] that was performed by the Southwest Oncology Group enrolled 54 patients with cholangiocarcinoma and 25 patients with GBC and reported that the 2-year OS that was used as the primary endpoint was 56% in GBC. The local recurrence in this study was 8% in GBC, while the 2-year DFS was 48%, and the rate of distant metastasis at 2 years in patients with cholangiocarcinoma was similar to that in patients with GBC. These results suggest local therapy when used as an adjuvant setting for GBC might be beneficial similar to that seen for cholangiocarcinoma.

How to Select the Candidates for Adjuvant Radiation Therapy?

The analysis of the surgical management of GBC based on one of the largest multi-institutional databases in the US showed that adjuvant chemotherapy or chemoradiotherapy was utilized in 36% of patients [12].

To identify potential candidates for adjuvant radiotherapy, the patterns of initial failure

Table 1 Summary of clinical investigations of radiotherapy with or without chemotherapy in adjuvant settings

References and year of publication	Study design	Number of patients	Clinical stage	Radiotherapy	Concurrent chemotherapy	Outcomes
Park et al. (2010[10])	Retrospective	61 GBC (CT: 28, RT: 7, CRT: 8)	IIB	45 Gy (36–50 Gy) tumor bed and local-regional LNs	5-FU	3y-OS (CT: 78%, RT: 36%, CRT: 36% versus non adj: 64%, p = 0.180), 3y-DFS (CT: 69%, RT: 14%, CRT: 47% versus non adj: 56%, p = 0.033)
Ben-Josef et al. (2015[11])	Phase II inter-group trial (SWOG S0809)	EHCC 54, GBC 25	GBC (n = 25) II: 9, IIIA: 6, IIIb: 8, IV: 2	3D-CRT or IMRT regional LNs: 45 Gy/25 fr tumor bed: 54 Gy/30 fr–59.4 Gy/33 fr	Capecitabine (after gemcitabine + capecitabine)	GBC (2y-OS 56%, 2y-DFS 48%, local recurrence 8%)
Kim et al. (2016[12])	Retrospective multi-institutional analysis	291 GBC (non Adj: 186, CT: 61, CRT: 44)	T2: 46.2%, T3: 38.6% LN metastasis: 37.8%	N/A	N/A	1y-OS: 76.7%, 3y-OS: 42.2%, 5y-OS: 33.0%, OS (CT, HR 0.38; CRT, HR 0.26; p < 0.001) DFS (CT, HR 0.61; CRT, HR 0.43; p < 0.05)
Mantripragada et al. (2017[13])	Retrospective NCDB	4775 GBC Adj CT 1373 (CRT 646)	T2-3 or LN positive	Median total dose 50.4 Gy (45–54 Gy)	N/A	3y-OS 39.9% (Adj CT/CRT, HR 1.01)
Gold et al. (2009[14])	Retrospective	73 GBC Adj CRT 25	I (T1-2N0M0): 59% II (T3N0M0 or T1-T3N1M0): 41%	Median total dose 50.4 Gy/28 fr	5-FU	mOS: Adj CRT 4.8y versus non Adj 4.2y (p = 0.56) (HR 0.3, p = 0.004 after adjusting PF)

SWOG: Southwest Oncology Group, NCDB: National Cancer Database
GBC: gallbladder cancer, EHCC: extrahepatic cholangiocarcinoma, Adj: adjuvant, CT: chemotherapy, RT: radiotherapy, CRT: chemoradiotherapy, 5-FU: 5-fluorouracil, LN: lymph node
OS: overall survival, DFS: disease-free survival, PF: prognostic factors, fr: fractions
3D-CRT: three-dimensional conformal radiotherapy, IMRT: intensity-modulated radiotherapy

in 70 patients who underwent curative-intent surgery between 2000 and 2016 were evaluated [16]. Adjuvant chemotherapy with 5-FU, gemcitabine, cisplatin, or capecitabine with a single or combination regimen was administered to 19 patients (27.1%), although there were no patients that received adjuvant RT. All the patients who underwent R2 resection and/or patients with ≥ T2 disease who did not undergo radical resection after a previous simple cholecystectomy were excluded in this study. After these exclusions, the 1-year OS was 84.5%, while the 3-year OS was 61.4%. Locoregional recurrence, which was defined as the first failure of any component, occurred in 29 patients (41.4%), with relapse at the locoregional area without concomitant distant metastasis observed in 13 patients (18.6%). Independent prognostic factors for locoregional recurrence were ≥ T2 disease (HR, 5.510; 95% confidence interval [CI], 1.260–24.094; $p = 0.023$) and R1 resection (HR, 6.981: 95% CI, 2.387–20.491; $p < 0.001$). The authors of this study concluded that patients with pT2 disease or R1 resection might benefit from adjuvant radiotherapy.

Wang et al. suggested using a nomogram built from a parametric survival model from the SEER-Medicare database for predicting the benefit of adjuvant chemoradiotherapy for resected GBC [17]. Based on this nomogram, certain subsets of patients with at least T2 or N1 disease may gain a survival benefit from adjuvant chemoradiotherapy.

Routine Practices and the Use of RT for GBC

As previously described, RT is considered to be a local treatment for locally advanced GBC, as it can contribute to not only relief of symptoms, but also to prolongation of the survival period in a certain proportion of patients. However, normal organs, such as the duodenum and large intestine, which are in close proximity, are highly radiosensitive and prone to adverse events. Thus, this often makes it difficult to treat with sufficient doses for tumor control. Furthermore, although the development of stereotactic irradiation has enabled high-dose irradiation, efforts to minimize the effects of radiation on the liver parenchyma will always be required when the tumor diameter increases.

Currently, the use of 3D treatment planning systems makes it possible for radiation oncologists to recognize the dose distribution as organ volume. These dose–volume data have been accumulated for various parameters being able to predict tumor control and adverse events during the treatment planning [18].

In the text that follows, we present an outline of an actual radiation treatment planning method.

Radiation Treatment Planning for GBC

The International Commission on Radiation Units and Measurements (ICRU) defined some target volumes in Report 50 in 1993 [19]. These were well suited for conformal radiotherapy, and further refined in the definition stated in Report 62 in 1999 [20], which expanded upon the concepts presented in Report 50. Currently, we are conducting dose assessments of tumors and surrounding organs in line with the definitions of both Reports 50 and 62.

First, gross tumor volume (GTV) is defined as a tumor that is visible either directly or on images such as CT and MRI. GTV also includes metastatic lymph nodes. The clinical target volume (CTV) is the volume that includes the extent of the microscopic tumor growth, which is defined based on the assumption that the tumor cells exist outside the gross range pathologically. While the GTV is usually added with a margin of about 5 to 10 mm as CTV, this margin is often increased or decreased based on the clinical decision according to the tumor invasiveness or histotropic affinity. In cases of adjuvant RT after complete resection, the gallbladder fossa should be defined as the CTV.

Depending on the types of cancer, the area of the regional lymph nodes may be added to the CTV as an elective nodal irradiation (ENI). However, there has yet to be any research that has established the benefits of ENI for regional LNs for GBC. Kim et al. evaluated initial recurrence patterns in patients who underwent curative-intent surgery [16]. Based on their results, they suggested that LNs of the caudal half-hepatoduodenal ligament, on the posterior surface of the pancreatic head, along the common hepatic artery, around the celiac artery, and around the abdominal aorta between the origin of the celiac artery and the origin of the inferior mesenteric artery should be included in the CTV with regard to the adjuvant radiotherapy setting. However, they said in their report, "they should be included, assuming that the target volume includes regions with a recurrence frequency of 10% or more". In fact, the larger the irradiation field is, the more attention that needs to be paid to the effects on normal organs, especially on the intestines. The benefits and disadvantages need to be weighed by comparing the expected effects with the possible adverse events. As for unresectable locally advanced GBC, one method that is used is to irradiate the primary tumor with the area of ENI with 40–50 Gy and followed by a boost of 10–20 Gy to the visible tumor alone. However, it remains controversial as to how much survival benefits ENI can provide when it is difficult to control the primary tumor itself. Thus, omitting ENI helps to minimize the adverse effects on the surrounding organs and, thereby, makes it possible to increase the dose to the primary tumor. This might be a more reasonable strategy.

Once the CTV is determined, the irradiation field for administering the prescribed dose can be set. However, CTV does not include uncertainties that could occur during irradiation, such as patient movements and organ motion. Therefore, additional margins need to be added to ensure that the target dose is delivered to the CTV. Currently, the margin added to the CTV is defined as an internal margin (IM), and the volume obtained by adding the IM to the CTV is defined as an internal target volume (ITV). In addition, a set-up margin (SM) is established in order to compensate for the uncertainty of the patient position reproducibility that may occur throughout the period from the time of treatment planning to the end of the treatments. The volume obtained by adding the IM and SM to the CTV is considered to be the volume which the prescribed dose is to be administered, and thus, is defined as the planning target volume (PTV).

Challenges of Radiation Therapy for Abdominal Tumors with Motion

Setting the PTV in conjunction with the addition of the IM and SM ensures that the CTV will be covered by sufficient doses. However, the PTV will contain a significant amount of volume of normal organs, which can result in adverse events. The above-mentioned IGRT is a useful method for suppressing the SM, and is an indispensable technique for securing safety especially when a single dose is large, such as in stereotactic irradiation. At the present, various IGRT methods have been developed and mounted on therapeutic devices, and are being studied for each facility or individual cases.

However, a major problem that needs to be solved in the abdominal region involves the respiratory motion, which is the largest component of the IM. Analysis from fluoroscopic, ultrasonographic, MRI studies, and four-dimensional computed tomography (4D-CT), which reconstructs images for each respiratory phase, has shown that the peak-to-peak magnitude of respiratory motion of abdominal organs was as large as 20–30 mm [21–27]. In an organ having a large motion due to respiration, this means a large IM must be set, which also can have a serious effect on normal organs, and thus, may possibly affect the outcome of the treatments.

Furthermore, range and path of intrafractional tumor motion or breathing rhythms may change during radiation therapy. If such changes cannot be managed in real time, the accuracy of the radiation therapy cannot be ensured [28]. IMRT, which can create an ideal dose distribution, is considered to be particularly advantageous in the liver and gallbladder, where highly radiosensitive normal organs such as the intestinal tract, kidney, and lung are close to each other. However, the interplay between the motion of the MLC and the motion of the targets or surrounding organs can create unexpected high or low dose areas. This means that the use of IMRT could lead to a decrease in the local control rate and/or an increase in adverse events in areas with respiratory motion [29]. In fact, this is one of the reasons why IMRT still does not play a large role in the treatment of GBC.

At the present time, there have been many attempts made to address these respiratory motion issues. Methods that have been used for a relatively long time include forced shallow breathing by abdominal compression with some restrictive devices placed above or around the abdomen or chest or active breathing control (ABC) using a special device to control breathing movement [30]. In addition, four-dimensional radiation treatment systems in which a time axis has been added to conventional 3D radiation treatments have been developed and applied clinically. These include the breath-hold irradiation method, tumor-tracking systems or respiratory-gated irradiation systems. With regard to the respiratory-gated irradiation method, several devices have been developed and investigated in the lung, liver, pancreas, and some thoracoabdominal organ tumors, for example, with a sensor attached to the body surface in order to monitor the abdominal or chest wall displacement. With this type of sensor, the abdominal or chest motion signals are captured as respiratory signals in order to substitute or predict tumor motion in the body. As for tumor-tracking systems, some devices have been developed that can monitor the motion of the fiducial markers implanted close to the tumors in the body or the tumor itself in real time, with previous results showing these to be effective strategies when trying to compensate for respiratory tumor motion [31–34]. After the introduction of these systems, new developments for the use of RT in abdominal organ malignancies are expected.

Quality Assurance (QA)

In high-precision RT, we usually perform patient-specific quality assurance (QA) to verify the feasibility of a treatment plan. One common QA method for RT involves using irradiation based on a treatment plan that is performed on a phantom, followed by a subsequent verification that confirms there is no difference between the radiation dose measured by a dosimeter inserted in the phantom and the calculated value at the time of treatment planning. The phantom, which is a model that simulates the human body as a tissue equivalent to water, is designed so that it can be used to estimate the absorbed dose of radiation in the human body.

In tumor-tracking RT cases, further accuracy is required, and special QA is needed. One method that can be used is to obtain the tumor respiratory motion log file from the tracking devices in each patient that is loaded into a motion phantom. This is a device that can replay the movement of the tumor accompanying the respiratory motion of the human body [35]. Thus, the planned tumor-tracking irradiation is performed on the motion phantom, with the point dose determined by the ionization chamber dosimeter and the dose distribution on the film then measured. As a result, the prescribed dose and the measured value can then be compared and verified.

In recent years, researchers have advocated for the development of a motion phantom that can more accurately and three-dimensionally reproduce the movement of a tumor.

Conclusion

The role of RT is primarily a local treatment for unresectable GBC or adjuvant therapy after surgery. Although clinical studies to establish definitive treatment regimens of RT or chemoradiotherapy have not been performed, retrospective promising results have been reported and recurrence patterns of GBC suggest local control with ablative radiotherapy doses is a reasonable strategy even for unresectable advanced GBC. RT technology has significantly progressed over past decade. Creation of more sophisticated irradiation systems for high-precision RT such as SBRT, IMRT, and IGRT has made it possible to deliver higher radiation doses with higher conformity, and furthermore they have combined with new technologies that can respond to organ motion. Therefore, the role of RT for GBC is expected to significantly change in the future.

References

1. Macdonald OK, Crane CH. Palliative and postoperative radiotherapy in biliary tract cancer. Surg Oncol Clin N Am. 2002;11:941–54.
2. Verma V, Surkar SM, Brooks ED, Simone CB II, Lin C. Chemoradiotherapy versus chemotherapy alone for unresected nonmetastatic gallbladder cancer: national practice patterns and outcomes. J Natl Compr Canc Netw. 2018;16:59–65.
3. Jaffray DA, Langen KM, Mageras G. Safety consideration for IGRT: executive summery. Pract Radiat Oncol. 2018;3(3):167–70.
4. Houry S, Barrier A, Huguer M. Irradiation therapy for gallbladder carcinoma: recent advances. J Hepatobiliary Pancreat Surg. 2001;8:518–24.
5. Engineer R, Wadasadawala T, Mehta S, Mahantshetty U, Purandare N, Rangarajan V, et al. Chemoradiation for unresectable gall bladder cancer: time to review historic nihilism? J Gastrointest Canc. 2011;42:222–7.
6. Crane CH, Macdonald KO, Vauthey JN, Yehuda P, Brown T, Curley S, et al. Limitation of conventional doses of chemoradiation for unresectable biliary cancer. Int Radiat Oncol Biol Phys. 2002;53:969–74.
7. Tao R, Krishnan S, Bhosale PR, Javle MM, Aloia TA, Shroff RT, et al. Ablative radiotherapy doses lead to a substantial prolongation of survival in patients with inoperable intrahepatic cholangiocarcinoma: a retrospective dose response analysis. J Clin Oncol. 2016;34:219–26.
8. Pan CC, Kavanagh BD, Dawson LA, Li XA, Das SK, Miften M, et al. Radiation-associated liver injury. J Radiat Oncol Biol Phys. 2010;76(3 Suppl):S94–100.
9. Glazer ES, Liu P, Abdalla EK, Vauthey JN, Curley SA. Neither neoadjuvant nor adjuvant therapy increases survival after biliary tract cancer resection with wide negative margins. J Gastrointerest Surg. 2012;16:1666–71.
10. Park HS, Lim JY, Yoon DS, Park JS, Lee DK, Lee SJ, et al. Outcome of adjuvant therapy for gallbladder cancer. Oncology. 2010;79:168–73.
11. Ben-Joseph E, Guthrie KA, El-Khoueiry AB, Corless CL, Zaluoski MM, Lowy AM, et al. SWOG S0809: a phase II intergroup trial of adjuvant capecitabine and gemcitabine followed by radiotherapy and concurrent capecitabine in extrahepatic cholangiocarcinoma and gallbladder carcinoma. J Clin Oncol. 2015;33(24):2617–22.
12. Kim Y, Amini N, Wilson A, Margonis GA, Ethun CG, Poultsides G, et al. Impact of chemotherapy and external beam radiation therapy on outcomes among patients with resected gallbladder cancer: a multi-institutional analysis. Ann Surg Oncol. 2016;23:2998–3008.
13. Mantripragada KC, Hamid F, Shafqat H, Olszewski AJ. Adjuvant therapy for resected gallbladder cancer: analysis of the national cancer data base. J Natl Cancer Inst. 2017;109:djw202.
14. Gold DG, Miller RC, Haddock MG, Gunderson LL, Quevedo F, Donohue JH, et al. Adjuvant therapy for gallbladder carcinoma: the Mayo clinic experience. Int J Radiat Oncol Biol Phys. 2009;75:150–5.
15. Kim BH, Kwon J, Chie EK, Kim K, Kim YH, Seo DW, et al. Adjuvant chemoradiotherapy is associated with improved survival for patients with resected gallbladder carcinoma: a systematic review and meta-analysis. Ann Surg Oncol. 2018;25:255–64.
16. Kim GT. Patterns of initial failure after resection for gallbladder cancer: implications for adjuvant radiotherapy. Radiat Oncol J. 2017;35:359–67.
17. Wang SJ, Lemieux A, Kalpathy-Cramer J, Ord CB, Walker GV, Fuller CD, et al. Nomogram for predicting the benefit of adjuvant chemoradiotherapy for resected gallbladder cancer. J Clin Oncol. 2011;29(35):4627–32.
18. Bentzen SM, Constine LS, Deasy JO, Eisbruch A, Jackson A, Marks LB, et al. Quantitative analyses of normal tissue effects in the clinic (QUANEC): an introduction to the scientific issues. Int J Radiat Oncol Biol Phys. 2010;76(3 Suppl):S3–9.
19. International Commission on Radiation Units and Measurements (ICRU) Report 50, Prescribing, Recording and Reporting Photon Beam Therapy. Bethesda, ICRU Publications, 1993.
20. International Commission on Radiation Units and Measurements (ICRU) Report 62, Prescribing, Recording and Reporting Photon Beam Therapy (Supplement to ICRU Report 50). Bethesda, ICRU Publications, 1999.
21. Bryan PJ, Custar S, Haaga JR, Balsara V. Respiratory movement of the pancreas: an ultrasonic study. J Ultrasound Med. 1984;3(7):317–20.
22. Suramo I, Paivansalo M, Myllyla V. Cranio-caudal movements of the liver, pancreas and kidneys in respiration. Acta Radiol Diagn. 1984;25(2):129–31.
23. Gierga DP, Chen GT, Kung JH, Betke M, Lombardi J, Willett CG. Quantification of respiration-induced abdominal tumor motion and its impact on IMRT dose distributions. Int J Radiat Oncol Biol Phys. 2004;58(5):1584–95.

24. Bussels B, Goethals L, Feron M, Bielen D, Dymarkowski S, Suetens P, et al. Respiration-induced movement of the upper abdominal organs: a pitfall for the three-dimensional conformal radiation treatment of pancreatic cancer. Radiother Oncol. 2003;68(1):69–74.
25. Feng M, Balter JM, Normolle D, Adusumilli S, Cao Y, Chenevert TL, et al. Characterization of pancreatic tumor motion using cine MRI: surrogates for tumor position should be used with caution. Int J Radiat Oncol Biol Phys. 2009;74(3):884–91.
26. Shiinoki T, Shibuya K, Nakamura M, Nakamura A, Matsuo Y, Nakata M, et al. Interfractional reproducibility in pancreatic position based on four-dimensional computed tomography. Int J Radiat Oncol Biol Phys. 2011;80(5):1567–72.
27. Langen KM, Jones DT. Organ motion and its management. Int J Radiat Oncol Biol Phys. 2002;50(1):265–78.
28. Ge J, Santanam L, Noel C, Parikh PJ. Planning 4-dimensional computed tomography (4DCT) cannot adequately represent daily intrafractional motion of abdominal tumors. Int J Radiat Oncol Biol Phys. 2013;85:999–1005.
29. Bortfeld T, Jokivarsi K, Goitein M, Kung J, Jiang SB. Effects of intra-fraction motion on IMRT dose delivery: statistical analysis and simulation. Phys Med Biol. 2002;47:2203–20.
30. Dawson LA, Brock KK, Kazanjian S, Fitch D, McGinn CJ, Lawrence TS, et al. The reproducibility of organ position using active breathing control (ABC) during liver radiotherapy. Int J Radiat Oncol Biol Phys. 2001;51(5):1410–21.
31. Shirato H, Shimizu S, Shimizu T, Nishioka T, Miyasaka K. Real-time tumor-tracking radiotherapy. Lancet. 1999;353(9161):1331–2.
32. Hanazawa H, Takahashi S, Shiinoki T, Park SC, Yuasa Y, Koike M, et al. Clinical assessment of coiled fiducial markers as internal surrogates for hepatocellular carcinomas during gated stereotactic body radiotherapy with a real-time tumor-tracking system. Radiother Oncol. 2017;123:43–8.
33. Kamino Y, Takayama K, Kokubo M, Narita Y, Hirai E, Kawawda N, et al. Development of a four-dimensional image-guided radiotherapy system with a gimbaled X-ray head. Int Radiat Oncol Biol Phys. 2006;66:271–8.
34. Iizuka Y, Matsuo Y, Ishihara Y, Akimoto M, Tanabe H, Takayama K, et al. Dynamic tumor-tracking radiotherapy with real-time monitoring for liver tumors using a gimbal mounted linac. Radiother Oncol. 2015;117:496–500.
35. Shiinoki T, Kawamura S, Uehara T, Yuasa Y, Kamomae T, Kotakebayashi T, et al. Quality assurance for respiratory-gated radiotherapy using the real-time tumor-tracking radiotherapy system. Int J Med Phys Clin Eng Radiat Oncol. 2014;3(3):125–32.

Patterns of Recurrence and Its Effective Treatment

Junji Furuse

Introduction

Gallbladder cancer is classified in biliary tract cancer, which also includes biliary duct and ampulla of Vater cancers. Most of gallbladder cancer is pathologically classified to adenocarcinoma. In the Japan national survey, tumor stage of gallbladder cancer was classified Stage I (19.8%), Stage II (29.4%), Stage IIIA (13.8%), Stage IIIB (14.4%), and Stage IVA (3.9%). Stage IVB (18.6%), by the classification of biliary tract cancers Japanese Society of Hepato-Biliary-Pancreatic Surgery: 3rd English edition [1, 2]. Thus, more than 20% patients with gallbladder cancer are diagnosed as advanced stage of Stage IVA, locally advanced disease (T4) with tumor invasion to the celiac axis, common hepatic artery, or superior mesenteric artery, or Stage IVB, metastatic disease. The prognosis in patients with advanced gallbladder cancer is still poor, especially the 5-year survival rate in stage IV is less than 10% [1].

While surgery remains the only potentially curative treatment, the curative resection rate remains low. Most patients, furthermore, develop recurrence even after curative surgery. Therefore, it is required to establish effective systemic treatments including chemotherapy to improve the prognosis.

Patterns of Metastases and Recurrence of Gallbladder Cancer

Spread patterns of gallbladder cancer was classified as (1) lymphatic, (2) vascular, (3) intraperitoneal seeding, (4) neural, (5) intraductal, or (6) by direct extension [3]. Barreto et al. [4] reported the spread patterns in patients who underwent re-resection for incidental gallbladder cancer. 127 of 163 patients underwent successful radical re-resection for incidental gallbladder cancer detected by cholecystectomy. The remaining 36 patients had evidence of metastatic disease, 21 (58%) of peritoneal or omental deposits (peritoneal seeding), 13 (36%) of extensive lymph node, 8 (22%) of extensive local liver infiltration (direct extension), 7 (19%) of distant liver metastases plus port-site invasion due to liver metastases (vascular).

In a phase III trial of systemic chemotherapy comparing gemcitabine (GEM) plus S-1 with GEM plus cisplatin conducted by Japan Clinical Oncology Group (JCOG), lymph nodes, liver, and peritoneum were identified as major metastatic sites of gallbladder cancer (unpublished data). Although there are some differences in spread patterns by primary tumor sites,

J. Furuse (✉)
Department of Medical Oncology,
Kyorin University Faculty of Medicine, 6-20-2,
Shinkawa, Mitaka-Shi, Tokyo 181-8611, Japan
e-mail: jfuruse@ks.kyorin-u.ac.jp

J. B. Chung and K. Okazaki (eds.), *Diseases of the Gallbladder*,
https://doi.org/10.1007/978-981-15-6010-1_23

lymphatic, liver via vascular, and peritoneal seeding are major metastatic ways in biliary tract cancer (Table 1).

Treatment Strategy for Metastatic Disease and Recurrence

Chemotherapy and/or radiotherapy are applied to unresectable diseases including metastatic disease and recurrence of gallbladder cancer, according to tumor condition. To assess the efficacy of chemotherapy in patients with advanced biliary tract cancer, some small randomized controlled trials (RCTs) comparing it with supportive treatment alone have been conducted (Table 2) [5–7]. Glimelius et al. reported a comparative study between chemotherapy and supportive care in patients with unresectable pancreatic cancer and biliary tract cancer. As a result, chemotherapy using fluorouracil (FU) plus leucovorin or FU plus leucovorin plus etoposide demonstrated the prolongation of survival was compared with supportive care group [5]. In only the patients with biliary tract cancer, no significant difference in survival between the two groups was noted, due to the small number of patients (n=37), and the survival in the two groups was similar (6.5 months in the chemotherapy group and 2.5 months in the supportive care group; P=0.1). Sharma et al. [7] conducted a comparative study of GEM plus oxaliplatin (GEMOX) or FU/folinic acid (FA), comparing with the best supportive care in patients with unresectable gallbladder cancer. The GEMOX yielded statistically significantly higher response rate, progression-free survival, and overall survival as compared with both FU/FA chemotherapy and best supportive care.

Table 1 Metastatic sites in patients with unresectable biliary tract cancer who were enrolled in the JCOG 1113 study

	Intrahepatic (n=80)	Hilar (n=42)	Distal (n=19)	Gallbladder (n=125)	Ampulla (n=10)
With metastasis	61	18	17	107	10
Metastatic site					
Liver	–	8 (44.4%)	6 (35.3%)	51 (47.7%)	5 (50%)
Lymph nodes	49 (80.3%)	11 (55.6%)	11 (64.7%)	75 (70.1%)	6 (60%)
Lung	12 (19.7%)	1 (5.6%)	4 (23.5%)	12 (11.2%)	0
Peritoneum	17 (27.9%)	3 (16.7%)	1 (5.9%)	25 (23.4%)	1 (10%)
Others	13 (21.3%)	1 (5.6%)	2 (11.8%)	9 (8.4%)	0

JCOG, Japan Clinical Oncology Group

Table 2 Randomized controlled trials between chemotherapy and supportive care in patients with unresectable biliary tract cancer

	n	Median OS	P-value	Author (year)
FU/leucovorin or FU/leucovorin/etoposide	47	6.0 months	<0.01	Glimelius (1996) [5]
Supportive care	43	2.5 months		
FU/doxorubicin/mitomycin C	42	4.96 months	0.283	Takada (1998) [6]
Control	41	4.7 months		
Gemcitabine/oxaliplatin	27[a]	9.5 months	0.039	Sharma (2010) [7]
FU/folinic acid	28[a]	4.6 months		
Best supportive care	27[a]	4.5 months		

OS, overall survival; FU, fluorouracil
[a]only patients with gallbladder cancer

On the other hand, some clinical trials using chemoradiotherapy or radiotherapy have conducted, but the efficacy of radiotherapy or chemoradiotherapy has not been confirmed, compared with chemotherapy alone. Phelip et al. [8] reported that chemotherapy using GEMOX demonstrated better progression-free survival (PFS) and overall survival (OS) in patients with locally advanced biliary tract cancer including gallbladder cancer, compared with chemoradiotherapy in a small randomized phase II study; the median PFS and OS were 11.0 months and 19.9 months in chemotherapy arm and 5.0 months and 13.5 months in chemoradiotherapy arm, respectively. Pollom et al. [9] reported that no difference in OS in patients with unresectable biliary tract cancer by radiotherapy was shown in evaluation using the SEER-Medicare database; the median OS was 10.0 months in radiotherapy group and 9.3 months in non-radiotherapy group. Thus, to date, the role of radiation therapy remains unclear in the treatment of locally advanced but non-metastatic biliary tract cancer including gallbladder cancer [10].

Thus, chemotherapy demonstrated the prolongation of survival in patients with unresectable biliary tract cancer, some guidelines recommended systemic chemotherapy as the first treatment of choice for unresectable biliary tract cancer [10–12].

Chemotherapy for Gallbladder Cancer

Although chemotherapy achieves the prolongation of the survival compared with supportive care, no standard chemotherapy was not established until a phase III trial comparing GEM plus cisplatin with GEM alone (ABC-02) demonstrated statistically significant longer survival. A randomized phase II and phase III trials (ABC-01, 02) comparing gemcitabine alone with gemcitabine plus cisplatin were conducted in the UK. The ABC-01 demonstrated superior 6-month progression-free survival (57.1% versus 45.5%) with acceptable toxicity in the gemcitabine 1000 mg/m^2 plus cisplatin 25 mg/m^2 group as compared with that in the gemcitabine 1000 mg/m^2-alone group [13]. Furthermore, the ABC-02 revealed a statistically significant improvement in the overall survival in the gemcitabine plus cisplatin group as compared with that in the gemcitabine-alone group (Table 3) [14]. The BT22 trial was conducted in parallel with the ABC-02 in Japan, and similar results to those of the ABC-02 were demonstrated in Japanese patients with biliary tract cancer (Table 3) [15]. Thus, chemotherapy using GEM plus cisplatin (GC therapy) has been recognized as a standard of care for unresectable biliary tract cancer.

Biliary tract cancer includes cholangiocarcinoma, gallbladder cancer, and ampullary cancer, and it was often controversial whether the efficacy of chemotherapy was different by primary tumor site in biliary tract cancer. A meta-analysis of two randomized trials of individual patient-level data, the ABC-02 and BT22 to confirm the efficacy of the GC therapy and carried out exploratory subgroup analyses. As a result, GC therapy resulted in improved PFS and OS for intra- and extra-hepatic cholangiocarcinomas, gallbladder cancer, and ampullary cancer [16].

Although various combinations of chemotherapy with GC therapy or GEMOX have been investigated, no regimen demonstrated survival benefits over GC therapy or GEMOX until recent phase III trials reported from Japan (Table 3). Two-phase IIII trials have demonstrated to meet the primary endpoint of overall survival in patients with unresectable biliary tract cancer. The FUGA trial (JCOG1113), which compared GEM plus S-1 (GS therapy) with the GC therapy, demonstrated non-inferiority of the GS therapy to the GC therapy in OS [23]. The MITSUBA trial (KHBO1401), which compared S-1 addition on the GC therapy regimen (GCS therapy) with the GC therapy, demonstrated superiority of the GCS therapy to the GC therapy in OS [24]. Thus, The GS and GCS therapies are also alternative treatment options for unresectable biliary tract cancer in Japan.

Since most patients who received the first-line chemotherapy of GC therapy have disease progression, development of a second-line

Table 3 Randomized controlled trials of chemotherapy for unresectable biliary tract cancer

Regimen	n	Response rate (%)	Median PFS	Median OS	Hazard ratio (95% CI)	p-value	Author (year)
Gemcitabine	44	22.6	4.0 months	–	–	–	Valle et al. (2010) [13]
Gemcitabine/cisplatin	42	27.8	8.0 months	–	–		
Gemcitabine	206	15.5	5.0 months	8.1 months	0.64 (0.52–0.80)	<0.001	Valle et al. (2010) [14]
Gemcitabine/cisplatin	204	26.1	8.0 months	11.7 months			
Gemcitabine	42	11.9	3.7 months	7.7 months	0.69 (0.42–1.13)	–	Okusaka et al. (2010) [15]
Gemcitabine/cisplatin	41	19.5	5.8 months	11.2 months			
Gemcitabine/oxaliplatin	133	16	4.2 months	9.5 months	0.93 (0.69–1.25)	0.611	Lee et al. (2012) [17]
Gemcitabine/oxaliplatin/erlotinib	135	30	5.8 months	9.5 months			
S-1	50	17.4	4.2 months	9.0 months	0.859 (0.543–1.360)	0.52	Morizane et al. (2013) [18]
Gemcitabine/S-1	51	36.4	7.1 months	12.5 months			
Gemcitabine/oxaliplatin	74	23	5.5 months	12.4 months	–	–	Malka et al. (2014) [19]
Gemcitabine/oxaliplatin/cetuximab	76	24	6.1 months	11.0 months			
Gemcitabine/oxaliplatin	60	15	4.1 months	9.8 months	–	0.91	Chen et al. (2013) [20]
Gemcitabine/oxaliplatin/cetuximab	62	27	6.7 months	10.6 months			
Gemcitabine/cisplatin	62	19	7.4 months	11.9 months	0.86 (0.58–1.27)	0.44	Valle et al. (2015) [21]
Gemcitabine/cisplatin/cediranib	62	44	8.0 months	14.1 months			
Gemcitabine/oxaliplatin	44	18.2	4.4 months	10.2 months	0.83 (0.53–1.3)	0.42	Leone et al. (2016) [22]
Gemcitabine/oxaliplatin/panitumumab	45	26.7	5.3 months	9.9 months			
Gemcitabine/cisplatin	175	32.4	5.8 months	13.4 months	0.95 (0.78–1.15)[a]	0.046[b]	Morizane et al. (2019) [23]
Gemcitabine/S-1	179	29.8	6.8 months	15.1 months			
Gemcitabine/cisplatin	123	15.0	5.5 months	12.6 months	0.791 (0.628–0.996)[a]	0.046	Sakai et al. (2018) [24]
Gemcitabine/cisplatin/S-1	123	41.5	7.4 months	13.5 months			

PFS, progression-free survival; OS, overall survival; CI, confidence interval
[a]90%CI; [b]non-inferiority

Part IV Current issues

IV-1 Polypoid lesions and wall thickening of the gallbladder therapy would be explored to improve the survival in patients with unresectable biliary tract cancer. To date, however, no standard of second-line therapy has been established. Le et al. [25] reported solid tumors with mismatch repair deficiency were sensitive to immune checkpoint blockade with antibodies to programmed death receptor–1 (PD-1). Pembrolizumab, anti-PD-1 blockade, is approved to solid tumors with mismatch repair deficiency, including biliary tract cancer. It is recommended that mismatch repair or microsatellite instability testing should be performed on tumor tissue [12], and it may be done during the first-line chemotherapy.

Future Perspectives

GEM-based therapy has been established as a standard of care for unresectable biliary tract cancer, including gallbladder cancer. However, very limited number of agents are available for biliary tract cancer, and various challenges are under investigation to develop new promising agents to improve the survival. One is to identify targeted driver mutations or overexpression of biomarkers by multiplex diagnosis using next-generation sequencing (NGS). the Food and Drug Administration has approved two tests, FoundationOne® CDx genome profiling test and MSK-IMPACT Tumor Profiling Test, to identify genetic alterations in tumors. FoundationOne® CDx and OncoGuide™ NCC Oncopanel system have also been approved as genome profiling test in Japan. Some clinically relevant and/or potentially targetable mutations or abnormal expression of molecular targets are identified in biliary tract cancer, and there are some differences in expression of biomarkers by primary tumor site of biliary tract [26, 27]. Some clinical trials of agents targeting specific biomarker using the NGS are under ongoing for biliary tract cancer including gallbladder cancer, such as HER2/neu overexpression and fibroblast growth factor receptor 2 (FGFR2) gene rearrangement.

Immune checkpoint inhibitors have recently been demonstrated to prolong the survival in patients with various advanced cancers. Two types of immune checkpoint inhibitors, namely, anti-cytotoxic T-lymphocyte-associated protein 4 (CTLA-4) antibody and anti-programmed cell death (PD)-1 or PD ligand 1 (PD-L1) antibody, have been developed and been administered as monotherapy or combination therapy. Nivolumab, anti-PD-1 antibody, was investigated as monotherapy in patients previously treated with GEM-based chemotherapy in monotherapy cohort, and in combined therapy cohort with the GC therapy in the first-line in biliary tract cancer; 30 patients were treated in each cohort. Only one patient had response to nivolumab in the monotherapy cohort, but the patient had Lynch syndrome, which is characterized by high microsatellite instability status. The objective response rate was 37%, median PFS was 4.2 months, and median OS was 15.4 months in the combined therapy cohort [28]. Analysis of PD-L1 expression in tumor or tumor-associated immune cells suggested a possible relationship between PD-1 expression and response to anti-PD-1 antibody treatment in patients with advanced biliary tract cancer. Various clinical trials of anti-PD-1 or PD-L1 antibodies are currently under ongoing in biliary tract cancer.

While biliary tract cancer is a common cause of cancer-related death in Asia, including Japan, and Latin America, it is relatively rare cancer type in Western countries. Furthermore, gallbladder cancer is a small patient number, and it is difficult to conduct a clinical trial limited in gallbladder cancer. In development of systemic therapy for biliary tract cancer, clinical trials have been conducted for all primary tumor sites of biliary tract. In the era of precision medicine, it would be appropriate to conduct a clinical trial according to expression of biomarker such as gene mutation or rearrangement. And it is required to conduct a clinical trial in global collaboration.

Acknowledgements The data in Table 1 is provided by the Japan Clinical Oncology Group (JCOG). I am grateful to the members of the Hepatobiliary and Pancreatic Oncology Group and the Data Center of the JCOG.

References

1. Ishihara S, Horiguchi A, Miyakawa S, Endo I, Miyazaki M, Takada T. Biliary tract cancer registry in Japan from 2008 to 2013. J Hepatobiliary Pancreat Sci. 2016;23(3):149–57.
2. Miyazaki M, Ohtsuka M, Miyakawa S, Nagino M, Yamamoto M, Kokudo N, et al. Classification of biliary tract cancers established by the Japanese Society of Hepato-Biliary-Pancreatic Surgery: 3rd English edition. J Hepatobiliary Pancreat Sci. 2015;22(3):181-96.
3. Fahim RB, Mc DJ, Richards JC, Ferris DO. Carcinoma of the gallbladder: a study of its modes of spread. Ann Surg. 1962;156:114–24.
4. Barreto SG, Pawar S, Shah S, Talole S, Goel M, Shrikhande SV. Patterns of failure and determinants of outcomes following radical re-resection for incidental gallbladder cancer. World J Surg. 2014;38(2):484–9.
5. Glimelius B, Hoffman K, Sjödén PO, Jacobsson G, Sellström H, Enander LK, et al. Chemotherapy improves survival and quality of life in advanced pancreatic and biliary cancer. Ann Oncol. 1996;7:593–600.
6. Takada T, Nimura Y, Katoh H, Nagakawa T, Nakayama T, Matsushiro T, et al. Prospective randomized trial of 5-fluorouracil, doxorubicin, and mitomycin C for non-resectable pancreatic and biliary carcinoma: multicenter randomized trial. Hepatogastroenterology. 1998;45:2020–6.
7. Sharma A, Dwary AD, Mohanti BK, Deo SV, Pal S, Sreenivas V, et al. Best supportive care compared with chemotherapy for unresectable gall bladder cancer: a randomized controlled study. J Clin Oncol. 2010;28(30):4581–6.
8. Phelip JM, Vendrely V, Rostain F, Subtil F, Jouve JL, Gasmi M, et al. Gemcitabine plus cisplatin versus chemoradiotherapy in locally advanced biliary tract cancer: Fédération Francophone de Cancérologie Digestive 9902 phase II randomised study. Eur J Cancer. 2014;50(17):2975–82.
9. Pollom EL, Alagappan M, Park LS, Whittemore AS, Koong AC, Chang DT. Does radiotherapy still have a role in unresected biliary tract cancer? Cancer Med. 2017;6(1):129–41.
10. Valle JW, Borbath I, Khan SA, Huguet F, Gruenberger T, Arnold D. ESMO Guidelines Committee. Biliary cancer: ESMO Clinical Practice Guidelines for diagnosis, treatment and follow-up. Ann Oncol. 2016;27(suppl 5):v28-v37.
11. Miyazaki M, Yoshitomi H, Miyakawa S, Uesaka K, Unno M, Endo I,et al. Clinical practice guidelines for the management of biliary tract cancers 2015: the 2nd English edition. J Hepatobiliary Pancreat Sci. 2015;22(4):249–73.
12. NCCN Clinical Practice Guidelines in Oncology. Hepatobiliary Cancers. Veron 3. 2019. https://www.nccn.org/professionals/physician_gls/pdf/hepatobiliary.pdf.
13. Valle JW, Wasan H, Johnson P, Jones E, Dixon L, Swindell R, et al. Gemcitabine alone or in combination with cisplatin in patients with advanced or metastatic cholangiocarcinomas or other biliary tract tumours: a multicentre randomised phase II study - The UK ABC-01 Study. Br J Cancer. 2009;101(4):621–7.
14. Valle J, Wasan H, Palmer DH, Cunningham D, Anthoney A, Maraveyas A, et al. ABC-02 Trial Investigators. Cisplatin plus gemcitabine versus gemcitabine for biliary tract cancer. N Engl J Med. 2010;362(14):1273–81.
15. Okusaka T, Nakachi K, Fukutomi A, Mizuno N, Ohkawa S, Funakoshi A, et al. Gemcitabine alone or in combination with cisplatin in patients with biliary tract cancer: a comparative multicentre study in Japan. Br J Cancer. 2010;103(4):469–74.
16. Valle JW, Furuse J, Jitlal M, Beare S, Mizuno N, Wasan H, et al. Cisplatin and gemcitabine for advanced biliary tract cancer: a meta-analysis of two randomised trials. Ann Oncol. 2014;25(2):391–8.
17. Lee J, Park SH, Chang HM, Kim JS, Choi HJ, Lee MA, et al. Gemcitabine and oxaliplatin with or without erlotinib in advanced biliary-tract cancer: a multicentre, open-label, randomised, phase 3 study. Lancet Oncol. 2012;13(2):181–8.
18. Morizane C, Okusaka T, Mizusawa J, Takashima A, Ueno M, Ikeda M, et al. Randomized phase II study of gemcitabine plus S-1 versus S-1 in advanced biliary tract cancer: a Japan Clinical Oncology Group trial (JCOG 0805). Cancer Sci. 2013;104(9):1211–6.
19. Malka D, Cervera P, Foulon S, Trarbach T, de la Fouchardière C, Boucher E, et al. BINGO investigators. Gemcitabine and oxaliplatin with or without cetuximab in advanced biliary-tract cancer (BINGO): a randomised, open-label, non-comparative phase 2 trial. Lancet Oncol. 2014;15(8):819–28.
20. Chen JS, Hsu C, Chiang NJ, Tsai CS, Tsou HH, Huang SF, et al. Taiwan Cooperative Oncology Group. A KRAS mutation status-stratified randomized phase II trial of gemcitabine and oxaliplatin alone or in combination with cetuximab in advanced biliary tract cancer. Ann Oncol. 2015;26(5):943–9.
21. Valle JW, Wasan H, Lopes A, Backen AC, Palmer DH, Morris K, et al. Cediranib or placebo in combination with cisplatin and gemcitabine chemotherapy for patients with advanced biliary tract cancer (ABC-03): a randomised phase 2 trial. Lancet Oncol. 2015;16(8):967–78.

22. Leone F, Marino D, Cereda S, Filippi R, Belli C, Spadi R, et al. Panitumumab in combination with gemcitabine and oxaliplatin does not prolong survival in wild-type KRAS advanced biliary tract cancer: A randomized phase 2 trial (Vecti-BIL study). Cancer. 2016;122(4):574–81.
23. Morizane C, Okusaka T, Mizusawa J, Katayama H, Ueno M, Ikeda M, et al.Combination gemcitabine plus S-1 versus gemcitabine plus cisplatin for advanced/recurrent biliary tract cancer: The FUGA-BT (JCOG1113) Randomized phase IIIclinical trial. Ann Oncol 2019;30(12):1950–8.
24. Sakai D, Kanai M, Kobayashi S, Eguchi H, Baba H, Seol S, et al: Randomized phase III study of gemcitabine, cisplatin plus S-1 (GCS) versus gemcitabine, cisplatin (GC) for advanced biliary tract cancer (KHBO1401-MITSUBA). 2018 ESMO annual meeting. #6150.
25. Le DT, Durham JN, Smith KN, Wang H, Bartlett BR, Aulakh LK, et al. Mismatch repair deficiency predicts response of solid tumors to PD-1 blockade. Science. 2017;357(6349):409–13.
26. Lee H, Ross JS. The potential role of comprehensive genomic profiling to guide targeted therapy for patients with biliary cancer. Therap Adv Gastroenterol. 2017;10(6):507–20.
27. Morizane C, Ueno M, Ikeda M, Okusaka T, Ishii H, Furuse J. New developments in systemic therapy for advanced biliary tract cancer. Jpn J Clin Oncol. 2018;48(8):703–11.
28. Ueno M, Ikeda M, Morizane C, Kobayashi S, Ohno I, Kondo S, et al. Nivolumab alone or in combination with cisplatin plus gemcitabine in Japanese patients with unresectable or recurrent biliary tract cancer: a non-randomised, multicentre, open-label, phase 1 study. Lancet Gastroenterol Hepatol. 2019;4(8):611–21.

Current Issues: Polypoid Lesions and Wall Thickening of the Gallbladder

Differential Diagnosis of Benign and Malignant Lesions with Imaging

Yong Eun Chung

Introduction

With the exception of advanced gallbladder cancer, the differential diagnosis of gallbladder lesions is still considered challenging. However, differentiating benign polypoid lesions from neoplastic lesions is essential. Although the incidence of benign polypoid lesions is much higher than neoplastic lesions, especially for smaller lesions less than 1.0 ~ 1.5 in size, neoplastic lesions have to be identified because gallbladder cancer has poor prognosis. In addition, when gallbladder wall thickening is present, benign lesions such as adenomyomatosis or xanthogranulomatous cholecystitis and early-stage gallbladder cancer should also be differentiated. The gallbladder is a superficially located organ that is rarely in the abdomen. Hence, US plays an important role in differential diagnosis along with MR and CT. This chapter discusses the types of diseases that require differential diagnosis and characteristic imaging findings of each.

Y. E. Chung (✉)
Department of Radiology, Yonsei University College of Medicine, Seoul, South Korea
e-mail: yelv2000@gmail.com

Differential Diagnosis of Polypoid Lesions in the Gallbladder

Gallbladder polypoid lesions can be defined as lesions that protrude into the gallbladder lumen [1]. Differential diagnoses of polypoid lesions include gallbladder stones, cholesterol polyps, adenomyomatosis, inflammatory polyps, adenomas, carcinomas in situ and other rare lesions such as leiomyomas, lipomas, neurofibromas, and carcinoids [2]. Definite mass-like lesions should be classified as gallbladder cancer rather than gallbladder polypoid lesions [1]. Cholesterol polyps, adenomyomatosis, and inflammatory polyps are also called pseudotumors or pseudopolyps [1, 2]. Cholesterol polyps account for two-thirds of the polypoid lesions in the gallbladder, while only about 4% of these lesions are adenomas (Table 1) [2].

Imaging for the Differential Diagnosis of Gallbladder Polypoid Lesions

Gallbladder stones can easily be differentiated from polyps when acoustic shadowing is observed in the posterior aspect of the lesion (Fig. 1). However, acoustic shadowing might not be seen in obese patients or when stones are deeply set in the gallbladder neck. [3]. In

J. B. Chung and K. Okazaki (eds.), *Diseases of the Gallbladder*,
https://doi.org/10.1007/978-981-15-6010-1_24

Table 1 Incidence of polypoid lesions in the gallbladder [2]

Cholesterol polyps	60%
Adenomyomatosis	25%
Inflammatory polyps	10%
Adenomas	4%
Rare miscellaneous polyps	1%

this case, changing the patient's position from supine to the left or right decubitus is helpful because stones usually move to the dependent part, while true polypoid lesions do not (Fig. 2). Using the ultrasound probe to induce abdominal movement can also nudge sticky stones or sludge balls to move that did not with just position change. Neoplastic polyps with stalks can also appear to move after position changes, so the radiologist needs to confirm that they have moved completely from their original position (Fig. 3)

With the exception of gallbladder stones, it is important to differentiate benign polypoid lesions and neoplastic lesions. This is because the incidence of gallbladder polyps is relatively

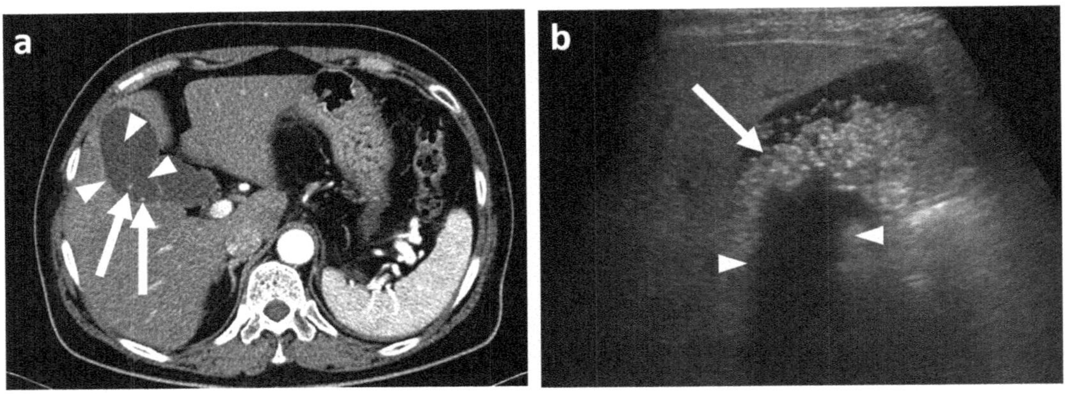

Fig. 1 Gallbladder stone and sludge. **a** On CT, several small high attenuating lesions are seen in the gallbladder (arrows). Iso- to slightly high attenuating material surrounds the gallbladder stone (arrowheads). **b** On US, sludge is noted in the gallbladder (arrow). Acoustic shadowing is also seen (arrowheads), which suggests combined gallbladder stones

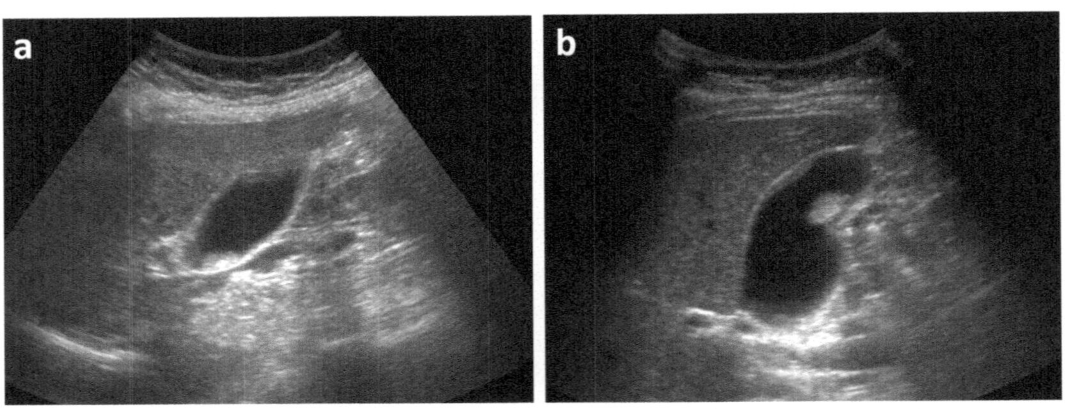

Fig. 2 Gallbladder stone without acoustic shadowing. **a** Stone was initially located around the GB neck. **b** After the patient changed from the supine position to the left decubitus, the stone moved to the fundus

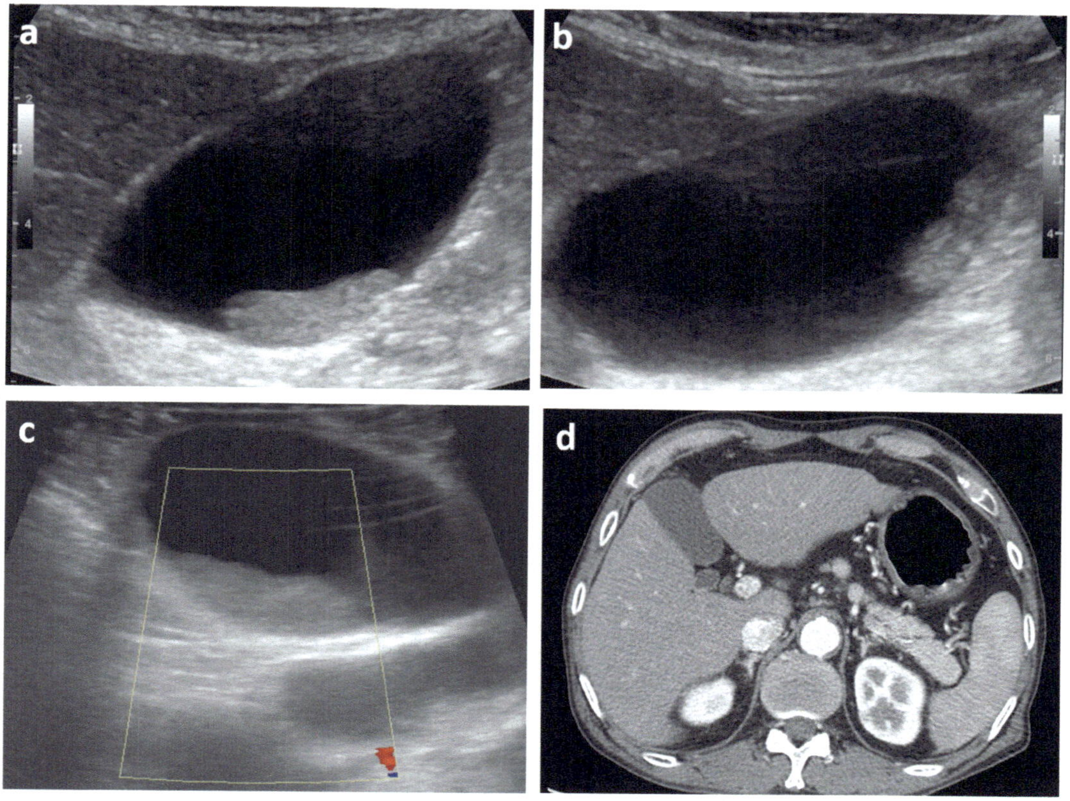

Fig. 3 Gallbladder adenoma. **a**, **b** After position change, the polypoid lesion appeared to move on US. **b** On Doppler US, no blood flow signal is observed within the lesion. **d** On CT, the polypoid lesion is not detected within the gallbladder. The first impression of this lesion was sludge or stone, but it was confirmed as adenoma after cholecystectomy

high at approximately 4–7% in healthy subjects [4, 5], and the prognosis for gallbladder malignancy is devastating. According to previous studies, risk factors for neoplastic polyps are larger lesion size (>10–15 mm), accompanying stones, single lesion, older age (>50 years old), sessile shape, rapid growth, and presence of associated symptoms [4, 6–13]. Based on these clinical parameters, most guidelines recommend cholecystectomy for gallbladder polyps with associated symptoms and those larger than 1 cm or more in size [1, 2, 14]. However, these criteria might not be sufficient to indicate cholecystectomy because approximately 50–70% of gallbladder polypoid lesions larger than 1.5 cm have been confirmed as benign [4]. Furthermore, past studies have found the incidence of some cancers including hepato-biliary, pancreatic, and colon cancer to increase after cholecystectomy [15–17], making the non-invasive diagnosis of gallbladder polyps increasingly more important as cholecystectomy might be avoided for benign polypoid lesions. US is usually used for the detection and differential diagnosis of gallbladder polypoid lesions. On US, cholesterol polyps may be high- to iso-echogenic compared to the most lateral layer of the gallbladder wall, and tiny hyperechogenic foci which represent cholesterol crystals (Fig. 4). Adenomyomatosis usually shows multiple microcysts which are Rokitansky–Aschoff sinuses in the thickened wall (Fig. 5). Comet tail artifacts on US or twinkling artifacts on Doppler US can accompany adenomyomatosis, whereas neoplastic

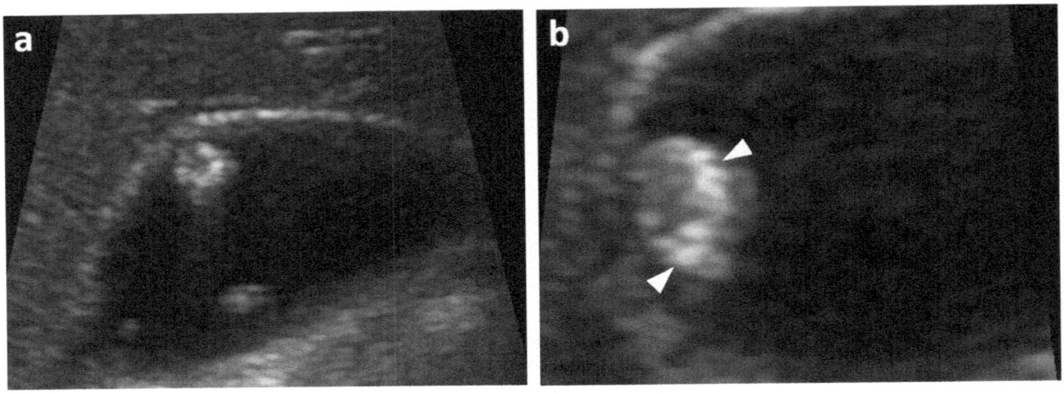

Fig. 4 Cholesterol polyp. **a**, **b** The echogenicity of the polyp is similar to the most lateral layer of the gallbladder wall. There are also multiple high echogenic foci within the polyp (arrowheads)

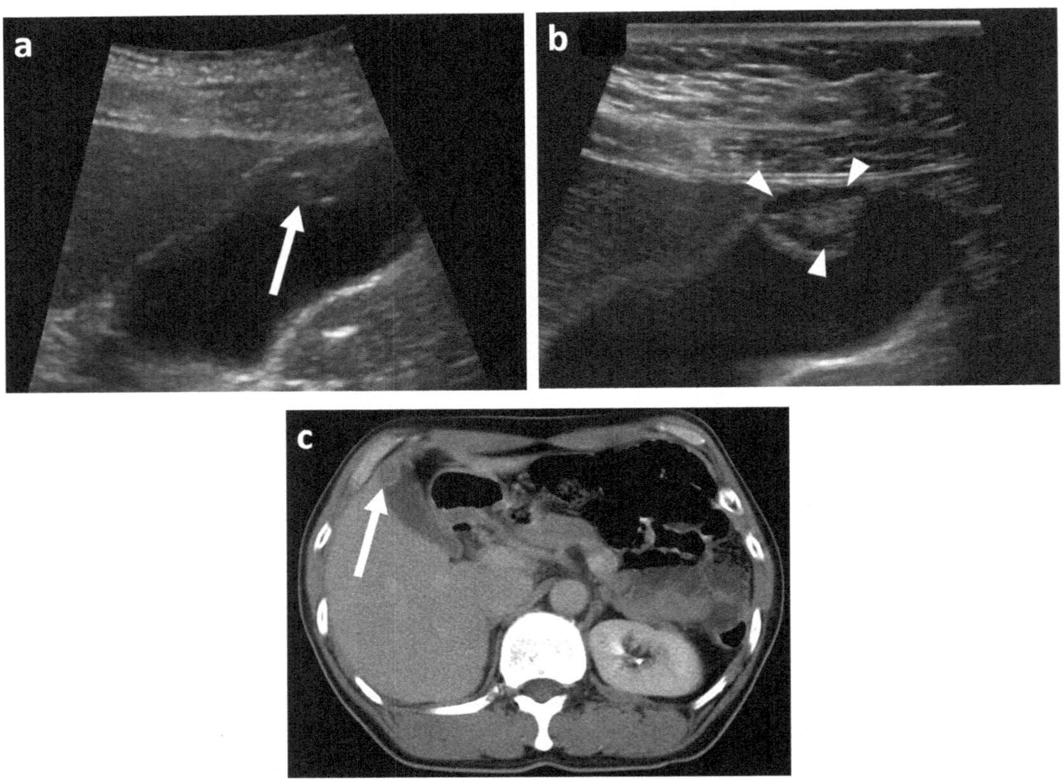

Fig. 5 Adenomyomatosis. **a** A polypoid lesion is noted in the gallbladder fundus (arrow). **b** Multiple microcysts which suggest Rokitansky–Aschoff sinuses are seen within the polypoid lesion. **c** On CT, an oval-shaped lesion is noted in the gallbladder fundus (arrow). This lesion was confirmed as adenomyomatosis

polyps show homogeneous hypo- to iso-echogenic internal echoes with nodular surfaces [18–20] (Figs. 6, 7 and 8). Traditionally, EUS has shown better diagnostic performance for the differentiation of benign and neoplastic polypoid lesions (sensitivity and specificity: 78–92%

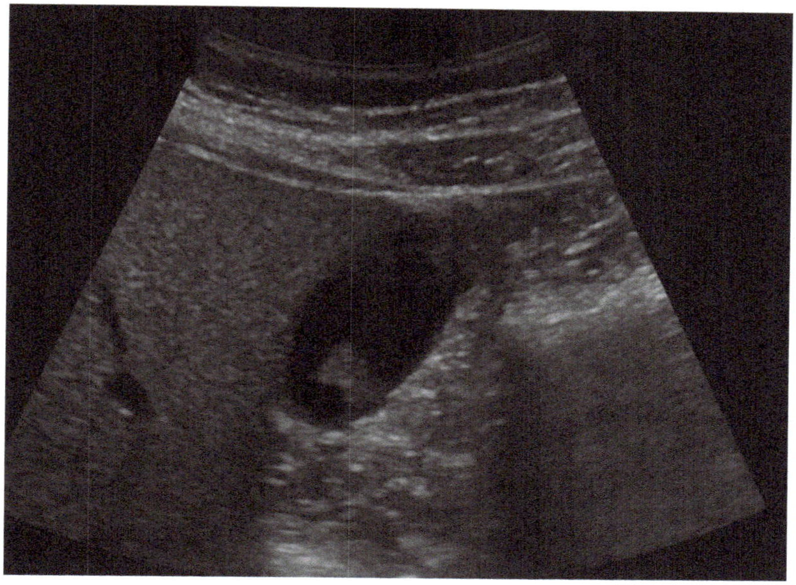

Fig. 6 Gallbladder adenoma. A low echogenic polypoid lesion is noted near the gallbladder neck

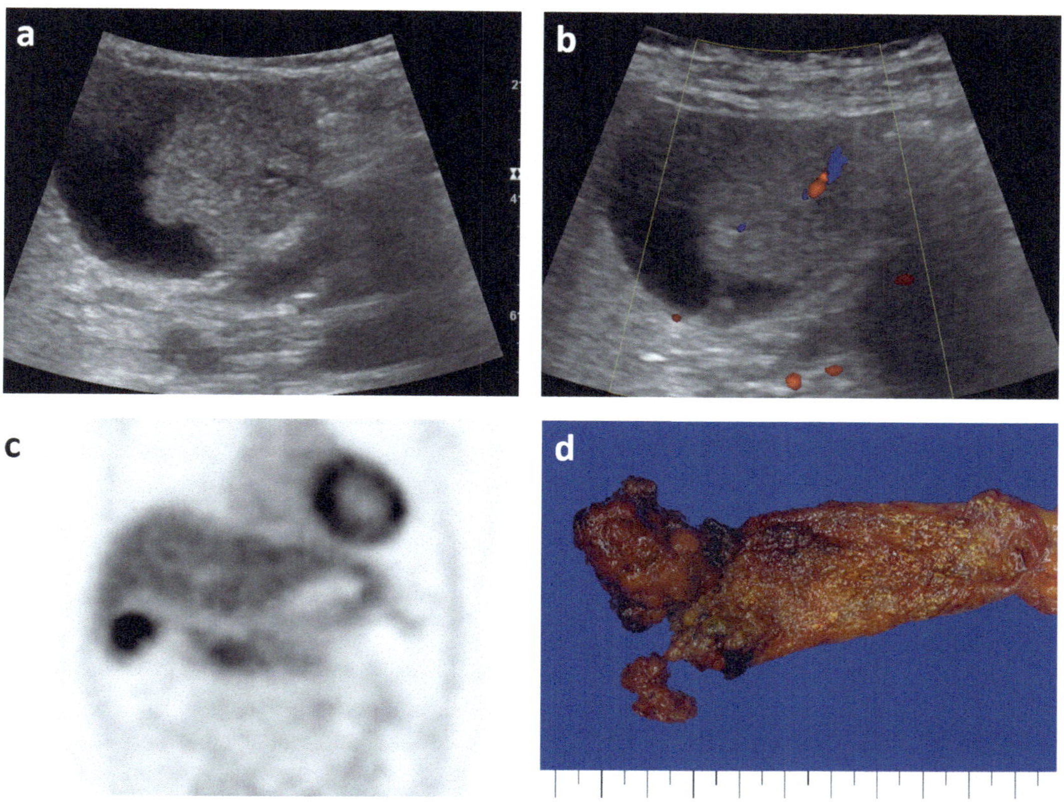

Fig. 7 Gallbladder cancer. **a** On US, a polypoid lesion is seen in the gallbladder. Gallbladder wall discontinuity is noted. **b** On Doppler US, a blood vessel is detected in the stalk. **c** On PET scan, increased 18F-FDG uptake can be observed in the polypoid lesion. **d** This lesion was confirmed as adenocarcinoma with invasion of the perimuscular connective tissue (T2)

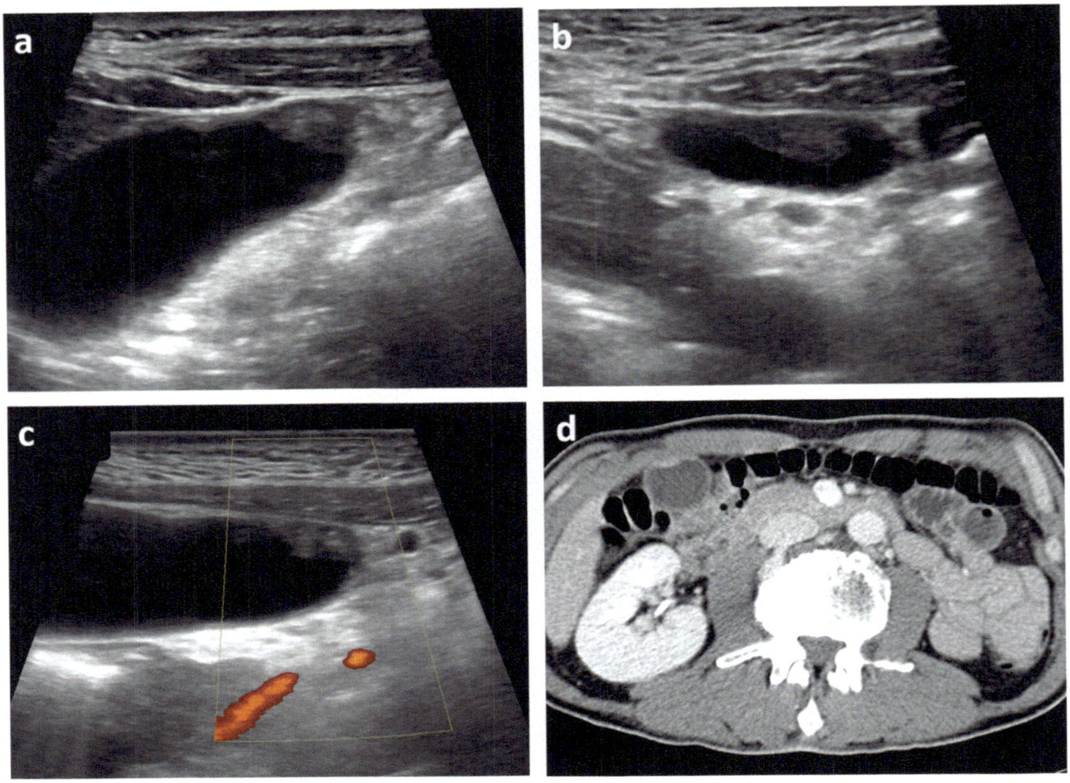

Fig. 8 Pyloric gland adenoma. **a**, **b** On US, focal wall thickening or a polypoid lesion is noted in the gallbladder fundus. Microcysts are not seen within the lesion. **c** On Doppler US, there is no blood flow or twinkling artifacts within the lesion. **d** On CT, focal wall thickening is noted in the gallbladder fundus. The initial impression was fundal adenomyomatosis, but the lesion was confirmed as pyloric gland adenoma

and 83–88%) than transabdominal US (54%, 54%) [19, 20]. However, a recent meta-analysis showed that transabdominal US can successfully detect gallbladder polyps with a pooled sensitivity of 84% and specificity of 96% along with sufficient diagnostic accuracy, but found it to be less accurate (sensitivity, specificity: 79%, 89%) compared with EUS (86%, 92%) for the differential diagnosis of benign and neoplastic polyps [21]. The recently introduced high-resolution gallbladder US is performed with a high-resolution linear probe rather than a low-frequency convex probe, showing the highest sensitivity (90%) for the diagnosis of neoplastic polyps, followed by EUS (86%) and CT (72%) [5].

Contrast-enhanced US (CEUS) has also been attempted for the differentiation of benign and neoplastic gallbladder polypoid lesions. Homogeneous enhancement and an intact GB wall might suggest a benign lesion, whereas heterogeneous enhancement, disruption of the gallbladder wall beneath the lesion, and wider stalk width are more common in neoplastic polypoid lesions [22–25]. According to previous studies, presence of vascularity or certain vessel types such as branched or linear intralesional vessels can suggest neoplastic polyps [3, 22], whereas another study stated that vascular types cannot be used as a differential point between benign and neoplastic polyps [25]. Although, there

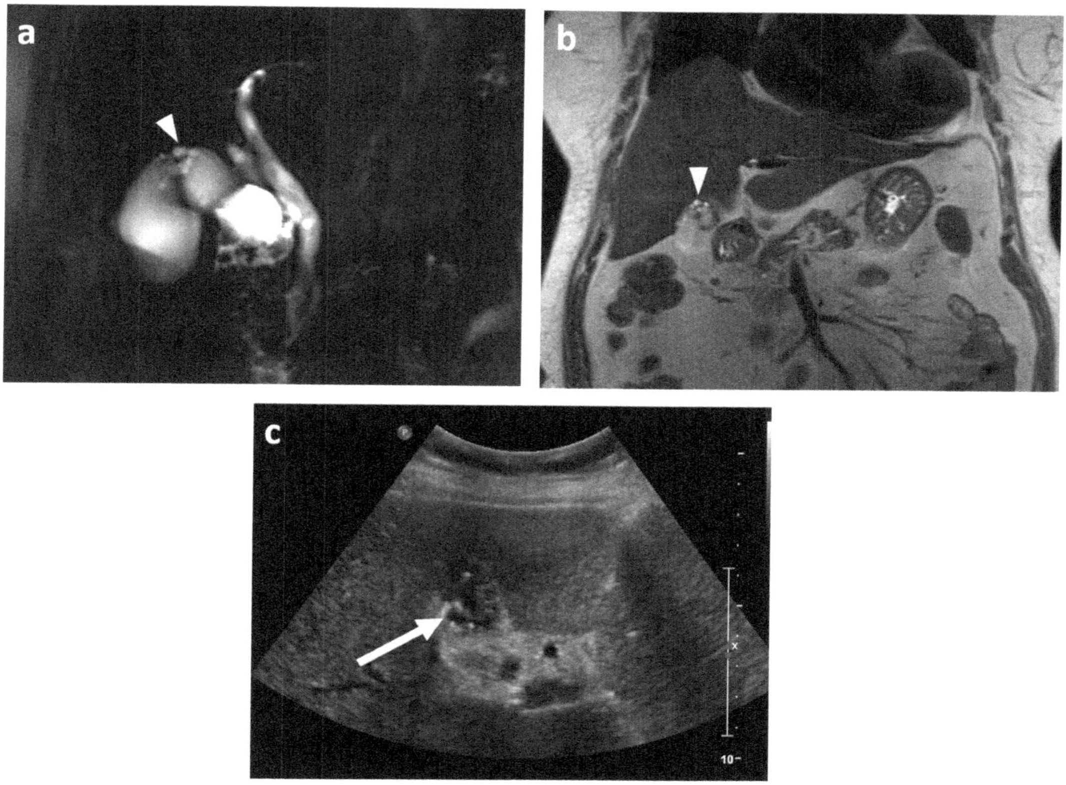

Fig. 9 Segmental adenomyomatosis. On MR cholangiography (**a**) and a coronal T2-weighted image (**b**), there are multiple microcysts arranged in a round shape (arrowheads). (**c**) On US, microcysts are noted within the thickened gallbladder wall (arrow)

have been reports that enhancement pattern and washout time differ between benign and neoplastic polyps [25, 26], these are relative rather than absolute findings and care should be taken in their application. CEUS is reported to have a sensitivity of 75–100% and a specificity of 67–87% for differentiating benign and neoplastic lesions [23].

Differential Diagnosis of Gallbladder Wall Thickening

For gallbladder wall thickening, a differential diagnosis is needed to distinguish early gallbladder cancer and diffuse or segmental type adenomyomatosis and to distinguish between xanthogranulomatous cholecystitis and locally advanced gallbladder cancer. Early gallbladder cancer and segmental or diffuse adenomyomatosis can be present as uniform and mild gallbladder wall thickening. Adenomyomatosis can be diagnosed when small round foci with T2 high signal intensity are observed within the thickened gallbladder wall (i.e., pearl neckless sign) which are due to Rokitansky–Aschoff sinuses on MR cholangiography or T2-weighted images (Fig. 9) [27]. On US, symmetric wall thickening, intramural cysts, and intramural echogenic foci which are cholesterol crystals and twinkling artifacts may suggest

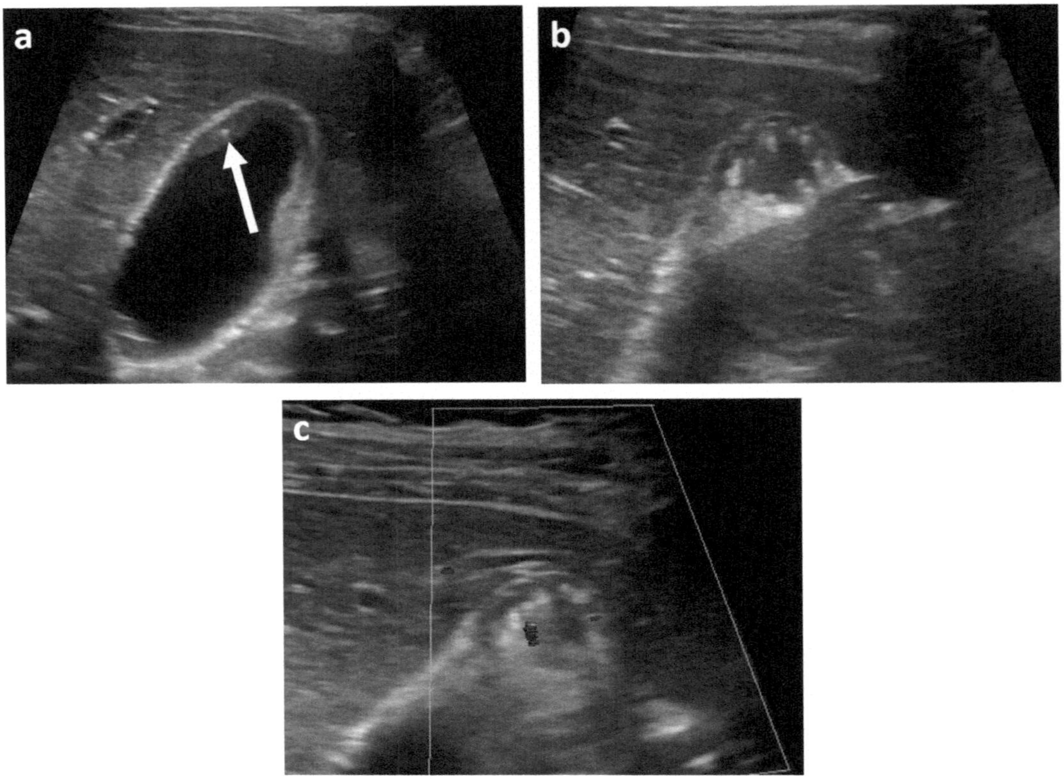

Fig. 10 Adenomyomatosis. (**a**) On US, an intramural echogenic dot is seen within the thickened wall (arrow). Multiple comet tail artifacts on US (**b**) and twinkling artifacts on Doppler US (**c**) are seen, suggesting adenomyomatosis

adenomyomatosis (Fig. 10), whereas gallbladder wall disruption or discontinuity and loss of multilayer pattern may suggest gallbladder cancer [28, 29].

Irregular wall thickening with accompanying stones are frequently noted in xanthogranulomatous cholecystitis, which makes it difficult to reach a differential diagnosis from gallbladder cancer. If a hypoechogenic nodule sits in the thickened wall on US, an intramural low attenuating nodule with continuous linear mucosal enhancement on CT may suggest xanthogranulomatous cholecystitis (Fig. 11). On MR, a signal drop in the opposed phase compared to the in-phase can be seen in the thickened wall due to the fat content [30]. Xanthogranulomatous inflammation or abscesses can be seen in high signal intensity foci on T2-weighted images [29, 30].

Conclusion

It is important to make a differential diagnosis between benign and neoplastic gallbladder lesions because treatment plans and prognosis are quite different for the two lesions. Although there are still a lot of gray zones left to interpretation, several helpful findings have been suggested for accurate differential diagnosis. Gallbladder stones can be diagnosed with accompanying posterior acoustic shadowing or position change made by the patient. High- to iso-echogenic polypoid lesions with tiny hyperechogenic foci might suggest cholesterol

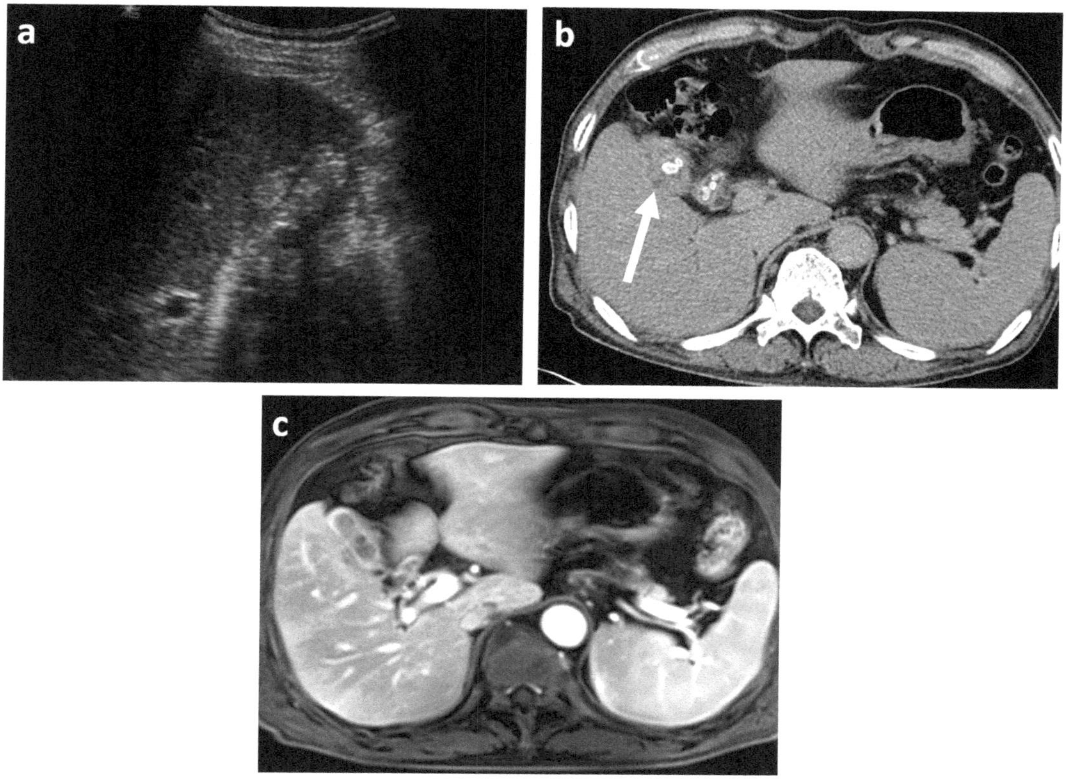

Fig. 11 Xanthogranulomatous cholecystitis. **a** On US, irregular gallbladder wall thickening with multiple impacted stones is noted. **b** On non-contrast CT, a focal low attenuating area is noted within the thickened wall (arrow). **c** On contrast-enhanced T1-weighted MR, gallbladder mucosa shows continuous linear enhancement

polyps and multiple microcysts in the thickened wall with comet tail artifacts or twinkling artifacts might suggest adenomyomatosis. On the other hand, hypo- to iso-echogenic polyps with nodular surfaces and larger than 1 cm in size might suggest neoplastic polyps. For gallbladder wall thickening, the pearl neckless sign on T2-weighted MR images is a specific finding for adenomyomatosis, whereas discontinuity or loss of gallbladder wall layers suggest gallbladder cancer. If there is a hypoechogenic nodule in the thickened wall on US or an intramural low attenuating nodule on CT, the findings would suggest xanthogranulomatous cholecystitis rather than gallbladder cancer. Careful imaging evaluation of the gallbladder enables accurate diagnosis of gallbladder lesions and can reduce unnecessary cholecystectomies.

References

1. Wiles R, Thoeni RF, Barbu ST, Vashist YK, Rafaelsen SR, Dewhurst C, et al. Management and follow-up of gallbladder polyps: joint guidelines between the European Society of Gastrointestinal and Abdominal Radiology (ESGAR), European Association for Endoscopic Surgery and other Interventional Techniques (EAES), International Society of Digestive Surgery—European Federation (EFISDS) and European Society of Gastrointestinal Endoscopy (ESGE). Eur Radiol. 2017;27(9):3856–66.
2. Gallahan WC, Conway JD. Diagnosis and management of gallbladder polyps. Gastroenterol Clin North Am. 2010;39(2):359–67.
3. Mellnick VM, Menias CO, Sandrasegaran K, Hara AK, Kielar AZ, Brunt EM, et al. Polypoid lesions of the gallbladder: disease spectrum with pathologic correlation. Radiographics. 2015;35(2):387–99.

4. Park JK, Yoon YB, Kim YT, Ryu JK, Yoon WJ, Lee SH, et al. Management strategies for gallbladder polyps: is it possible to predict malignant gallbladder polyps? Gut Liver. 2008;2(2):88–94.
5. Jang JY, Kim SW, Lee SE, Hwang DW, Kim EJ, Lee JY, et al. Differential diagnostic and staging accuracies of high resolution ultrasonography, endoscopic ultrasonography, and multidetector computed tomography for gallbladder polypoid lesions and gallbladder cancer. Ann Surg. 2009;250(6):943–9.
6. Sun X-J, Shi J-S, Han Y, Wang J-S, Ren H. Diagnosis and treatment of polypoid lesions of the gallbladder: report of 194 cases. Hepatobiliary Pancreat Dis Int. 2004;3(4):591–4.
7. Yeh CN, Jan YY, Chao TC, Chen MF. Laparoscopic cholecystectomy for polypoid lesions of the gallbladder: a clinicopathologic study. Surg Laparosc Endosc Percutan Tech. 2001;11(3):176–81.
8. Terzi C, Sökmen S, Seçkin S, Albayrak L, Uğurlu M. Polypoid lesions of the gallbladder: report of 100 cases with special reference to operative indications. Surgery. 2000;127(6):622–7.
9. Mainprize KS, Gould SW, Gilbert JM. Surgical management of polypoid lesions of the gallbladder. Br J Surg. 2000;87(4):414–7.
10. Collett JA, Allan RB, Chisholm RJ, Wilson IR, Burt MJ, Chapman BA. Gallbladder polyps: prospective study. J Ultrasound Med. 1998;17(4):207–11.
11. Kubota K, Bandai Y, Noie T, Ishizaki Y, Teruya M, Makuuchi M. How should polypoid lesions of the gallbladder be treated in the era of laparoscopic cholecystectomy? Surgery. 1995;117(5):481–7.
12. Yang HL, Sun YG, Wang Z. Polypoid lesions of the gallbladder: diagnosis and indications for surgery. Br J Surg. 1992;79(3):227–9.
13. Kim JS, Lee JK, Kim Y, Lee SM. US characteristics for the prediction of neoplasm in gallbladder polyps 10 mm or larger. Eur Radiol. 2016;26(4):1134–40.
14. Boulton RA, Adams DH. Gallbladder polyps: when to wait and when to act. Lancet. 1997;349(9055):817.
15. Kao WY, Hwang CY, Su CW, Chang YT, Luo JC, Hou MC, et al. Risk of hepato-biliary cancer after cholecystectomy: a nationwide cohort study. J Gastrointest Surg. 2013;17(2):345–51.
16. Lin G, Zeng Z, Wang X, Wu Z, Wang J, Wang C, et al. Cholecystectomy and risk of pancreatic cancer: a meta-analysis of observational studies. Cancer Causes Control. 2012;23(1):59–67.
17. Shao T, Yang YX. Cholecystectomy and the risk of colorectal cancer. Am J Gastroenterol. 2005;100(8):1813–20.
18. Akatsu T, Aiura K, Shimazu M, Ueda M, Wakabayashi G, Tanabe M, et al. Can endoscopic ultrasonography differentiate nonneoplastic from neoplastic gallbladder polyps? Dig Dis Sci. 2006;51(2):416–21.
19. Sadamoto Y, Oda S, Tanaka M, Harada N, Kubo H, Eguchi T, et al. A useful approach to the differential diagnosis of small polypoid lesions of the gallbladder, utilizing an endoscopic ultrasound scoring system. Endoscopy. 2002;34(12):959–65.
20. Azuma T, Yoshikawa T, Araida T, Takasaki K. Differential diagnosis of polypoid lesions of the gallbladder by endoscopic ultrasonography. Am J Surg. 2001;181(1):65–70.
21. Wennmacker SZ, Lamberts MP, Di Martino M, Drenth JP, Gurusamy KS, van Laarhoven CJ. Transabdominal ultrasound and endoscopic ultrasound for diagnosis of gallbladder polyps. Cochrane Database Syst Rev. 2018;8(8):CD012233.
22. Liu L-N, Xu H-X, Lu M-D, Xie X-Y, Wang W-P, Hu B, et al. Contrast-enhanced ultrasound in the diagnosis of gallbladder diseases: a multi-center experience. PLoS One. 2012;7(10):e48371-e.
23. Park CH, Chung MJ, Oh TG, Park JY, Bang S, Park SW, et al. Differential diagnosis between gallbladder adenomas and cholesterol polyps on contrast-enhanced harmonic endoscopic ultrasonography. Surg Endosc. 2013;27(4):1414–21.
24. Kumagai Y, Kotanagi H, Ishida H, Komatsuda T, Furukawa K, Yamada M, et al. Gallbladder adenoma: report of a case with emphasis on contrast-enhanced US findings. Abdom Imaging. 2006;31(4):449–52.
25. Fei X, Lu WP, Luo YK, Xu JH, Li YM, Shi HY, et al. Contrast-enhanced ultrasound may distinguish gallbladder adenoma from cholesterol polyps: a prospective case-control study. Abdom Imaging. 2015;40(7):2355–63.
26. Yuan H-X, Cao J-Y, Kong W-T, Xia H-S, Wang X, Wang W-P. Contrast-enhanced ultrasound in diagnosis of gallbladder adenoma. Hepatobiliary Pancreat Dis Int. 2015;14(2):201–7.
27. Haradome H, Ichikawa T, Sou H, Yoshikawa T, Nakamura A, Araki T, et al. The pearl necklace sign: an imaging sign of adenomyomatosis of the gallbladder at MR cholangiopancreatography. Radiology. 2003;227(1):80–8.
28. Joo I, Lee JY, Kim JH, Kim SJ, Kim MA, Han JK, et al. Differentiation of adenomyomatosis of the gallbladder from early-stage, wall-thickening-type gallbladder cancer using high-resolution ultrasound. Eur Radiol. 2013;23(3):730–8.
29. van Breda Vriesman AC, Engelbrecht MR, Smithuis RH, Puylaert JB. Diffuse gallbladder wall thickening: differential diagnosis. AJR Am J Roentgenol. 2007;188(2):495–501.
30. Singh VP, Rajesh S, Bihari C, Desai SN, Pargewar SS, Arora A. Xanthogranulomatous cholecystitis: What every radiologist should know. World J Radiol. 2016;8(2):183–91.

Role of EUS

Jae Hee Cho

Introduction

Endoscopic ultrasonography (EUS) is a significantly more sensitive, accurate, and effective diagnostic tool than computed tomography or transabdominal ultrasonography (TAUS) for evaluating gallbladder (GB) disease [1–4]. Because EUS includes a high-frequency ultrasound transducer at the tip of the echoendoscope, when it is placed within the gastric or duodenal lumen, we can obtain more detailed pancreatobiliary images. EUS uses high ultrasound frequencies (5–20 MHz) to create high-resolution gray-scale color Doppler and contrast-enhanced images. The underlying principle of ultrasound and echogenic properties of GB polyp are the same as those for TAUS. However, because EUS can provide close contact with the GB, we can identify its three layers—mucosa (inner layer), muscularis propria (middle layer of muscular tissue), and sub-serosa (outer layer of connective tissue)—as well as the detailed morphologic variables of polypoid lesions including shape, lobulation, irregular surface, and echogenic characteristics.

In this chapter, we describe the diagnostic value of EUS for GB polypoid lesions and wall thickening.

Role of EUS for Diagnosis of Gallbladder Diseases

Differential Diagnosis of GB Polypoid Lesions

With advances in radiologic imaging, the diagnosis of GB polyps is increasing. Most are harmless and referred to as non-neoplastic polyps. The remaining are neoplastic polyps that can be adenomatous with or without dysplasia or cancerous. Because adenomatous polyps can turn cancerous, the decision to perform cholecystectomy is made according to GB polyp size on TAUS and/or EUS. If they grow to be more than 1 cm, laparoscopic cholecystectomy is considered; however, even after surgery, it is not rarely found to be benign polyps. Because the preoperative differential diagnosis remains very difficult in many cases of GB polyps, especially those smaller than 20 mm in diameter, many EUS studies have been conducted to achieve an accurate diagnosis prior to surgery. Several reports showed widely varying incidence rates of neoplastic pathologic conditions in 10–20-mm (26–88%) and 6–10-mm polyps (19–25%) [5–8]. Thus, an accurate imaging assessment to

J. H. Cho (✉)
Department of Internal Medicine, Yonsei University College of Medicine, Gangnam Severance Hospital, 211, Eonju-Ro Gangnam-Gu, Seoul 06273, Republic of Korea
e-mail: jhcho9328@yuhs.ac

J. B. Chung and K. Okazaki (eds.), *Diseases of the Gallbladder*,
https://doi.org/10.1007/978-981-15-6010-1_25

differentiate neoplastic from non-neoplastic GB polyps is required to overcome the limitations of size criteria alone [9].

The great majority of polyps are composed of cholesterol and less often neoplastic. Cholesterol polyps are usually less than 10 mm in diameter, whereas adenomatous polyps can be up to 20 mm. Both appear as polypoid or sessile-shaped echogenic non-shadowing small masses like lesions adherent to the GB wall, often in a non-dependent portion. The first step of the differential diagnosis of GB polyp involves excluding small gallstones, which are most commonly GB disease (Fig. 1a). When detected on a careful EUS examination, gallstones have a posterior acoustic shadowing that appears as a subtle, thin, echo-free line under polypoid lesions. A lack of mobility favors a polyp rather than gallstone.

Single polyps are no more likely to be neoplastic than multiple polyps. If the estimated polyp growth rate was more 2 mm per year, neoplasticity is highly likely to develop and a cholecystectomy is recommended [10]. In terms of typical EUS findings of polypoid lesions, previous EUS studies showed that, neoplastic polyps had an internal heterogenous iso/hypoechoic echogenicity (Fig. 1b). With advances in EUS imaging, we can distinguish relatively hypoechoic central portions from peripheral iso/hyperechogenic GB polyps. This is called hypoechoic foci, which is compatible with a

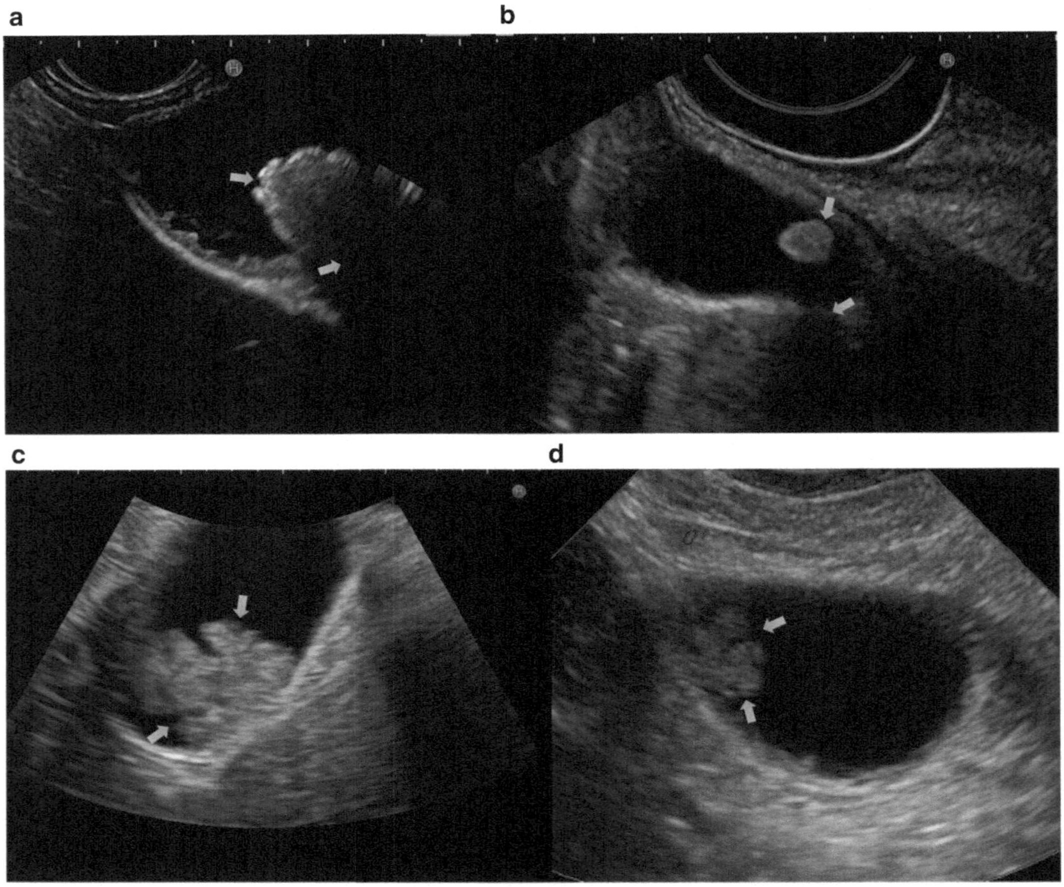

Fig. 1 EUS shows a gallstone with a posterior acoustic shadowing under hyperechoic polypoid lesion (**a**, **b**) and adenomatous polyp which have internal heterogenous iso/hypo-echogenicity (**c**, **d**)

microscopically loose core structure containing the dilated cystic gland and prominent vessels, and can be considered a predictive EUS variable of neoplastic polyps (Fig. 2a) [7]. Meanwhile, regarding cholesterol polyps, focal or diffuse cholesterol-laden macrophages in the lamina propria represented the iso-hyperechoic texture on EUS. They usually have homogenous echogenicity and the presence of hyperechoic spots, which are aggregates of many tiny hyperechoic dots in the inner part of the polyp, and it is considered a simple predictive variable for cholesterol polyps (Fig. 2b) [7, 11]. Furthermore, the presence of multiple microcysts, which are usually composed of 2–8-mm anechoic round lesions with the comet tail sign of V-shaped reverberation ultrasound artifact, was a strong predictive factor for focal adenomyomatosis (Fig. 2c) [7, 11]. Besides, although true malignant polyps such as adenocarcinoma are rare, local disruption of the adjacent GB wall on EUS is a strong predictor of malignant GB polyp (Fig. 2d).

Nevertheless, evidence of the effectiveness of an EUS diagnosis remains limited because EUS examinations are subjectively and highly influenced by endoscopist's skill [12]. Therefore, two additional EUS scoring systems have been proposed to predict neoplastic GB polyps. Choi et al. [13] suggested a scoring system according to layer structure, echo patterns, margins, stalks, and number of polyps. At a cutoff score of 6, the sensitivity and specificity for the risk of neoplastic polyps were 84.6% and 84.6%, respectively.

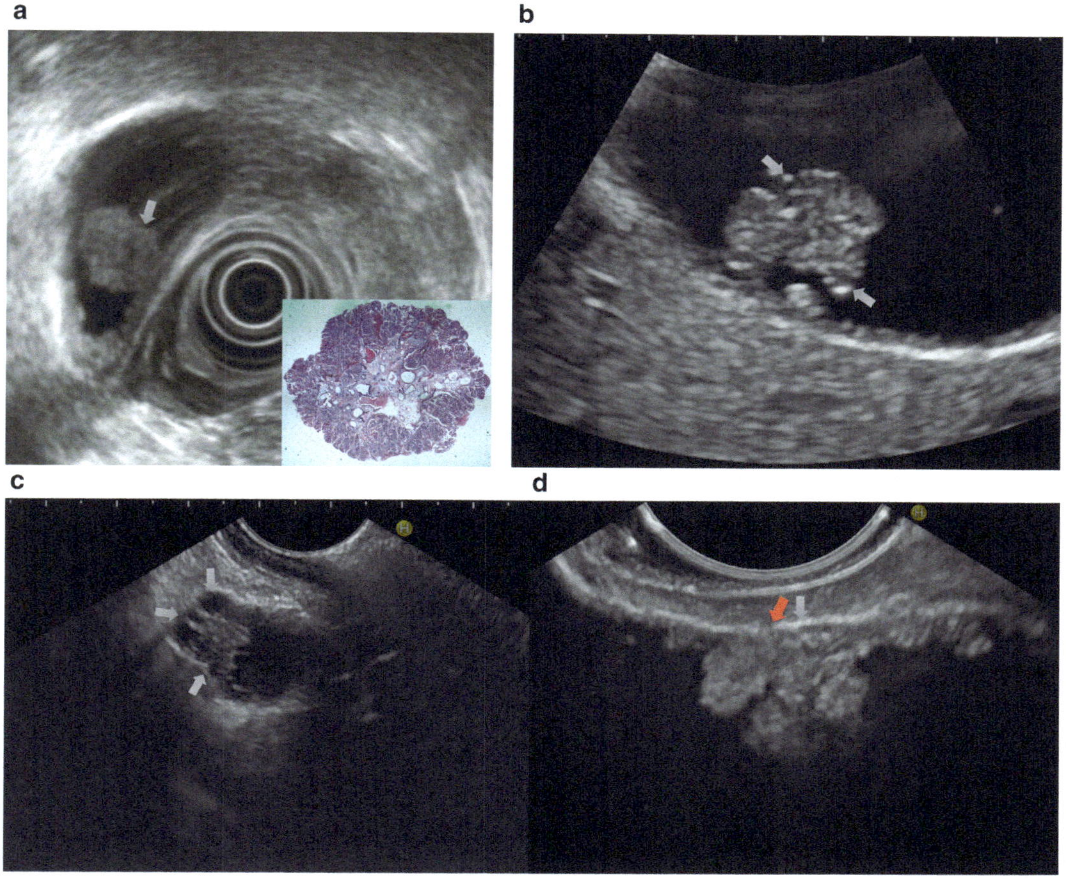

Fig. 2 EUS shows adenomatous polyp with hypoechoic foci (**a**), cholesterol polyp with hyperechoic spot (**b**), localized adenomyomatosis with microcysts (**c**), and adenocarcinoma with inner hyperechoic wall layer disruption (**d**)

Sadamoto et al. [14] suggested another EUS formula: maximum diameter (in millimeters), internal echo pattern score (heterogeneous 4, homogenous 0), hyperechoic spot (5). Using this system, the sensitivity, and specificity of the risk of neoplastic polyps with scores ≥12 were 77.8% and 82.7%, respectively. However, the clinical application of these formulae remains limited because of their uncertain utility and complexity.

In addition, the following novel methods are currently being studied. Contrast-enhanced harmonic EUS (CEH-EUS) is useful for observing microvascular structures and providing additional enhancement pattern images of GB polyps; therefore, its use could improve the differential diagnostic accuracy of neoplastic and non-neoplastic GB polyps [15, 16] The presence of irregular intratumoral vessels or perfusion defects on CEH-EUS was considered a sensitive and accurate predictor of malignant GB polyps. However, the distribution of contrast in polyps occurs over a very short interval; therefore, enhancement and perfusion images can only be observed during a brief window. Because it might be impossible to make an immediate diagnosis in a short period of CEH-EUS perfusion time, additional post-recording analyses are required to reach the correct diagnosis of GB polyps during CEH-EUS.

Color Doppler flow (CDF) within a polypoid echogenic lesion can also differentiate GB polyps from gallstones by documenting their internal vascular structures. A recent prospective study was conducted to distinguish between non-neoplastic and neoplastic polyps using CDF-EUS. Because cholesterol polyps are mainly composed of lipid-laden foamy macrophages deposited within the lamina propria, microvessel frequency and size appear to be relatively low and immature compared to neoplastic polyps. Kim et al. [17] reported that the presence of a vascular core, which reflects a strong Doppler flow, was more significant in neoplastic GB polyps with relatively good specificity, accuracy, and diagnostic discrimination with high reliability (Fig. 3).

Differential Diagnosis of GB Wall Thickening

Localized or diffuse thickening of the GB wall can be associated with myriad disorders. When diffuse wall thickening and perivesicular fluid are present, the differentiation of cholecystitis

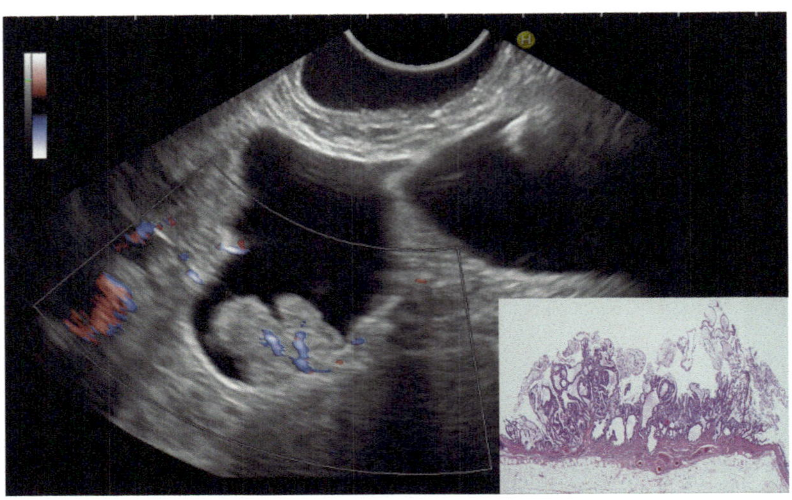

Fig. 3 Color Doppler flow endoscopic ultrasonography image shows a strong continuous flow in adenomatous polyp which is compatible with prominent small feeding arterioles in gallbladder polyp

from other diseases including liver cirrhosis, hepatitis, ascites, and hypalbuminemia can be difficult. Therefore, it is necessary to evaluate first, the clinical presentations. In terms of localized, focal, or segmental GB wall thickening, it can be difficult to differentiate benign diseases from GB cancer. In fact, most cases are ultimately diagnosed with benign diseases such as chronic cholecystitis or adenomyomatosis with a hyperechoic wall with a preserved layer structure; however, we should always try to discern GB cancer due to its unfavorable prognosis.

Adenomyomatosis of the GB is generally considered a benign condition associated with segmental or diffuse wall thickening along with the presence of small cysts, which usually represent intramural diverticula (dilated Rokitansky–Aschoff sinuses). On EUS, the layers of a thickened GB wall are usually preserved, but there are microcysts with bright echoes arising from the cystic spaces (comet tail sign). According to involvement extent and site, adenomyomatosis can be classified as fundal (most common), segmental (usually in mid-body), or diffuse type. Xanthogranulomatous cholecystitis (XGC) is an uncommon disease involving chronic inflammation of the GB. Its clinical presentation is like that of cholecystitis, making it very difficult to distinguish from GB cancer. EUS can sometimes visualize hyperechoic nodules in the GB wall, probably representing xanthogranulomas (Fig. 4).

The role of EUS in the diagnosis of GB wall thickening remains poorly defined. Mizuguchi et al. [18] compared EUS, conventional ultrasonography, computed tomography, and magnetic resonance imaging in the differential diagnosis of GB wall thickening. The multiple-layer pattern was demonstrated more effectively by EUS than by other imaging modalities. Loss of multiple-layer patterns of the GB wall demonstrated by EUS was the most specific finding in diagnosing GB cancer (Fig. 2) [19]. Nevertheless, it is not pathognomonic, as this finding can also be seen in XGC. Furthermore, the utility of CEH-EUS was recently evaluated in 36 patients with a thickened GB wall. The overall sensitivity, specificity, and accuracy for diagnosing malignant GB wall thickening of conventional and CEH-EUS were 83% versus 90%, 65% versus 98% ($P<0.001$), and 73% vs. 94% ($P<0.001$), respectively, indicating an additive role of contrast enhancement that can be helpful for the differential diagnosis of malignant GB wall thickening [20]. EUS-guided fine-needle aspiration has played an increasing role in providing histological diagnosis of GB wall thickening and GB tumors.

Conclusion

EUS provides a better image than TAUS, which helps distinguish GB disease such as gallstone/sludge, non-neoplastic, and neoplastic lesions. Because those are very difficult to differentiate preoperatively; some physicians argue against the utility of EUS because of its invasiveness, need for sedation, and unclear diagnostic superiority compared to TAUS [12, 21, 22]. However, because EUS provides the most precise real-time image of GB and recent advances in technology of imaging processors and endoscopic systems make it safer and easier than before, EUS is considered the best diagnostic method for GB disease. It could be more helpful in the preoperative assessment of patients with GB polyps suspected to be neoplastic, especially those, 7–20 mm in size. In cases of uncertainty on other imaging modalities, it could be more practical to develop a treatment strategy for polypoid lesions and wall thickening of GB. Furthermore, EUS has several additional advantages of fine-needle aspiration for tissue diagnosis and the potentially therapeutic application of biliary drainage.

In conclusion, EUS findings of GB including hypoechoic foci, hyperechoic spots, microcysts, Doppler flow, and CEH images aid in the preoperative diagnosis of GB polyps. GB wall layer disruptions on EUS are characteristic of GB cancer. As there are still limitations of EUS for GB disease, further research is required in line with technological advances in EUS to improve the diagnostic accuracy of GB disease.

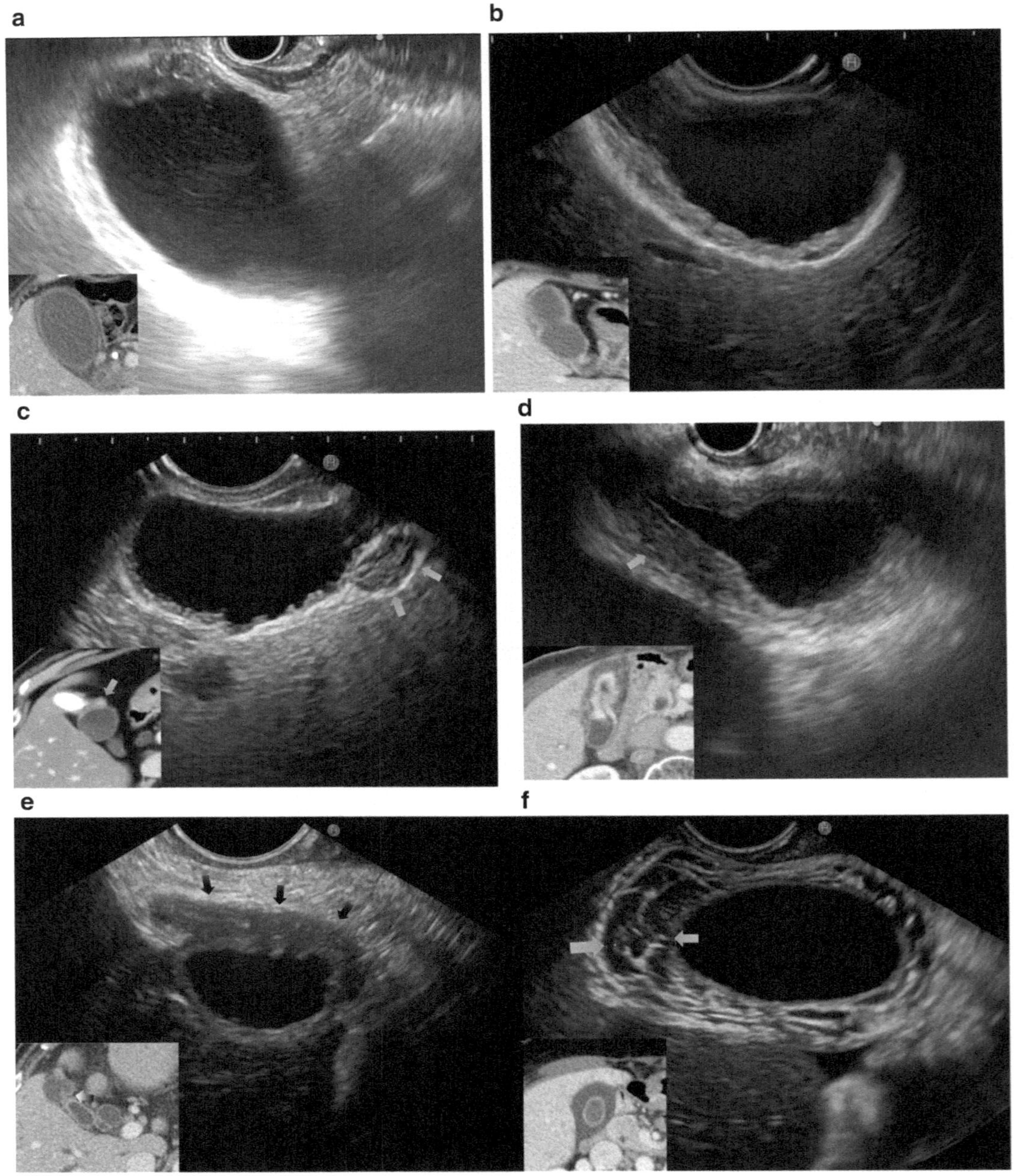

Fig. 4 EUS shows gallbladder wall thickening caused by primary gallbladder diseases including acute cholecystitis (**a**), chronic cholecystitis (**b**), segmental adenomyomatosis (**c**), adenocarcinoma (**d**) and xanthogranulomatous cholecystitis (**e**). And secondary diffuse GB wall thickening is also developed from other diseases such as pelvic inflammatory disease (**f**)

References

1. Sugiyama M, Xie XY, Atomi Y, Saito M. Differential diagnosis of small polypoid lesions of the gallbladder: the value of endoscopic ultrasonography. Ann Surg. 1999;229(4):498–504.
2. Azuma T, Yoshikawa T, Araida T, Takasaki K. Differential diagnosis of polypoid lesions of the gallbladder by endoscopic ultrasonography. Am J Surg. 2001;181(1):65–70.
3. Sugiyama M, Atomi Y, Yamato T. Endoscopic ultrasonography for differential diagnosis of polypoid gall bladder lesions: analysis in surgical and follow up series. Gut. 2000;46(2):250–4.
4. Wennmacker SZ, Lamberts MP, Di Martino M, Drenth JP, Gurusamy KS, van Laarhoven CJ. Transabdominal ultrasound and endoscopic ultrasound for diagnosis of gallbladder polyps. Cochrane Database Syst Rev. 2018;8:CD012233.
5. Kubota K, Bandai Y, Noie T, Ishizaki Y, Teruya M, Makuuchi M. How should polypoid lesions of the gallbladder be treated in the era of laparoscopic cholecystectomy? Surgery. 1995;117(5):481–7.
6. Myers RP, Shaffer EA, Beck PL. Gallbladder polyps: epidemiology, natural history and management. Can J Gastroenterol. 2002;16(3):187–94.
7. Cho JH, Park JY, Kim YJ, Kim HM, Kim HJ, Hong SP, et al. Hypoechoic foci on EUS are simple and strong predictive factors for neoplastic gallbladder polyps. Gastrointest Endosc. 2009;69(7):1244–50.
8. Bhatt NR, Gillis A, Smoothey CO, Awan FN, Ridgway PF. Evidence based management of polyps of the gall bladder: A systematic review of the risk factors of malignancy. Surgeon. 2016;14(5):278–86.
9. Kimura K, Fujita N, Noda Y, Kobayashi G, Ito K. Differential diagnosis of large-sized pedunculated polypoid lesions of the gallbladder by endoscopic ultrasonography: a prospective study. J Gastroenterol. 2001;36(9):619–22.
10. Wiles R, Thoeni RF, Barbu ST, Vashist YK, Rafaelsen SR, Dewhurst C, et al. Management and follow-up of gallbladder polyps: joint guidelines between the European Society of Gastrointestinal and Abdominal Radiology (ESGAR), European Association for Endoscopic Surgery and other Interventional Techniques (EAES), International Society of Digestive Surgery—European Federation (EFISDS) and European Society of Gastrointestinal Endoscopy (ESGE). Eur Radiol. 2017;27(9):3856–66.
11. Akatsu T, Aiura K, Shimazu M, Ueda M, Wakabayashi G, Tanabe M, et al. Can endoscopic ultrasonography differentiate nonneoplastic from neoplastic gallbladder polyps? Dig Dis Sci. 2006;51(2):416–21.
12. Cheon YK, Cho WY, Lee TH, Cho YD, Moon JH, Lee JS, et al. Endoscopic ultrasonography does not differentiate neoplastic from non-neoplastic small gallbladder polyps. World J Gastroenterol. 2009;15(19):2361–6.
13. Choi WB, Lee SK, Kim MH, Seo DW, Kim HJ, Kim DI, et al. A new strategy to predict the neoplastic polyps of the gallbladder based on a scoring system using EUS. Gastrointest Endosc. 2000;52(3):372–9.
14. Sadamoto Y, Oda S, Tanaka M, Harada N, Kubo H, Eguchi T, et al. A useful approach to the differential diagnosis of small polypoid lesions of the gallbladder, utilizing an endoscopic ultrasound scoring system. Endoscopy. 2002;34(12):959–65.
15. Choi JH, Seo DW, Choi JH, Park DH, Lee SS, Lee SK, et al. Utility of contrast-enhanced harmonic EUS in the diagnosis of malignant gallbladder polyps (with videos). Gastrointest Endosc. 2013;78(3):484–93.
16. Park CH, Chung MJ, Oh TG, Park JY, Bang S, Park SW, et al. Differential diagnosis between gallbladder adenomas and cholesterol polyps on contrast-enhanced harmonic endoscopic ultrasonography. Surg Endosc. 2013;27(4):1414–21.
17. Kim SY, Cho JH, Kim EJ, Chung DH, Kim KK, Park YH, et al. The efficacy of real-time colour Doppler flow imaging on endoscopic ultrasonography for differential diagnosis between neoplastic and non-neoplastic gallbladder polyps. Eur Radiol. 2018;28(5):1994–2002.
18. Mizuguchi M, Kudo S, Fukahori T, Matsuo Y, Miyazaki K, Tokunaga O, et al. Endoscopic ultrasonography for demonstrating loss of multiple-layer pattern of the thickened gallbladder wall in the preoperative diagnosis of gallbladder cancer. Eur Radiol. 1997;7(8):1323–7.
19. Kim HJ, Park JH, Park DI, Cho YK, Sohn CI, Jeon WK, et al. Clinical usefulness of endoscopic ultrasonography in the differential diagnosis of gallbladder wall thickening. Dig Dis Sci. 2012;57(2):508–15.
20. Imazu H, Mori N, Kanazawa K, Chiba M, Toyoizumi H, Torisu Y, et al. Contrast-enhanced harmonic endoscopic ultrasonography in the differential diagnosis of gallbladder wall thickening. Dig Dis Sci. 2014;59(8):1909–16.
21. Jang JY, Kim SW, Lee SE, Hwang DW, Kim EJ, Lee JY, et al. Differential diagnostic and staging accuracies of high resolution ultrasonography, endoscopic ultrasonography, and multidetector computed tomography for gallbladder polypoid lesions and gallbladder cancer. Ann Surg. 2009;250(6):943–9.
22. Lee JS, Kim JH, Kim YJ, Ryu JK, Kim YT, Lee JY, et al. Diagnostic accuracy of transabdominal high-resolution US for staging gallbladder cancer and differential diagnosis of neoplastic polyps compared with EUS. Eur Radiol. 2017;27(7):3097–103.

Diagnostic and Therapeutic Algorithm: Polypoid Lesions of the Gallbladder

Woojin Lee

Introduction

The term gallbladder polyp generally refers to any mucosal projection into the gallbladder lumen regardless of whether it is neoplasm or not [1]. Compared with'gallbladder polyps' or other terms, the morphological term 'polypoid lesions of the gallbladder' could be more comprehensive and clinically useful for this heterogeneous group of diseases, among which true gallbladder polyps are relatively rare.

Most gallbladder polyps are not neoplastic lesions. Actually, 70% of these elevated lesions are pseudopolyps, which include cholesterol polyps, cholesterol stones (crystal), cholesterolosis, or adenomyomatosis. Pseudopolyps do not in themselves have malignant potential. True gallbladder polyps can be benign or malignant. Benign true gallbladder polyps are most commonly adenomas while malignant polyps are usually adenocarcinomas.

Clinically, diagnosis, routine medical check-up, and follow-up of these elevated lesions are almost always performed by ultrasonography (US). Despite gallbladder polyps being common, only a few develop to carcinoma, which usually presents late in diagnosis and carries a poor prognosis. Prognosis of advanced gallbladder cancer is dismal (5-year survival rate less than 5%), but 5-year survival rate of T1 gallbladder cancer is reported 71–100%.

Although it is ideal to treat true gallbladder polyps early, after histological diagnosis, clinicians must decide to recommend cholecystectomy based on indirect information such as the radiographic appearance of the polyp, patient demographics, and symptoms. It may be difficult, therefore, for the practicing radiologist or clinician to know what to recommend when they encounter a gallbladder polyp. This was also suggested by the results from a survey that there is inhomogeneity of surgical practice in the management of gallbladder polyps [2].

The current literature lacks uniformity and a single consensus on gallbladder polyps because a majority of data was acquired by individual, observational, and retrospective studies which involved limited numbers of participants and might have been biased. Currently, larger gallbladder polyps, for example, larger than 1 cm, are recommended for surgical removal in view of the higher chance of malignancy. On the other hand, patients with smaller polyps usually require repeated US and follow-up. This policy not only imposes a certain degree of anxiety on the part of patients, but also carries with it significant economic cost to the health care system.

W. Lee (✉)
Department of Internal Medicine, National Cancer Center, Goyang-si, Gyeonggi-do, Korea
e-mail: lwj@ncc.re.kr

J. B. Chung and K. Okazaki (eds.), *Diseases of the Gallbladder*,
https://doi.org/10.1007/978-981-15-6010-1_26

Epidemiology

Due to the rising prevalence of gallbladder polyp and more frequent use of abdominal imaging modalities, the detection of gallbladder polyps has been increasing in past decades, affecting approximately 5–10% of the global adult population [3–6]. However, only 5% of these are considered to be "true" gallbladder polyps [7].

Most of the cases are diagnosed by abdominal US especially for periodic health examination. Otherwise, gallbladder polyps are often found incidentally during cholecystectomy. The frequency of resected gallbladder polyps in cholecystectomy specimens ranges from 2.6 to 12.1%; it seems to vary widely among reports and appears to be related to the indications for cholecystectomy, as well as to the study design [8].

Although the detection of gallbladder polyps has been increasing, the risk factors and natural history remain unclear. In contrast to the well-known risk factors for gallstones, no consistent relationship has been found between the formation of gallbladder polyps and sex, age, or medical conditions, such as diabetes, hyperlipidemia, and metabolic syndrome.

Histologic Type

Nonneoplastic polyps account for 95% and most of the neoplastic polyps are adenoma. Histological diagnostic terms are more scientific and accurate for each subtype of these lesions, but they could only be obtained postoperatively and therefore are difficult to be commonly used in clinical application and with imaging modalities. A worldwide, uniformly accepted classification is still lacking.

Cholesterol Polyps

Cholesterol polyps are the most common type (60%) of gallbladder polyp. Usually they are multiple, pedunculated, and less than 10 mm in diameter (Fig. 1) [9]. However, the sizes of these polyps vary quite widely, in some cases measuring over a centimeter. About 20% may be single lesions. They are not neoplastic polyps, but variants of cholesterolosis resulting from infiltration of lipid-laden foamy macrophages in the lamina propria.

The cholesterol in bile is absorbed by the gallbladder epithelium and taken up by macrophages and accumulates in the lamina propria. Cholesterol deposition within the lamina propria creates a mass and protrudes out of the mucosa into the lumen, and these masses are called cholesterol polyps. They are surrounded by vascular connective tissue and attached to the fibromuscular layer of the gallbladder wall protruding into the gallbladder lumen. They are covered with a single layer of epithelium enveloping a core of cholesterol filled macrophages. In cases where cholesterol deposits are tiny and diffuse, creating tiny, yellow excrescences on the surface of the gallbladder mucosa, having an almost strawberry-like appearance, the condition is referred to as cholesterolosis.

Diagnosis is easier in cases when there are multiple polyps. When there is one large cholesterol polyp, differentiation from the far less common adenoma is difficult (Fig. 2). Rarely, they may detach and behave clinically as gallstones, causing biliary colic, bile duct obstruction, or pancreatitis [10]. Cholesterol polyps have no malignant potential and no proven relation to gallstones. Surgery is not required unless the patient is symptomatic.

Adenomyoma

Adenomyomatosis of the gallbladder is characterized by excessive proliferation of the epithelium and hypertrophy of the muscle. This proliferation is associated with invagination of the proliferated epithelium into the muscularis propria. The invaginated epithelium forms an intramural diverticulum referred to as Rokitansky–Aschoff sinuses. In addition to mucosal hyperplasia, the smooth muscle layer is hypertrophied, both of these pathologic processes causing marked thickening of the

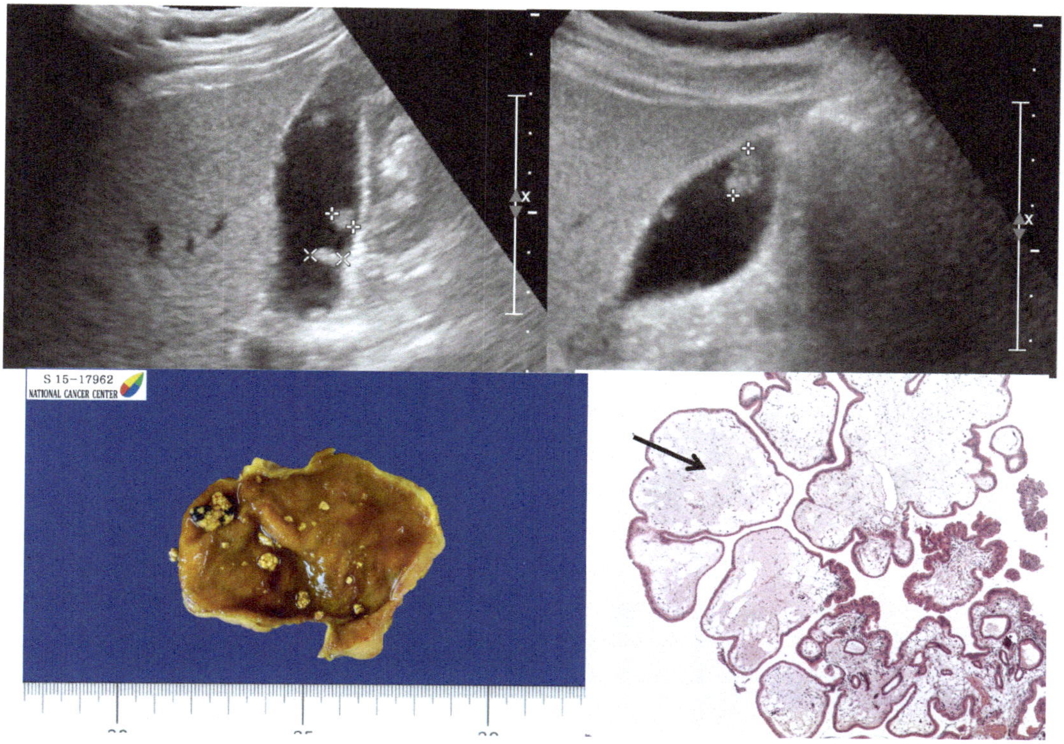

Fig. 1 Cholesterol polyp. **a** Sonographic view of multiple gallbladder polyps (0.8 cm, 0.6 cm size). **b** Sonographic view of another 1.1 cm-sized polyp. **c** Photograph of the gross pathologic specimen after cholecystectomy shows multiple yellowish cholesterol polyps. **d** H-E stain of the specimen demonstrating lipid-laden macrophages (arrow)

gallbladder wall. The Rokitansky–Aschoff sinus is usually confined to the thickened muscle, but in some cases, the sinus extends into the perimuscular connective tissue like a colonic diverticulum. Occasionally, Rokitansky–Aschoff sinuses are impacted with cholesterol crystals, debris, or fragments of stone.

There are three different types: the localized type, the segmental type, and the diffuse type. The focal type, the most common form, is referred to as adenomyoma. In the segmental type, there is a focal circumferential thickening of the gallbladder wall, often at the fundus or body. When it occurs at the body, there is a segmental narrowing of the gallbladder, dividing the gallbladder lumen into two separate compartments, mimicking an hour-glass. Segmental adenomyomatosis commonly occurs in the Phrygian cap and also gallstones are frequently entrapped in the cap. The diffuse form of adenomyomatosis causes diffuse thickening of the gallbladder wall and it may be difficult to distinguish adenomyomatosis from acute or chronic cholecystitis.

Localized form of gallbladder adenomyomatosis, confined to the fundus, may resemble a polyp. It is not neoplastic and confined to the gallbladder muscle layer. The average size is about 10–20 mm. Focal or segmental adenomyomatosis of the gallbladder fundus may be difficult to distinguish from intraluminal polyps or small carcinomas (Fig. 3). Surgery is not required unless it is symptomatic or indistinguishable from a tumor.

Inflammatory Polyps

Inflammatory polyps are small, sessile lesions, and the average size is about 5–10 mm, although

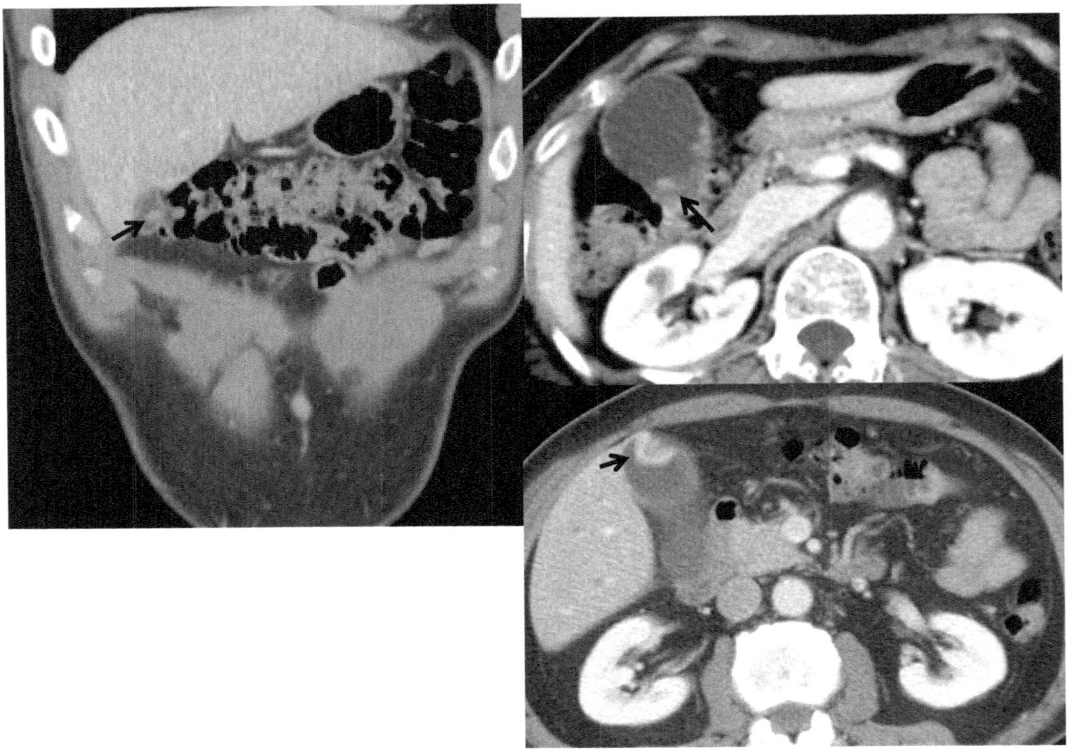

Fig. 2 CT view of single, large gallbladder polyp. **a** 1.4 cm-sized cholesterol polyp (after cholecystectomy). **b** 1.1 cm-sized gallbladder adenoma (after cholecystectomy). **c** 2.1 cm-sized gallbladder adenocarcinoma (after cholecystectomy)

inflammatory polyps larger than 1 cm have been described. These large polyps can be confused with gallbladder carcinoma [11]. About 50% may be single lesions. In about half, 2–5 lesions are observed. Surgery is not required and most are found incidentally during cholecystectomy.

Adenomas

Unlike other gastrointestinal adenomatous polyps, gallbladder adenoma is a rare lesion, found in only 0.15% of resected gallbladders [12]. Adenoma is characteristically a single lesion with a diameter of 5–20 mm (Fig. 4). Commonly, adenoma appears as sessile or pedunculated polypoid nodules. It can occur anywhere in the gallbladder. When multiple, as they are in approximately one-third of cases, 2–5 polyps are usually present. Adenomas may cause symptoms but are typically incidentally found. They are most frequently seen in patients with primary sclerosing cholangitis (PSC) and gastrointestinal polyposis syndromes, such as Peutz–Jegher and Gardner syndromes.

Histopathologically, adenomas are classified into tubular, papillary, and tubulopapillary types. Tubular adenomas are the most common and appear lobular, possessing smooth contours, while papillary adenomas appear cauliflower-like.

It is the only polyp in the gallbladder that has a premalignant potential. Several studies do support this potential progression [13, 14]. However, the frequency of progression from adenoma to carcinoma is much lower than that for colon polyps. Gallbladder cancer is 4 times more common than gallbladder adenoma. Furthermore, adenomas are rarely found around invasive gallbladder cancers, and adenomas are less frequently associated with gallstones than

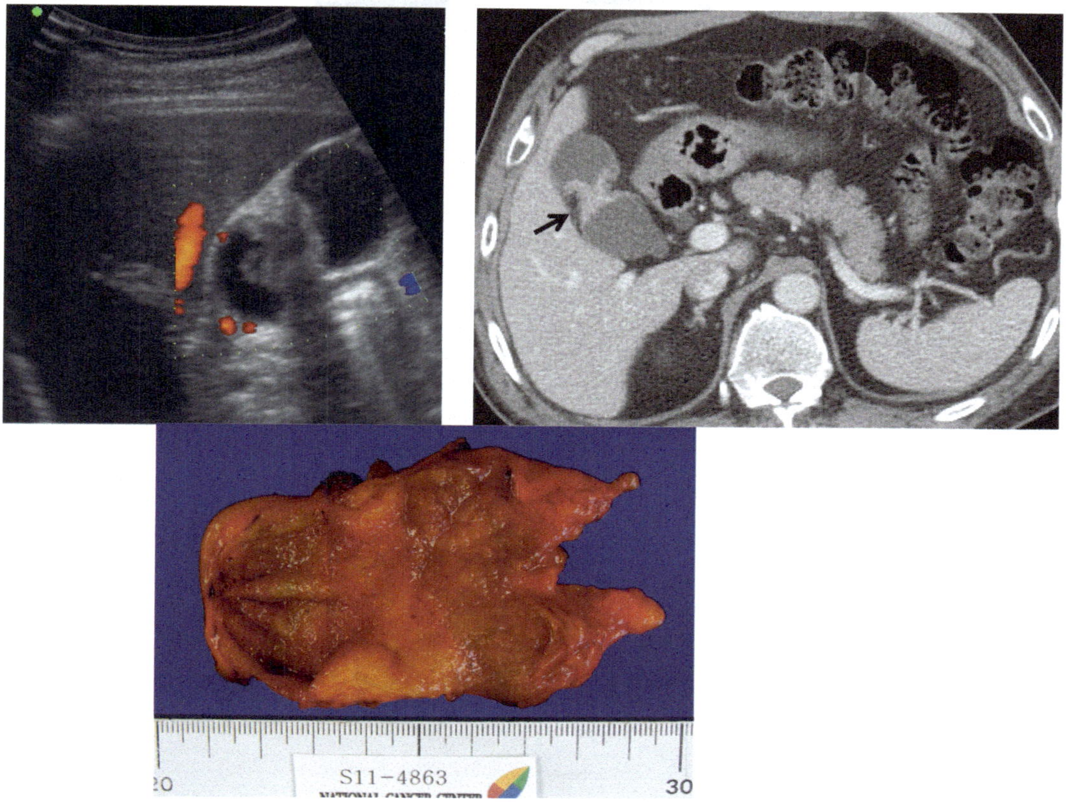

Fig. 3 Gallbladder cancer that mimicks segmental adenomyomatosis. **a**, **b** Sonographic and CT view of annular wall thickening of the gallbladder body. **c** Photograph of the gross pathologic specimen after cholecystectomy shows irregular wall thickening of the gallbladder body

gallbladder cancers. Therefore, this progression is not felt to be the predominant pathway of carcinogenesis in the gallbladder, and K-*ras* mutations have not been detected in gallbladder carcinomas associated with an adenoma. The frequency of transition from adenoma to cancer is unclear [13].

The pathologic diagnosis of adenoma or adenocarcinoma can only be made after cholecystectomy. In general, malignant tumors account for 3–8% of the gallbladder polyps. Virtually all adenomas with a focus of carcinoma are >12 mm in diameter; lesions <10 mm can be monitored with US. For lesions 10–18 mm in size, laparoscopic cholecystectomy should be considered in good surgical candidates. For lesions >18 mm in size, open rather than laparoscopic cholecystectomy should be considered because invasive cancer is more likely and extended resection may be required.

Other Polyps

Fibromas, leiomyomas, neurofibromas, carcinoids, and lipomas of the gallbladder have been reported, but are less than 0.1%. Pathology cannot be diagnosed before resection.

Clinical Features and Diagnosis

Because clinical findings alone cannot distinguish the histological types of gallbladder polyps, surgery is determined based on symptoms and image findings.

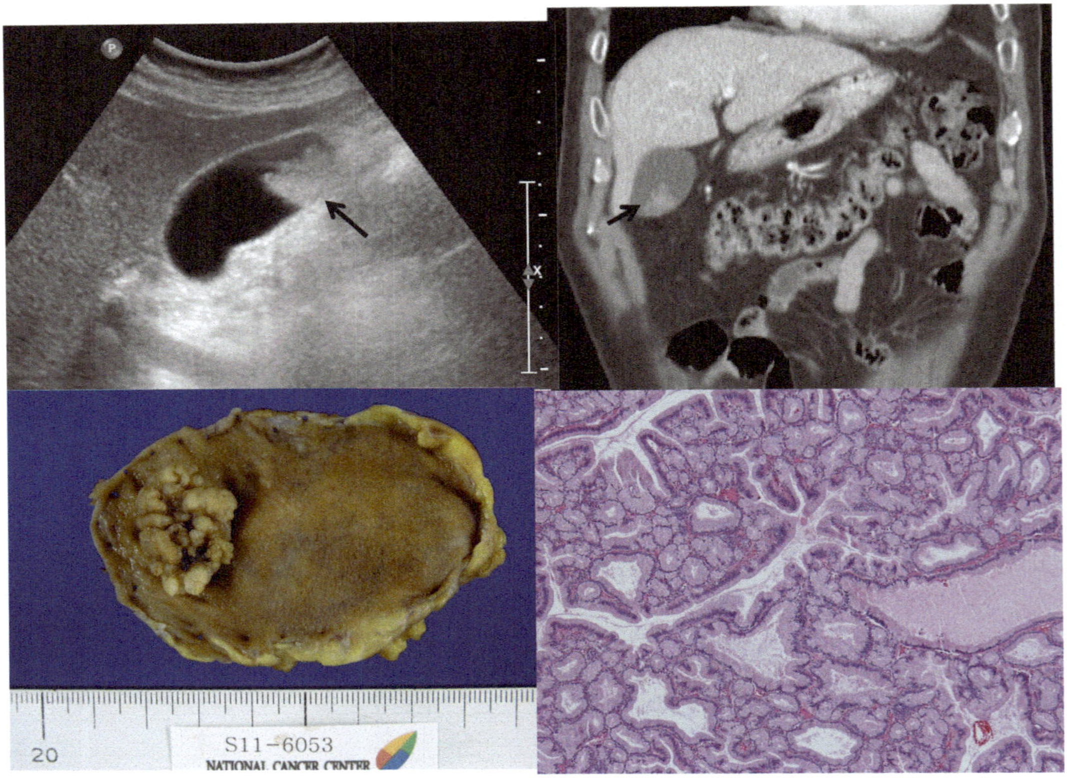

Fig. 4 Gallbladder adenoma. **a**, **b** Sonographic and CT view of 2.4 cm-sized solitary polypoid mass (arrow). **c** Photograph of the gross pathologic specimen after cholecystectomy shows lobulated polypoid mass. **d** H-E stain of the specimen demonstrating tubular adenoma, pyloric gland type

Most gallbladder polyps do not cause symptoms. Polyps can be found incidentally after cholecystectomy for the treatment of gallstone or by imaging studies performed for periodic health exams or other indications. Rarely, biliary pain may appear [15, 16]. Rare cases of acute acalculous cholecystitis and even hemobilia have been reported [17]. It is unclear whether the polyps primarily drive the symptoms, and it is difficult to distinguish the symptoms from those associated with gallstones. There is no sufficient evidence to show that tumor markers will assist in the decision-making process for gallbladder polyps.

Although imaging features of gallbladder polyps may, at times, indicate a specific diagnosis, there is a large degree of overlap in the appearances of benign and potentially malignant gallbladder lesions. About 85% of the polyps found by US are less than 5 mm in size. Only 2% are more than 10 mm in size.

Radiologic findings can be used to stratify gallbladder polyps into three groups: those that need no further follow-up, those that require follow-up, and those that should undergo cholecystectomy. In addition to the likelihood of malignancy on the basis of imaging findings, a surgeon's judgment on whether to perform cholecystectomy relies on clinical factors, such as patient age, medical comorbidities, and the presence of symptoms that are attributable to gallbladder disease.

US is the most commonly used and best available imaging modality because it is the simplest and sensitive diagnostic methods for the detection of gallbladder polyps. However, US is often limited by the body habitus of the patient, and technical limitations can lead to intraobserver variability in interpretation. It cannot reliably distinguish between non-neoplastic and neoplastic polyps (see chapter "Differential Diagnosis of Benign and Malignant Lesions with Imaging") [18]. On US, a gallbladder polyp is seen as an elevation of the gallbladder wall that protrudes into the lumen. It should not be mobile or demonstrate posterior acoustic shadowing (which would suggest it is more likely a calculus). It may be sessile or pedunculated. A clearly infiltrating or large mass should be treated as a gallbladder cancer rather than a polyp (Fig. 5). If there is clear reverberation or "comet tail" artifact present posterior to the lesion, this should be identified as a focal adenomyomatosis [19, 20]. The general sensitivity of US in detecting gallbladder polyp ranges from 36 to 90%, reaching 99% in patients without gallstones [21]. It was noted that gallstones mask the presence of polyps [22–24]. Besides, small polyps can also be obscured on US by thickened gallbladder wall [25].

Endoscopic ultrasound (EUS) is a more sensitive and specific method for diagnosing gallbladder polyps because of its use of high-frequency probes, which provide better resolution of small lesions (see chapter "Role of EUS"). EUS may be useful for identifying benign features of a polyp—such as cystic spaces or comet-tail artifact, which is associated with adenomyomatosis—that may not be visible with a transabdominal approach [26]. An EUS scoring system to predict malignancy in a gallbladder polyp on the basis of its size, its internal echo pattern, and the presence of hyperechoic spotting has been suggested, with sensitivity and specificity of 78% and 83%, respectively [20, 27, 28]. One study comparing

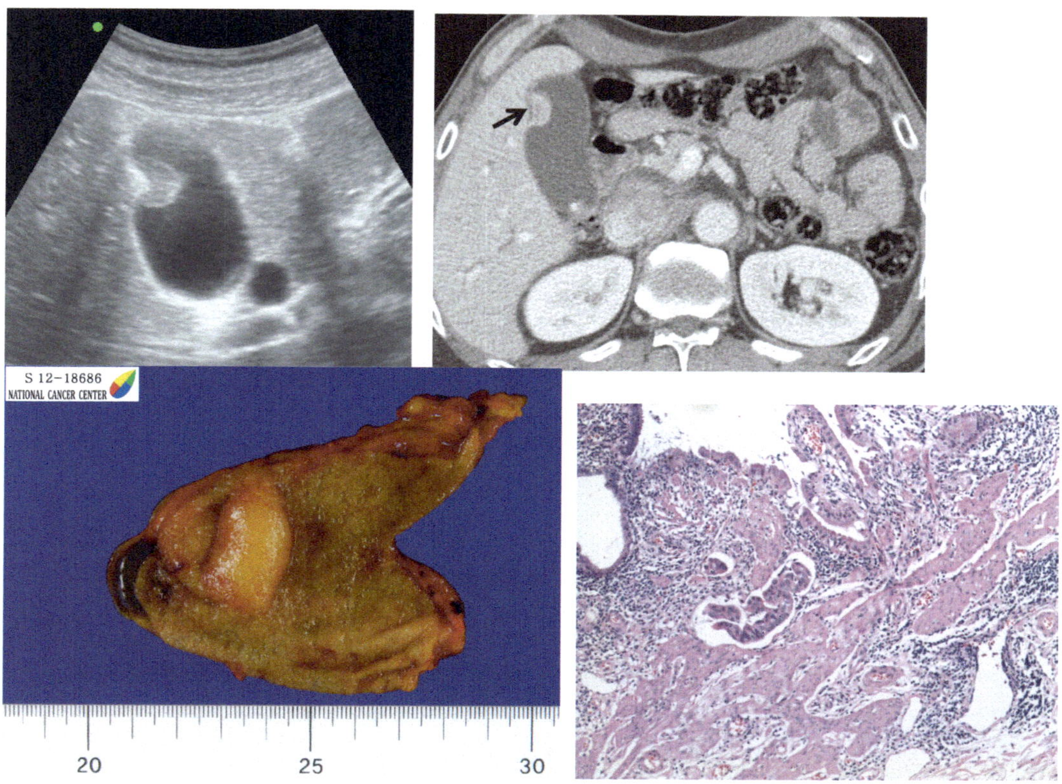

Fig. 5 Gallbladder adenocarcinoma. **a**, **b** Sonographic and CT view of 1.9 cm-sized, solitary polypoid mass (arrow). **c** Photograph of the gross pathologic specimen after cholecystectomy shows large, solid mass. **d** H-E stain of the specimen demonstrating adenocarcinoma

transabdominal US and EUS found that the diagnostic accuracy of EUS for differentiating polyp types exceeded 90% [20]. However, EUS alone is not sufficient to determine treatment plan in many cases. Also, it is limited due to the need for equipment and skilled endosonographers and the risk of adverse events.

High-resolution ultrasound (HRUS) operates at a higher frequency than conventional US (5–7 MHz) but a lower frequency than EUS (5–12 MHz) and therefore theoretically has a better diagnostic accuracy than US but is less accurate than EUS [29]. However, it does have the benefit over EUS, in that it is a noninvasive procedure. The diagnostic accuracy of HRUS has been shown to be comparable with EUS for the differential diagnosis of gallbladder polyps [30]. Perhaps most importantly, considering patient comfort and the lack of requirement for sedation, HRUS has real potential as an important diagnostic modality for the differential diagnosis and staging of malignant gallbladder polyps and early gallbladder cancer.

Contrast-enhanced ultrasound (CE-US) has also been used to assess gallbladder polyps. It was reported that CE-US may facilitate the detection of gallbladder polyps by helping to distinguish them from mural folds, gallbladder contents, or sludge and also to detect invasion into the liver and metastasis [31, 32]. Moreover, it may offer more useful information for distinguishing adenoma from cholesterol polyps compared with conventional US, especially in cases in which the polyp was larger than 1 cm [33, 34].

Computed tomography (CT) or magnetic resonance imaging (MRI) has been reported to be less sensitive than ultrasound and it has limitation in differential diagnosis of small gallbladder polyps (see chapter "Differential Diagnosis of Benign and Malignant Lesions with Imaging"). Enhanced helical CT could reveal gallbladder polyps larger than 5 mm and could differentiate neoplastic or nonneoplastic lesions [35, 36]. Attempts have also been made to predict the malignant potential of gallbladder polyps using MRI with diffusion weighted imaging [37]. If malignant polyps are suspected by abdominal US, additional abdominal CT or MRI is performed to detect the invasion into surrounding tissue, presence of lymphadenopathy, or distant metastasis.

Several cases in which preoperative 18-fluorodeoxyglucose positron emission tomography (PET) accurately predicted the presence of malignant tumor of the gallbladder in patients with gallbladder polyps have been reported (Fig. 6) [38]. However, it was applicable for the assessment of 1–2 cm gallbladder polyps and false-positive results may occur in the presence of acute cholecystitis, a limitation of FDG PET.

In summary, alternative imaging modalities, particularly EUS, may provide additional information in the diagnosis of gallbladder polyps. At present, however, there is insufficient data to suggest that they should be used ahead of conventional US in the investigation of gallbladder polyps. In addition, transabdominal US is a relatively low cost, low risk, and widely available technique. Some specific centers with sufficient resources and expertise may find the additional information available useful, especially in patients for whom cholecystectomy may have additional risk.

When gallbladder polyps are detected by imaging, such as US, they are sometimes not found in cholecystectomy specimen. Such false positive finding of gallbladder polyps on US ranges from 6 to 43% [22, 25, 39, 40]. Normal mucosal folds, sludge, or small stones impacted in the gallbladder wall can be misinterpreted as polyps. In addition, small polyps may fall off during processing of surgical specimens. Thus, patients should be informed before operation of the possibility of negative findings or of finding a gallstone instead.

Treatment

When a gallbladder polyp is identified on abdominal US, the two major questions are (1) is this causing any symptoms and (2) does this need to be removed? As discussed above, most polyps are generally thought to be asymptomatic. Therefore, the main role for the clinician in managing these polyps is recommending when to proceed with surgery and

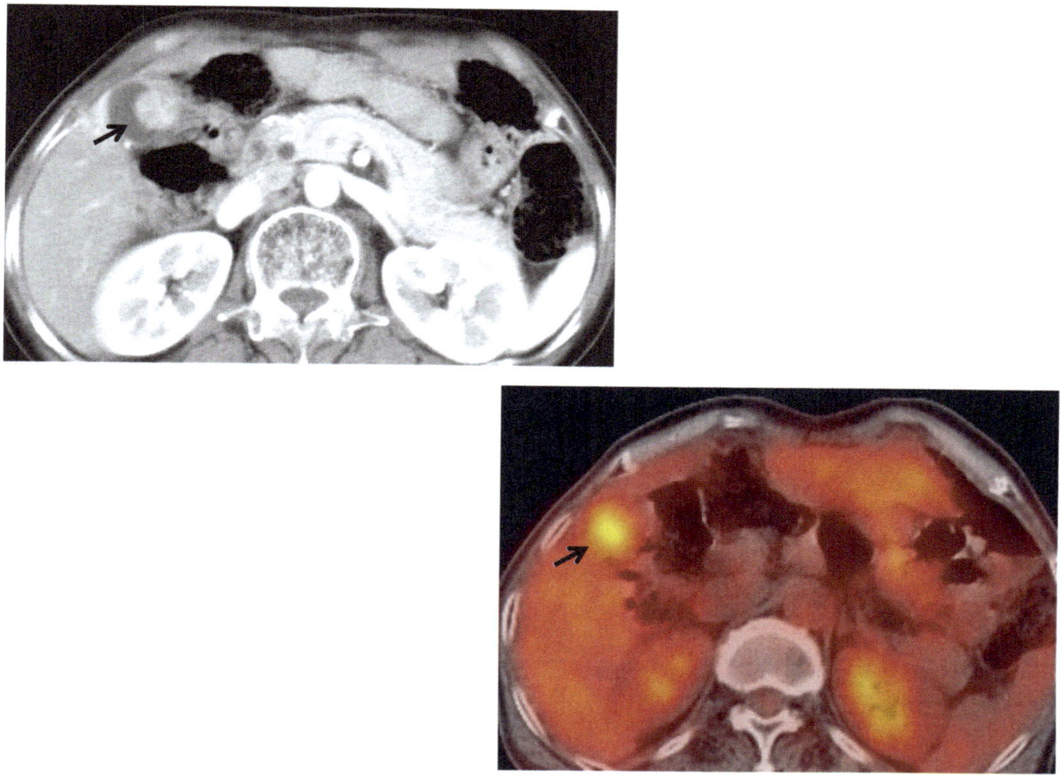

Fig. 6 Gallbladder adenocarcinoma. **a** CT view of 2 cm-sized, enhancing gallbladder polypoid mass (arrow). **b** PET view of the increased FDG-uptaken mass (arrow)

when to take a watchful waiting approach, recognizing that gallbladder cancer, while quite rare, carries a poor prognosis. The main concern in the management of gallbladder polyps is to identify and treat malignant lesions that are usually still at a relatively early stage and amendable to surgical cure. Currently, there remain controversies and challenges in many aspects of gallbladder polyps. It is difficult to differentiate benign lesions from malignant gallbladder polyps based on available diagnostic modalities. Prophylactic cholecystectomy is sometimes performed too early or is even absolutely unnecessary for well-functioning gallbladders with some subtypes of gallbladder polyps.

As mentioned earlier, the commonly reported rate of malignancy in gallbladder polyps is around 3 to 8%. Obviously, operation will be overdone if cholecystectomy is offered to every patient with gallbladder polyps. The issue is further complicated by the reliability of US which is usually the diagnostic tool used. The reported sensitivity and specificity of US in diagnosing gallbladder polyps is widely variable. Unnecessary operations would occur in case of false positive findings. The risks associated with surgery include damage to intra-abdominal structures during port insertion, bile duct injury (between 0.3 and 1%), and bile leak [41, 42]. Furthermore, endoscopic retrograde cholangio-pancreatography (ERCP) to manage a bile leak and bile duct injury are associated with significant adverse events [43, 44].

It is unlikely that small gallbladder polyps themselves cause patient's symptoms. There is evidence, however, that gallbladder polyps may be indicative of underlying inflammation or stone disease that may not have been detected on US [45]. The relationship between symptoms and risk of malignancy is not established.

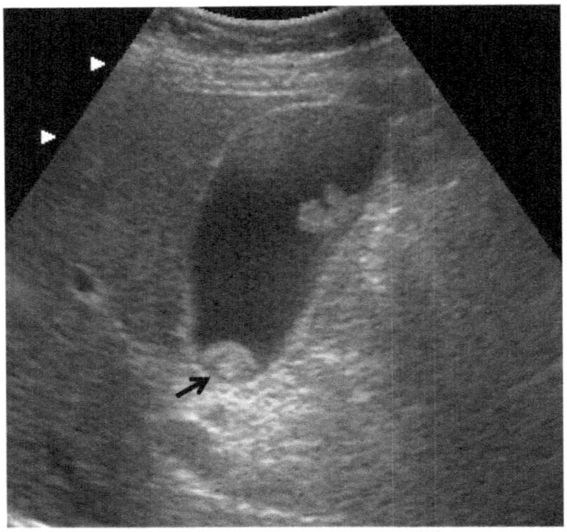

Fig. 7 Sonographic view of gallbladder polyp and gallbladder stone (arrow). After laparoscopic cholecystectomy, the diagnosis of the polyp reveals cholesterol polyp

Patients with biliary pain and US evidence of both polyps and stones in the gallbladder should undergo elective cholecystectomy (Fig. 7). The decision is more complicated for patients in whom gallbladder polyps without concurrent gallstones are discovered. For these patients, the decision to operate depends on the severity of symptoms, confidence of the clinician that the symptoms are biliary in origin, and US features (particularly the size) of the polyp.

Most polyps do not grow over time. About 7% of the polyps increase in size during follow-up (Fig. 8). Polyps less than 5 mm rarely grow. Sometimes (7–34%) polyps are reported to disappear [46–51].

Because polyps 10 mm in size or larger have a greater likelihood of being cancerous, elective laparoscopic cholecystectomy should be considered in acceptable surgical candidates with asymptomatic polyps of this size [45, 52, 53]. In a patient who is a poor surgical risk with a polyp that is 10 mm or larger, periodic monitoring for polyp growth (perhaps every 6 months) with US or additional characterization with EUS may be reasonable.

Polyps larger than 18 mm in diameter pose a significant risk of malignancy and should prompt cholecystectomy if possible. One study found that lesions of this size often contain advanced, invasive cancer that involves the serosal surface of the gallbladder and requires a more extensive dissection than can be accomplished by laparoscopy [54]. As a result, the investigators advocate open cholecystectomy for these large polypoid lesions of the gallbladder. Unfortunately, trials comparing these surgical approaches are not available. Thus, the ideal surgical approach for gallbladder polyps with suspicion of malignancy is unsettled.

How best to manage patients with polyps that are 6–9 mm in size is debated. Multiple polyps, pedunculated polyps, and those that are hyperechoic compared with the liver are usually cholesterol polyps, while solitary and sessile polyps that are isoechoic with the liver are more likely to be neoplastic. In this generally low-risk population, periodic surveillance for polyp growth or change may be prudent. One group of investigators has recommended transabdominal US evaluation 3–6 months after the initial discovery of such polyps to exclude a rapidly growing tumor, followed by ongoing surveillance at 6–12-month intervals. The optimal duration of surveillance is unknown. Two studies have suggested that the 10-mm cut-off value for cholecystectomy may be too high, as premalignant or malignant gallbladder lesions were found in persons with polyps that were initially 6–9 mm in size [49, 55]. So, some other investigators have advocated aggressive approach of performing cholecystectomy for polyps of this size given the small but possible risk of neoplasia such as increased size of polyp (>2 mm) [20], single [48, 56], sessile polyp (including focal gallbladder wall thickening >4 mm) [48, 57–68], Indian ethnicity [58] or old age [46, 56, 57, 60, 61]. As with most other cancers, the risk of a gallbladder polyp being malignant increases with increasing patient age. Currently, there is insufficient data to determine what the most appropriate threshold is. Also, there was insufficient evidence to include gallstones as a strong risk factor, but some of these patients are likely to be symptomatic and as such will undergo cholecystectomy anyway.

The best practice for gallbladder polyp surveillance needs clarification. Given the rarity of

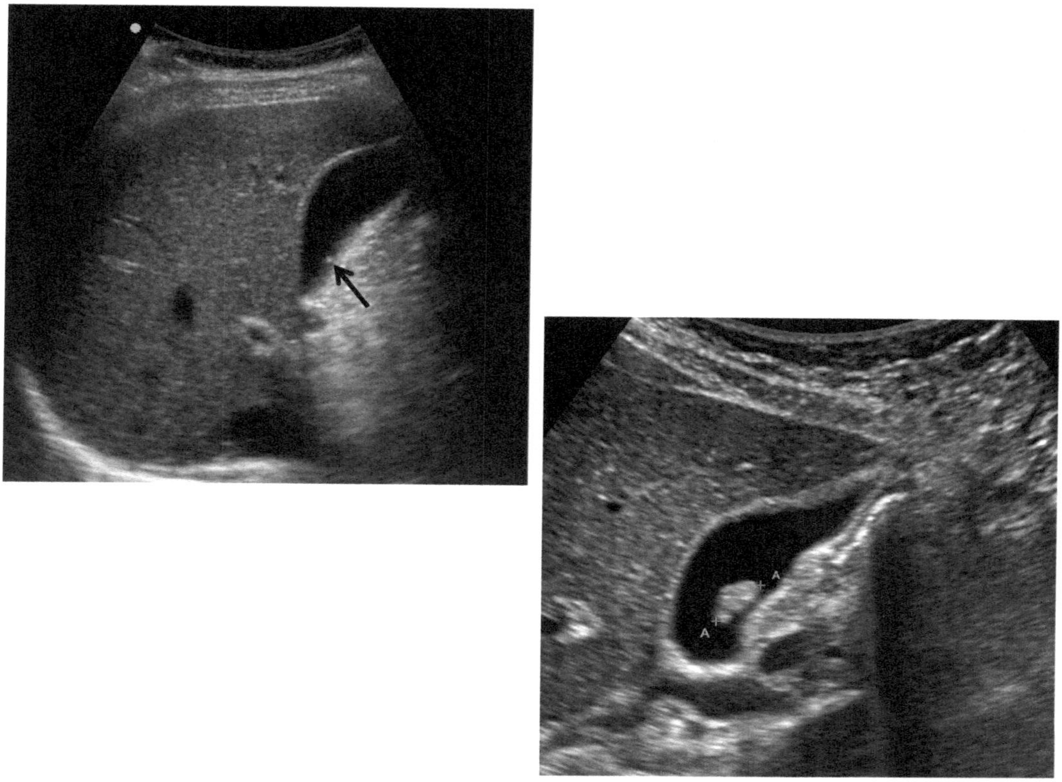

Fig. 8 **a**, **b** Sonographic view of increasing single gallbladder polyp (from 0.3 cm (arrow) to 1.1 cm) over 10 years. After laparoscopic cholecystectomy, the diagnosis reveals cholesterol polyp

gallbladder cancer, the cost of universal gallbladder polyp surveillance may not be justifiable; the cost-effectiveness might be improved by limiting surveillance to polyps between 5 and 10 mm in size because no study has reported neoplasia in an asymptomatic polyp less than 6 mm in size [50]. Polyps less than 6 mm in size are usually benign and most frequently represent cholesterolosis. However, although no malignant polyps have been shown to be below 4 mm, there is still a risk of adenomas and these polyps therefore would still require follow up but on a less frequent basis [46]. If the gallbladder polyp disappears, then it was likely a pseudopolyp and does not require further follow-up.

The recommendations for following small gallbladder polyps expectantly may not apply to patients with PSC, in whom the risk of malignancy in polypoid lesions of the gallbladder may be as high as 60% [62–65]. These patients should undergo a more intensive follow-up and have a lower threshold for cholecystectomy than non-PSC patients. In this high-risk population, cholecystectomy for polyps smaller than 10 mm should be considered. This, however, is challenged by observations that gallbladder cancer is seen only in polyps greater than 8 mm and that cholecystectomy in patients with PSC and cirrhosis is associated with high morbidity [65–67]. There was insufficient data to support cholecystectomy in all patients with PSC and a gallbladder polyp, because of the potential increased morbidity.

Recently, the European Society of Gastrointestinal and Abdominal Radiology (ESGAR) developed a consensus-based guideline. A summary of the recommendations is described in the algorithm (Fig. 9) [68].

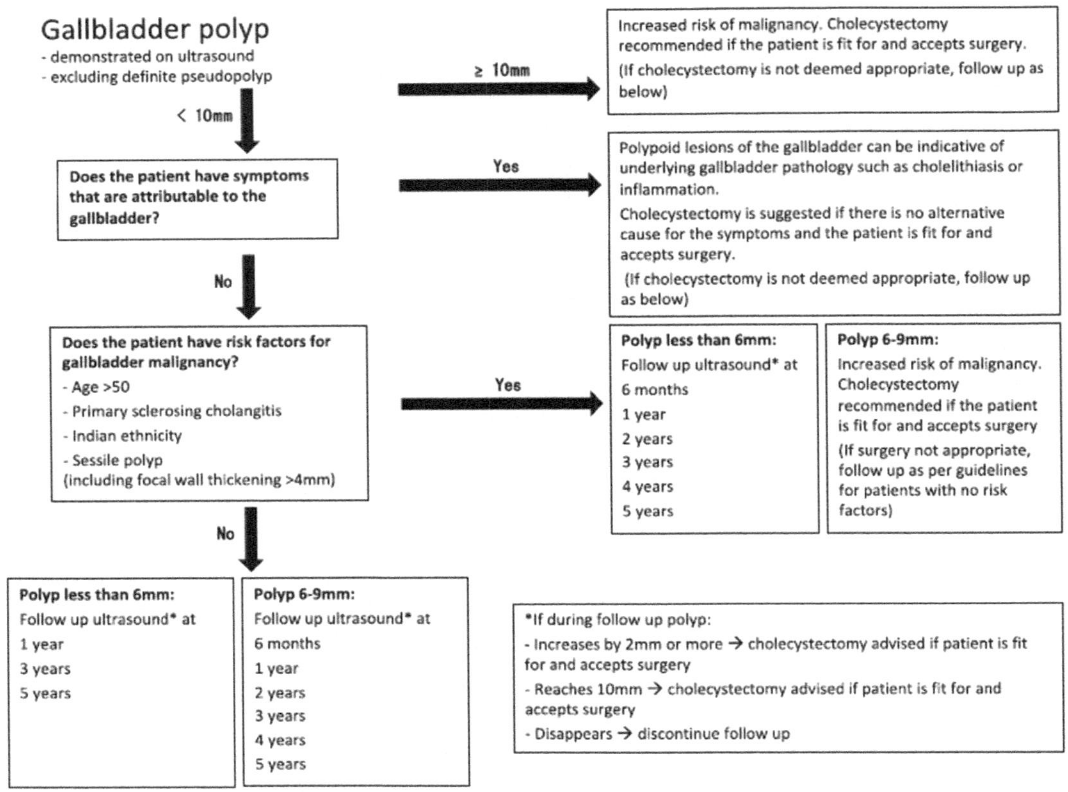

Fig. 9 Management algorithm of gallbladder polyp (Reproduced from Wiles et al. [68])

Conclusion

Currently, there remain controversies and challenges in many aspects of gallbladder polyps. It is difficult to differentiate benign lesions from malignant gallbladder polyps based on available diagnostic modalities. Patients with gallbladder polyps should be treated with personalized and differentiated strategies. Better understanding of the clinicopathologic characteristics, risk factors, classification and natural history of gallbladder polyps are necessary and larger prospective trials involving multiple centers should be conducted.

References

1. Okamoto M, Okamoto H, Kitahara F, Kobayashi K, Karikome K, Miura K, et al. Ultrasonographic evidence of association of polyps and stones with gallbladder cancer. Am J Gastroenterol. 1999;94:446–50.
2. Marangoni G, Hakeem A, Toogood GJ, Lodge JP, Prasad KR. Treatment and surveillance of polypoid lesions of the gallbladder in the United Kingdom. HPB (Oxford). 2012;14:435–40.
3. Lee YJ, Park KS, Cho KB, Kim ES, Jang BK, Chung WJ, et al. Shifting prevalence of gallbladder polyps in Korea. J Korean Med Sci. 2014;29:1247–52.
4. Choi YS, Do JH, Seo SW, Lee SE, Oh HC, Min YJ, et al. Prevalence and risk factors of gallbladder polypoid lesions in a healthy population. Yonsei Med J. 2016;57:1370–5.
5. Kratzer W, Schmid A, Akinli AS, Thiel R, Mason RA, Schuler A, et al. Gallbladder polyps: prevalence and risk factors. Ultraschall Med. 2011;32(Suppl 1):68–73.
6. Jørgensen T, Jensen K. Polyps in the gallbladder: a prevalence study. Scand J Gastroenterol. 1990;25:281–6.
7. Lin WR, Lin DY, Tai DI, Hsieh SY, Lin CY, Sheen IS, et al. Prevalence of and risk factors for gallbladder polyps detected by ultrasonography

among healthy Chinese: analysis of 34,669 cases. J Gastroenterol Hepatol. 2008;23:965–9.
8. Terzi C, Sökmen S, Seçkin S, Albayrak L, Uğurlu M. Polypoid lesions of the gallbladder: report of 100 cases with special reference to operative indications. Surgery. 2000;127:622–7.
9. Selzer DW, Dockerty MB, Stauffer MH, Priestley JT. Papillomas (so-called) in the non-calculous gallbladder. Am J Surg. 1962;103:472–6.
10. Parrilla Paricio P. Garcia Olmo D, Pellicer Franco E, Prieto González A, Carrasco González L, Bermejo López J. Gallbladder cholesterolosis: an aetioloaical factor in acute pancreatitis of uncertain origin. Br J Surg. 1990;77:735–6.
11. Maevama R, Yamaguchi K, Noshiro H, Takashima M, Chijiiwa K, Tanaka M. A large inflammatory polyp of the gallbladder masquerading as gallbladder carcinoma. J Gastroenterol. 1998;33:770–4.
12. Swinton N, Becker W. Tumors of the gallbladder. Surg Clin North Am. 1948;28:669–72.
13. Kozuka S, Tsubone N, Yasui A, Hachisuka K. Relation of adenoma to carcinoma in the gallbladder. Cancer. 1982;50:2226–34.
14. Farinon AM, Pacella A, Cetta F, Sianesi M. "Adenomatous polyps of the gallbladder" adenomas of the gallbladder. HPB Surg. 1991;3:251–8.
15. Mitty WF Jr, Rousselot LM. Cholesterosis of the gallbladder. Gastroenterology. 1957;32:910–6.
16. Kmiot WA, Perry EP, Donovan IA, Lee MJ, Wolverson RF, Harding LK, et al. Cholesterolosis in patients with chronic acalculous biliary pain. Br J Surg. 1994;81:112–5.
17. Cappell MS, Marks M, Kirschenbaum H. Massive hemobilia and acalculous cholecystitis due to benign gallbladder polyp. Dig Dis Sci. 1993;38:1156–61.
18. Akyürek N, Salman B, Irkörücü O, Sare M, Tatlicioğlu E. Ultrasonography in the diagnosis of true gallbladder polyps: the contradiction in the literature. HPB (Oxford). 2005;7:155–8.
19. Shapiro RS, Winsberg F. Comet-tail artifact from cholesterol crystals: observations in the postlithotripsy gallbladder and an in vitro model. Radiology. 1990;177:153–6.
20. Sugiyama M, Atomi Y, Yamato T. Endoscopic ultrasonography for differential diagnosis of polypoid gall bladder lesions: analysis in surgical and follow up series. Gut. 2000;46:250–4.
21. Chattopadhyay D1, Lochan R, Balupuri S, Gopinath BR, Wynne KS. Outcome of gall bladder polypoidal lesions detected by transabdominal ultrasound scanning: a nine year experience. World J Gastroenterol. 2005;11:2171–3.
22. Yang HL, Sun YG, Wang Z. Polypoid lesions of the gallbladder: diagnosis and indications for surgery. Br J Surg. 1992;79:227–9.
23. Rodríguez-Fernández A, Gómez-Río M, Medina-Benítez A, Moral JV, Ramos-Font C, Ramia-Angel JM, et al. Application of modern imaging methods in diagnosis of gallbladder cancer. J Surg Oncol. 2006;93:650–64.
24. Koga A, Watanabe K, Fukuyama T, Takiguchi S, Nakayama F. Diagnosis and operative indications for polypoid lesions of the gallbladder. Arch Surg. 1988;123:26–9.
25. Jones-Monahan KS, Gruenberg JC, Finger JE, Tong GK. Isolated small gallbladder polyps: an indication for cholecystectomy in symptomatic patients. Am Surg. 2000;66:716–9.
26. Sugiyama M, Xie XY, Atomi Y, Saito M. Differential diagnosis of small polypoid lesions of the gallbladder: the value of endoscopic ultrasonography. Ann Surg. 1999;229:498–504.
27. Sadamoto Y, Oda S, Tanaka M, Harada N, Kubo H, Eguchi T, et al. A useful approach to the differential diagnosis of small polypoid lesions of the gallbladder, utilizing an endoscopic ultrasound scoring system. Endoscopy. 2002;34:959–65.
28. Cheon YK, Cho WY, Lee TH, Cho YD, Moon JH, Lee JS, et al. Endoscopic ultrasonography does not differentiate neoplastic from non-neoplastic small gallbladder polyps. World J Gastroenterol. 2009;15:2361–6.
29. Kim JH, Lee JY, Baek JH, Eun HW, Kim YJ, Han JK, et al. High-resolution sonography for distinguishing neoplastic gallbladder polyps and staging gallbladder cancer. AJR Am J Roentgenol. 2015;204:W150–9.
30. Jang JY, Kim SW, Lee SE, Hwang DW, Kim EJ, Lee JY, et al. Differential diagnostic and staging accuracies of high resolution ultrasonography, endoscopic ultrasonography, and multidetector computed tomography for gallbladder polypoid lesions and gallbladder cancer. Ann Surg. 2009;250:943–9.
31. Meacock LM, Sellars ME, Sidhu PS. Evaluation of gallbladder and biliary duct disease using microbubble contrast-enhanced ultrasound. Br J Radiol. 2010;83:615–27.
32. Liu XS, Gu LH, Du J, Li FH, Wang J, Chen T, et al. Differential diagnosis of polypoid lesions of the gallbladder using contrast-enhanced sonography. J Ultrasound Med. 2015;34:1061–9.
33. Yuan HX, Cao JY, Kong WT, Xia HS, Wang X, Wang WP. Contrast-enhanced ultrasound in diagnosis of gallbladder adenoma. Hepatobiliary Pancreat Dis Int. 2015;14:201–7.
34. Choi JH, Seo DW, Choi JH, Park DH, Lee SS, Lee SK, et al. Utility of contrast-enhanced harmonic EUS in the diagnosis of malignant gallbladder polyps (with videos). Gastrointest Endosc. 2013;78:484–93.
35. Furukawa H, Kosuge T, Shimada K, Yamamoto J, Kanai Y, Mukai K, et al. Small polypoid lesions of the gallbladder: differential diagnosis and surgical indications by helical computed tomography. Arch Surg. 1998;133:735–9.
36. Lou MW, Hu WD, Fan Y, Chen JH, E ZS, Yang GF. CT biliary cystoscopy of gallbladder polyps. World J Gastroenterol. 2004;10:1204–7.
37. Irie H, Kamochi N, Nojiri J, Egashira Y, Sasaguri K, Kudo S. High b-value diffusion-weighted MRI in

differentiation between benign and malignant polypoid gallbladder lesions. Acta Radiol. 2011;52:236–40.
38. Koh T, Taniguchi H, Kunishima S, Yamagishi H. Possibility of differential diagnosis of small polypoid lesions in the gallbladder using FDG-PET. Clin Positron Imaging. 2000;3:213–8.
39. Ozdemir A, Ozenc A, Bozoklu S, Coskun T. Ultrasonography in the diagnosis of gallbladder polyps. Br J Surg. 1993;80:345.
40. Csendes A, Burgos AM, Csendes P, Smok G, Rojas J. Late follow-up of polypoid lesions of the gallbladder smaller than 10mm. Ann Surg. 2001;234:657–60.
41. Gurusamy KS, Koti R, Fusai G, Davidson BR. Early versus delayed laparoscopic cholecystectomy for uncomplicated biliary colic. Cochrane Database Syst Rev. 2013;(6):CD007196.
42. Krähenbühl L, Sclabas G, Wente MN, Schäfer M, Schlumpf R, Büchler MW. Incidence, risk factors, and prevention of biliary tract injuries during laparoscopic cholecystectomy in Switzerland. World J Surg. 2001;25:1325–30.
43. Gurusamy KS, Abu-Amara M, Farouk M, Davidson BR. Cholecystectomy for gallbladder polyp. Cochrane Database Syst Rev. 2009;(1):CD007052.
44. Christensen M, Matzen P, Schulze S, Rosenberg J. Complications of ERCP: a prospective study. Gastrointest Endosc. 2004;60:721–31.
45. Mainprize KS, Gould SW, Gilbert JM. Surgical management of polypoid lesions of the gallbladder. Br J Surg. 2000;87:414–7.
46. Babu BI, Dennison AR, Garcea G. Management and diagnosis of gallbladder polyps: a systematic review. Langenbecks Arch Surg. 2015;400:455–62.
47. Wiles R, Varadpande M, Muly S, Webb J. Growth rate and malignant potential of small gallbladder polyps–systematic review of evidence. Surgeon. 2014;12:221–6.
48. Bhatt NR, Gillis A, Smoothey CO, Awan FN, Ridgway PF. Evidence based management of polyps of the gall bladder: a systematic review of the risk factors of malignancy. Surgeon. 2016;14:278–86.
49. Park JY, Hong SP, Kim YJ, Kim HJ, Kim HM, Cho JH, et al. Long-term follow up of gallbladder polyps. J Gastroenterol Hepatol. 2009;24:219–22.
50. Cairns V, Neal CP, Dennison AR, Garcea G. Risk and cost-effectiveness of surveillance followed by cholecystectomy for gallbladder polyps. Arch Surg. 2012;147:1078–83.
51. Shin SR, Lee JK, Lee KH, Lee KT, Rhee JC, Jang KT, et al. Can the growth rate of a gallbladder polyp predict a neoplastic polyp? J Clin Gastroenterol. 2009;43:865–8.
52. Kubota K, Bandai Y, Otomo Y, Ito A, Watanabe M, Toyoda H, et al. Role of laparoscopic cholecystectomy in treating gallbladder polyps. Surg Endosc. 1994;8:42–6.
53. Sheth S, Bedford A, Chopra S. Primary gallbladder cancer: recognition of risk factors and the role of prophylactic cholecystectomy. Am J Gastroenterol. 2000;95:1402–10.
54. Kubota K, Bandai Y, Noie T, Ishizaki Y, Teruya M, Makuuchi M. How should polypoid lesions of the gallbladder be treated in the era of laparoscopic cholecystectomy? Surgery. 1995;117:481–7.
55. Zielinski MD, Atwell TD, Davis PW, Kendrick ML, Que FG. Comparison of surgically resected polypoid lesions of the gallbladder to their pre-operative ultrasound characteristics. J Gastrointest Surg. 2009;13:19–25.
56. Elmasry M, Lindop D, Dunne DF, Malik H, Poston GJ, Fenwick SW. The risk of malignancy in ultrasound detected gallbladder polyps: a systematic review. Int J Surg. 2016;33:28–35.
57. Park JK, Yoon YB, Kim Y-T, Ryu JK, Yoon WJ, Lee SH, et al. Management strategies for gallbladder polyps: is it possible to predict malignant gallbladder polyps? Gut Liver. 2008;2:88–94.
58. Aldouri AQ, Malik HZ, Waytt J, Khan S, Ranganathan K, Kummaraganti S, et al. The risk of gallbladder cancer from polyps in a large multiethnic series. Eur J Surg Oncol. 2009;35:48–51.
59. Choi SY, Kim TS, Kim HJ, Park JH, Park DI, Cho YK, et al. Is it necessary to perform prophylactic cholecystectomy for asymptomatic subjects with gallbladder polyps and gallstones? J Gastroenterol Hepatol. 2010;25:1099–104.
60. Gallahan WC, Conway JD. Diagnosis and management of gallbladder polyps. Gastroenterol Clin North Am. 2010;39:359–67.
61. Corwin MT, Siewert B, Sheiman RG, Kane RA. Incidentally detected gallbladder polyps: is follow-up necessary–Long-term clinical and US analysis of 346 patients. Radiology. 2011;258:277–82.
62. Karlsen T, Schrumpf E, Boberg K. Gallbladder polyps in primary sclerosing cholangitis: not so benign. Curr Opin Gastroenterol. 2008;24:395–9.
63. Said K, Glaumann H, Bergquist A. Gallbladder disease in patients with primary sclerosing cholangitis. J Hepatol. 2008;48:598–605.
64. Buckles DC, Lindor KD, Larusso NF, Petrovic LM, Gores GJ. In primary sclerosing cholangitis, gallbladder polyps are frequently malignant. Am J Gastroenterol. 2002;97:1138–42.
65. Eaton JE, Thackeray EW, Lindor KD. Likelihood of malignancy in gallbladder polyps and outcomes following cholecystectomy in primary sclerosing cholangitis. Am J Gastroenterol. 2012;107:431–9.
66. Razumilava N, Gores GJ, Lindor KD. Cancer surveillance in patients with primary sclerosing cholangitis. Hepatology. 2011;54:1842–52.
67. Schramm C, Lohse AW. Gallbladder polyps in primary sclerosing cholangitis: indication for early intervention. Hepatology. 2012;56:396.
68. Wiles R, Thoeni RF, Barbu ST, Vashist YK, Rafaelsen SR, Dewhurst C, et al. Management and follow-up of gallbladder polyps: Joint guidelines between the European Society of Gastrointestinal and Abdominal Radiology (ESGAR), European Association for Endoscopic Surgery and other Interventional Techniques (EAES), International Society of Digestive Surgery- European Federation (EFISDS) and European Society of Gastrointestinal Endoscopy (ESGE). Eur Radiol. 2017;27:3856–66.

Imaging Features of Gallbladder Lesions Manifesting Wall Thickening

Dai Inoue and Akira Izumozaki

Introduction

Various gallbladder diseases ranging from benign to malignant cause diffuse or focal wall thickening of the gallbladder (>3 mm). For favorable management of patients having gallbladder wall thickening, appropriate differential diagnosis is required. Ultrasonography (US) is a widely accepted imaging examination as an initial choice for screening and characterization of gallbladder wall thickening. With its high contrast resolution and accessibility, US is frequently applied for patients with abdominal symptoms or abnormal liver function. However, US diagnostic ability is somewhat operator dependent and can be affected by patient factors (e.g., obesity or intestinal gas). Therefore, additional imaging examinations including computed tomography (CT) or Magnetic resonance imaging (MRI) are sometimes needed to reach final diagnosis. CT is also frequently applied for evaluation of gallbladder lesions [1]. An advantage of CT is its high spatial resolution of less than 1 mm slice thickness. Especially, since multi-detector row CT (MDCT) has enabled the gathering of iso-voxel data of less than 1 mm, multi-directional evaluation by multi-planar reconstruction has been realized. MRI is also considered as a useful imaging modality to evaluate the pancreato-biliary system including the gall bladder [2]. With its high contrast resolution, it can sensitively describe small amounts of hemorrhaging or fat. Additionally, magnetic resonance cholangiopancreatography (MRCP) is able to describe the whole bile duct and the pancreatic duct non-invasively. Being familiar with imaging findings in each modality is a key step in the procedure for differential diagnosis of gallbladder lesions.

Non-neoplastic Lesions

Acute Cholecystitis

Acute cholecystitis is the most frequent inflammatory gall bladder disease, and it occurs in approximately one-third of patients who have gallstones. Most cases present with cholelithiasis in the gall bladder neck or cystic duct leading to obstruction of bile flow. Patients usually complain of right upper abdominal pain (Murphy sign) or fever elevation accompanied with evidence of inflammation in serum tests (WBC, CRP). US examinations describe cholelithiasis with diffuse wall thickening by focusing on the sonolucent layer reflecting

D. Inoue (✉) · A. Izumozaki
Department of Radiology, Kanazawa University Hospital, Kanazawa, Japan
e-mail: d-inoue@lake.ocn.ne.jp

A. Izumozaki
e-mail: aizumozaki@gmail.com

J. B. Chung and K. Okazaki (eds.), *Diseases of the Gallbladder*,
https://doi.org/10.1007/978-981-15-6010-1_27

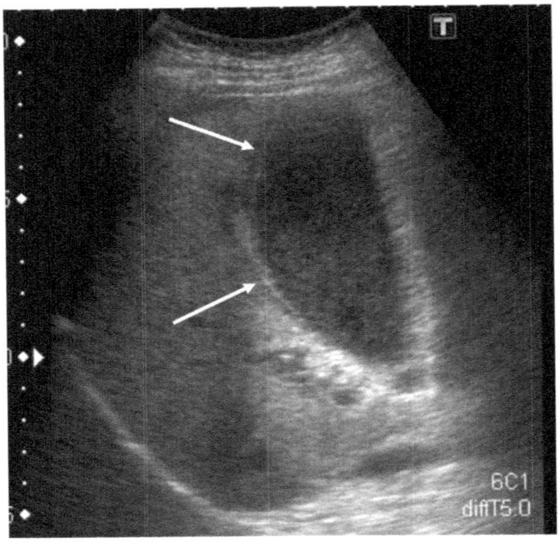

Fig. 1 US image of acute cholecystitis. US shows wall thickening of gallbladder with sonolucent layer (arrows)

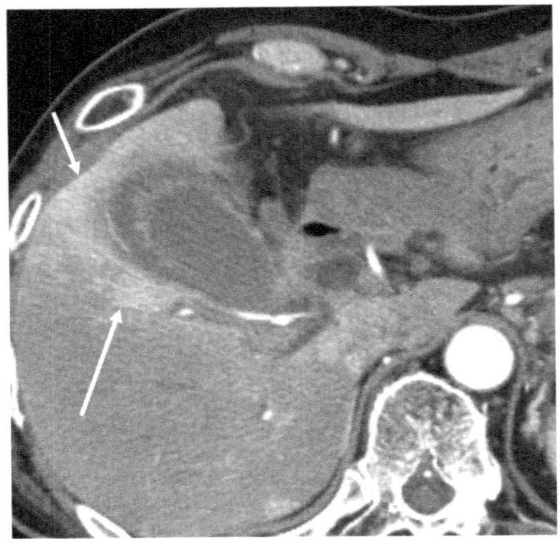

Fig. 2 Dynamic CT image of acute cholecystitis. Gallbladder wall thickening with edematous change is described. Transient staining of neighboring hepatic parenchyma is also demonstrated (arrows)

the submucosal edema (Fig. 1) [3]. Adding to these findings, a sonographic Murphy sign is also helpful for diagnosis of acute cholecystitis [4]. Although US examination is useful for diagnosis of acute cholecystitis, it should be noted that US sometimes has blind areas due to large cholelithiasis (acoustic shadow) or intestinal gas leading to less sensitive evaluation of gallbladder wall thickening or peri-cholecystic inflammation. On CT examinations, acute cholecystitis typically demonstrates diffuse low-attenuating wall thickening which accompanies the cholecystitis. On dynamic CT, transient staining in the hepatic parenchyma neighboring the gall bladder reflects the hyperemic state due to acute inflammation in the gallbladder (Fig. 2). This can be seen in arterial phase images, and layered wall structures are clearly depicted. CT is also useful to evaluate secondary findings such as peri-cholecystic fluid collection or fat stranding, and peri-portal edema [5, 6]. In MRI, a thickened gallbladder wall is shown as a hyper-intensity structure on T2-weighted images reflecting the edematous change [7]. MRI is usually not required for diagnosis of acute cholecystitis. However, it sometimes can depict small cholelithiasis or debris collection with greater sensitivity than US and the less invasive evaluation of bile duct anatomy in MRCP is helpful for presurgical planning [8]. When inflammation or infection of acute cholecystitis gets worse, it leads to more severe conditions including gangrenous cholecystitis or emphysematous cholecystitis. US examinations can describe linear hyper-echoic structures that represent sloughed epithelium due to necrosis (Fig. 3) [9]. Additionally, intraluminal hemorrhaging sometimes is shown as heterogeneous hyper-echoic shadows. Sloughed epithelium can be depicted as hyperattenuating linear structures on CT, and in some cases, necrotic epithelium or intra-mural hemorrhaging are described as hyper attenuation along with the gallbladder wall. On dynamic study, there is diffuse or partial lack of enhancement in the epithelial layer in both arterial and venous phase images (Fig. 4) [10]. This finding also corresponds to epithelial necrosis and useful findings suggesting gangrenous cholecystitis. Additionally, luminal protrusions or peri-cholecystic abscesses are also frequently seen in this condition (Fig. 5) [9, 11, 12]. For evaluation of the spread of abscesses, CT is superior to US. Emphysematous cholecystitis is another manifestation of severe acute cholecystitis that could

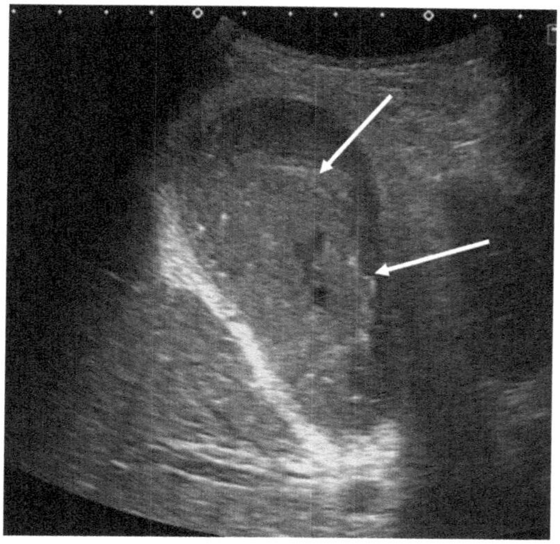

Fig. 3 US image of gangrenous cholecystitis. Liner hyper-echoic structures are described (suspected sloughed epithelium, arrows)

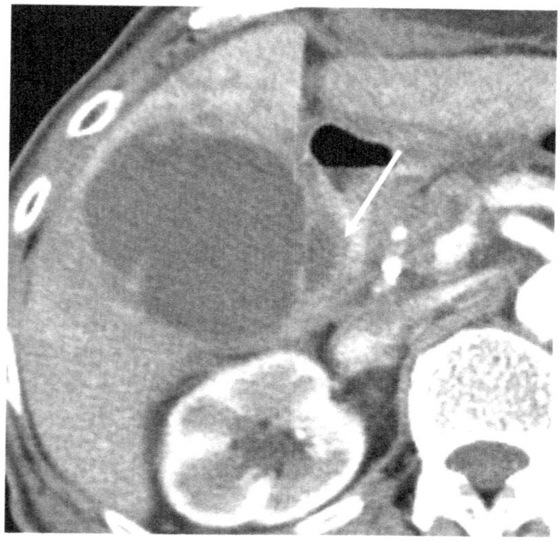

Fig. 5 Dynamic CT image of gangrenous cholecystitis. Luminal protrusion due to wall necrosis and perforation is demonstrated (arrow)

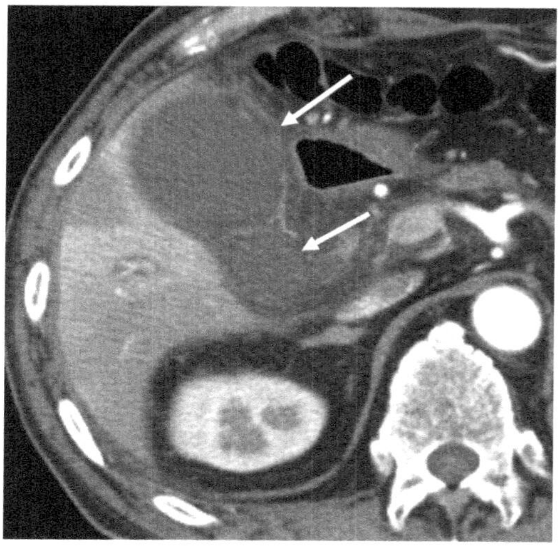

Fig. 4 Dynamic CT image of gangrenous cholecystitis. Thickened wall lacks enhancement due to necrosis (arrows)

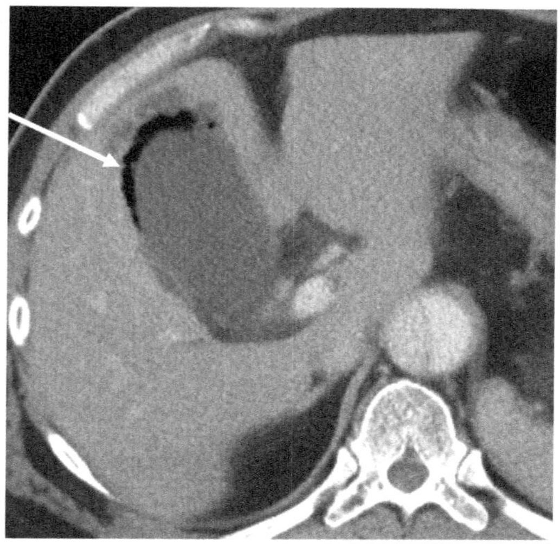

Fig. 6 Dynamic CT image of emphysematous cholecystitis. Intra-mural gas is clearly shown (arrow)

be lethal. Intra-mural gas is usually described as linear or heterogeneous echogenic structures along the gallbladder wall. CT can clearly demonstrate intra-mural gas directly (Fig. 6). Thus, when emphysematous cholecystitis is suspected in the clinical course or from US examination, we should consider CT to confirm the diagnosis [12].

Chronic Cholecystitis

Chronic cholecystitis is a condition usually accompanied by gall stones. Typical imaging findings are diffuse gallbladder wall thickening with delayed enhancement reflecting the fibrosis due to chronic inflammation in the gallbladder

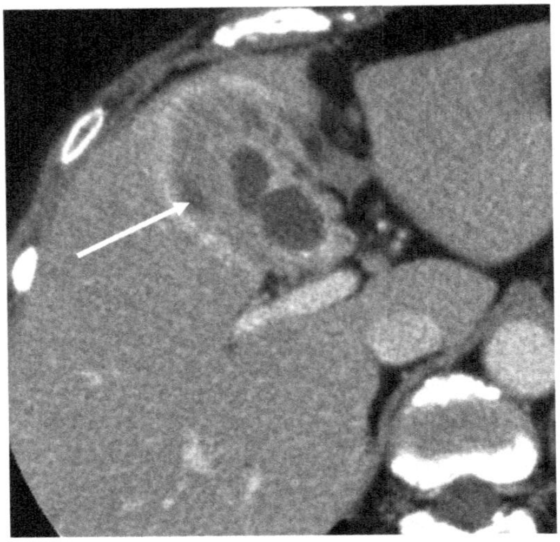

Fig. 7 Dynamic CT image of xanthogranulomatous cholecystitis. Gallbladder wall is remarkably thickened containing low-attenuating area (arrow). Luminal surface is relatively smooth

wall. Wall thickening can sometimes appear irregular although peri-cholecystic infiltration or peri-cholecystic fluid is usually absent. Edematous wall thickening is rarely seen. When wall thickening is focal or localized, it is extremely difficult to distinguish from gallbladder carcinoma [13]. Xanthogranulomatous cholecystitis is a rare form of chronic cholecystitis [14, 15]. Pathologically, it is characterized by intra-mural inflammation, the result of extravasation of bile juice through Rokitansky-Aschoff sinuses or infected epithelium. This intra-mural infection consists of inflammatory cell infiltration including lipid-laden macrophages and fibrosis. Given this pathological background, affected gallbladder walls show wall thickening containing hypoechoic areas. On dynamic CT, the thickened walls often demonstrate heterogeneous attenuation corresponding to the fibrous portion and hypercellular areas (Fig. 7) [15]. Multiple calcifications can also be seen in CT. When an inflammation penetrates the gallbladder wall structure, peri-cholecystic, or neighboring liver parenchymal inflammation can be seen leading to difficulty in differential diagnosis from carcinoma [14]. Several CT findings such as continuity of mucosal line, intra-mural low-density nodule, and lack of intra-hepatic bile duct dilatation have been reported as useful findings to distinguish this condition from gallbladder carcinoma though, discrimination still remains challenging for some cases [16]. The usefulness of MRI is controversial although lipid-rich portions sometimes can be described in T1-weighted images (chemical shift images) (Fig. 8) [17].

Adenomyomatosis

Adenomyomatosis is an acquired condition led by epithelial proliferation. The proliferated epithelium extends deep into the muscular layer forming Rokitansky-Aschoff sinuses (RAS). The affected gallbladder wall is thickened focally, segmentally, and diffusely [18]. Focal type is most commonly observed in fundus with segmental type in the body leading to a waisted shape (Fig. 9). Usually, this condition is asymptomatic and found incidentally. Typical US finding includes wall thickening with a comet-tail sign (representing the cholesterol crystals in RAS causing reverberation artifacts). This finding is considered as highly suggestive for the diagnosis of this condition (Fig. 10). RAS structures could be described as multiple cystic areas in the thickened wall lined by a hyper-enhanced layer (corresponding to the invaginated epithelium) on dynamic CT. Additionally, observing in multiple angles using MPR images make it easy to detect multiple focal lesions or describe waist-shaped gallbladder characteristics for segmental adenomyomatosis. However, in the cases of adenomyomatosis with small RAS structures, it is difficult to depict them on CT images, and they can be confused with other conditions causing gallbladder wall thickening. Calcifications are sometimes detected in the thickened wall. For typical cases, the role of MRI is limited. However, for atypical cases or indeterminate cases, high contrast resolution of MRI/MRCP is helpful to describe RAS structures in the thickened wall [19] (Fig. 11). RAS structures usually present hypo-signal intensity in T1 weighted images and hyper-intensity in T2 weighted

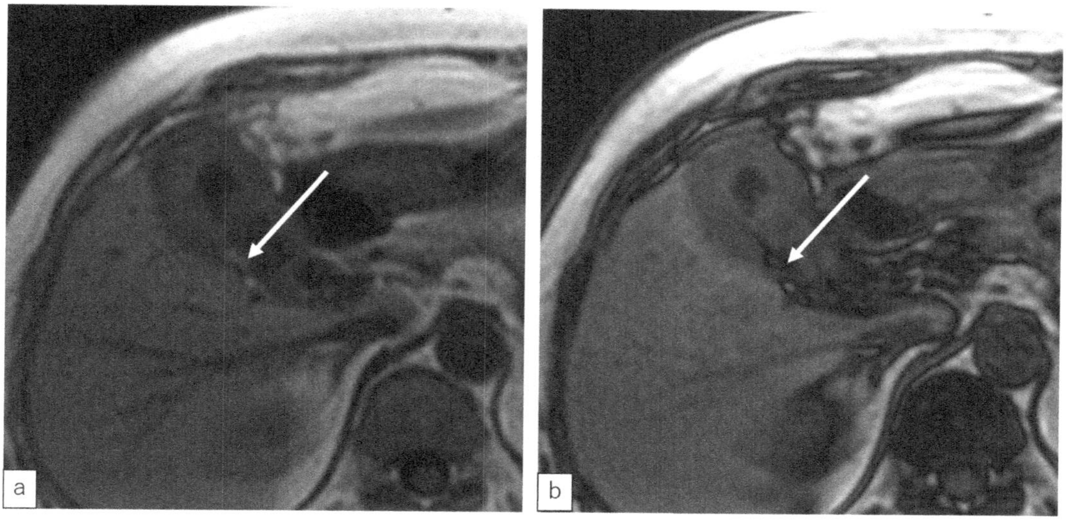

Fig. 8 MRI (**a** T1WI in phase, **b** T1WI out of phase) of xanthogranulomatous cholecystitis. Small nodular structure showing hyper-intensity in T1WI in phase image demonstrates signal drop in T1WI out of phase suggesting small amount of fat-containing portion (arrow)

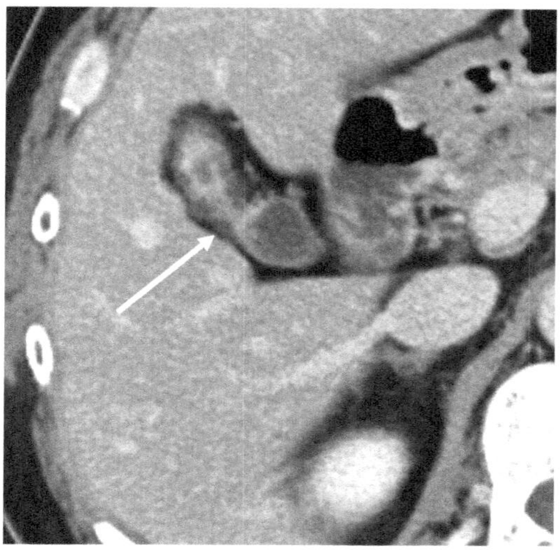

Fig. 9 Dynamic CT image of adenomyomatosis. Gallbladder shows waisted shape with multiple RAS structures (arrow)

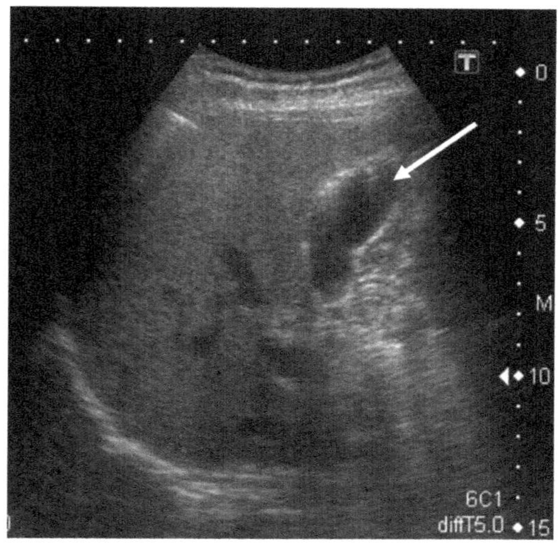

Fig. 10 US image of adenomyomatosis. US demonstrates comet-tail sign (arrow)

images reflecting the trapped bile in the RAS [20]. When viscosity of the bile in the RAS increases, RAS structures show hyper-intensity in T1 weighted images (Fig. 12). In diffuse-type adenomyomatosis, intra-mural multiple RAS structures appear like strings of pearls in MRCP (Pearl necklace sign) [21]. For any cases describing the RAS structures in the thickened wall, we should consider which modality is the best to depict them for patients in whom adenomyomatosis is suspected.

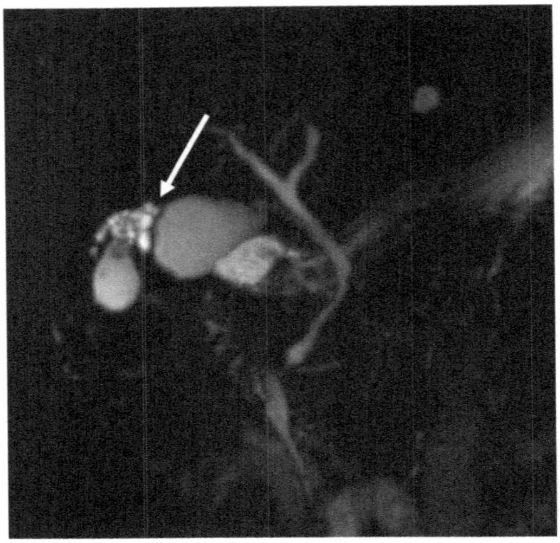

Fig. 11 MRCP of adenomyomatosis. MRCP clearly describes multiple RAS structures (arrow)

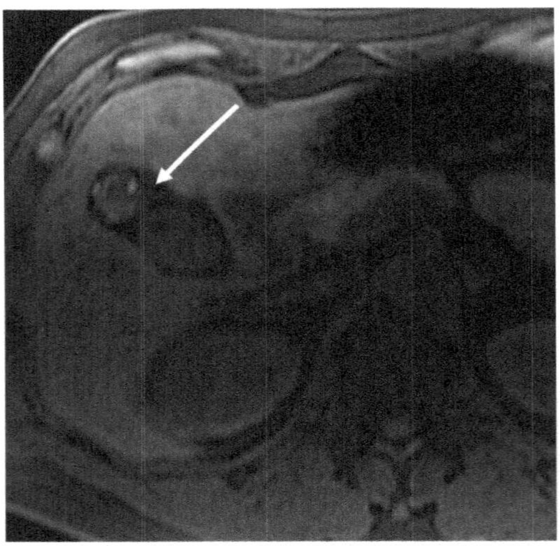

Fig. 12 T1WI of adenomyomatosis. Some RAS structures present hyper-intensity due to the increase of viscosity of the trapped bile (arrow)

IgG4-Related Cholecystitis

IgG4-related disease (IgG4-RD) is a recently established systemic disease. It is characterized by predominant occurrence in elderly males with serum IgG4 elevation, simultaneous or metachronous involvement systemic organs, and favorable response to steroid therapy. The organs frequently affected include lacrimal or salivary glands, lungs, pancreas, bile duct, kidneys, and the aorta [22]. In the biliary system, intra or extra bile ducts are known to be highly involved parts, although recent reports suggest that the gallbladder could also be a target organ of IgG4-RD. IgG4-related cholecystitis is pathologically characterized by lymphoplasmacytic infiltrations, obliterative phlebitis, and fibrosis [23]. Abundant IgG4-bearing cells are also found in the thickened walls. As with other organs like lung or pancreas, destructive change is rarely seen in IgG4-related cholecystitis and the epithelium layer is usually intact. Considering its pathological background, IgG4-related cholecystitis is described as wall thickening with a hyper-enhanced epithelium lining the luminal surface (Fig. 13) [24]. Usually, peri-cholecystic inflammation or intra-mural calcification is not observed. Additionally, this condition is usually observed as a gallbladder manifestation of systemic disease IgG4-RD. Detecting IgG4-related lesions in other organs is a key step to suggesting this condition in clinical practice. Thus, being familiar with imaging

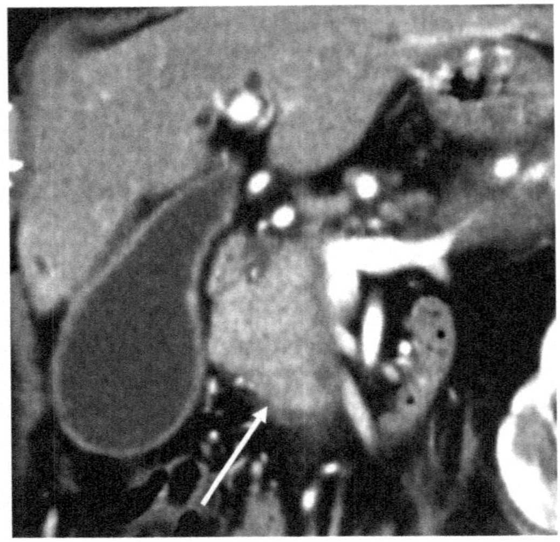

Fig. 13 Dynamic CT image (coronal image) of IgG4-related cholecystitis. Gallbladder wall thickening is homogeneous and luminal surface is totally smooth. Autoimmune pancreatitis (IgG4-related pancreatitis) is also shown (arrow)

features of IgG4-related lesions in frequently involved organs is crucial to make correct diagnosis of IgG4-related cholecystitis. At the same time, if IgG4-related cholecystitis is suspected, systemic screening using contrast-enhanced CT or FDG-PET and checking the serum IgG4 value would be helpful.

Systemic Disease or Condition

Gallbladder wall thickening can sometimes occur secondary to extra-gall bladder conditions. Acute hepatitis is well known to cause gall bladder wall thickening. On US and CT, diffuse edematous wall thickening is the typical imaging finding without gallbladder stones. Additionally, the gallbladder lumen is usually collapsed supposedly due to insufficient production of the bile juice [25]. Peri-cholecystic stranding is usually absent. Patients with acute hepatitis rarely have Murphy's symptom and they usually present abnormal elevation of liver enzymes higher than those seen in patients with acute cholecystitis. In acute hepatitis, liver parenchymal enlargement and edematous change in Glisson's sheath are frequently observed and this morphological change is depicted as peri-portal echogenicity in US examinations and hypo-density areas along with intra-hepatic portal veins. MRI, especially T2 weighted images, can describe peri-portal edema as hyper-intensity [26]. Thus, when there is diffuse edematous wall thickening of the gallbladder without distention or abdominal pain suggesting acute cholecystitis, acute hepatitis should be considered as a cause of wall thickening. Chronic liver diseases or liver cirrhosis are also causes of edematous gallbladder wall thickening without distention or acute symptoms [1]. In these conditions, portal hypertension and hypoalbuminemia are considered as the mechanism of wall thickening. US and CT findings are usually similar to those seen in acute hepatitis including diffuse edematous wall thickening, lack of peri-cholecystic inflammation, or distention (Fig. 14) [27]. Liver morphology (irregular edge, heterogeneous/multi-nodular parenchyma) or secondary signs for portal hypertension (collateral formations, varices, and splenomegaly) are also frequently seen.

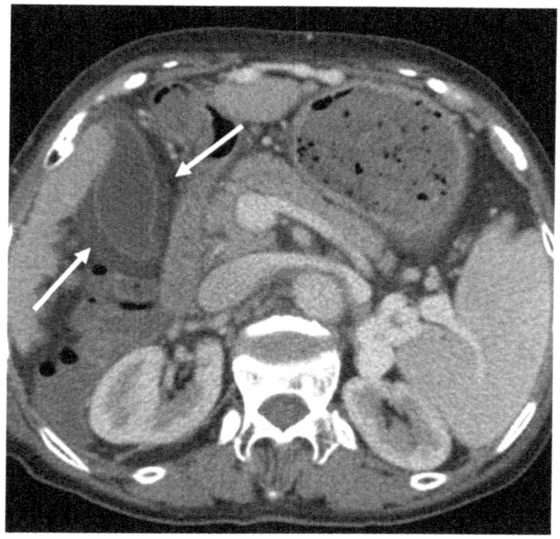

Fig. 14 Dynamic CT of liver cirrhosis. Gallbladder wall shows edematous change due to portal hypertension (arrow)

Other causes of diffuse edematous gallbladder wall thickening such as heart or renal failure should also be noted. In these conditions, portal hypertension due to elevation of venous pressure or decreased intravascular osmic pressure is suspected to be the mechanisms of wall thickening. Imaging findings of wall thickening due to other organ dysfunctions are usually non-characteristic (diffuse edematous wall thickening, lack of gallbladder stones or distention, less peri-cholecystic inflammation). Therefore, when we find diffuse edematous gallbladder wall thickening, it is important to consider the possibility of secondary wall thickening and check other organs to avoid diagnostic delay for these organ failures.

Secondary Involvement from Extracholecystic Inflammation

Gall bladder wall thickening can also be seen as being secondary to inflammation in other organs including acute pancreatitis [28], pyelonephritis

[29], and peritonitis. Usually, the wall thickening is caused by direct involvement from the inflammation's primary site. Identifying primary site/cause of inflammation is a key step to distinguishing this cause from acute cholecystitis or other organ dysfunctions noted above. Contrast-enhanced CT has an advantage over US in seeking the primary site due to its being less operator dependent as well as its spatial resolution.

Neoplastic Lesions

Primary Gallbladder Carcinoma

Gallbladder carcinoma is the most important differential diagnosis of gallbladder wall thickening, and maximum attention should be paid to this when gallbladder wall thickening is detected. Gallbladder stones are a well-known risk factor of gallbladder carcinoma and frequently coexist with carcinoma [30]. Gallbladder carcinoma can manifest various imaging features including focal or diffuse wall thickening and polypoid lesions. Concerning wall thickening types, typical imaging findings include irregular wall thickening with invasion to neighboring fat tissue or liver parenchyma [31–34]. On US, the affected wall usually shows pronounced and irregular wall thickening, and the gallbladder configuration usually has become asymmetric. Heterogeneity and mural irregularity are considered highly suggestive for gallbladder carcinoma [34]. Contrast-enhanced CT also shows irregular wall thickening with heterogeneous attenuation. Mural irregularity or extramural invasion to adjacent fat tissue or liver parenchyma are also seen (Fig. 15). Additionally, peri-cholecystic vascular invasion, lymph node enlargement, or peritoneal disseminations are suggestive for the diagnosis of gallbladder carcinoma [32]. The extent of liver parenchymal or hepatic hilar invasion or vascular invasion is more precisely evaluated in contrast-enhanced CT images by observing from multiple directions (Axial, sagittal, and coronal images) using MPR technique. As noted above, advanced gallbladder carcinoma is a relatively less difficult diagnosis to make, although early stage carcinomas often present only mild wall thickening without secondary signs like invasion to adjacent tissue or vascular invasion, which leads to diagnostic challenges. Unlike chronic

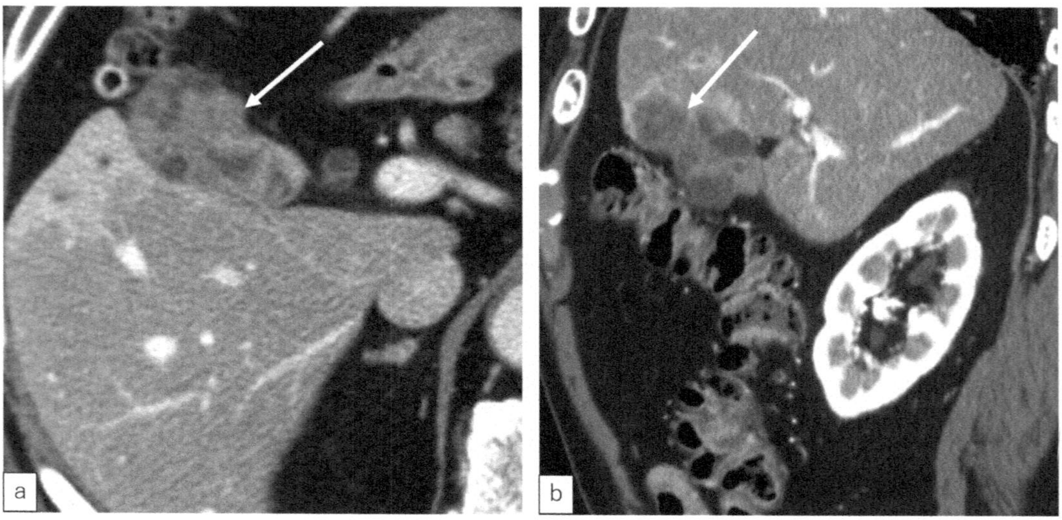

Fig. 15 Dynamic CT of Gallbladder carcinoma (**a** Axial, **b** Oblique image). Gallbladder wall is heterogeneously thickened (**a** arrow). Hepatic parenchymal invasion is also noted (**b** arrow)

cholecystitis, carcinoma more frequently demonstrates mural irregularity even in the early stage [32, 34]. Thus, detailed evaluation of the lining epithelium layer or gallbladder configuration by US or CT is essential for early diagnosis of non-advanced gallbladder carcinoma.

Other Malignancies

Malignant lymphoma or metastatic tumors can be seen in the gallbladder, but they are extremely rare and characteristic imaging features have not been established. Metastatic tumors are more often found as nodular lesions rather than wall thickening ones [35]. Imaging features are similar to those in primary tumors. Hyper-vascular tumors like hepatocellular carcinoma or renal cell carcinoma are well-known primary sites, and likewise metastatic tumors in the gallbladder also demonstrate hyper-vascular lesions [36].

Conclusion

As noted in this chapter, various conditions including acute or chronic inflammation, systemic disease, and malignancies occur in the gall bladder as demonstrated by wall thickening. We explained characteristic imaging findings for each of various conditions sharing demonstrable figures, although they have large overlaps and it is sometimes challenging to reach the correct diagnosis in clinical practice. Thus, for adequate management for patients with gallbladder wall thickening, making diagnosis through a comprehensive approach including clinical, imaging, and pathological examinations should be mandatory.

References

1. Zissin R, Osadchy A, Shapiro-Feinberg M, Gayer G. CT of a thickened-wall gall bladder. Br J Radiol. 2003;76(902):137–43.
2. Jung SE, Lee JM, Lee K, Rha SE, Choi BG, Kim EK, et al. Gallbladder wall thickening: MR imaging and pathologic correlation with emphasis on layered pattern. Eur Radiol. 2005;15(4):694–701.
3. Huffman JL, Schenker S. Acute acalculous cholecystitis: a review. Clin Gastroenterol Hepatol. 2010;8(1):15–22.
4. Ralls PW, Colletti PM, Lapin SA, Chandrasoma P, Boswell WD Jr, Ngo C, et al. Real-time sonography in suspected acute cholecystitis. Prospective evaluation of primary and secondary signs. Radiology. 1985;155(3):767–71.
5. Yamashita K, Jin MJ, Hirose Y, Morikawa M, Sumioka H, Itoh K, et al. CT finding of transient focal increased attenuation of the liver adjacent to the gallbladder in acute cholecystitis. AJR Am J Roentgenol. 1995;164(2):343–6.
6. Fidler J, Paulson EK, Layfield L. CT evaluation of acute cholecystitis: findings and usefulness in diagnosis. AJR Am J Roentgenol. 1996;166(5):1085–8.
7. Adusumilli S, Siegelman ES. MR imaging of the gallbladder. Magn Reson Imaging Clin N Am. 2002;10(1):165–84.
8. Park MS, Yu JS, Kim YH, Kim MJ, Kim JH, Lee S, et al. Acute cholecystitis: comparison of MR cholangiography and US. Radiology. 1998;209(3):781–5.
9. Teefey SA, Baron RL, Radke HM, Bigler SA. Gangrenous cholecystitis: new observations on sonography. J Ultrasound Med. 1991;10(11):603–6.
10. Bennett, G.L., Rusinek H, Lisi V, Israel GM, Krinsky GA, Slywotzky CM, et al. CT findings in acute gangrenous cholecystitis. AJR Am J Roentgenol. 2002;178(2):275–81.
11. Kane RA. Ultrasonographic diagnosis of gangrenous cholecystitis and empyema of the gallbladder. Radiology. 1980;134(1):191–4.
12. Grayson DE, Abbott RM, Levy AD, Sherman PM. Emphysematous infections of the abdomen and pelvis: a pictorial review. Radiographics. 2002;22(3):543–61.
13. Levy AD, Murakata LA, Abbott RM, Rohrmann CA Jr. From the archives of the AFIP. Benign tumors and tumorlike lesions of the gallbladder and extrahepatic bile ducts: radiologic-pathologic correlation. Armed Forces Institute of Pathology. Radiographics. 2002;22(2):387–413.
14. Chun KA, Ha HK, Yu ES, Shinn KS, Kim KW, Lee DH, et al. Xanthogranulomatous cholecystitis: CT features with emphasis on differentiation from gallbladder carcinoma. Radiology. 1997;203(1):93–7.
15. Parra JA, Acinas O, Bueno J, Güezmes A, Fernández MA, Fariñas MC. Xanthogranulomatous cholecystitis: clinical, sonographic, and CT findings in 26 patients. AJR Am J Roentgenol. 2000;174(4):979–83.
16. Goshima S, Chang S, Wang JH, Kanematsu M, Bae KT, Federle MP. Xanthogranulomatous cholecystitis: diagnostic performance of CT to differentiate from gallbladder cancer. Eur J Radiol. 2010;74(3):e79–83.
17. Hatakenaka M, Adachi T, Matsuyama A, Mori M, Yoshikawa Y. Xanthogranulomatous cholecystitis:

importance of chemical-shift gradient-echo MR imaging. Eur Radiol. 2003;13(9):2233–5.
18. Rosenthal SJ, Cox GG, Wetzel LH, Batnitzky S. Pitfalls and differential diagnosis in biliary sonography. Radiographics. 1990;10(2):285–311.
19. Yoshimitsu K, Honda H, Jimi M, Kuroiwa T, Hanada K, Irie H, et al. MR diagnosis of adenomyomatosis of the gallbladder and differentiation from gallbladder carcinoma: importance of showing Rokitansky-Aschoff sinuses. AJR Am J Roentgenol. 1999;172(6):1535–40.
20. Kim MJ, Oh YT, Park YN, Chung JB, Kim DJ, Chung JJ, et al. Gallbladder adenomyomatosis: findings on MRI. Abdom Imaging. 1999;24(4):410–3.
21. Haradome H, Ichikawa T, Sou H, Yoshikawa T, Nakamura A, Araki T, et al. The pearl necklace sign: an imaging sign of adenomyomatosis of the gallbladder at MR cholangiopancreatography. Radiology. 2003;227(1):80–8.
22. Inoue D, Yoshida K, Yoneda N, Ozaki K, Matsubara T, Nagai K, et al. IgG4-related disease: dataset of 235 consecutive patients. Medicine (Baltimore). 2015;94(15):e680.
23. Zen Y. The pathology of IgG4-related disease in the bile duct and pancreas. Semin Liver Dis. 2016;36(3):242–56.
24. Vlachou PA, Khalili K, Jang HJ, Fischer S, Hirschfield GM, Kim TK. IgG4-related sclerosing disease: autoimmune pancreatitis and extrapancreatic manifestations. Radiographics. 2011;31(5):1379–402.
25. Maresca G, De Gaetano AM, Mirk P, Cauda R, Federico G, Colagrande C. Sonographic patterns of the gallbladder in acute viral hepatitis. J Clin Ultrasound. 1984;12(3):141–6.
26. Ito K, Mitchell DG, Gabata T. Enlargement of hilar periportal space: a sign of early cirrhosis at MR imaging. J Magn Reson Imaging. 2000;11(2):136–40.
27. Kaftori JK, Pery M, Green J, Gaitini D. Thickness of the gallbladder wall in patients with hypoalbuminemia: a sonographic study of patients on peritoneal dialysis. AJR Am J Roentgenol. 1987;148(6):1117–8.
28. Somer K, Kivisaari L, Standertskjöld-Nordenstam CG, Kalima TV. Contrast-enhanced computed tomography of the gallbladder in acute pancreatitis. Gastrointest Radiol. 1984;9(1):31–4.
29. Zissin R, Kots E, Rachmani R, Hadari R, Shapiro-Feinberg M. Hepatic periportal tracking associated with severe acute pyelonephritis. Abdom Imaging. 2000;25(3):251–4.
30. Lowenfels AB, Lindström CG, Conway MJ, Hastings PR. Gallstones and risk of gallbladder cancer. J Natl Cancer Inst. 1985;75(1):77–80.
31. Franquet T, Montes M, Ruiz de Azua Y, Jimenez FJ, Cozcolluela R. Primary gallbladder carcinoma: imaging findings in 50 patients with pathologic correlation. Gastrointest Radiol. 1991;16(2):143–8.
32. Lane J, Buck JL, Zeman RK. Primary carcinoma of the gallbladder: a pictorial essay. Radiographics. 1989;9(2):209–28.
33. Yeh HC. Ultrasonography and computed tomography of carcinoma of the gallbladder. Radiology. 1979;133(1):167–73.
34. Weiner SN, Koenigsberg M, Morehouse H, Hoffman J. Sonography and computed tomography in the diagnosis of carcinoma of the gallbladder. AJR Am J Roentgenol. 1984;142(4):735–9.
35. Barretta ML, Catalano O, Setola SV, Granata V, Marone U, Gallipoli AD. Gallbladder metastasis: spectrum of imaging findings. Abdom Imaging. 2011;36(6):729–34.
36. Chatterjee A, Lopes Vendrami C, Nikolaidis P, Mittal PK, Bandy AJ, Menias CO, et al. Uncommon intraluminal tumors of the gallbladder and biliary tract: spectrum of imaging appearances. Radiographics. 2019;39(2):388–412.

Current Issues: Prophylactic Cholecystectomy

Prophylactic Cholecystectomy in Patients with Concomitant Gallstones After Removal of CBD Stones by ERCP

Byung Kyu Park

Introduction

Endoscopic retrograde cholangiopancreatography (ERCP) and stone removal are the current standard treatments for common bile duct (CBD) stones. CBD stones predominantly originate in the gallbladder (GB) and migrate to the CBD, or may primarily form in the CBD. The remaining GB stones after ERCP stone removal may later migrate to the CBD and cause complications such as biliary obstruction, acute cholangitis, and gallstone pancreatitis. Moreover, GB stones themselves cause biliary colic and acute cholecystitis. Therefore, cholecystectomy seems a reasonable method for reducing CBD stone recurrence and its complications when GB stones are present.

Prospective studies of patients with concomitant GB stones who underwent ERCP stone removal have shown that cholecystectomy reduces the risk of recurrent biliary events compared to the wait-and-see policy [1, 2]. In addition, several retrospective studies recommend cholecystectomy after ERCP stone removal [3–6]. However, other studies have shown that elective cholecystectomy after ERCP stone removal does not reduce the incidence of recurrent biliary complications [7–11]. In recent years, after endoscopic CBD stone removal, prophylactic cholecystectomy in patients with GB stones is generally recommended to reduce biliary complications. However, the necessity of cholecystectomy is frequently debated.

Endoscopic sphincterotomy (ES) is generally required for CBD stone removal. In this procedure, the biliary orifice is widened so that the subsequent small CBD stone or sludge can pass spontaneously into the duodenum without causing an obstruction. Additionally, ES can reduce recurrent pancreatitis by separating the biliary and pancreatic orifice, eliminating common channels [12]. ES alone may reduce recurrent biliary complications.

Laparoscopic cholecystectomy is preferred over open cholecystectomy as surgical treatment because it has a lower morbidity and requires a shorter hospital stay. However, 3–20% of laparoscopic cholecystectomies require conversion to open cholecystectomy because of technical difficulties such as bleeding and adhesions [13, 14]. Furthermore, elderly patients, who make up the majority of patients with complicated gallstone disease, have a higher incidence of comorbidity, an increased conversion rate to open cholecystectomy, and higher morbidity and

B. K. Park (✉)
Division of Gastroenterology, Department of Internal Medicine, National Health Insurance Service Ilsan Hospital, Yonsei University College of Medicine, Goyang-si, Gyeonggi-do, Korea
e-mail: bkpark@nhimc.or.kr

J. B. Chung and K. Okazaki (eds.), *Diseases of the Gallbladder*,
https://doi.org/10.1007/978-981-15-6010-1_28

mortality than do younger patients. Therefore, the wait-and-see policy without cholecystectomy can be considered in elderly or surgically high-risk patients [15, 16]. In addition, optimal timing of cholecystectomy after ERCP stone removal is important to reduce recurrent biliary events and the conversion rate to open cholecystectomy; however, there is no consensus on this.

Biliary Complications After ERCP Stone Removal

After successful removal of CBD stones, biliary complications such as recurrent CBD stones and cholecystitis occur in 7–47% of patients within 2.5–15 year follow-up periods [17–21]. The risk factors for the development of biliary complications include GB stones, dilated CBD, mechanical lithotripsy, periampullary diverticulum, and bile duct strictures [11, 17, 20, 22–25].

Considering CBD stone recurrence, its incidence after ERCP stone removal has found to be 2–22% in follow-up studies [17–21, 24–27] and 11.3% in a population-based study [28]. Recurrence of CBD stones after ERCP stone removal is caused by a number of mechanisms. Migration of the GB stone into the CBD is an important mechanism. Moreover, reflux of duodenal contents into the bile duct, stricture at the ES site, and dilated CBD lead to bile stasis and bacterial infection with consequent sludge and stone formation in the CBD.

Acute cholecystitis is another concern in patients who have undergone CBD stone removal, especially in patients with GB stones. The risk of acute cholecystitis has been suggested to be increased after ES. Dysfunction of the biliary sphincter after ES might be a cause of reflux of duodenal contents into the bile duct and biliary infection, leading to infection of the GB and subsequent cholecystitis [3].

The development of acute cholecystitis is a definite indication of cholecystectomy. A study of 100 patients who had their CBD stone removed without cholecystectomy reported that acute cholecystitis occurred in 17% and CBD stone recurred in 15% of the patients. The risk factors of acute cholecystitis include nondilated CBD (<11 mm) and absence of jaundice (serum total bilirubin < 1.3 mg/dL) at the time of CBD stone removal [29]. Small CBD stones in association with a nondilated CBD are more likely to originate from the GB. If cholecystectomy is not performed in such patients, development of acute cholecystitis due to cystic duct obstruction by a small gallstone is a risk during passage of gallstones.

Prophylactic Cholecystectomy

Several retrospective, prospective, and population-based studies of cholecystectomies performed after ERCP stone removal have been conducted. Each study differs in design, including sample size, follow-up duration, age of the patients studied, and whether only patients with GB stones or those with intact GB are included (Table 1).

Patients Without GB Stones

Patients without GB stones have a lower recurrence rate of CBD stone than do patients with GB stones [3, 4, 19]. Furthermore, CBD stone recurrence rate was lower in patients with acalculous GB in situ than in patients who had previously undergone a cholecystectomy [4]. Theoretically, because GB stone migration from the GB is a possible mechanism of CBD stone recurrence, a patient without GB stones is not considered a surgical candidate. It has also been reported that a GB without stones after ERCP stone removal does not increase the risk of acute cholecystitis [3]. A GB without gallstones after ERCP stone removal helps to wash away bile and prevent new stone formation or flush out newly produced gallstones [30]. Therefore, prophylactic cholecystectomy after ERCP stone removal is not generally recommended in patients without GB stones in terms of its preventive effect on recurrent CBD stones.

Table 1 Studies of prophylactic cholecystectomy in patients who underwent ERCP stone removal

Study	Year	Country	Design	Subgroups of patients	No. of patients	Follow-up duration (yrs)	Recommendation of cholecystectomy
Hammarstrom et al. [8]	1996	Sweden	Retrospective	Intact GB	265	5.8	No
Pereira-Lima et al. [5]	1998	Germany	Retrospective	Intact GB	203	6.2	Yes
Lai et al. [9]	1999	China	Retrospective	Intact GB	140	3.6	No
Boerma et al. [1]	2002	Netherlands	Prospective, RCT	With GB stones	120	2.0	Yes
Schreurs et al. [10]	2004	Netherlands	Retrospective	With GB stones	242	5.9	No
Lau et al. [2]	2006	China	Prospective, RCT	≥60 yrs, with GB stones	178	5.0	Yes
Kageoka et al. [4]	2009	Japan	Retrospective	With GB stones	175	5.1	Yes
Lai et al. [6]	2012	Taiwan	Retrospective	With GB stones	183		Yes
Cui et al. [3]	2013	Korea	Retrospective	Intact GB	232	6.1	Equivocal
Heo et al. [7]	2015	Korea	Prospective, RCT	With GB stones	90	3.4	No
Song et al. [11]	2016	Korea	Retrospective	Intact GB	317	2.1	No
Nakai et al. [43]	2016	Japan	Retrospective	EPBD, with GB stones	294	4.2	Yes
Elmunzer et al. [37]	2017	United States	Population-based	≥65 yrs, intact GB	11,808	6.0	Yes
Huang, et al. [32]	2017	United States	Population-based	Intact GB	4,516	–	Yes
Young et al. [36]	2017	Taiwan	Population-based	≥70 yrs, gallstone pancreatitis	670	–	Yes
Park et al. [28]	2018	Korea	Population-based	With GB stones	16,910	4.2	Yes
Khan et al. [31]	2018	–	Meta-analysis	–	916	–	Yes

RCT, randomized controlled trial; GB, gallbladder; yrs, years

Patients with GB Stones

Patients with GB stones are considered to have an increased risk of recurrent CBD stone secondary to stone migration from the GB and subsequent acute cholecystitis. There has been much research on the prophylactic effect of cholecystectomy after ERCP stone removal. Some studies recommended cholecystectomy, while others do not. Most of these studies had had small sample sizes, short follow-up durations, and retrospective chart reviews; moreover, there is a lack of large randomized studies.

Schreurs et al. conducted a large cohort study of 447 patients with symptomatic GB and CBD stones. Of these patients, 164 underwent

ERCP stone removal and no additional cholecystectomy, and 78 underwent cholecystectomy after ERCP stone removal. Of the patients who underwent only ERCP stone removal, 27 (16%) developed recurrent biliary complications. Specifically, 12 had recurrent CBD stones, 3 developed cholangitis, and 1 had papillary stenosis. Of these 27 patients, 13 underwent cholecystectomy. Of the cholecystectomized patients, 6 (7.6%) developed recurrent biliary complications. In patients who did not undergo cholecystectomy, the risk of biliary complications was similar to that in the normal population with silent stones. The authors concluded that when CBD stones are successfully removed and the patient is asymptomatic, routine prophylactic cholecystectomy is not required [10].

Boerma et al. conducted a randomized, prospective study that evaluated 120 patients with GB stones who underwent ERCP stone removal. All patients underwent ERCP and were randomized to a wait-and-see policy arm (64 patients) versus laparoscopic cholecystectomy (56 patients). They found that 47% of the wait-and-see group developed recurrent biliary symptoms compared with 2% of the laparoscopic cholecystectomy group, and 22 of 27 (81%) patients in the wait-and-see arm subsequently underwent cholecystectomy for recurrent biliary symptoms. The conversion rate to open cholecystectomy was 55% in the wait-and-see group and 23% in the laparoscopic cholecystectomy group. The authors concluded that a wait-and-see policy after ERCP stone removal in patients with concomitant GB stones cannot be recommended as standard treatment given the high rate of recurrent biliary symptoms and high conversion rate to open cholecystectomy [1].

In another prospective study, further biliary events after ERCP stone removal developed more frequently in patients with GB in situ than in cholecystectomized patients (24% versus 7%). The most common biliary event in both groups was cholangitis, for which the authors recommended cholecystectomy, just as in the previous report [2]. However, in a recent prospective study, cholecystectomy after CBD stone removal failed to reduce additional recurrent cholangitis, and the authors suggested that cholecystectomy should be limited to patients with symptomatic GB stones [7]. Furthermore, several retrospective studies show different results on this issue [3–6, 8, 9, 11].

A recent meta-analysis of 7 randomized control trials with 916 patients showed no difference in mortality between patients who underwent cholecystectomy after ERCP stone removal and patients who did not. In addition, there was no difference in the rate of acute pancreatitis between the two groups. However, pooled relative risk (RR) for occurrence of biliary colic and cholecystitis in the wait-and-see policy patients was 9.82 (4.27–22.59) compared to prophylactic cholecystectomy patients, and the RR for cholangitis and recurrent jaundice was 2.16 (1.14–4.07). Therefore, the author recommended laparoscopic cholecystectomy because of the lower rates of subsequent recurrent cholecystitis, cholangitis, and biliary colic, even in high-risk surgical patients [31].

A Korean population-based study reported different CBD stone recurrence rates in patients with GB stones who underwent cholecystectomy after ERCP stone removal and those who did not. During the follow-up period, CBD stone recurrence occurred in 7.92% (920/11,617) in the cholecystectomy group and in 14.60% (773/5,293) in the no-cholecystectomy group. The recurrence rate of CBD stone in the no-cholecystectomy group was about two times than that in the cholecystectomy group (RR = 1.961, 95% CI = 1.783–2.158, $p < 0.0001$). The RR for CBD stone recurrence in the no-cholecystectomy group compared with the cholecystectomy group was 3.198 in patients aged < 50 years, 2.371 in patients aged 50–59 years, 1.618 in patients aged 60–69 years, and 1.262 in patients aged ≥ 70 years. The RR for CBD stone recurrence in the no-cholecystectomy group was higher in younger patients. As age increased, the RR decreased. The authors recommended cholecystectomy in patients aged < 70 years with GB stone to reduce the risk of CBD stone recurrence as well as cholecystitis, and it was strongly recommended for relatively younger patients [28].

In addition, Huang et al. reported that the cumulative incidence of recurrent biliary events 60 days after discharge was 10.3% in the no-cholecystectomy group, 1.4% in the early cholecystectomy group, and 1.3% in the delayed cholecystectomy group. Prophylactic cholecystectomy within 60 days after ERCP was associated with 87–88% RR reduction for recurrent biliary events compared to the no-cholecystectomy group [32].

Elderly Patients

Due to comorbidities and low-performance status, elderly patients are thought to be at risk of increased perioperative morbidity and mortality. A systemic review demonstrated that early cholecystectomy for acute cholecystitis in patients aged ≥70 years is associated with a perioperative morbidity of 24% and a mortality of 3.5% [33]. These rates are higher than those in non-elderly patients, which have been investigated in a meta-analysis, being approximately 15% and <1%, respectively [34].

Some investigators do not recommend cholecystectomy after ERCP stone removal in elderly patients with GB stones [15, 16]. In a cost-effectiveness analysis, cholecystectomy was not recommended in elderly patients considering economic and survival benefits [15]. According to a Japanese study, in very elderly patients (those older than 80), the incidence of acute cholecystitis is low even when GB is preserved after ERCP stone removal, with a similar risk of CBD stone recurrence. The author does not recommend cholecystectomy after ERCP stone removal in very elderly patients [16]. GB contractile function in very elderly patients might decline, and they rarely develop acute cholecystitis. The low incidence of acute cholecystitis in very elderly patients might be explained by the decreased preference for fatty foods by older patients, which can trigger the development of cholecystitis [35].

In a previous Korean population-based study, the RR reported for CBD stone recurrence in the no-cholecystectomy group was only 1.262 for patients over 70 years old. The authors recommended to decide the cholecystectomy for patients over 70, considering the risk of operation and the comorbid illnesses [28].

Young et al. conducted a propensity score matching population-based study of 670 patients over 70 years of age to evaluate the preventive effect of cholecystectomy against recurrent pancreatitis. The incidence rate of recurrent pancreatitis was 12.39 per 1000 person-year in the cholecystectomy cohort and 23.94 per 1000 person-year in the control cohort. The risk of recurrent pancreatitis was significantly lower in the cholecystectomy cohort (hazard ratio [HR] = 0.56, 95% CI = 0.59–0.95, p = 0.021). The HR for all-cause mortality among the cholecystectomy cohort was 0.75 (95% CI = 0.59–0.95; p = 0.016) compared with the control cohort. The authors concluded that prophylactic cholecystectomy should be recommended in these elderly patients [36].

Furthermore, in a population-based study of patients over 65 years of age, prophylactic cholecystectomy was significantly associated with a 50–70% RR reduction in recurrent CBD stones, cholangitis, and gallstone pancreatitis compared to only ES. This benefit was preserved in patients over the age of 75 and in those with serious comorbidities such as cancer and heart failure, and did not appear to be outweighed by surgical complications [37].

Endoscopic Balloon Biliary Dilatation

Endoscopic papillary balloon dilation (EPBD) can be another alternative to ES in selected patients, such as those with an altered anatomy or at bleeding risk. Several studies have shown that EPBD alone or in combination with small ES and lithotripsy can be used for the management of difficult biliary stones [38–40]. The advantage of EPBD is that it can preserve the biliary sphincter function, which prevents duodeno-biliary reflux and bacterial contamination [41].

In a prospective multicenter randomized controlled trial that compared the early outcomes after ES and EPBD, the overall incidence of late biliary complications in the EPBD group was significantly lower than that in the ES group (10.1% versus 25.0%, p=0.016). The biliary sphincter dysfunction after ES results in additional late complications [42].

However, according to a propensity score-based cohort study that compared cholecystectomy and the wait-and-see approach after EPBD, the rates of late biliary complications were 5.4 and 25.2% in the cholecystectomy and wait-and-see groups, respectively. Recurrent CBD stones rates were 4.1 and 19.0%, and cholecystitis rates were 0.7 and 6.1%, respectively. The majority of late complications in the group with GB left in situ with stones was CBD stone recurrence, which had likely migrated from the GB. Preserved papillary function after EPBD had no impact on the prevention of CBD stone recurrence in this group. The authors recommended prophylactic cholecystectomy to all surgically fit patients after EPBD for CBD stones with concomitant GB stones [43].

Decision of Prophylactic Cholecystectomy in the Real World

Taken together, the results of previous retrospective and prospective studies showed equivocal outcomes of recommendations for cholecystectomy [1–11, 43]. However, several large-scale population-based studies and meta-analyses recommend cholecystectomy [28, 31, 32, 36, 37].

The decision to perform cholecystectomy in patients who undergone ERCP stone removal should be considered in two ways. One is the effect on the prevention of recurrent biliary complications, and the other is the burden on morbidity, mortality, and health care expenditure associated with cholecystectomy. Unless patients are at high risk for cholecystectomy, it is reasonable to recommend cholecystectomy for patients with GB stones after ERCP stone removal regardless of age. However, in reality, cholecystectomy is not always performed in line with patients' preferences or comorbidities in elderly patients. In retrospective population-based cohort studies, the proportion of patients who underwent no-cholecystectomy after ERCP stone removal was 48% in the United States [32] and 78.8% in Taiwan [44]. The rate of laparoscopic cholecystectomy was over 95% in Australia and 90% in the United States [32]. In contrast, the population-based study in Taiwan found that the proportion of patients undergoing laparoscopic cholecystectomy was only 51.16%. In addition, the durations of hospital stay were longer in the open surgery group. This is one reason for the relatively low rate of prophylactic cholecystectomy in Taiwanese patients [44]. Whether cholecystectomy is performed in the actual clinical field, is influenced by hospital factors such as volume and location, and patient factors such as race and insurance status.

Timing of Prophylactic Cholecystectomy

The timing of cholecystectomy following ERCP is also important. Traditionally, surgeons have been reluctant to perform early cholecystectomy because of concerns about inflammation, which may increase the risk of surgical complications. Generally, a cholecystectomy after ERCP stone removal is classified as early cholecystectomy if performed during index admission, delayed cholecystectomy if performed within 60 days of discharge, and no-cholecystectomy if not performed within 60 days of discharge [32, 44–46]. Early cholecystectomy is also often defined as a cholecystectomy performed within 72 hours, 7 days, 14 days, or 6 weeks after ERCP [47–50]. In the literature, the proportion of early cholecystectomy in patients who underwent cholecystectomy after ERCP stone removal was 28.6–79.1%, varying by country or medical institution [32, 44, 45, 47, 48, 50].

In a retrospective study of patients awaiting delayed cholecystectomy (a delayed median of 7 weeks) following ERCP for CBD stone, 20% of all patients had recurrent biliary events during the waiting period. The median time between ERCP and the development of recurrent complications was 22 days. These recurrent complications were associated with a significantly longer hospital stay [51]. Another retrospective study of patients with mild biliary pancreatitis requiring ERCP found a strong protective effect of early cholecystectomy against biliary complications compared to delayed cholecystectomy [48]. Reinders et al. performed a randomized trial of 96 patients with GB stones who underwent ERCP stone removal. Patients were randomly assigned to groups that underwent early cholecystectomy (within 72 hours after ES, n=49) or delayed cholecystectomy (after 6–8 weeks, n=47). During the waiting period for cholecystectomy, 17 (36.2%) patients in the delayed group developed recurrent biliary events compared with 1 patient in the early group ($p<0.001$) [49]. In addition, early cholecystectomy is important because it can reduce morbidity during the waiting period for elective cholecystectomy, hospital stay, and operating time [52].

A retrospective cohort study in the United States demonstrated practice patterns for performing cholecystectomy following ERCP for CBD stones in 4,516 patients. Of these patients, 41.2% underwent early cholecystectomy (at the index admission), 10.9% underwent delayed cholecystectomy (within 60 days of discharge), and 48.0% underwent no-cholecystectomy. Early cholecystectomy reduced RR of recurrent biliary events within 60 days by 92% compared with delayed or no-cholecystectomy ($p<0.001$) [32]. On the other hand, a recent Taiwanese population-based study found that early cholecystectomy had no effect on reducing the interval recurrent biliary event, but delayed cholecystectomy reduced medical expenses [44].

Delayed cholecystectomy can increase the conversion rate to open cholecystectomy. This is thought to be due to local inflammation related to biliary complications and progression of subsequent scarring as these factors make delayed laparoscopic cholecystectomy more difficult. Prior randomized studies have demonstrated a higher rate of open cholecystectomy when surgery is delayed [1, 2]. Open cholecystectomy is associated with increased postoperative pain, more pulmonary complications and wound infections, and a lengthened hospital stay [53–55]. A study specifically considering the timing of laparoscopic cholecystectomy after ERCP in relation to the conversion rate found that it was significantly higher when laparoscopic cholecystectomy was performed 2–6 weeks after ERCP than when the operation was performed within 2 weeks after ERCP [56]. In a systemic review of 14 studies with 1,930 patients, the conversion rate increased when the delay between ERCP and laparoscopic cholecystectomy increased. The conversion rate was 4.2% when laparoscopic cholecystectomy was performed within 24 hours of ERCP, and it was 7.6% for 24–76 hours' delay, 12.3% within 2 weeks, 12.3% after 2–6 weeks, and 14% after more than 6 weeks [57]. Recently, however, there are reports suggesting that early cholecystectomy is not associated with the conversion rate [45, 47, 50].

The rate of complications increases when cholecystectomy is delayed. Li et al. reported that intra-operative and postoperative complications were higher if surgery was delayed for more than 6 weeks after cholangitis [47]. In addition, in a recent study by Discolo et al., intra-operative, postoperative, and overall complications were higher in the delayed cholecystectomy group than early cholecystectomy group [45].

In the United States population-based study, a low-volume facility is associated with delayed cholecystectomy. Hispanics, Asian races, the availability of Medicaid insurance, and no insurance were associated with early cholecystectomy [32]. In a retrospective population-based study, there was wide variability in the rates of early cholecystectomy among census areas (range 0–96%) and health regions (range 20–66%) [48]. The reasons for disparity may be multifactorial. Individual hospitals use a variety of approaches in deciding when to operate on a patient. The culture of hospitals also has a significant impact on the timing of surgery. In addition, the availability of acute surgery at the institution, the experience of the surgeon, the communication between surgeons and endoscopists, and the aggressiveness of endoscopic management are factors to be considered [45, 48, 50].

Conclusion

Prophylactic cholecystectomy is recommended to reduce recurrent biliary complications in patients with GB stones who have undergone CBD stone removal. Although this recommendation applies to patients who are very old or with comorbid diseases, it is necessary to determine whether to perform the operation considering the surgical risk and the patient's comorbid illness. When cholecystectomy is delayed, recurrent biliary complications, the rate of conversion to open surgery, and postoperative complications may increase. Therefore, it is advisable to perform early cholecystectomy during the index admission period, if possible. However, in practice, whether and when cholecystectomy is performed, varies between countries, regions, and institutions.

References

1. Boerma D, Rauws EAJ, Keulemans YCA, Janssen IMC, Bolwerk CJM, Timmer R, et al. Wait-and-see policy or laparoscopic cholecystectomy after endoscopic sphincterotomy for bile-duct stones: A randomised trial. Lancet. 2002;360:761–5.
2. Lau JYW, Leow C, Fung TMK, Suen B, Yu L, Lai PBS, et al. Cholecystectomy or gallbladder in situ after endoscopic sphincterotomy and bile duct stone removal in chinese patients. Gastroenterology. 2006;130:96–103.
3. Cui ML, Cho JH, Kim TN. Long-term follow-up study of gallbladder in situ after endoscopic common duct stone removal in Korean patients. Surg Endosc. 2013;27:1711–6.
4. Kageoka M, Watanabe F, Maruyama Y, Nagata K, Ohata A, Noda Y, et al. Long-term prognosis of patients after endoscopic sphincterotomy for choledocholithiasis. Dig Endosc. 2009;21:170–5.
5. Pereira-Lima JC, Jakobs R, Winter UH, Benz C, Martin WR, Adamek HE, et al. Long-term results (7 to 10 years) of endoscopic papillotomy for choledocholithiasis. multivariate analysis of prognostic factors for the recurrence of biliary symptoms. Gastrointest Endosc. 1998;48:457–64.
6. Lai J, Wang H, Chang W, Chu C, Shih S, Lin S. Recurrent cholangitis after endoscopic lithotripsy of common bile duct stones with gallstones in situ: predictive factors with and without subsequent cholecystectomy. J Laparoendosc Adv Surg Tech A. 2012;22:324–9.
7. Heo J, Jung MK, Cho CM. Should prophylactic cholecystectomy be performed in patients with concomitant gallstones after endoscopic sphincterotomy for bile duct stones? Surg Endosc. 2015;29:1574–9.
8. Hammarstrom LE, Holmin T, Stridbeck H. Endoscopic treatment of bile duct calculi in patients with gallbladder in situ: long-term outcome and factors. Scand J Gastroenterol. 1996;31:294–301.
9. Lai KH, Lin LF, Lo GH, Cheng JS, Huang RL, Lin CK, et al. Does cholecystectomy after endoscopic sphincterotomy prevent the recurrence of biliary complications? Gastrointest Endosc. 1999;49:483–7.
10. Schreurs WH, Vles WJ, Stuifbergen, W. H. N. M., Oostvogel HJM. Endoscopic management of common bile duct stones leaving the gallbladder in situ. A cohort study with long-term follow-up. Dig Surg. 2004;21:60–4.
11. Song ME, Chung MJ, Lee DJ, Oh TG, Park JY, Bang S, et al. Cholecystectomy for prevention of recurrence after endoscopic clearance of bile duct stones in Korea. Yonsei Med J. 2016;57:132–7.
12. da Costa DW, Schepers NJ, Römkens TEH, Boerma D, Bruno MJ, Bakker OJ. Endoscopic sphincterotomy and cholecystectomy in acute biliary pancreatitis. Surgeon. 2016;14:99–108.
13. Bingener J, Richards ML, Schwesinger WH, Strodel WE, Sirinek KR. Laparoscopic cholecystectomy for elderly patients: gold standard for golden years? Arch Surg. 2003;138:531–6.
14. Bratzler DW, Murray CK. Laparoscopic cholecystectomy in older medicare patients. J Am Geriatr Soc. 1997;45:1157–8.
15. Drake BB, Arguedas MR, Kilgore ML, Hawn MT, Wilcox CM. Economical and clinical outcomes of alternative treatment strategies in the management of common bile duct stones in the elderly: wait and see or surgery? Am J Gastroenterol. 2006;101:746–52.
16. Yasui T, Takahata S, Kono H, Nagayoshi Y, Mori Y, Tsutsumi K, et al. Is cholecystectomy necessary after endoscopic treatment of bile duct stones in patients older than 80 years of age? J Gastroenterol. 2012;47:65–70.
17. Ando T, Tsuyuguchi T, Okugawa T, Saito M, Ishihara T, Yamaguchi T, et al. Risk factors for recurrent bile duct stones after endoscopic papillotomy. Gut. 2003;52:116–21.
18. Costamagna G, Tringali A, Shah SK, Mutignani M, Zuccalà G, Perri V. Long-term follow-up of patients after endoscopic sphincterotomy for choledocholithiasis, and risk factors for recurrence. Endoscopy. 2002;34:273–9.
19. Tanaka M, Takahata S, Konomi H, Matsunaga H, Yokohata K, Takeda T, et al. Long-term consequence of endoscopic sphincterotomy for bile duct stones. Gastrointest Endosc. 1998;48:465–9.
20. Sugiyama M, Atomi Y. Risk factors predictive of late complications after endoscopic sphincterotomy for bile duct stones: long-term (more than 10 years) follow-up study. Am J Gastroenterol. 2002;97:2763–7.

21. Prat F, Malak NA, Pelletier G, Buffet C, Fritsch J, Choury AD, et al. Biliary symptoms and complications more than 8 years after endoscopic sphincterotomy for choledocholithiasis. Gastroenterology. 1996;110:894–9.
22. Cheon YK, Lehman GA. Identification of risk factors for stone recurrence after endoscopic treatment of bile duct stones. Eur J Gastroenterol Hepatol. 2006;18:461–4.
23. Kim DI, Kim MH, Lee SK, Seo DW, Choi WB, Lee SS, et al. Risk factors for recurrence of primary bile duct stones after endoscopic biliary sphincterotomy. Gastrointest Endosc. 2001;54:42–8.
24. Jakobs R, Hartmann D, Kudis V, Eickhoff A, Schilling D, Weickert U, et al. Risk factors for symptomatic stone recurrence after transpapillary laser lithotripsy for difficult bile duct stones using a laser with a stone recognition system. Eur J Gastroenterol Hepatol. 2006;18:469–73.
25. Keizman D, Ish Shalom M, Konikoff FM. Recurrent symptomatic common bile duct stones after endoscopic stone extraction in elderly patients. Gastrointest Endosc. 2006;64:60–5.
26. Bergman JJ, van der Mey S, Rauws EA, Tijssen JG, Gouma DJ, Tytgat GN, et al. Long-term follow-up after endoscopic sphincterotomy for bile duct stones in patients younger than 60 years of age. Gastrointest Endosc. 1996;44:643–9.
27. Kim KY, Han J, Kim HG, Kim BS, Jung JT, Kwon JG, et al. Late complications and stone recurrence rates after bile duct stone removal by endoscopic sphincterotomy and large balloon dilation are similar to those after endoscopic sphincterotomy alone. Clin Endosc. 2013;46:637–42.
28. Park BK, Seo JH, Jeon HH, Choi JW, Won SY, Cho YS, et al. A nationwide population-based study of common bile duct stone recurrence after endoscopic stone removal in Korea. J Gastroenterol. 2018;53:670–8.
29. Lee JK, Ryu JK, Park JK, Yoon WJ, Lee SH, Lee KH, et al. Risk factors of acute cholecystitis after endoscopic common bile duct stone removal. World J Gastroenterol. 2006;12:956–60.
30. Frossard JL, Hadengue A, Amouyal G, Choury A, Marty O, Giostra E, et al. Choledocholithiasis: a prospective study of spontaneous common bile duct stone migration. Gastrointest Endosc. 2000;51:175–9.
31. Khan MA, Khan Z, Tombazzi CR, Gadiparthi C, Lee W, Wilcox CM. Role of cholecystectomy after endoscopic sphincterotomy in the management of choledocholithiasis in high-risk patients: a systematic review and meta-analysis. J Clin Gastroenterol. 2018;52:579–89.
32. Huang RJ, Barakat MT, Girotra M, Banerjee S. Practice patterns for cholecystectomy after endoscopic retrograde cholangiopancreatography for patients with choledocholithiasis. Gastroenterology. 2017;153:762–71.
33. Loozen CS, van Ramshorst B, van Santvoort HC, Boerma D. Early cholecystectomy for acute cholecystitis in the elderly population: a systematic review and meta-analysis. Dig Surg. 2017;34:371–9.
34. Cao AM, Eslick GD, Cox MR. Early cholecystectomy is superior to delayed cholecystectomy for acute cholecystitis: a meta-analysis. J Gastrointest Surg. 2015;19:848–57.
35. Iso H, Date C, Noda H, Yoshimura T, Tamakoshi A. Frequency of food intake and estimated nutrient intake among men and women: the JACC study. J Epidemiol. 2005;15(Suppl 1):S24–42.
36. Young S, Peng Y, Lin X, Chen Y, Luo J, Wang Y, et al. Cholecystectomy reduces recurrent pancreatitis and improves survival after endoscopic sphincterotomy. J Gastrointest Surg. 2017;21:294–301.
37. Elmunzer BJ, Noureldin M, Morgan KA, Adams DB, Coté GA, Waljee AK. The impact of cholecystectomy after endoscopic sphincterotomy for complicated gallstone disease. Am J Gastroenterol. 2017;112:1596–602.
38. Disario JA, Freeman ML, Bjorkman DJ, Macmathuna P, Petersen BT, Jaffe PE, et al. Endoscopic balloon dilation compared with sphincterotomy for extraction of bile duct stones. Gastroenterology. 2004;127:1291–9.
39. Ersoz G, Tekesin O, Ozutemiz AO, Gunsar F. Biliary sphincterotomy plus dilation with a large balloon for bile duct stones that are difficult to extract. Gastrointest Endosc. 2003;57:156–9.
40. Itoi T, Itokawa F, Sofuni A, Kurihara T, Tsuchiya T, Ishii K, et al. Endoscopic sphincterotomy combined with large balloon dilation can reduce the procedure time and fluoroscopy time for removal of large bile duct stones. Am J Gastroenterol. 2009;104:560–5.
41. Natsui M, Honma T, Genda T, Nakadaira H. Effects of endoscopic papillary balloon dilation and endoscopic sphincterotomy on bacterial contamination of the biliary tract. Eur J Gastroenterol Hepatol. 2011;23:818–24.
42. Yasuda I, Fujita N, Maguchi H, Hasebe O, Igarashi Y, Murakami A, et al. Long-term outcomes after endoscopic sphincterotomy versus endoscopic papillary balloon dilation for bile duct stones. Gastrointest Endosc. 2010;72:1185–91.
43. Nakai Y, Isayama H, Tsujino T, Hamada T, Kogure H, Takahara N, et al. Cholecystectomy after endoscopic papillary balloon dilation for bile duct stones reduced late biliary complications: a propensity score-based cohort analysis. Surg Endosc. 2016;30:3014–20.
44. Wang C, Tsai M, Wang Y, Yang T, Chen H, Sung W, et al. Role of cholecystectomy in choledocholithiasis patients underwent endoscopic retrograde cholangiopancreatography. Sci Rep. 2019;9(1):2168. https://doi.org/10.1038/s41598-018-38428-z.
45. Discolo A, Reiter S, French B, Hayes D, Lucas G, Tan L, et al. Outcomes following early versus delayed cholecystectomy performed for acute cholangitis. Surg Endosc. 2019. https://doi.org/10.1007/s00464-019-07095-0. (Epub ahead of print).

46. Mador BD, Panton ONM, Hameed SM. Early versus delayed cholecystectomy following endoscopic sphincterotomy for mild biliary pancreatitis. Surg Endosc. 2014;28:3337–42.
47. Li VKM, Yum JLK, Yeung YP. Optimal timing of elective laparoscopic cholecystectomy after acute cholangitis and subsequent clearance of choledocholithiasis. Am J Surg. 2010;200:483–8.
48. Mador BD, Nathens AB, Xiong W, Panton ONM, Hameed SM. Timing of cholecystectomy following endoscopic sphincterotomy: a population-based study. Surg Endosc. 2017;31:2977–85.
49. Reinders JSK, Goud A, Timmer R, Kruyt PM, Kruijt PM, Witteman BJM, et al. Early laparoscopic cholecystectomy improves outcomes after endoscopic sphincterotomy for choledochocystolithiasis. Gastroenterology. 2010;138:2315–20.
50. Severance SE, Feizpour C, Feliciano DV, Coleman J, Zarzaur BL, Rozycki GF. Timing of cholecystectomy after emergent endoscopic retrograde cholangiopancreatography for cholangitis. Am Surg. 2019;85:895–9.
51. Schiphorst AHW, Besselink MGH, Boerma D, Timmer R, Wiezer MJ, van Erpecum KJ, et al. Timing of cholecystectomy after endoscopic sphincterotomy for common bile duct stones. Surg Endosc. 2008;22:2046–50.
52. Gurusamy KS, Koti R, Fusai G, Davidson BR. Early versus delayed laparoscopic cholecystectomy for uncomplicated biliary colic. Cochrane Database Syst Rev. 2013;(6):CD007196. https://doi.org/10.1002/14651858.cd007196.pub3.
53. Hasukić S, Mesić D, Dizdarević E, Keser D, Hadziselimović S, Bazardzanović M. Pulmonary function after laparoscopic and open cholecystectomy. Surg Endosc. 2002;16:163–5.
54. Hendolin HI, Pääkönen ME, Alhava EM, Tarvainen R, Kemppinen T, Lahtinen P. Laparoscopic or open cholecystectomy: a prospective randomised trial to compare postoperative pain, pulmonary function, and stress response. Eur J Surg. 2000;166:394–9.
55. Neugebauer E, Troidl H, Spangenberger W, Dietrich A, Lefering R. Conventional versus laparoscopic cholecystectomy and the randomized controlled trial. cholecystectomy study group. Br J Surg. 1991;78:150–4.
56. de Vries A, Donkervoort SC, van Geloven AAW, Pierik EGJM. Conversion rate of laparoscopic cholecystectomy after endoscopic retrograde cholangiography in the treatment of choledocholithiasis: does the time interval matter? Surg Endosc. 2005;19:996–1001.
57. Friis C, Rothman JP, Burcharth J, Rosenberg J. Optimal timing for laparoscopic cholecystectomy after endoscopic retrograde cholangiopancreatography: a systematic review. Scand J Surg. 2018;107:99–106.

Current Issues: Drainage of the Gallbladder: PTGBD Versus Endoscopic Drainage

Percutaneous Transhepatic Gallbladder Drainage (PTGBD)

Kwang-Hun Lee

Introduction

PTGBD was first reported in 1743 but was not used clinically until the late nineteenth century [1]. PTGBD was not widely practiced due to fear of peritonitis caused by bile leakage during and after the procedure, bradycardia and hypotension caused by vagus nerve stimulation. By 1980, PTGBD and other percutaneous intervention became popular [2, 3].

Nowadays, PTGBD has been widely performed as a treatment for the acute cholecystitis. PTGBD has been useful in patients who cannot tolerate surgical cholecystectomy due to other clinical problems and has been used as a conservative or curative treatment for critically ill patients [4–9].

Anatomy of Gallbladder

Histologically, the gallbladder consists of a columnar epithelial mucosa, a muscular coat, a subserosa, and serosa. Unlike ordinary intraperitoneal organs, there is no submucosa. The gallbladder is a thin-walled pear-shaped organ with a bile bile capacity of about 50–70 mL. However, in the case of cystic duct obstruction, it has the potential to grow into very large volumes. Both sides and back of the gallbladder are completely enclosed by the peritoneum. The front surface of the gallbladder is connected to the liver by fibroareolar tissue and forms a bare area. The gallbladder is sometimes surrounded by the colon and freely moves when connected by the mesentery. Sometimes it is completely located in the liver parenchyma [10]. Since the location of normal gallbladder changes in relation to other organs according to the tumor, hepatomegaly, and liver atrophy, it is important to identify these anatomical variations using ultrasound or CT images for safe percutaneous intervention [11, 12]. Because the area around the gallbladder neck is fixed to the portal part and it is not exposed to the peritoneum, this area is used as a main puncture route. If the puncture near the gallbladder neck is difficult due to anatomical variation, try to get as close as possible to the area. The puncture should be avoided as close as possible to the gallbladder fundus derived for peritoneum. Avoid puncturing near gallbladder fundus exposed to the peritoneum.

Indication of PTGBD

In the case of acute calculous cholecystitis, surgical cholecystectomy is scheduled after stabilizing the patient by PTGBD first when the

K.-H. Lee (✉)
Department of Radiology, Division of Intervention, Gangnam Severance Hospital, Yonsei University College of Medicine, 211, Eonju-ro, Gangnam-gu, Seoul 06273, Republic of Korea
e-mail: DOCTORLKH@yuhs.ac

J. B. Chung and K. Okazaki (eds.), *Diseases of the Gallbladder*,
https://doi.org/10.1007/978-981-15-6010-1_29

patient's general condition is severe or when emergency surgery cannot be performed, such as an elderly patient over 75 years old. Because acalculous cholecystitis does not require surgery, PTGBD may be the ultimate treatment. In addition, there are cases of empyema, hydrops, perforation, and transcholecystic biliary intervention [3–9, 13].

Contraindication of PTGBD

Absolute contraindications are those with a tendency to bleed, platelets below 50,000/cm^3, or prothrombin times above 15 seconds. A relative contraindication is when there is a large amount of ascites since is a risk of peritonitis following bile leakage or hemoperitoneum.

Puncture Route (Transhepatic vs. Transperitoneal)

The advantage of the transhepatic route is that, unlike the fundus of the gallbladder, the drainage tube is inserted into the gallbladder that is attached to the liver and has less movement. Therefore, the bile leakage can be prevented because it is easy to puncture and can be pressed by the liver if there is a bile leakage. The disadvantage is the potential risk of hepatic arterial bleeding complications.

The transperitoneal route is a direct puncture of the gallbladder fundus without passing through the liver. It is difficult to puncture the fundus of the gallbladder due to severe movement, and if the transverse colon covers the gallbladder, there is a possibility of perforation. In addition, it is hard to insert a drainage tube. Chemical peritonitis may occur due to bile leakage during the procedure.

Technique of Procedure

First, when the CT is available, the anatomic location of the gallbladder and surrounding structures should be assessed, then puncture point is determined under ultrasound guidance, local anesthesia is performed, and the skin is incised 2–3 mm.

The puncture of gallbladder is performed with an 18G needle with internal stylet. After removing the stylet of the 18G puncture needle, confirm the proper puncture by aspiration of gallbladder content and injecting contrast media under the fluoroscopy guidance. Then, insert the 0.035" guide wire. After removing 18G puncture needle while remaining 0.035" guide wire, dilate the liver parenchymal tract with a dilator (usually 8Fr). Finally, insert the locking pigtail drainage tube (7–10 Fr, usually 8–8.5 Fr) over the 0.035" guide wire [14–17]. All procedures are careful not to bend the guide wires or tools under the fluoroscopy guidance in the transhepatic route and GB entrance. Finally, contrast medium is injected to confirm the location of the drainage tube, aspiration of all the bile to confirm the function of the drainage tube and at the same time gallbladder decompression (Fig. 1a–e). The number of instruments used is reduced and the procedure time is shortened. Therefore, there is an advantage of reducing pain and peritonitis due to bile leakage occurring during the procedure.

Management of Drainage Tube

Drainage tube should be washed three times a day with about 10 mL of saline solution to increase the opening period. The drainage tube should be removed at least two weeks later. Two weeks are required for the maturation of the transhepatic route, because removing the drainage tube before this may cause the bile leakage into the peritoneal space [18].

Complications

PTGBD is an image-guided (ultrasound and fluoroscopy) procedure, so the rate of complication is very low. The incidence of PTGBD complications is 0–8%, which is very low compared to about 24% of surgical cholecystostomy. The

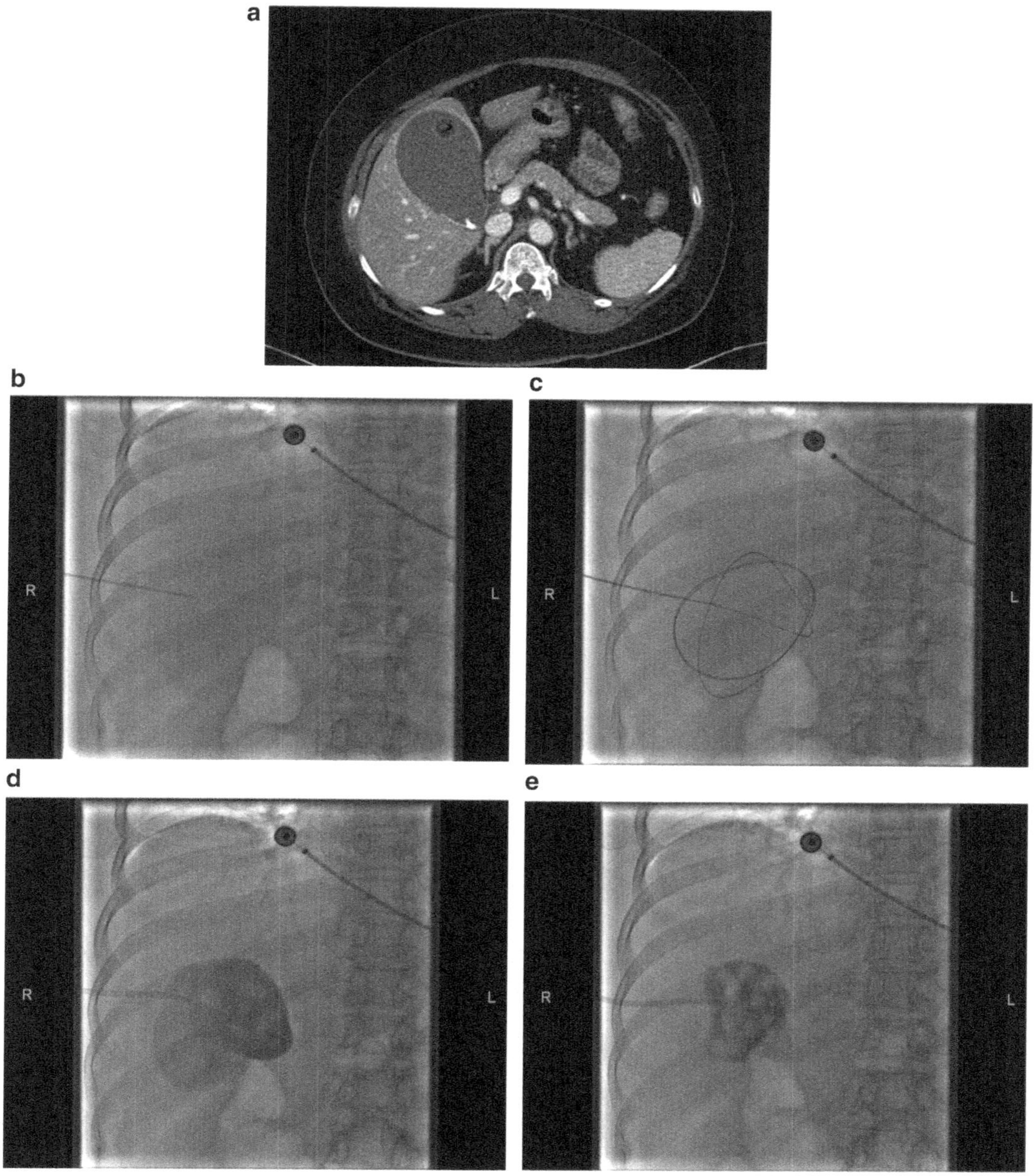

Fig. 1 **a** A 56-year old female with acute calculous cholecystitis. Note tense gallbladder and gallstone. **b** A transhepatic puncture of inflamed gallbladder with 18G needle. In case of gallbladder puncture, the puncture plane is usually parallel to the vertebral body, unlike parallel to the rib course in case of bile duct puncture. **c** A 0.035" guide wire was inserted through the puncture needle. **d** A 8.5 Fr locking pigtail drainage tube was inserted into the gallbladder. Contrast media filling the gallbladder confirmed the position of the drainage tube and multiple filling defects of gallstones. **e** Decompression status of the gallbladder after aspiration of the inflamed gallbladder content. Note multiple filling defects of the gallstones

main complications are bleeding (hepatic artery or cystic artery), bradycardia, and hypotension due to vagus nerve stimulation, and peritonitis due to bile leakage [19, 20]. In about 5%, the gallbladder is not attached to the liver but may be wrapped in the peritoneum or suspended by the intestinal mesentery. In those cases, there is a possibility of bile leakage. If a bile leakage is suspected, antibiotics should be administered and the patient closely monitored. If the patient's condition is not stable, laparoscopy, or laparotomy is required. Some physicians insist on the use of atropine before the procedure to prevent bradycardia and hypotension caused by vagus nerve stimulation. For the authors, it is not used preemptively and is injected only during the procedure when the bradycardia occurs.

Conclusion

PTGBD is the simplest and fastest way to quickly normalize a patient's condition in cases of acute cholecystitis [21, 22]. In order to prevent the complications of the procedure, it is important to determine the puncture point and the route by CT or ultrasound, and to finish the procedure in the shortest time using the minimum possible instrument.

References

1. Glenn F, Grafe WR Jr. Historical events in biliary tract surgery. Arch Surg. 1966;93:848–52.
2. Elyaderani MK, McDowell DE, Gabriele OF. A preliminary report of percutaneous cholecystostomy under ultrasonography and fluoroscopy guidance. J Clin Gastroenterol. 1983;5:277–81.
3. Pearse DM, Hawkins IF Jr, Shaver R, Vogel S. Percutaneous cholecystostomy in acute cholecystitis and common duct obstruction. Radiology. 1984;152:365–7.
4. Vogelzang RL, Nemcek AA Jr. Percutaneous cholecystostomy: diagnostic and therapeutic efficacy. Radiology. 1988;168:29–34.
5. Werbel GB, Nahrwold DL, Joehl RJ, Vogelzang RL, Rege RV. Percutaneous cholecystostomy in the diagnosis and treatment of acute cholecystitis in the high-risk patient. Arch Surg. 1989;124:782–5.
6. Van Steenbergen W, Rigauts H, Ponette E, Peetermans W, Pelemans W, Fevery J. Percutaneous transhepatic cholecystostomy for acute complicated calculous cholecystitis in elderly patients. J Am Geriatr Soc. 1993;41(2):157–62.
7. Lee MJ, Saini S, Brink JA, Hahn PF, Simeone JF, Morrison MC, et al. Treatment of critically ill patients with sepsis of unknown cause: value of percutaneous cholecystostomy. AJR Am J Roentgenol. 1991;156:1163–6.
8. Jang WS, Lim JU, Joo KR, Cha JM, Shin HP, Joo SH. Outcome of conservative percutaneous cholecystostomy in high-risk patients with acute cholecystitis and risk factors leading to surgery. Surg Endosc. 2015;29:2359–64.
9. Boland GW, Lee MJ, Leung J, Mueller PR. Percutaneous cholecystostomy in critically ill patients: early response and final outcome in 82 patients. AJR Am J Roentgenol. 1994;163:339–42.
10. Chuang VP. The aberrant gallbladder: angiographic and radioisotopic considerations. AJR Am J Roentgenol. 1976;127:417–21.
11. Gore RM, Ghahremani GG, Joseph AE, Nemcek AA Jr, Marn CS, Vogelzang RL. Acquired malposition of the colon and gallbladder in patients with cirrhosis: CT findings and clinical implications. Radiology. 1989;171:739–42.
12. Warren LP, Kadir S, Dunnick NR. Percutaneous cholecystostomy: anatomic considerations. Radiology. 1988;168:615–6.
13. Ginat D, Saad WE. Cholecystostomy and transcholecystic biliary access. Tech Vasc Interv Radiol. 2008;11:2–13.
14. McGahan JP. A new catheter design for percutaneous cholecystostomy. Radiology. 1988;166:49–52.
15. Little MW, Briggs JH, Tapping CR, Bratby MJ, Anthony S, Phillips-Hughes J, et al. Percutaneous cholecystostomy: the radiologist's role in treating acute cholecystitis. Clin Radiol. 2013;68:654–60.
16. Akhan O, Akinci D, Ozmen MN. Percutaneous cholecystostomy. Eur J Radiol. 2002;43:229–36.
17. Tseng LJ, Tsai CC, Mo LR, Lin RC, Kuo JY, Chang KK, et al. Palliative percutaneous transhepatic gallbladder drainage of gallbladder empyema before laparoscopic cholecystectomy. Hepatogastroenterology. 2000;47:932–6.
18. D'Agostino HB, vanSonnenberg E, Sanchez RB, Goodacre BW, Casola G. Imaging of the percutaneous cholecystostomy tract: observations and utility. Radiology. 1991;181:675–8.
19. van Sonnenberg E, D'Agostino HB, Goodacre BW, Sanchez RB, Casola G. Percutaneous gallbladder puncture and cholecystostomy: results, complications, and caveats for safety. Radiology. 1992;183:167–70.
20. Nghiem DD. Bile leakage after fracture of a percutaneous transhepatic biliary drainage catheter. JAMA. 1984;251:892.

21. Ke CW, Wu SD. Comparison of emergency cholecystectomy with delayed cholecystectomy after percutaneous transhepatic gallbladder drainage in patients with moderate acute cholecystitis. J Laparoendosc Adv Surg Tech A. 2018;28:705–12.

22. Abe K, Suzuki K, Yahagi M, Murata T, Sako H, Ishii Y. The efficacy of PTGBD for acute cholecystitis based on the Tokyo Guidelines 2018. World J Surg. 2019;43:2789–96.

Endoscopic Drainage of the Gallbladder: Endoscopic Transpapillary Gallbladder Drainage and Endoscopic Ultrasonography-Guided Gallbladder Drainage

Kenjiro Yamamoto and Takao Itoi

Introduction

Among the gallbladder diseases, acute cholecystitis (AC) is one of the most common inflammatory diseases of gastrointestinal (GI) infections. Early or emergency cholecystectomy has been proposed as the gold standard of treatment for patients with AC who do not respond to initial conservative treatment based on the latest guideline of AC [1, 2],

Although cholecystectomy is relatively safe, the morbidity and mortality rates of cholecystectomy still remain high in patients at high risk due to comorbid conditions [3, 4]. In addition, cholecystectomy cannot be always performed under several situations such as few surgery-related staff particularly at night. Therefore, high-risk patients with AC need an alternative nonsurgical gallbladder decompressions such as percutaneous transhepatic gallbladder drainage (PTGBD), endoscopic transpapillary gallbladder drainage (ETGBD), and endoscopic ultrasonography-guided gallbladder drainage (EUS-GBD).

PTGBD is traditionally considered as a safe alternative procedure of early cholecystectomy, especially in critically ill patients with AC [5]. The latest guidelines demonstrate that PTGBD should be recommended as a first alternative to surgical intervention in such cases [1, 2]. However, there are several contraindications to PTGBD for AC as follows: (1) patients showing the presence of severe coagulopathy or thrombocytopenia; (2) patients with anatomically inaccessible gallbladder locations such as those with Chilaiditi syndrome; and (3) patients showing the presence of a large amount of ascites.

Therefore, endoscopic drainages such as ETGBD and EUS-GBD appear to be suitable in patients in whom PTGBD is contraindicated. Hereafter, we describe a standard endoscopic drainage technique "ETGBD" and the advanced endoscopic drainage method and "EUS-GBD" for surgically high-risk patients with AC.

K. Yamamoto · T. Itoi (✉)
Departments of Gastroenterology and Hepatology, Tokyo Medical University, Tokyo, Japan
e-mail: itoi@tokyo-med.ac.jp

K. Yamamoto
e-mail: ken.yamamoto5544@gmail.com

J. B. Chung and K. Okazaki (eds.), *Diseases of the Gallbladder*,
https://doi.org/10.1007/978-981-15-6010-1_30

Endoscopic Nasogallbladder Drainage (ENGBD) or Endoscopic Gallbladder Stenting (EGBS)

ETGBD via the cystic duct has been used for approximately 35 years [6], which can be divided into two different methods: ENGBD and EGBS. The detailed techniques for ENGBD procedure are as follows. After successful bile duct cannulation, a 0.025- or 0.035-inch guidewire is advanced into the cystic duct (Fig. 1a) and subsequently into the gallbladder (Fig. 1b). Next, the catheter is withdrawn and the guidewire remains in the gallbladder, and a 5-Fr to 8.5-Fr pigtail nasogallbladder drainage tube is inserted into the gallbladder (Fig. 1c). By contrast, EGBS

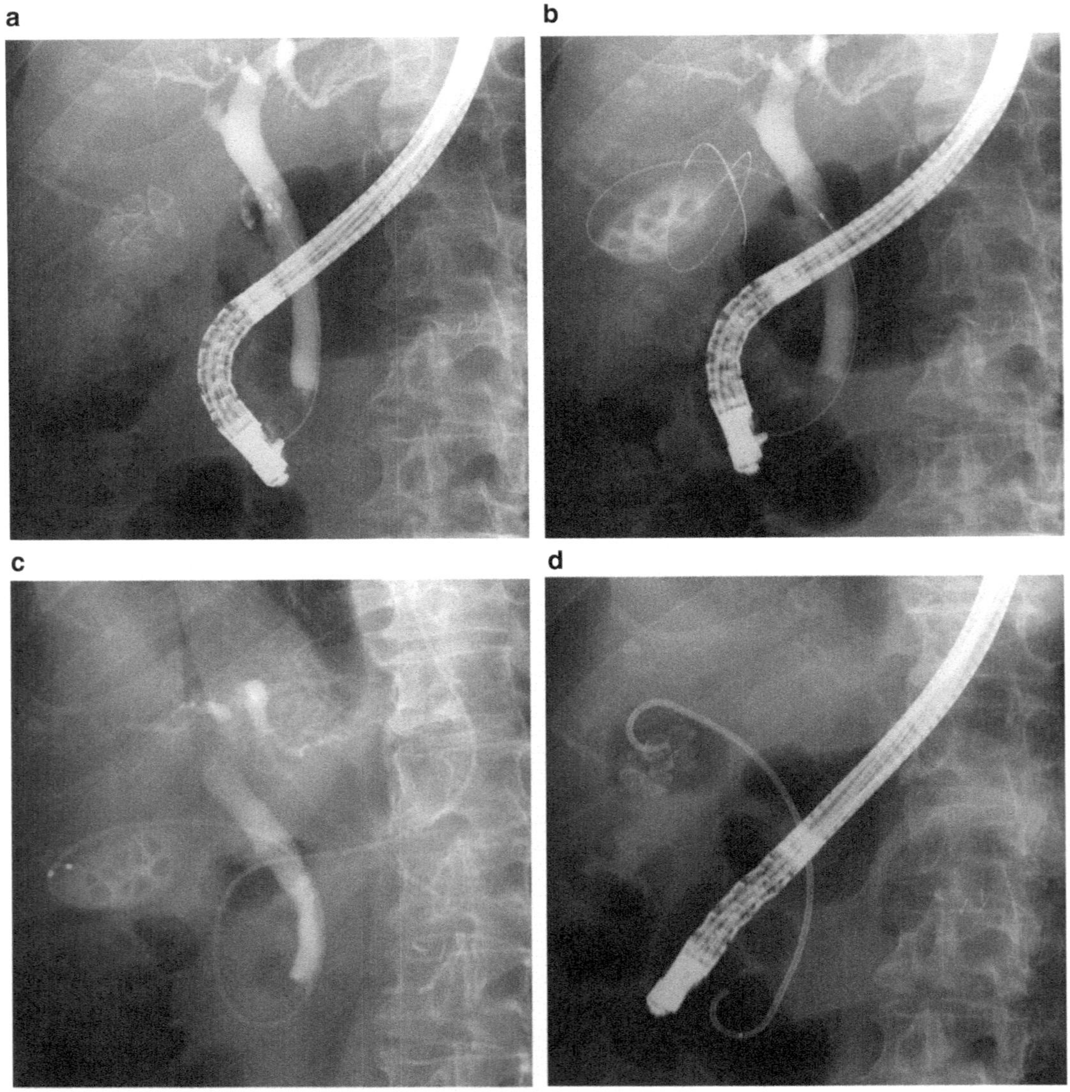

Fig. 1 Endoscopic nasogallbladder drainage (ENGBD). **a** A guidewire is advanced into the cystic duct after successful bile duct cannulation. **b** A guidewire is advanced subsequently into the gallbladder. **c** A nasogallbladder drainage tube is inserted into the gallbladder. **d** An internal stent is placed in the gallbladder

procedure is the same as for ENGBD, but a 6–10-Fr internal stent is placed in the gallbladder (Fig. 1d).

ETGBD is another alternative procedure to early cholecystectomy for patients whom PTGBD is contraindicated as mentioned above. In addition, ETGBD has other advantages over PTGBD as follows: (1) provides a physiological approach and avoids procedure-related adverse events such as bile leakage and bleeding that can occur after PTGBD; (2) possibility of earlier discharge than PTGBD, which requires at least 2 weeks to create a fistula; (3) endoscopic biliary drainage and bile duct stone removal can be performed during the same session with the treatment of cholangitis; and (4) better tolerated and less painful than PTGBD.

Although ETGBD as well as PTGBD is thought to be suboptimal treatment of AC for patients who cannot undergo emergency cholecystectomy, there are no comparative studies between these procedures. Recently an international multicenter study has been published that ETGBD showed similar clinical efficacy compared with PTGBD without significant differences of adverse event rate for the treatment of AC [7].

On the other hand, two RCTs as for the comparison of ENGBD and EGBS [8, 9] showed there are no significant difference in technical and clinical success or adverse event rates. Note that there are advantages and disadvantages of each drainage method. Firstly, ENGBD has the advantage of irrigating the gallbladder via the transnasal tube and performing the bile cytological examination. However, ENGBD involves the risk of the tube removal by patients themselves because of its discomfort. In contrast, no surprisingly EGBS has no discomfort and no risk of stent removal owing to an internal drainage, but carries a risk of stent obstruction. Consequently, either ENGBD or EGBS should be considered for gallbladder drainage based on the patient's background.

ETGBD requires skillful techniques because prolonged or unsuccessful procedures may lead to serious and occasionally fatal complications such as post-ERCP pancreatitis and perforation of a cystic duct or gallbladder. Therefore, endoscopists should acquire accurate knowledge and technical skills including selective biliary cannulation and appropriate guidewire techniques.

Endoscopic Ultrasonography-Guided Gallbladder Drainage (EUS-GBD)

EUS-GBD is a transenteric drainage technique, in which the gallbladder is directly punctured from the body or antrum of the stomach or duodenal bulb under EUS visualization. EUS-GBD using a double pigtail stent was first reported by Baron and Topazian in 2007 [10]. Although self-expandable metal stent and double pigtail stent have been used in EUS-GBD, these stents were not entirely suitable for translumenal applications and adverse events such as bile leakage and stent migration were concerned problems. Meanwhile, newly lumen-apposing metal stents (LAMS) with diameters ranging from 10 to 15 mm have been developed. LAMS is theoretically suitable for EUS-GBD, which requires large target and a short access route. After Itoi et al. published the study on EUS-GBD using LAMS in 2012 [11], several studies and case series on EUS-GBD using LAMS have been published [12, 13].

However, EUS-GBD required multiple steps and instruments for the access, tract dilation, and stent deployment. In addition, repeated instrument exchanges over a guidewire can result in increased risk of adverse events. Under those circumstances, LAMS with a novel cautery-tipped stent delivery system has been developed to allow single-step EUS-GBD from puncture to deployment of the stent with a single maneuver [14]. Thus, EUS-GBD appears as the most effective and safest procedure for treating AC.

The detailed techniques for EUS-GBD procedure using LAMS with a cautery-tipped stent delivery system are as follows. After confirming no blood vessels through the puncture route, a delivery system including the LAMS was transgastrically and directly advanced into the enlarged gallbladder under EUS guidance (Fig. 2a). The distal flange was deployed under EUS and fluoroscopic guidance (Fig. 2b) and then the proximal flange was deployed under endoscopic and fluoroscopic guidance (Fig. 2c) and during the process a small amount of infected bile juice flowed out from gallbladder to stomach through the LAMS.

In a meta-analysis and systematic review, Khan et al. showed that the technical and clinical success rates of EUS-GBD were superior to those of ETGBD [15]. Furthermore, EUS-GBD using LAMS appears to be a potential alternative to surgical intervention because it allows not only gallbladder drainage but also stone removal from the gallbladder (Fig. 3).

Although PTGBD and ETGBD have been used for the treatment of AC patients, they are not always successful because of anatomical and technical issues. EUS-GBD may be useful for such patients in hospitals with EUS expertise as salvage therapy. EUS-GBD will become widely used among skilled endosonographers in the near future.

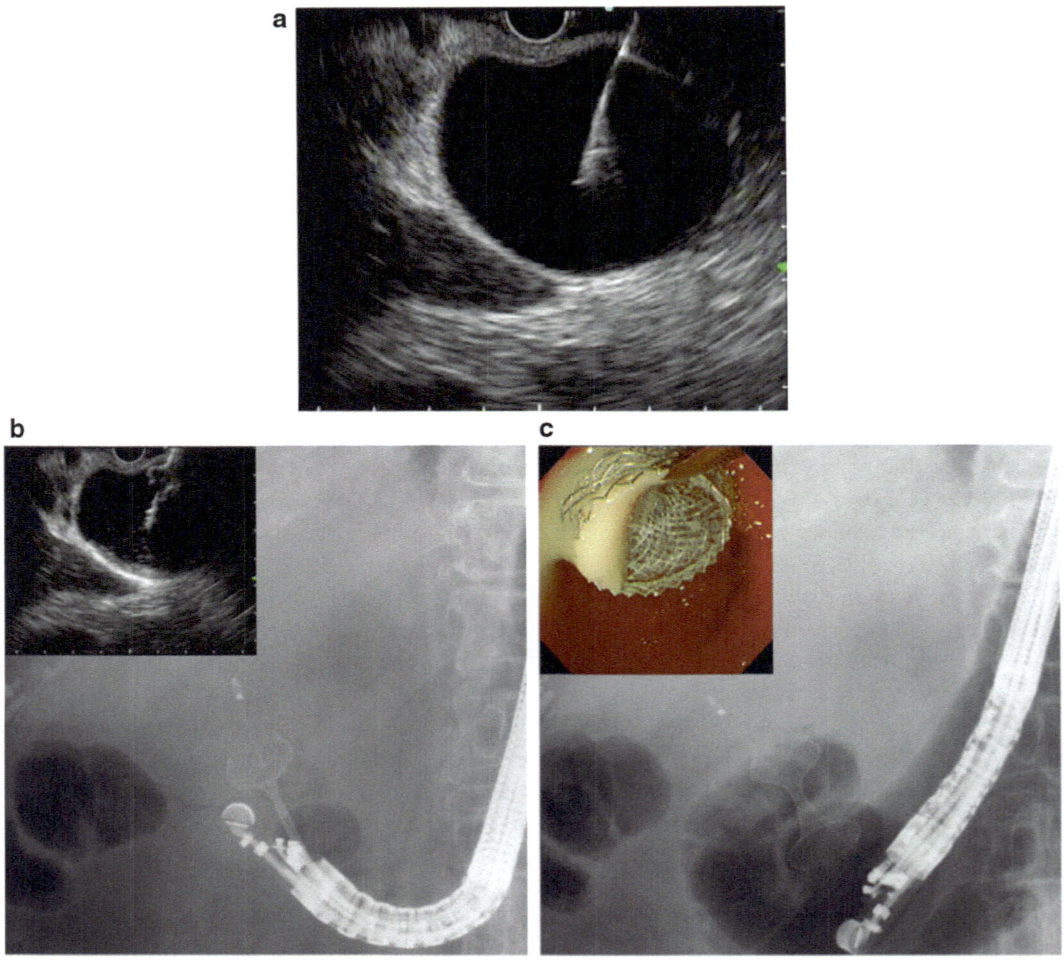

Fig. 2 EUS-GBD procedure using LAMS. **a** A delivery system including the LAMS was transgastrically and directly advanced into the enlarged gallbladder under EUS guidance. **b** The distal flange was deployed under EUS and fluoroscopic guidance. **c** The proximal flange was deployed under endoscopic and fluoroscopic guidance

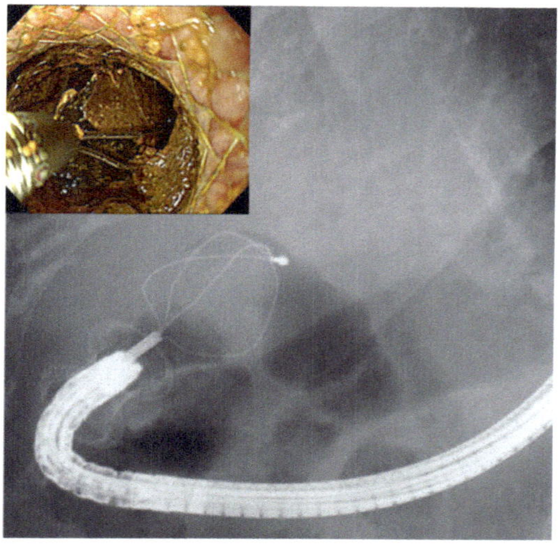

Fig. 3 Stone extraction was performed through the LAMS

Conclusion

ETGBD is the promising drainage technique for the treatment of AC that does not have inferiority than PTGBD. And also EUS-GBD is the advanced endoscopic drainage method for AC with the superiority over other gallbladder drainages.

References

1. Miura F, Takada T, Strasberg SM, Solomkin JS, Pitt HA, Gouma DJ, et al. TG13 Flowchart for management of acute cholangitis and cholecystitis. J Hepatobiliary Pancreat Sci. 2013;20:47–54.
2. Yamashita Y, Takada T, Strasberg SM, Pitt HA, Gouma DJ, Garden OJ, et al. TG13 surgical management of acute cholecystitis. J Hepatobiliary Pancreat Sci. 2013;20:89–96.
3. Houghton PWG, Jenkinson LR, Donaldson LA. Cholecystectomy in the elderly: a prospective study. Br J Surg. 1985;72:220–2.
4. Frazee RC, Nagorney DM, Mucha P Jr. Acute calculus cholecystitis. Mayo Clin Proc. 1989;64:163–7.
5. Yamada K, Yamashita Y, Yamada T, Takeno S, Noritomi T. Optimal timing for performing percutaneous transhepatic gallbladder drainage and subsequent cholecystectomy for better management of acute cholecystitis. J Hepatobiliary Pancreat Sci. 2015;22:855–61.
6. Kozarek RA. Selective cannulation of the cystic duct at the time of ERCP. J Clin Gastroenterol. 1984;6:37–40.
7. Itoi T, Takada T, Hwang TL, Endo I, Akazawa K, Miura F, et al. Percutaneous and endoscopic gallbladder drainage for acute cholecystitis: international multicenter comparative study using propensity score-matched analysis. J Hepatobiliary Pancreat Sci. 2017;24:362–8.
8. Yang MJ, Yoo BM, Kim JH, Hwang JC, Baek NH, Kim SS, et al. Endoscopic naso-gallbladder drainage versus gallbladder stenting before cholecystectomy in patients with acute cholecystitis and a high suspicion of choledocholithiasis: a prospective randomised preliminary study. Scand J Gastroenterol. 2016;51:472–8.
9. Itoi T, Kawakami H, Katanuma A, Irisawa A, Sofuni A, Itokawa F, et al. Endoscopic nasogallbladder tube or stent placement in acute cholecystitis: a preliminary prospective randomized trial in Japan (with videos). Gastrointest Endosc. 2015;81:111–8.
10. Baron TH, Topazian MD. Endoscopic transduodenal drainage of the gallbladder: implications for endoluminal treatment of gallbladder disease. Gastrointest Endosc. 2007;65:735–7.
11. Itoi T, Binmoeller KF, Shah J, Sofuni A, Itokawa F, Kurihara T, et al. Clinical evaluation of a novel lumen-apposing metal stent for endosonography-guided pancreatic pseudocyst and gallbladder drainage (with videos). Gastrointest Endosc. 2012;75:870–6.
12. Walter D, Teoh AY, Itoi T, Pérez-Miranda M, Larghi A, Sanchez-Yague A, et al. EUS-guided gall bladder drainage with a lumen-apposing metal stent: a prospective long-term evaluation. Gut. 2016;65:6–8.
13. Moon JH, Choi HJ, Kim DC, Lee YN, Kim HK, Jeong SA, et al. A newly designed fully covered metal stent for lumen apposition in EUS-guided drainage and access: a feasibility study (with videos). Gastrointest Endosc. 2014;79:990–5.
14. Teoh AY, Binmoeller KF, Lau JY. Single-step EUS-guided puncture and delivery of a lumen-apposing stent for gallbladder drainage using a novel cautery-tipped stent delivery system. Gastrointest Endosc. 2014;80:1171.
15. Khan MA, Atiq O, Kubiliun N, Ali B, Kamal F, Nollan R, et al. Efficacy and safety of endoscopic gallbladder drainage in acute cholecystitis: is it better than percutaneous gallbladder drainage? Gastrointest Endosc. 2017;85(76–87):e3.

Future Perspective

Future Perspective

Jae Bock Chung, Jae Uk Chong, Jin-Young Choi, and Kazuichi Okazaki

Introduction

Most of the patients with gallbladder diseases come to hospital with RUQ pain or discomfort. We can diagnose most diseases of the GB (gallstone, inflammation, and cancer) by laboratory examinations and imaging (ultrasonography, CT, and MRI) with endoscopic ultrasonography. However, early diagnosis of gallbladder cancer (GBC) is still difficult.

Our knowledge on the genetics and pathogenesis of gallstones has expanded recently; however, surgery is the cornerstone of treatment currently, and there is no effective preventive strategies for gallstone.

The most important factor of current guideline for operation of GB polyp is the size, but this is based on limited evidence. Adjuvant and neoadjuvant chemotherapy for GBC seems to be beneficial; however, the prognosis of GBC is still dismal, and the biomarker-driven therapeutic trials using targeted agents and immunotherapy trials in GBC are rare.

Operative approach to gallbladder has been in a state of constant evolution with the advancement of surgical techniques and tools.

In this chapter, we will describe the future perspective of diagnosis and management of diseases of the gallbladder.

Laboratory Findings

Bile

Currently, bile examinations can be used for the diagnosis of diseases of the GB: microscopic examination of bile for diagnosis of cholecystolithiasis and prediction of gallstone composition, bile cytology using endoscopic transpapillary gallbladder drainage (ETGD) for diagnosis of GBC, and gram-stained smear and culture of GB bile from percutaneous aspiration of the GB in patients with acute cholecystitis (Chap. 2)

J. B. Chung (✉)
Department of Internal Medicine, NHIS Ilsan Hospital, Yonsei University College of Medicine, 100 Ilsanro, Ilsandong-gu, Goyang-si, Gyeonggi-do 10444, Korea
e-mail: jbchung@yuhs.ac

J. U. Chong
Department of Surgery, NHIS Ilsan Hospital, Yonsei University College of Medicine, 100 Ilsanro, Ilsandong-gu, Goyang-si, Gyeonggi-do 10444, Korea
e-mail: jaeuk1216@nhimc.or.kr

J.-Y. Choi
Department of Radiology, Severance Hospital, Yonsei University College of Medicine, 50-1, Yonseiro, Seodaemun-du, Seoul 03722, Korea
e-mail: gafield2@yuhs.ac

K. Okazaki
The Third Department of Internal Medicine, Division of Gastroenterology and Hepatology, 2-3-1 Shinmachi, Hirakata, Osaka 573-1191, Japan
e-mail: okazaki@hirakata.kmu.ac.jp

J. B. Chung and K. Okazaki (eds.), *Diseases of the Gallbladder*,
https://doi.org/10.1007/978-981-15-6010-1_31

[1–10]. However, bile examination is not widely used clinically due to complexity in sampling and relatively poor clinical benefits.

Recently, circulating tumor DNA (ctDNA) in bile was detected by next-generation sequencing (NGS) of GBC. 57.1% of DNA samples from tumor tissue were positive for a mutation, and among these patients, 87.5% of the bile ctDNA samples had same mutation. The concordance rate between bile ctDNA and tissue DNA samples was 85.7%. The sensitivity of liquid biopsy of bile was higher than the cytology (58.1% and 45.8%, respectively), and the concordance rate between cytology and bile ctDNA analyses was 87.5% [11].

Composition and content of bile in the GB may be related to various diseases of the GB, and therefore serial changes of bile may show clues to identify the causes of diseases. Further efforts in improving the various methods for examination of bile and discovery of novel targets in bile may be useful for diagnosis and treatment of diseases of the GB.

Tumor Markers

Carbohydrate antigen 19-9 and carcinoembryonic antigen are tumor markers most commonly utilized in the diagnosis of GBC [12–16], however the sensitivity and specificity are unsatisfactory.

There are several reports investigating neutrophil/lymphocyte ratio (NLR), platelet/lymphocyte ratio (PLR), GPS (Glasgow prognostic score), absolute neutrophil count, and absolute lymphocyte count in patients with GBC as a prognostic indicator (Chap. 2) [17–20].

Currently, many tumor diagnostic, prognostic, predictive, and therapeutic biomarkers are being evaluated for clinical applications (Chap. 2) [21–26].

Imaging

Appropriate evaluation and choice of management for gallbladder diseases require a multidisciplinary approach because each imaging modality has its own advantage and no single imaging tool is perfect. Imaging methods for gallbladder diseases have improved remarkably, however unmet needs still remain.

Ultrasound and CT are commonly used imaging modalities for evaluating gallbladder abnormalities. MRI is used as a secondary or problem-solving exam to obtain more information when a diagnosis cannot be reached by ultrasound or CT (Chap. 4) [27]. Various imaging techniques in addition to conventional ultrasonography such as CT and MRI methods in diseases of the gallbladder have been studied.

The new imaging techniques to discover the small or minute lesion of the wall and epithelium need to be developed to assist differential diagnosis and early detection of the gallbladder diseases (Chap. 4) [27]. To overcome the limitation of conventional transabdominal ultrasound, high-resolution ultrasound, three-dimensional ultrasound, or contrast-enhanced ultrasound have been developed and used. High-resolution US is an emerging modality for staging gallbladder cancer due to its high resolution and non-invasiveness. Contrast-enhanced US has been used to improve the diagnostic accuracy of identifying gallbladder malignancy. Three-dimensional US continues to evolve toward better image resolution [28].

In staging of GBC, CT and MRI can provide fairly good accuracy, particularly for T factor. Adding PET or ADC (apparent diffusion coefficient) information may enhance the diagnosis when CT or MRI findings are equivocal, particularly for N and M factors (Chap. 17) [29]. Specifically, ADC or SUV information may not only enhance the diagnosis when conventional CT or MRI findings are equivocal, but also be independent biomarkers to predict the prognosis of gallbladder cancer (Chap. 17) [29]. The ADC value of GBCs was significantly correlated with tumor differentiation as well as AJCC stage. In addition, it predicted long-term outcomes after surgery in patients with GBC [30].

Addition of diffusion-weighted imaging (DWI) to conventional MRI is also used in improving diagnostic accuracy such as discrimination between xanthogranulomatous cholecystitis and the wall-thickening type of GBC [31], and sensitivity for distinguishing GB cancers from benign GB diseases with wall thickening [32, 33].

Multidetector-row computed tomography (MDCT) is a reliable diagnostic method for differentiating malignantly thickened gallbladder wall [34]. Dual energy CT, which enabled the concurrent acquisition of data with two different X-ray energy spectra at high and low voltage peaks and postprocessing techniques, has the potential to facilitate improved detection and characterization of gallbladder carcinoma. With the iodine content highlighted, carcinoma can be visualized more easily when compared with benign entities [35].

Deep learning and radiomics approaches seem to hold promise in enhancing the performance of imaging, especially if collaborative multidisciplinary teams are involved in the gallbladder diseases. The goal of radiomics for gallbladder diseases is to develop decision-supporting tools, by incorporating radiomics signatures and other morphologic features in predictive model [36]. For example, a radiomics model may provide a noninvasive and convenient tool for preoperative individualized prediction of nodal metastasis in biliary tract cancer that helps to define subsets of patients who would benefit most from surgery [37].

Ultimately, to achieve personalized medicine, personalized imaging must be involved and deep learning and radiomics may help pave the road to personalized medicine.

Endoscopy

Endoscopic ultrasonography is important for specific diagnosis of polypoid gallbladder lesions and gallbladder wall thickening. EUS is also useful in staging of gallbladder carcinoma. Recent advances in contrast-enhanced EUS are expected to contribute further to diagnosis of gallbladder lesions. Additionally, EUS has shown promise in diagnosing gallbladder microlithiasis in patients with grossly clear biliary colic and normal transabdominal ultrasonography results (Chap. 5) [38].

Although EUS-FNA of the gallbladder is useful for diagnosing gallbladder tumors, it is not the initial method of choice because of associated risks of bile leakage and needle tract seeding. Large clinical studies, including randomized controlled clinical trials, are necessary to test the efficacy and safety of EUS-FNA in patients with gallbladder tumors (Chap. 7) [39].

Endoscopic transpapillary gallbladder drainage (ETGD) for bile cytologic examination revealed high diagnostic accuracy rate [8].

Peroral cholecystoscopy can be performed after dilatation of the cystic duct ranging from 8.5 to 10.0 mm in diameter, permitting passage of a 4.5 mm diameter baby scope for endoscopic lithotripsy, or after placement of lumen-apposing metal stents (LAMS) during EUS-guided gallbladder drainage (EUS-GBD). The large diameter of LAMS acts as a portal for endoscopic access to the gallbladder [40–42].

While techniques such as chromoendoscopy and conventional magnification endoscopy try to predict histology from mucosal patterns, confocal laser endomicroscopy (CLE) actually allows intravital microscopy of the human gastrointestinal tract during ongoing endoscopy, enabling real-time optical biopsy [43, 44].

A variety of endoscopy for image-enhancing modalities for the evaluation of gallbladder mucosa can be performed after EUS-GBD using LAMS [45, 46]. Chan et al. [41, 42] carried out peroral cholecystoscopy after EUS-GBD using LAMS. They performed several endoscopic procedures, such as magnifying endoscopy, confocal endomicroscopy, and biopsy. Furthermore, interventional procedures for gallstone removal and polypectomy could be done without difficulty.

In the future, various endoscopic methods, such as peroral cholecystoscopy and CLE will be widely used as an important diagnostic methods for diseases of the GB. Moreover, endoscopic treatment of gallbladder lesions can become a simple procedure, as in the gastrointestinal tract, in the near future.

Gallstone

Our knowledge on the genetics and pathogenesis of gallstones has expanded recently (Chap. 8) [47]. Although surgery is currently the cornerstone of treatment for gallstone disease, much more emphasis should be given to the prevention of gallstone [48].

In the general population, a major intervention should include lifestyle changes. Healthy lifestyle and food, regular physical activity, and maintenance of an ideal body weight might prevent cholesterol gallbladder stones and symptomatic gallstones. Pharmacological prevention of gallstones is not advisable in the general population due to the lack of strong evidence of effectiveness [48–50].

Accurate stratification according to individual risk for gallstones might be possible with methodical profiling of genetic and environmental risk factors. Defining the high-risk group will allow screening for early diagnosis and preventive drugs may be beneficial [48].

In situations associated with rapid weight loss (e.g., very low calorie diet, bariatric surgery), temporary ursodeoxycholic acid (at least 500 mg per day until body weight has stabilized) is an evidence-based preventive measure for gallstones [48, 51, 52]. Most of the ABCB4-deficient patients benefit from prophylactic or long-term therapy with UDCA (15 mg/kg body weight and day) [49, 51, 53, 54]. In patients on long-term therapy with somatostatin or analogues, concomitant treatment with ursodeoxycholic acid can be considered to prevent cholesterol gallstone formation [49]. Other therapeutic options are promising but not yet supported by strong evidence [50].

Experimental and clinical studies are absolutely needed to clarify the real efficacy of various innovative and potentially preventive tools in selected groups of gallstone [50].

GB Polyp

Current guidelines recommend cholecystectomy for gallbladder polyps sized 10 mm and greater. This threshold is lowered when other risk factors are identified, or size increased by more than 2 mm at follow-up transabdominal ultrasonography [28].

There are controversies and challenges in many aspects of gallbladder polyps. It is difficult to differentiate benign lesions from malignant gallbladder polyp based on available diagnostic modalities (Chap. 26) [55].

Although polyps of 10 mm and greater are more likely to be true polyps, this cutoff will overlook a significant number of true polyp below this threshold and cholecystectomy will also be performed unnecessarily for pseudopolyps when they are greater than 10 mm [28].

There is a lack of evidence comparing growth pattern between pseudopolyps and true polyps, and small individual studies have shown that both can undergo growth [56, 57].

Patients with gallbladder polyps should be treated with personalized and differentiated strategies. Better understanding of the clinicopathologic characteristics, risk factors, classification, and natural history of gallbladder polyps are necessary and large retrospective and prospective trials involving international multiple centers should be conducted (Chap. 26) [55].

GB Cancer

Gallbladder cancers are rare and aggressive tumors, with a paucity of clinical trials using biomarker-guided targeted treatment [58].

The main associated risk factors of gallbladder cancer (GBC) identified so far include cholelithiasis (especially untreated chronic symptomatic gallstones), obesity, reproductive factors, chronic infections of the gallbladder, and environmental exposure to specific chemicals (Chap. 15) [59, 60].

GBC is enriched with multiple mutations, from germline mutations such as genetic susceptibility of *DCC* and *ABCB4* variants to somatic mutations including TP53, KRAS, PI3K/AKT/mTOR pathway, chromatin-remodeling pathway, and ErbB pathway genes in GBC tissues (Chap. 16) [61].

Currently, CT and MRI can provide fairly good accuracy in staging GBC, particularly for T factor. Adding PET or ADC (apparent diffusion coefficient) information may not only enhance the diagnosis when CT or MRI findings are equivocal, particularly for N and M factors, but also be independent biomarkers to predict the prognosis of GBC patients (Chap. 17) [62].

Adjuvant chemotherapy for GBC seems to be beneficial, especially in cases of node-positive and/or positive resection margin. However, further validation, in terms of the most effective regimen and chemotherapy itself as the adjuvant treatment for gallbladder cancer, is necessary. Neoadjuvant chemotherapy can be considered in locoregionally advanced GBC (Chap. 21) [63].

Various challenges are under investigation to develop new promising agents to improve the survival. One is to identify targeted driver mutations or overexpression of biomarkers by multiplex diagnosis using next-generation sequencing (NGS). Some clinical trials of agents targeting specific biomarker using the NGS are ongoing for biliary tract cancer including gallbladder cancer, such as HER2/neu overexpression and fibroblast growth factor receptor 2 (FGFR2) gene rearrangement. In addition, immune checkpoint inhibitors have recently been demonstrated to prolong the survival in patients with various advanced cancers (Chap. 23) [64].

Indications and the appropriate combination of drug for chemotherapy require further validation. Additionally, most appropriate therapeutic modality among chemotherapy, chemoradiation, and radiation therapy alone should be evaluated. In terms of indication for neoadjuvant therapy, more studies should evaluate feasibility even for earlier staged GBC (Chap. 21) [63].

In the era of precision medicine, it would be appropriate to conduct a clinical trial according to expression of biomarker such as gene mutation or arrangement. And it is required to conduct a clinical trial involving global collaboration (Chap. 23) [64].

Early GB Cancer

Early diagnosis and identification of high-risk cases of GBC, and providing prophylactic cholecystectomy could offer a potential cure for patients [65].

The great majority of in situ carcinomas of the GB are grossly indistinguishable from cholecystitis and can easily be overlooked on macroscopic examination. The only in situ carcinoma that can be recognized grossly with some degree of certainty is the papillary type, but this variety represents only a small group [66, 67].

For early detection of carcinoma of the gallbladder, watchful attention to mild mucosal changes is essential, as more than 50% of early cancer did not show apparently protruding lesions [68]. Peroral cholecystoscopy may be a useful diagnostic method for early detection of GBC in the near future. Cytologic examination and liquid biopsy of bile may also be a useful method to diagnose GBC early [8, 11].

It is necessary to make a diagnostic and therapeutic algorithm in high-risk groups of GBC (Chap. 19) [69] and discuss a need for mass screening for GBC among population [65].

Surgery

Operative approach to gallbladder has been in a state of constant evolution with the advancement of surgical techniques and tools. The demand for safer and less-invasive interventions continues to promote innovations in the management of gallbladder diseases [70].

Laparoscopic cholecystectomy has been the treatment of choice for cholelithiasis since 1992 [71]. Further efforts to reduce operative scars led to introduction of single-incision laparoscopic cholecystectomy (SILC) using three ports from a single incision made at the umbilicus in 1996 [72]. However, ergonomic difficulties of standard instruments prevented wide adaptation. Introduction of the single-site robotic cholecystectomy (SSRC) in 2011 revolutionized single-incision surgery. Technical limitations of SILC, such as ergonomics, internal and external instrument clashing, and image instability, were overcome. SSRC allows for the shorter learning curve and has potential to increase safety [73]. However, higher cost associated with SSRC remains a hurdle to overcome [74]. With the robotic system evolving continuously and more companies currently developing new systems, cost issue might be resolved in the near future.

In an effort to eliminate all abdominal scars after surgery, natural orifice translumenal endoscopic surgery (NOTES) has also been proposed. Use of natural orifices, such as transgastric and transvaginal, for the removal of the diseased organ has potential advantages for patients. Recent prospective, randomized evaluation of NOTES showed that transvaginal cholecystectomy is safe with non-inferior clinical results and superior cosmesis compared to laparoscopic cholecystectomy [75]. Transvaginal approach to cholecystectomy is now no longer considered experimental.

Most feared complication following cholecystectomy is bile duct injury with the risk estimated at 0.4% [76]. There is always some substantial risk of bile duct injury whenever minimally invasive cholecystectomy is performed. To reduce such complication, real-time indocyanine green (ICG) fluorescence cholangiography has been introduced. ICG cholangiography during minimally invasive cholecystectomy enables a better visualization and identification of biliary tree [77]. Enhanced understanding of biliary tree anatomy consequently increases safety of operation with reduced risk of bile duct injury.

In gallbladder cancer (GBC), laparoscopic surgery for T1b or greater tumor has been contraindicated due to risk of tumor dissemination [78]. Although the evidence is limited, selected patients with T1, T2 GBC have shown favorable long-term oncologic outcomes using laparoscopic cholecystectomy including lymphadenectomy [79]. Although extended cholecystectomy is recommended for T1b or greater GBC, evaluation of tumor depth under frozen section examination can be difficult.

Recent study evaluating the tumor depth used an ultrasound with 18 MHz transducer on the removed gallbladder specimen [80]. Results showed only moderate accuracy of tumor depth evaluation. Nevertheless, direct application of a higher frequency transducer on the resected gallbladder specimen can enhance the diagnostic accuracy for the depth of invasion. The combined use of intraoperative ultrasound and frozen section examination could assist surgeons in deciding the extent of cholecystectomy. Better diagnostic definition may extend the use of laparoscopic surgery in GBC patients in the future.

Surgical management of gallbladder diseases is still open for innovation and continuous effort to overcome the limitation of minimally invasive surgery by surgeon's endeavor and development of groundbreaking technology are essential.

Conclusion

Bile examination is not widely used clinically due to complexity in sampling with relatively poor clinical benefits. However, in the future, cytology, liquid biopsy, and discovery of novel targets in bile may prove to be useful for diagnosis and treatment of diseases of the GB.

The new imaging techniques to discover the small lesion of the wall and epithelium need to be developed to help differentiate GB cancer for early detection. Ultimately, to achieve personalized medicine, personalized imaging must be involved, and deep learning and radiomics may help pave the road to personalized medicine.

Various endoscopic methods, such as peroral cholecystoscopy and confocal laser endomicroscopy, will be widely used as important diagnostic methods for the diseases of the GB.

Accurate stratification according to individual risk for gallstones might be possible with methodical profiling of genetic and environmental risk factors. Defining the high-risk group will allow screening for early diagnosis and preventive drugs may be beneficial in the near future.

Patients with GB polyps should be treated with personalized and differentiated strategies based on clinicopathologic characteristics, risk factors, classification, and natural history of GB polyps.

Early diagnosis of GB cancer is essential to improve survival. It is necessary to make a diagnostic and therapeutic algorithm in high-risk groups of GB cancer and discuss a need for mass screening for GB cancer among population.

Surgical management of gallbladder diseases is still open for innovation and continuous effort to overcome the limitation of minimally invasive surgery by surgeon's endeavor and development of groundbreaking technology are essential.

References

1. Chung JB, Chong JU. Laboratory examinations of diseases of the gallbladder. In: Chung JB, Okazaki K, editors. Diseases of the gallbladder. Springer Nature Singapore Pte Ltd. 2020. Chapter 2.
2. Lyon BBV. Diagnosis and treatment of diseases of the gallbladder and bile ducts. JAMA. 1919;73:980–2.
3. Juniper K Jr, Burson EN Jr. Biliary tract studies. II. The significance of biliary crystals. Gastroenterology. 1957;32(2):175–208.
4. Goodman AJ, Neoptolemos JP, Carr-Locke DL, Finlay DB, Fossard DP. Detection of gallstones after acute pancreatitis. Gut. 1985;26:125–32.
5. Marks JW, Bonorris G. Intermittency of cholesterol crystals in duodenal bile from gallstone patients. Gastroenterology. 1984;87(3):622–7.
6. Agarwal DK, Choudhuri G, Saraswat VA, Negi TS, Kapoor VK, Saxena R. Duodenal bile examination in identifying potential non-responders to bile salt treatment and its comparison with gall bladder bile examination. Gut. 1994;35(1):112–6.
7. Dahan P, Andant C, Levy P, Amouyal P, Amouyal G, Dumont M, et al. Prospective evaluation of endoscopic ultrasonography and microscopic examination of duodenal bile in the diagnosis of cholecystolithiasis in 45 patients with normal conventional ultrasonography. Gut. 1996;38(2):277–81.
8. Itoi T, Sofuni A, Itokawa F, Kurihara T, Tsuchiya T, Moriyasu F, et al. Preoperative diagnosis and management of thick-walled gallbladder based on bile cytology obtained by endoscopic transpapillary gallbladder drainage. Gastrointest Endosc. 2006;64(4):512–9.
9. McGahan JP, Lindfors KK. Acute cholecystitis: diagnostic accuracy of percutaneous aspiration of the gallbladder. Radiology. 1988;167(3):669–71.
10. Manolis EN, Filippou DK, Papadopoulos VP, Katostaras T, Christianakis E, Bonatsos G, et al. The culture site of the gallbladder affects recovery of bacteria in symptomatic cholelithiasis. J Gastrointestin Liver Dis. 2008;17(2):179–82.
11. Kinugasa H, Nouso K, Ako S, Dohi C, Matsushita H, Matsumoto K, et al. Liquid biopsy of bile for the molecular diagnosis of gallbladder cancer. Cancer Biol Ther. 2018;19(10):934–8.
12. Shukla VK, Gurubachan, Sharma D, Dixit VK, Usha. Diagnostic value of serum CA 242, CA 19-9, CA 15-3 and CA 125 in patients with carcinoma of the gallbladder. Trop Gastroenterol. 2006;27(4):160–5.
13. Chaube A, Tewari M, Singh U, Shukla HS. CA 125: a potential tumor marker for gallbladder cancer. J Surg Oncol. 2006;93:665–9.
14. Rana S, Dutta U, Kochhar R, Rana SV, Gupta R, Pal R, et al. Evaluation of CA 242 as a tumor marker in gallbladder cancer. J Gastrointest Cancer. 2012;43:267–71.
15. Srivastava K, Srivastava A, Mittal B. Potential biomarkers in gallbladder cancer: present status and future directions. Biomarkers. 2013;18(1):1–9.
16. Tunan Y, Hong Y, Xiujun C. Preoperative prediction of survival in resectable gallbladder cancer by a combined utilization of CA 19-9 and carcinoembryonic antigen. Chin Med J. 2014;127(12):2299–303.
17. Zhang Y, Jiang C, Li J, Sun J, Qu X. Prognostic significance of preoperative neutrophil/lymphocyte ratio and platelet/lymphocyte ratio in patients with gallbladder carcinoma. Clin Transl Oncol. 2015;17:810–8.
18. Zhang L, Wang R, Chen W, Xu X, Dong S, Fan H, et al. Prognostic significance of neutrophil to lymphocyte ratio in patients with gallbladder carcinoma. HPB (Oxford). 2016;18:600–7.
19. Wu X-S, Shi L-B, Li M-L, Ding Q, Weng H, Wu WG, et al. Evaluation of two inflammation-based prognostic scores in patients with resectable gallbladder carcinoma. Ann Surg Oncol. 2014;21: 449–57.
20. Zhnag Y, Ma C, Wang M, Hou H, Cui L, Jiang C, et al. Prognostic significance of immune cell in the tumor microenvironment and peripheral blood of gallbladder carcinoma patients. Clin Transl Oncol. 2017;19:477–88.
21. Zhang X, Niu Y, Wang X, Liu ZP, Liu T, Wang RT. Mean platelet volume and platelet distribution width are associated with gallbladder cancer. Asian Pac J Cancer Pre. 2018;19(2):351–5.
22. Xu WY, Zhang HH, Xiong JP, Yang XB, Bai Y, Kin JZ, et al. Prognostic significance of the fibrinogen-to-albumin ratio in gallbladder cancer patients. World J Gastroenterol. 2018;24(29): 3281–92.
23. Vinocha A, Grover RK, Deepak R. Clinical significance of interleukin-6 in diagnosis of lung, oral, esophageal, and gallbladder carcinomas. J Cancer Res Ther. 2018;14(Suppl):S758–60.
24. Kumara S, Husain N, Agarwal A, Neyaz A, Gupta S, et al. Daignostic value of circulating free DNA integrity and global methylation status in gallbladder carcinoma. Pathol Oncol Res. 2018. https://doi.org/10.1007/s12253-017-0380-6.
25. Letelier P, Riquelme I, Hernandez AH, Guzman N, Farias JG, Roa JG. Circulating microRNAs as biomarkers in biliary tract cancers. Int J Mol Sci. 2016;17:791. https://doi.org/10.3390/ijms17050791.
26. Hu J, Yin B. Advances in biomarkers of biliary tract cancers. Biomed Pharmacother. 2016;81:128–35.

27. Choi JY, Chang DR. Imaging diagnosis of diseases of the gallbladder. In: Chung JB, Okazaki K, editors. Diseases of the gallbladder. Springer Nature Singapore Pte Ltd. 2020. Chapter 4.
28. McCain RS, Diamond A, Jones C, Coleman HG. Current practices and future prospects for the management of gallbladder polyps: a topical review. World J Gastroenterol. 2018;24(26):2844–52.
29. Yoshimitsu K. Gallbladder cancer: Staging by radiologic imaging. In: Chung JB, Okazaki K, editors. Diseases of the gallbladder. Springer Nature Singapore Pte Ltd. 2020. Chapter 17.
30. Min JH, Kang TW, Cha DI, Kim SH, Shin KS, Lee JE, et al. Apparent diffusion coefficient as a potential marker for tumor differentiation, staging and long-term clinical outcomes in gallbladder cancer. Eur Radiol. 2019;29(1):411–21.
31. Kang TW, Kim SH, Park HJ, Lim S, Jang KM, Choi D, Lee SJ. Differentiating xanthogranulomatous cholecystitis from wall thickening type of gallbladder cancer: add value of diffusion-weighted MRI. Clin Radiol. 2013;68(10):992–1001.
32. Kim SJ, Lee JM, Kim H, Yoon JH, Han JK, Choi BI. Role of diffusion-weighted magnetic resonance imaging in the diagnosis of gallbladder cancer. J Magn Reson Imaging. 2013;38(1):127–37.
33. Lee NK, Kim S, Kim TU, Kim DU, Seo HI, Jeon TY. Diffusion-weighted MRI for differentiation of benign from malignant lesions in the gallbladder. Clin Radiol. 2014;69(2):e78–85.
34. Tongdee R, Maroongroge P, Suthikeree W. The value of MDCT scans in differentiation between benign and malignant gallbladder wall thickening. J Med Assoc Thai. 2011;94(5):592–600.
35. Ratanaprasatporn L, Uyeda JW, Wortman JR, Richardson I, Sodickson AD. Multimodality imaging, including dual-energy CT, in the evaluation of gallbladder diseases. Radiographics. 2018;38(1):75–89.
36. Gillies RJ, Kinahan PE, Hricak H. Radiomics: images are more than pictures, they are data. Radiology. 2016;278(2):563–77.
37. Ji GW, Zhang YD, Zhang H, Zhu FP, Wnag K, Xia YX, et al. Biliary tract cancer at CT: a radiomics-based model to predict lymph node metastasis and survival outcomes. Radiology. 2019;290(1):90–8.
38. Inui K, Miyoshi H, Yamamoto S. EUS of diseases of the gallbladder. In: Chung JB, Okazaki K, editors. Diseases of the gallbladder. Springer Nature Singapore Pte Ltd. 2020. Chapter 5.
39. Kitano M, Tamura T. Tissue acquisition of diseases of the gallbladder: EUS-guided biopsy. In: Chung JB, Okazaki K, editors. Diseases of the gallbladder. Springer Nature Singapore Pte Ltd. 2020. Chapter 7.
40. Fujita R, Hirata N, Fujita Y. Peroral cholecystoscopy. Endoscopy. 1989;21(Suppl 1):378–80.
41. Chan SM, Teoh AYB, Yip HC, Wong VWY, Chiu PWY, Nq EKW. Feasibility of per-oral cholecystoscopy and advanced gallbladder interventions after EUS-guided gallbladder stenting (with video). Gastrointest Endosc. 2017;85:1225–32.
42. Chan JHY, Teoh AYB. The development of peroral cholecystoscopy and advanced gallbladder interventions. Endosc Ultrasound. 2018;7(2):85–8.
43. Goetz M, Watson A, Kiesslich R. Confocal laser endomicroscopy in gastrointestinal diseases. J Biophotonics. 2011;4(7–8):498–508.
44. Goetz M. Confocal laser endomicroscopy: current indications and future perspectives in gastrointestinal diseases. Endoscopia. 2012;24:67–74.
45. Ogura T, Higuchi K. Endoscopic ultrasound-guided gallbladder drainage: current status and future prospects. Dig Endosc. 2019;31(Suppl 1):55–64.
46. Teoh Anthony YB, Chan AW, Chiu PW, Lau JY. *In vivo* appearances of gallbladder carcinoma under magnifying endoscopy and probe-based confocal laser endomicroscopy after endosonographic gallbladder drainage. Endoscopy. 2014;46(Suppl 1):E13–4.
47. Lee DK, Jang SI. Pathogenesis and treatment of gallbladder stone. In: Chung JB, Okazaki K, editors. Diseases of the gallbladder. Springer Nature Singapore Pte Ltd. 2020. Chapter 8.
48. Lammert F, Gurusamy K, Ko CW, Miquel JF, Mendez-Sanchez N, Portincasa P, et al. Gallstones. Nat Rev Dis Primers. 2016;2:16024. https://doi.org/10.1038/nrdp.2016.24.
49. Lammert F, Acalovschi M, Ercolani G, van Erpecum K, Gurusamy KS, van Laarhoven CJ. EASL Clinical Practice Guidelines on the prevention, diagnosis and treatment of gallstones. J Hepatol. 2016;65:146–81.
50. Di Ciaula A, Portincasa P. Recent advances in understanding and managing cholesterol gallstones. F1000Research. 2018;7:1529. https://doi.org/10.12688/f1000research.15505.1.
51. Scherber PR, Lammert F, Glanemann M. Gallstone disease: Optimal timing of treatment. J Hepatol. 2017;67:645–7.
52. Sugerman HJ, Brewer WH, Shiffman ML, Brolin RE, Fobi MA, Linner JH, et al. A multicenter, placebo-controlled, randomized, double-blind, prospective trial of prophylactic ursodiol for the prevention of gallstone formation following gastric-bypass-induced rapid weight loss. Am J Surg. 1995;169(1):91–6; discussion 96–7.
53. Poupon R, Rosmorduc O, Boelle PY, Chretien Y, Corpechot C, Chazouilleres O, et al. Genotype-phenotype relationships in the low-phospholipid-associated cholelithiasis syndrome: a study of 156 consecutive patients. Hepatology. 2013;58:1105–10.
54. Frider B, Castillo A, Gordo-Gilart R, Bruno A, Amante M, Alvarez L, et al. Reversal of advanced fibrosis after long-term ursodeoxycholic acid therapy in a patient with residual expression of MDR3. Ann Hepatol. 2015;14:745–51.
55. Lee WJ. Diagnostic and therapeutic algorithm: polypoid lesions of the gallbladder. In: Chung JB, Okazaki K, editors. Diseases of the gallbladder. Springer Nature Singapore Pte Ltd. 2020. Chapter 26.

56. Andren-Sandberg A. Diagnosis and management of gallbladder polyps. N Am J Med Sci. 2012;4(5):203–11.
57. Inui K, Yoshino J, Miyoshi H. Diagnosis of gallbladder tumors. Intern Med. 2011;50:1133–6.
58. Sicklick JK, Fanta PT, Shimabukuro K, Kurzrock R. Genomics of gallbladder cancer: the case for biomarker-driven clinical trial design. Cancer Metastasis Rev. 2016;35(2):263–75.
59. Seo JH. Gallbladder cancer: Risk factors. In: Chung JB, Okazaki K, editors. Diseases of the gallbladder. Springer Nature Singapore Pte Ltd. 2020. Chapter 15.
60. Lazcano-Ponce EC, Miquel JE, Munoz N, Herrero R, Ferrecio C, Wistuba II, et al. Epidemiology and molecular pathology of gallbladder cancer. CA Cancer J Clin. 2001;51:349–64.
61. Lee HS, Park SW. Gallbladder cancer: Gene mutations and its clinical significance. In: Chung JB, Okazaki K, editors. Diseases of the gallbladder. Springer Nature Singapore Pte Ltd. 2020. Chapter 16.
62. Yoshimitsu K. Gallbladder cancer: Staging by radiological imaging. In: Chung JB, Okazaki K, editors. Diseases of the gallbladder. Springer Nature Singapore Pte Ltd. 2020. Chapter 17.
63. Bang S. Gallbladder cancer: Neoadjuvant and adjuvant chemotherapy. In: Chung JB, Okazaki K, editors. Diseases of the gallbladder. Springer Nature Singapore Pte Ltd. 2020. Chapter 21.
64. Furuse J. Gallbladder cancer: Patterns of recurrences and its effective treatment. In: Chung JB, Okazaki K, editors. Diseases of the gallbladder. Springer Nature Singapore Pte Ltd. 2020. Chapter 23.
65. Vijayakumar A, Vijayakumar A, Patil V, Mallikarjuna MN, Shivaswamy BS. Early diagnosis of gallbladder carcinoma: an algorithm approach. ISRN Radiology. 2012 Oct 18;2013:239424. https://doi.org/10.5402/2013/239424. eCollection 2013.
66. Black WC, Key CR, Carmany TB, Herman D. Carcinoma of the gallbladder in a population of Southwestern American Indians. Cancer. 1977;39:1267–79.
67. Albores-Saavedra J, Alcantra-Vazquez A, Cruz-Ortiz H, Herrera-Goepfert R. The precursor lesions of invasive gallbladder carcinoma. Hyperplasia, atypical hyperplasia and carcinoma in situ. Cancer. 1980;45(5):919–27.
68. Tsuchiya Y. Early carcinoma of the gallbladder: macroscopic features and US findings. Radiology. 1991;179(1):171–5.
69. Hirooka Y. Gallbladder cancer: Diagnostic strategies of early gallbladder cancer. In: Chung JB, Okazaki K, editors. Diseases of the gallbladder. Springer Nature Singapore Pte Ltd. 2020. Chapter 19.
70. Baron TH, Grimm IS, Swanstrom LL. Interventional approaches to gallbladder disease. N Engl J Med. 2015;373:357–65.
71. National Institutes of Health (US). Office of Medical Applications of Research. NIH Consensus Statement, vol. 10. National Institutes of Health, Office of Medical Applications of Research;1992.
72. Donini A, Petri R, Terrosu G, Pasqualucci A, Prati M. cautero N, et al. Trans-umbilical cholecystectomy: a new laparoscopic cholecystectomy technique. Description of the technique and preliminary results. Ann Ital Chir. 1996;67(4):475–8.
73. Pietrabissa A, Sbrana F, Morelli L, Badessi F, Pugliese L, Vinci A, et al. Overcoming the challenges of single-incision cholecystectomy with robotic single-site technology. Arch Surg. 2012;147(8):709–14.
74. Sun N, Zhang JL, Zhang CS, Li XH, Shi Y. Single-incision robotic cholecystectomy versus single-incision laparoscopic cholecystectomy: a systematic review and meta-analysis. Medicine. 2018;97(36):e12103.
75. Schwaitzberg SD, Roberts K, Romanelli JR, Desilets DJ, Earle D, Horgan S, et al. The NOVEL trial: natural orifice versus laparoscopic cholecystectomy-a prospective, randomized evaluation. Surg Endosc. 2018;32(5):2505–16.
76. Waage A, Nilsson M. Iatrogenic bile duct injury: a population-based study of 152 776 cholecystectomies in the Swedish Inpatient Registry. Arch Surg. 2006;141(12):1207–13.
77. Ambe PC, Plambeck J, Fernandez-Jesberg V, Zarras K. The role of indocyanine green fluoroscopy for intraoperative bile duct visualization during laparoscopic cholecystectomy: an observational cohort study in 70 patients. Patient Saf Surg. 2019;13(1):2. https://doi.org/10.1186/s13037-019-0182-8. eCollection 2019.
78. Lundberg O, Kristoffersson A. Open versus laparoscopic cholecystectomy for gallbladder carcinoma. J Hepatobiliary Pancreat Surg. 2001;8(6):525–9.
79. Yoon YS, Han HS, Cho JY, Choi Y, Lee W, Jang JY, et al. Is laparoscopy contraindicated for gallbladder cancer? A 10-year prospective cohort study. J Am Coll Surg. 2015;221(4):847–53.
80. Park JH, Kim YH, Kim H, Yoon YS, Choi YR, Cho JY, et al. Determining the extent of cholecystectomy using intraoperative specimen ultrasonography in patients with suspected early gallbladder cancer. Surg Endosc. 2016;30(10):4229–38.

Index

J. B. Chung and K. Okazaki (eds.), *Diseases of the Gallbladder*,
https://doi.org/10.1007/978-981-15-6010-1

The manufacturer's authorised representative in the EU is Springer Nature Customer Service Centre GmbH, Europaplatz 3, 69115 Heidelberg, Germany. If you have any concerns regarding our products, please contact ProductSafety@springernature.com

Printed and bound by CPI Group (UK) Ltd, Croydon, CR0 4YY
30/09/2026
02225299-0015